Noninvasive Mechanical Ventilation

Antonio M. Esquinas
Editor

Noninvasive Mechanical Ventilation

Theory, Equipment, and Clinical Applications

Second Edition

Springer

Editor
Antonio M. Esquinas
Murcia
Spain

ISBN 978-3-319-79357-3 ISBN 978-3-319-21653-9 (eBook)
DOI 10.1007/978-3-319-21653-9

Springer Cham Heidelberg New York Dordrecht London

Softcover re-print of the Hardcover 2nd edition 2016

Printed on acid-free paper

Springer International Publishing AG Switzerland is part of Springer Science+Business Media (www.springer.com)

To my wife Rosario

Preface

Despite significant technological advances in medicine today, the reality of everyday practice continues to reveal that not everyone can apply and know the limits of the technologies used in the treatment of respiratory failure.

Nowadays, in the treatment of acute respiratory failure in various medical specialties, the use of noninvasive mechanical ventilation continues to show a positive end result. There are few hospitals that have the necessary equipment to make its implementation possible. However, as we will see in this second edition, there are still several points of controversy, and important advances continue to be made, not only in new indications but also in the equipment (mechanical ventilator, interfaces) and patient–ventilator interaction. This gives scope for improving our understanding and maintains a growing interest in new possibilities.

In this second edition, we have analyzed the impact of published studies on the effects of potential, new noninvasive ventilation treatments and clinical practice, described by well-known researchers as well as other emerging groups of young researchers.

Experience and new insights make this book a basic reference to understanding and encouraging new ideas.

Personally, I want to thank all authors for trusting and contributing their time and efforts in the development of this book. Finally, if I wanted to point out that we must not stop this research inertia on noninvasive mechanical ventilation, knowing communicate well their knowledge and limits, and never forget that our end reference points problems and circumstances that our patients during noninvasive mechanical ventilation raising to us day to day.

This technique is still a life-saving treatment, relieves pain for many patients, and gives encouragement. However, many aspects need to be reinvestigated and research is necessary to resolve open controversies which indicate the failures of noninvasive ventilation, methodology, and therapy. The question of what are the limits of noninvasive ventilation and where needs to be addressed.

As *Albert Einstein* said, "We cannot solve our problems with the same thinking we used when we created them." We hope that this second edition becomes a useful reference that serves this modest reflection.

Murcia, Spain Antonio M. Esquinas, MD, PhD, FCCP

Contents

Part IV Hospital Critical Care Applications: Acute Chronic Exacerbations

Part V Hospital Critical Care Applications: Critical Care Acute Hypoxemic Respiratory Failure

Part I

Rational, Interface, Equipment and Ventilatory Modes of Non Invasive Mechanical Ventilation

Rationale of Noninvasive Ventilation

1

Nicolino Ambrosino

Contents

1.1 Stable Hypercapnic Chronic Obstructive Pulmonary Disease

The hypothesized but not proven mechanisms of action of long-term noninvasive positive pressure ventilation (NPPV) in stable hypercapnic patients with chronic obstructive pulmonary disease (COPD) are

1. Reverting hypoventilation
2. Respiratory muscle unloading
3. Respiratory center reset
4. Cardiovascular effects

These mechanisms may work alone or in synergy.

N. Ambrosino
Pulmonary Rehabilitation and Weaning Unit, Auxilium Vitae, Volterra, Italy
e-mail: nico.ambrosino@gmail.com

A.M. Esquinas (ed.), *Noninvasive Mechanical Ventilation: Theory, Equipment, and Clinical Applications*, DOI 10.1007/978-3-319-21653-9_1

1.1.1 Correction of Hypoventilation

Physiological studies have shown that, in stable hypercapnic COPD patients, NPPV in pressure support mode is able to improve alveolar ventilation by increasing the tidal volume and reducing the respiratory rate [1].

1.1.2 Respiratory Muscle Unloading

There is evidence that noninvasive inspiratory pressure is able to unload the inspiratory muscles, whereas the application of positive end-expiratory pressure (PEEP) counteracts the intrinsic PEEP (PEEPi) associated with hyperinflation in these patients [2], an effect more evident in acute exacerbations.

1.1.3 Reset of the Respiratory Centers

There is evidence that, compared with long-term oxygen therapy (LTOT) alone, addition of NPPV at night resulted in significant improvements in daytime arterial oxygen (PaO_2) and carbon dioxide ($PaCO_2$) tension, total sleep time, sleep efficiency, and overnight $PaCO_2$. Quality of life with LTOT plus NPPV was significantly better than with LTOT alone. The degree of improvement in daytime $PaCO_2$ was significantly correlated with an improvement in mean overnight $PaCO_2$ [3].

1.1.4 Cardiovascular Effects

Night-time NPPV applied over 3 months may improve heart rate variability, reduce circulating natriuretic peptide levels, and enhance the functional performance of patients with advanced but stable COPD, suggesting that nocturnal NPPV may reduce the impact of cardiac comorbidities in COPD patients [4].

1.2 Acute COPD Exacerbations

In acute exacerbations of COPD leading to acute respiratory failure (ARF), the work of breathing (WOB is) increased as a result of the increase in airway resistances. Because of lung hyperinflation, the respiratory muscles are less effective and, if the underlying pathology does not reverse in a relatively short time, they are at risk of failure and fatigue. Despite an increase in respiratory drive, rapid shallow breathing may lead to reduction in alveolar ventilation, even when minute ventilation is normal or even increased. Respiratory muscles progressively become unable to maintain adequate alveolar ventilation, resulting in an increase of $PaCO_2$. When $PaCO_2$ is severely increased for a prolonged time, the level of consciousness is generally impaired.

1.3 How Does NPPV Work in Acute Exacerbations of COPD?

When the cause of ARF is reversible, medical treatment works to maximize lung function and reverse the precipitating cause, whereas the aim of ventilatory support is [5]

- To buy time for the treatment of the cause of ARF to work
- To decrease the work of breathing (WOB)
- To reverse life-threatening hypoxemia and respiratory acidosis

In these circumstances, inspiratory support works to increase alveolar ventilation by increasing tidal volume and to unload inspiratory muscles by decreasing WOB. The addition of an external PEEP may further reduce WOB by counterbalancing the PEEPi.

Such patients may require intubation for airway protection in addition to ventilatory assistance, unless the hypercapnia can be reversed within minutes. It has been shown that NPPV may avoid most of the complications associated with invasive mechanical ventilation, ensuring at the same time a similar degree of efficacy [6]. The early use of NPPV in COPD patients may prevent further deterioration and thus avoid endotracheal intubation, improving survival compared with standard medical therapy. As a consequence, NPPV is considered as the first-line treatment of acute exacerbations of COPD.

The early use of NPPV is mandatory because success rate decreases with disease progression. On the other hand, NPPV may be useless or even a problem for the patient when applied in mild exacerbations that can be treated only by medical therapy [7]. In other words, as in other fields of medicine, this therapeutic tool should be applied during a therapeutic window: not too early, not too late. In practice, arterial blood gases, and signs (tachypnea or increased accessory muscle use) and symptoms (dyspnea) of increased WOB should be used as markers to start NPPV in these conditions [8]. When NPPV is started early, those patients not in danger (pH not lower than 7.30) can be managed outside of the intensive care unit (ICU), eventually even in a ward with an adequately skilled team [9]. In addition, dedicated units such as high-dependency respiratory intensive care should be encouraged to deliver NPPV to most but not all patients. For these patients, these units may offer noninvasive monitoring systems and higher nurse-to-patient ratios than in general wards with less burden but similar success rates as in ICUs [10].

Key Points

- Possible mechanisms of action of long-term NPPV in stable hypercapnic COPD patients are correction of hypoventilation, respiratory muscle unloading, reset of the respiratory centers, and inducing positive cardiovascular effects.
- The goals of ventilatory support in ARF are to buy time for the treatment of the cause of ARF to work, to decrease the WOB, and to reverse life-threatening hypoxemia and respiratory acidosis.
- NPPV may avoid most of complications associated with invasive mechanical ventilation, ensuring at the same time a similar degree of efficacy.
- NPPV in acute COPD exacerbation must be applied during an appropriate therapeutic window.
- The location of NPPV must be related to timing and severity of disease.

References

1. Ambrosino N, Nava S, Bertone P, et al. Physiologic evaluation of pressure support ventilation by nasal mask in patients with stable COPD. Chest. 1992;101:385–91.
2. Nava S, Ambrosino N, Rubini F, et al. Effect of nasal pressure support ventilation and external PEEP on diaphragmatic activity in patients with severe stable COPD. Chest. 1993;103:143–50.
3. Meecham Jones DJ, Paul EA, Jones PW, et al. Nasal pressure support ventilation plus oxygen compared with oxygen therapy alone in hypercapnic COPD. Am J Respir Crit Care Med. 1995;152:538–44.
4. Sin DD, Wong E, Mayers I, et al. Effects of nocturnal noninvasive mechanical ventilation on heart rate variability of patients with advanced COPD. Chest. 2007;131:156–63.
5. Tobin MJ. Advances in mechanical ventilation. N Engl J Med. 2001;344:1986–96.
6. Ambrosino N, Vagheggini G. Noninvasive positive pressure ventilation in the acute care setting: where are we? Eur Respir J. 2008;31:874–86.
7. Barbè F, Togores B, Rubi M, et al. Noninvasive ventilator support does not facilitate recovery from acute respiratory failure in chronic obstructive pulmonary disease. Eur Respir J. 1996;9:1240–5.
8. Keenan SP, Powers CE, McCormack DG. Noninvasive positive-pressure ventilation in patients with milder chronic obstructive pulmonary disease exacerbations: a randomized controlled trial. Respir Care. 2005;50:610–6.
9. Plant PK, Owen JL, Elliott MW. A multicenter randomized controlled trial of the early use of non-invasive ventilation in acute exacerbation of chronic obstructive pulmonary disease on general respiratory wards. Lancet. 2000;355:1931–5.
10. Nava S, Hill N. Non-invasive ventilation in acute respiratory failure. Lancet. 2009;374:250–9.

Cardiopulmonary Function Interactions during Noninvasive Mechanical Ventilation: Key Topics and Clinical Implications

2

Angelo Petroianni

Contents

Abbreviations

CO	Cardiac output
COPD	Chronic obstructive pulmonary disease
FRC	Functional residual volume
ITP	Intrathoracic pressure
LV	Left ventricle
MV	Mechanical ventilation
NIV	Noninvasive ventilation
P_A	Alveolar pressure
P_a	Arterial pressure
PEEP	Positive end-expiratory pressure
PH	Pulmonary hypertension
P_{pl}	Pleural pressure

A. Petroianni, MD, PhD, FCCP
Respiratory Diseases Unit, Department of Cardiovascular and Respiratory Diseases, Polyclinic Umberto I, Sapienza University of Rome, Viale del Policlinico 155, Rome 00100, Italy
e-mail: angelo.petroianni@uniroma1.it

A.M. Esquinas (ed.), *Noninvasive Mechanical Ventilation: Theory, Equipment, and Clinical Applications*, DOI 10.1007/978-3-319-21653-9_2

PPV	Positive pressure ventilation
P_{tm}	Transmural pressure
P_v	Venous pressure
PVR	Pulmonary vascular resistance
RV	Right ventricle
TLC	Total lung capacity
V/Q	Ventilation/perfusion ratio
VI	Ventricular interdependence
WOB	Work of breathing

2.1 Introduction

The thoracic cavity contains the lungs, with pulmonary vasculature divided into intra- and extra-alveolar vessels, and the heart, with the great veins and thoracic aorta. The dynamic mechanical properties of the thoracic organs are variable and conditioned by their volume and elasticity. Changes in lung volume and pleural pressure (P_{pl}) influence cardiac function even during spontaneous breathing.

The intrathoracic cardiovascular system is described as two pumps (right and left ventricles) connected in series and separated from each other by the pulmonary and systemic circulation. Output of the right ventricle (RV) provides the input (venous return) for the left ventricle (LV) through the pulmonary circulation with a lag time of two beats [1].

Cardiopulmonary interactions can be substantially understood on the basis of the effects of changes in intrathoracic pressure (ITP) and lung volume on the determinants of cardiovascular performance: atrial preload, ventricular afterload, myocardial contractility, and heart rate. Changes in ITP are transmitted to the intrathoracic structures: the heart and pericardium, the great arteries and veins [2]. These interactions are observable in health and can be increased or modified in the presence of diseases or mechanical ventilation (MV).

The effects of spontaneous ventilation on the circulation were first documented in 1733 by Stephen Hales, showing that the blood pressure of healthy people fell during spontaneous inspiration. Over a century later, Kussmaul described the *pulsus paradoxus* (inspiratory absence of the radial pulse) in patients with tuberculous pericarditis [3].

2.1.1 Basic Physiological Concepts in Cardiopulmonary Interactions

A brief definition of some basic physiological concepts involved in cardiopulmonary interactions is essential before illustrating their effects during noninvasive ventilation (NIV).

- *Pulmonary compliance* defines the change in lung volume due to changes in transpulmonary pressure applied to the lung ($\Delta V/\Delta P$). It is a measure of the ability of the lungs to be stretched and expanded. The transpulmonary pressure is determined by the difference between pleural pressure (P_{pl}) or ITP and alveolar pressure (P_A). P_{pl} is normally a subatmospheric pressure (−5 cmH_2O) and P_A (force of airflow into and out of the lungs) is <0 cmH_2O in inspiration and >0 in expiration. The compliance is highest at moderate lung volumes, near functional residual capacity (FRC), with a normal value of 200 ml/cmH_2O, and much lower at very low volumes (toward residual volume) or very high volumes (toward total lung capacity). However, if the lung is more rigid (as in restrictive diseases), pulmonary compliance decreases, moving the pressure-volume curve to the right, whereas increases in conditions with less rigidity (emphysema) move the pressure-volume curve to the left. This concept is important when NIV is applied. Lung and chest wall compliance constitutes the total compliance of the system. In the supine position, the pressure-volume curve of the lung does not change compared with the orthostatic position, but the curve of the chest wall moves to the right because it is more difficult to stretch the chest [4].
- *Transmural* pressure (P_{tm}), also called distending pressure, is the difference between the pressure within a chamber or vessel (intramural stress or P_{in}) and the pressure around it (extramural stress or P_{ex}). The P_{tm} (=P_{in}–P_{ex}) describes the complex effects of changes in ITP or blood volume on the cardiac chambers. Respiration induces phasic fluctuations in cardiac P_{tm}, and inspiratory P_{pl} is lowered by the respiratory muscles during spontaneous breathing and is increased during the application of positive pressure ventilation (PPV). The resultant variation of P_{pl} determines a change in P_{ex} in the heart with a direct influence on LV and RV volume and function. The rise in P_{tm}, consequent to a fall in P_{pl}, promotes ventricular filling and impedes ejection [4].
- *Ventricular interdependence* (VI) is the influence of the RV on the LV. Anatomically, the LV and RV share a common pericardial sac, with limited volume and compliance, and a common interventricular septum [4]. The filling of one ventricle can directly influence the function of the other: an increase in RV volume during spontaneous inspiration leads to a reduction in LV compliance and, hence, LV filling. VI is considered the major cause of *pulsus paradoxus* in patients with a restrictive pericardium as a result of tamponade. This effect becomes greater as P_{pl} becomes more negative or with a fluid bolus that acutely fills the RV. The application of positive end-expiratory pressure (PEEP) can be beneficial in these conditions [4].
- *Cardiac output* (CO) is the volume of blood pumped by the LV or RV in 1 min. An average resting CO is 5.6 l/min for a male and 4.9 l/min for a female [5]. Respiration with its ITP variations influences diastolic heart filling and, hence, CO. During NIV, these respiratory changes are particularly important. CO is measured at a defined phase of the respiratory cycle, usually at end-expiration [5].
- *Ventilation/perfusion ratio* (V/Q) is not uniform in all the zones of the lung. V/Q inequalities in the lung were proposed by Permutt in 1962 and 2 years later by

West et al. [6]. In the erect position, the perfusion increases from the top to the bottom of the lung. This is a result of hydrostatic forces combined with the different effect of airway pressure. In theory, the lung is divided into three vertical regions, based on the relationship between the pressure in the alveoli (P_A), in the arteries (P_a), and the veins (P_v). *Zone 1* ($P_A > P_a > P_v$) is a region at the top of the lung in which P_a falls below P_A. It is not observed in the normal healthy human lung, because P_a exceeds P_A in all parts of the lung. This is generally observed in marked hypotension or during NIV. In these circumstances, capillaries remain collapsed and low perfusion occurs (dead space). In zone 1, V/Q is the highest. *Zone 2* ($P_a > P_A > P_v$) is the part of the lung about 3 cm above the heart, where pulmonary P_a is greater than P_A, but P_v remains below P_A. In this region, blood flows in pulses. *Zone 3* ($P_a > P_v > P_A$) includes the majority of the lung in health. In this zone, both P_a and P_v exceed P_A, producing continuous blood flow throughout the cardiac cycle.

- *Pulmonary vascular resistance* (PVR) is the flow resistance that must be overcome to push blood through the vasculature of the lungs. The total resistance of the pulmonary circulation depends on the balance in the vascular tone of its two components: the *alveolar vessels* and the *extra-alveolar* or *parenchymal vessels*. PVR is closely related to lung volume, rising at both extremes of lung volume variations (Fig. 2.1). PVR is minimal at FRC. When the lungs are inflated above FRC toward total lung capacity (TLC), alveolar vessels become compressed as a result of alveolar distension or hyperinflation. As lung volume falls from FRC toward residual volume, extra-alveolar vessels become progressively more tortuous and tend to collapse and terminal airway collapse at low volumes causing

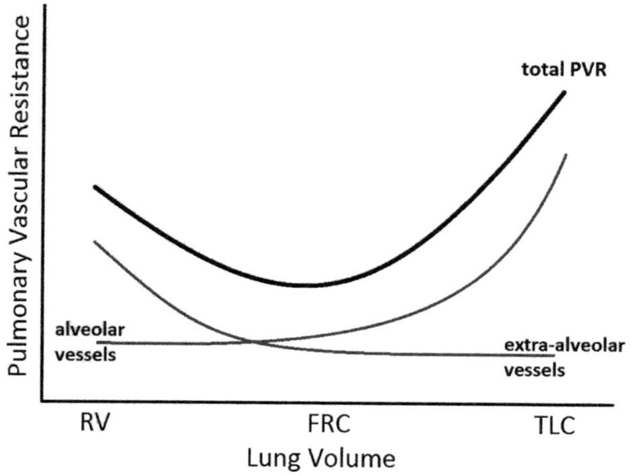

Fig. 2.1 Schematic representation of the relation between lung volumes and pulmonary vascular resistance (*PVR*). Alveolar and extra-alveolar resistance determine the PVR. As lung volume increase from residual volume (*RV*) to total lung capacity (*TLC*), the alveolar vessels become compressed by distending alveoli and their resistance increases, whereas the extra-alveolar vessels become less tortuous with a fall of their resistance. At functional residual capacity (*FRC*) PVR is lowest

alveolar hypoxia. *Hypoxic pulmonary vasoconstriction* independently increases PVR. In addition, lower pH leads to increased pulmonary vasoconstriction.

Hereafter, these concepts will be applied to the interactions in cardiopulmonary function in spontaneous breathing, during NIV, and in the presence of respiratory and cardiac diseases.

2.1.2 Cardiopulmonary Interaction During Spontaneous Breathing

In spontaneous breathing, the contractions of the diaphragm and intercostal muscles reduce ITP, leading to a greater pressure gradient according to the values of atmospheric and airway pressure. The decrease in ITP is transmitted to the intrathoracic organs, resulting in a fall in cardiac P_{ex} and a rise in P_{tm}. The increase in P_{tm} promotes RV diastolic filling. Consequently, RV increases stroke volume via the Frank-Starling mechanism [5]. The subsequent rise in pulmonary flow increases LV pressure load and its end-diastolic volume. Also, LV P_{ex} falls and P_{tm} rises during inspiration, increasing LV afterload during the systole. As a result, LV stroke volume and systolic blood pressure fall and LV end-systolic volume rises [5]. Thus, the main consequences of the decrease in ITP during spontaneous breathing are an increase in LV afterload and an increase in RV preload (Table 2.1).

In healthy subjects, spontaneous inspiration is usually associated with a slight fall in systolic blood pressure (<10 mmHg). During spontaneous inspiration, both P_{pl} and intravascular aortic pressure fall, but the fall in P_{pl} is relatively greater than the fall in aortic pressure, increasing P_{tm} and resulting in an increased LV afterload and a reduction in LV stroke volume.

Table 2.1 Different effects on lung and heart function

Spontaneous breathing	Noninvasive ventilation
↓ *ITP (negative)*	↑↑ *ITP (positive)*
↓ Blood systemic pressure inspiration	↓↓ Blood systemic pressure inspiration
÷ PVR	↑ PVR
↑ P_{tm}	↓ P_{tm}
↑ Venous return RA	↓↓ Venous return RA
↑ RA preload	↓ RA preload
↑ RV afterload	↑ RV afterload
↑ RV cardiac output	↓ RV cardiac output
↑ LV afterload	↓ LV afterload
↓ LV cardiac output	↑ LV cardiac output
	↑ Myocardial O_2 consumption RV
	↓ Myocardial O_2 consumption LV

ITP intrathoracic pressure, *PVR* pulmonary vascular resistance, *Ptm* transmural pressure, *RA* right atrium, *RV* right ventricle, *LV* left ventricle

Increased respiratory efforts with a greater variation of P_{pl} and P_{tm}, as in asthma and pulmonary edema, or increased sensitivity to changes in P_{tm} in the heart, as in hypovolemia and congestive cardiac failure, leads to a decrease in systolic blood pressure during inspiration more than 10 mmHg, creating pulsus paradoxus [3].

The effect of spontaneous breathing on pulmonary blood vessels is generally irrelevant and hardly ever causes a significant drop in systolic pressure. In addition, changes in lung volumes during spontaneous ventilation rarely determine an increase in PVR.

Neurohumoral processes probably play a primary role in the long-term effects of ventilation on the cardiovascular system. However, most of the immediate effects of ventilation on the heart are secondary to changes in autonomic tone. The lungs are richly enervated with somatic and autonomic fibers that mediate different homeostatic processes and instantaneously alter the cardiovascular function. The most common of these are the vagally mediated heart rate changes during ventilation [7]. Inflation of the lung to normal tidal volumes (<10 ml/kg) induces vagal-tone withdrawal, accelerating heart rate. This phenomenon is known as respiratory sinus arrhythmia and can be used to document normal autonomic control, especially in patients with diabetes who are at risk for peripheral neuropathy [7]. Inflation to larger tidal volumes (>15 ml/kg) decreases heart rate by a combination of both increased vagal tone and sympathetic withdrawal. Sympathetic withdrawal also determines arterial vasodilation. This inflation/vasodilation response can reduce LV contractility in healthy subjects and, as reported below, in ventilator-dependent patients with the initiation of high-frequency ventilation or hyperinflation [7].

2.2 Interactions on Cardiopulmonary Function in NIV

Mechanical ventilation, applying a positive pressure on inspiration and increasing ITP, produces physiological effects that are directly opposite from normal spontaneous ventilation. The positive ITP is transmitted to the alveoli and the interstitial tissues. Intrapulmonary and interstitial pressures remain positive in inspiration and return toward atmospheric pressure on expiration. If a PEEP is added, ITP remains positive even in expiration. As in spontaneous breathing, MV is associated with an inspiratory fall in aortic flow and systolic blood pressure, but the mechanism is considerably different [8].

In the 1940, Cournand et al. [9] studied the physiological effects of a PPV on cardiac function, demonstrating a variable reduction in CO in healthy subjects receiving PPV. Cournand showed that RV filling was inversely related to ITP, and as this became more positive the RV preload fell, producing an evident fall in CO.

PPV determines a simultaneous rise in ITP and in lung volumes. The increase in lung volume plays a significant role in the hemodynamic changes during NIV: tidal volumes are often higher than those in spontaneous breathing.

The interactions with cardiopulmonary function during NIV are complex and may depend on baseline cardiopulmonary function and, in a certain way, differences in the mode of ventilation.

The main hemodynamic effects of PPV include a decrease in venous return of RV and LV, an increase in VI, an increase in PVR, an increase in central venous pressure, and a decrease in LV afterload (Table 2.1).

The positive ITP decreases venous return and alters RV and LV ejection. Increased lung volume enlarges RV size by raising PVR, causing intraventricular cardiac septum shift and decreasing LV filling. In addition, augmented ITP reduces LV afterload, increasing ejection of blood from LV. These effects are proportional to the amount of positive pressure, inspiratory volume, and value of PEEP [4].

The decrease in preload and blood pressure essentially depends on the volume status of the patient and is more pronounced in conditions of reduced venous return (hypovolemia and vasodilation). This is primarily due to the influence of ITP on venous return of RV, leading to a fall in left heart output. Considering ventilation modalities, the decrease in preload and blood pressure can be greater with controlled modes of MV with high tidal volume and high airway pressure. Thus, the application of assisted MV modalities (CPAP, BiPAP, PSV), maintaining a spontaneous inspiratory effort, is favored in these cases [10].

Conversely, patients with fluid overload and congestive heart failure considerably benefit from PEEP or PPV and may radically improve after its application. Because ITP is higher during NIV, volume infusion stabilizes the relationship between venous return and CO.

The intrathoracic cardiovascular system is often described as two sections (RV and LV) connected in series. Therefore, it is clinically more practical to consider the effects of NIV on right and left heart (Table 2.1).

- *Effects of NIV on right heart*: the effects on right heart are mainly characterized by a decrease in venous return (RA preload), an increase of RV afterload, and a decrease in RV coronary flow. PVR is the main determinant of RV afterload and is directly affected by changes in lung volume (Fig. 2.1). PVR rises during NIV, determining increased work for the right heart and decreased filling for the left heart.

  The decrease of venous return, especially in patients with hypovolemia (real or relative), determines a complex compensatory sympathetic response with tachycardia, vasoconstriction, oliguria, and retention of water and NaCl [4]. Increased RV afterload, especially when using high tidal volumes, results in an increase of RV work and O_2 consumption. For this reason, the use of low tidal volumes is preferable in patients with acute cor pulmonale.
- *Effects of NIV on left heart*: the effects on the left heart include a decrease in LA preload, the reduction of LV afterload, an increase in stroke volume, decrease in O_2 consumption, and increase of CO. The reduction of LV afterload is the most relevant effect during NIV, restoring the hemodynamics to a more favorable position on the Starling curve: P_{tm} (distending pressure) decreases with a high ITP ($P_{tm} = P_{in} - \text{ITP}$). Therefore, patients with left heart failure show a functional improvement during NIV, even if limited by the decrease in venous return for high levels of PEEP.

Extrinsic PEEP ($PEEP_e$), increasing mean P_A and also P_{pl}, is commonly used to recruit alveoli, defend end-expiratory lung volume, and improve oxygenation during MV. Some data support the neurohumoral-mediated effects of PEEP on cardiac function in addition to its mechanical effects [10]. The achievement of the best value of PEEP is based on the balance between the respiratory benefits of PEEP and its adverse cardiovascular and respiratory effects.

Physiologically, V/Q inequalities coexist in the different zones of the lung. Alveolar recruitment is essential for the efficacy of NIV. The state of the airways, their resistance, and the alveolar compliance determine the effect of the pressure in different regions of the lung. These factors define the individual *time constant* of the different regions. Positive pressure preferentially aerates high compliance areas at the expense of lower compliance areas, whereas collapsed alveoli may require higher constant pressure to be opened. The variation in time constants between alveoli and lung regions precludes a single pressure as suitable for all lung regions [11].

Dyspnea is the imbalance between breathing effort and chest displacement. The patient's strategy to maintain alveolar ventilation that minimizes the work of breathing (WOB) is the breathing pattern balancing the elastic and resistive ventilation forces. Increased inspiratory effort produces a large negative P_{pl} that increases LV afterload and may lead to respiratory muscle fatigue and respiratory acidosis. A positive inspiratory pressure-assist favors the reduction of patient's WOB, inspiratory effort, and dyspnea [11].

NIV does not directly depress cardiac contractility. The presence of PEEP promotes the release of cardiodepressive humoral factors. Furthermore, the alteration between O_2 demand and supply for increased RV afterload can justify a reduction in contractility, rather than the LV, where the decrease in preload and afterload reduces wall stress and O_2 demand.

In summary, conditions that can accentuate the hemodynamic effects of MV include hypovolemia and venodilation (decrease in venous return), use of large tidal volume or high $PEEP_e$ (increase in mean ITP), and anesthesia and sedatives (reduction of compensatory sympathetic reflexes). The use of volume expansion to restore LV preload, assisted modes of ventilation to reduce P_{pl}, and the avoidance of high ITP occurring with a high minute volume, high inspiratory flow, or $PEEP_e$ are efficient strategies to minimize these effects.

2.2.1 NIV and Clinical Implications in Respiratory and Cardiovascular Diseases

In patients with cardiovascular or pulmonary diseases, the application of NIV requires special consideration.

- *Cardiac diseases* are frequent in patients requiring MV. These have important hemodynamic effects during NIV depending on the type and severity of the disease. As described above, the main physiological determinants of CO are preload, contractility, afterload, and heart rate. Changes in CO are the result of the increase in ITP, which causes a decrease in preload and afterload [11].

In cases of hypovolemia, restrictive cardiomyopathy, tamponade, or valvular stenosis, where CO is *dependent on venous return*, PPV can cause a further reduction in CO. In coronary heart disease, heart diseases with fibrosis, or hypertrophy, characterized by *reduced ventricular compliance*, increased ITP during NIV reduces LV afterload and increases CO.

In ischemic diastolic LV dysfunction with pulmonary edema, characterized by the *increase in preload and afterload*, increased intrathoracic blood volume, a positive ITP, or simply the use of PEEP can improve CO by limiting venous return and lowering LV afterload. In addition, PEEP helps to maintain alveolar patency and lung volume in these patients at risk of secondary atelectasis as a result of edema. In cases of coronary artery disease and *impaired LV contractility*, the heart is not able to compensate for the increased O_2 need and increased effort for breathing, which can increase up to 20 times and can sometimes result in cardiorespiratory arrest [2]. In LV failure, an increase in preload and afterload also increases O_2 demand of the myocardium, leading to a negative myocardial O_2 balance. The application of MV may have a favorable effect on preload and afterload reduction of LV, and reduces the need for O_2 with the correction of hypoxia and metabolic acidosis. PEEP determines improvements in oxygenation and in lung volume toward FRC and can also have a beneficial effect on RV afterload.

The effect of PPV on the RV is not so favorable. The increase in ITP and PEEP increases PVR and impairs RV function by reducing preload and increasing afterload. In subjects with pulmonary hypertension (PH), acute pulmonary embolism, COPD, or RV infarction, characterized by *afterload-induced RV dysfunction*, MV may affect the balance of RV supply and demand of oxygen. The treatment of reversible pulmonary vasoconstriction by hypoxia or acidosis and the defense of coronary perfusion pressure with pressor agents can be beneficial [8].

In heart failure secondary to RA stretch, circulating levels of natriuretic peptides increase. These hormones promote sodium and water diuresis. PPV and persistent hyperinflation decrease RA stretch mimicking hypovolemia. During PPV, plasma norepinephrine and rennin increase, whereas atrial natriuretic peptide decreases [4].

- *Pulmonary diseases* determine pathological changes in lung mechanics affecting lung volume and elasticity, airflow resistance, WOB, and RV impedance [10].

  Conditions altering lung volume, with a *reduction in lung compliance and volume*, are the result of bronchial obstruction (inflammation, secretions), an increase in lung elastance (pulmonary edema, pneumonia, acute respiratory distress syndrome (ARDS)), a reduction in FRC (anesthesia, supine posture, abdominal and thoracic trauma), or an increase in closing volume.

  Any variation in lung volume increases PVR (Fig. 2.1) and increases RV load.

  A reduction in lung volume increases the resistance in extra-alveolar pulmonary vessels due to hypoxic vasoconstriction, structural distortion, and vasoconstrictor mediators (thromboxanes). This condition also increases the dependence and interaction of LV function on the RV.

The prevention of acute right heart failure due to excessive increase in PVR can be achieved by avoiding NIV with large volumes and high pressure. Alveolar recruitment and reversal of hypoxia and acidosis are important efforts to reduce PVR. After the initiation of MV in patients with severe lung diseases, assisted ventilation modes are recommended utilizing fluid therapy to improve LV preload and inotropic agents to support CO.

Pulmonary diseases with *increased airway resistance* (asthma, COPD) prolong the expiratory time and oppose alveolar deflation resulting in dynamic hyperinflation and creating intrinsic PEEP ($PEEP_i$). $PEEP_i$ is the lowest P_A that must be overcome by the inspiratory muscles to initiate inspiratory gas flow. As already mentioned, increased lung volume reduces venous return of RV and LV. Dynamic hyperinflation and inspiratory airflow limitation both increase the inspiratory effort to maintain alveolar ventilation. Consequently, the increased ITP at expiration increases LV afterload and reduces venous return, producing a greater fall in systolic blood pressure and increasing the possibility of paradoxical pulse. Extreme expiratory effort with increase in WOB can cause respiratory arrest and sudden death in severe bronchospasm [2]. Hence, MV may further increase dynamic hyperinflation and P_{pl} in presence of severe airflow limitation. Ventilatory settings must carefully avoid further air trapping, using a long expiratory time and avoiding large tidal volume, high frequency, and prolonged inspiratory time. In these patients, assisted modes of ventilation, reducing the threshold work and inspiratory effort and improving minute volume, minimize the hemodynamic effects of MV. Although $PEEP_e$ reduces WOB, it is recommended to avoid $PEEP_e$ in excess of $PEEP_i$ [11].

Most pulmonary diseases are associated with an increase in minute volume and an *increase in respiratory effort per breath* (*WOB*). High minute volume demand may result from an elevation in metabolic rate or deterioration in gas exchange. The metabolic cost of breathing, normally only 1–2 % of total body O_2 consumption, may rise to as much as 20 % in acute respiratory failure. MV has therapeutically beneficial effects on WOB by reducing O_2 consumption and preserving cardiac function. Significant negative deflections in both esophageal and transdiaphragmatic pressure characterize chronic lung diseases with elevated spontaneous WOB. Applying a PEEP, NIV reduces WOB by counterbalancing $PEEP_i$, reducing the threshold load to inspiration, and by increasing respiratory-system compliance, reducing the elastic load to inspiration. In general, an inspiratory pressure-support level of 15 cmH_2O and a PEEP of 5 cmH_2O reduce most measures of WOB and inspiratory effort toward normal [11].

In pulmonary diseases with *increased RV impedance* (afterload), *increase in lung volume* progressively increases alveolar vessel resistance. Hyperinflation can cause considerable hemodynamic compromise and create significant PH and precipitate acute cor pulmonale and RV ischemia. PH is a frequent complication of pulmonary embolism, acute exacerbation of chronic lung disease, ARDS, and chronic pulmonary disease. PH increases RV afterload and induces acute RV dilatation and progressive RV failure. This may significantly reduce pulmonary flow and LV preload and precipitate systemic hypotension. The combination of systemic hypotension and PH has an unfavorable effect on RV myocardial O_2 supply and demand. In addition, most inotropic agents have pulmonary vasoconstrictor properties. In these cases, noradrenaline appears to have the best profile by producing less pulmonary vasoconstriction for comparable levels of inotropic effect and support of myocardial perfusion [4]. Appropriate ventilatory management in PH aims at avoiding factors that exacerbate pulmonary vasoconstriction: hypoxia, hypercapnia or acidosis, atelectasis, and excessive changes in lung volume. MV reduces pulmonary vasomotor tone by counteracting hypoxic pulmonary vasoconstriction, increasing O_2 alveolar partial pressure, PEEP recruitment of collapsed alveoli, and small lung volume toward FRC, and reducing respiratory acidosis and central sympathetic output, which decreases the stress of breathing.

ARDS is characterized by markedly increased lung elastance, alveolar collapse, airflow limitation, pulmonary hypertension, and elevated metabolic rate and WOB. Humoral inflammatory mediators can produce pulmonary vasoconstriction, myocardial depression, and systemic hypotension. During MV in ARDS, a greater inspiratory airway pressure is required to maintain adequate alveolar ventilation, and high levels of PEEP are often utilized to prevent airway collapse and aid recruitment of alveoli. Moreover, RV dysfunction during MV is due to the combined effects of positive ITP and presence of elevated PVR. In ARDS, maintenance of RV preload (volume loading), RV contractility (inotropic agents), and systemic blood pressure (pressor agents) with clinical and hemodynamic assessment is essential. The requirement for an ideal MV mode in ARDS, without adverse respiratory and cardiac side effects, has lead to the proposal of the use of high-frequency ventilation, inverse ratio ventilation, extracorporeal oxygenation, inhaled pulmonary vasodilators, and prone ventilation [4].

Finally, the evaluation of *fluid status* during the initiation of PPV is crucial. An acute reduction in systemic venous return is one of the most commonly observed cardiopulmonary interactions. The inflation-vasodilatation response due to vagal overstimulation can further aggravate it. This can be particularly dramatic in hypovolemic patients and in vasodilated patients with systemic sepsis. The respiratory variation in arterial pressure induced by MV, initially described as reversed pulsus paradoxus, is currently considered a predictor of fluid responsiveness and not an indicator of blood volume [10].

Conclusions

Respiration and circulation are complementary physiological processes that interact with each other during spontaneous breathing. The introduction of MV and the presence of pulmonary and cardiac diseases increase the complexity of this interaction. ITP decreases during spontaneous inspiration and increases during PPV. Thus, the different hemodynamic responses during spontaneous and positive-pressure breathing are related to the changes in ITP and the energy necessary to produce these changes. Spontaneous inspiration increases RV preload and LV afterload. MV with a positive pressure decreases RV preload and reduces LV preload and afterload. Therefore, NIV can alter the cardiovascular function by altering lung volume and ITP and increasing metabolic demands. Preexisting cardiac and respiratory conditions and the mode of ventilation modulate the influence of MV on the cardiopulmonary system. Mechanisms involved in these interactions include mechanical (pressure and volume), neural, and humoral processes.

In a normal heart, CO is principally preload dependent. The application of PEEP typically causes a reduction in CO by the Frank-Starling mechanism through a decrease in venous return and LV filling. This is particularly true in hypovolemic patients.

In cardiac failure, CO is more responsive to changes in afterload than preload. In MV, LV function improves for the better LV filling and the reduction of afterload and O_2 consumption.

In addition, NIV reduces WOB in direct proportion to the level of inspiratory pressure-assist and also by the ability of applied PEEP to counter $PEEP_i$. Modes and parameters of ventilation to minimize cardiovascular effects depend upon the pulmonary pathophysiological status and may change over time in the same subject. An accurate consideration of cardiopulmonary interactions in NIV helps to treat appropriately the different pathological conditions.

Key Recommendations

- Spontaneous breathing with a negative ITP leads to increased venous return (RV preload) and a rise in LV afterload. Conversely, PPV increases ITP and lung volume leading to a reduction in venous return (RV preload) and a decrease of LV afterload.
- NIV determines cardiopulmonary effects through mechanical, neural, and humoral mechanisms. The increase in ITP and lung volume affect venous return, RV and LV filling and afterload, and heart rate. Consequently, CO is reduced by increase of PVR, reduced preload, VI, and changes in contractility.
- In presence of LV or RV dysfunctions, MV determines different effects on CO and O_2 consumption: functional improvement in left heart failure or impaired RV function in cor pulmonale.
- Pulmonary diseases with different lung volume and elasticity, airflow resistance, WOB, and RV impedance may require appropriate modes of ventilation to reduce the negative cardiopulmonary effects of NIV.
- An adequate blood volume minimizes the negative effects of PPV on venous return. A significant decrease in venous return is observed in hypovolemic status, whereas an improved LV ejection, increased CO, and reduced myocardial O_2 demand can result in patients with hypervolemic heart failure.

References

1. Pinsky MR. Clinical applications of cardiopulmonary interactions. J Physiol Pharmacol. 1997;48:587–603.
2. Shekerdemian L, Bohn D. Cardiovascular effects of mechanical ventilation. Arch Dis Child. 1999;80:475–80.
3. Wise RA, Robotham JL, Summer WR. Effects of spontaneous ventilation on the circulation. Lung. 1981;159:175–86.
4. Gomez H, Pinsky MR. Effect of mechanical ventilation on heart-lung interactions. In: Principles and practice of mechanical ventilation. 3rd ed. New York: MacGrawHill; 2012. p. 821–49.
5. Guyton AC, John E. Textbook of medical physiology. 11th ed. Philadelphia: Elsevier Inc; 2006. p. 161–80; 471–90.
6. West J, Dollery C, Naimark A. Distribution of blood flow in isolated lung; relation to vascular and alveolar pressures. J Appl Physiol. 1964;19:713–24.
7. Pinsky MR. Recent advances in the clinical application of heart-lung interactions. Curr Opin Crit Care. 2002;8:26–31.
8. Pinsky MR. The hemodynamic consequences of mechanical ventilation: an evolving story. Intensive Care Med. 1997;23:493–503.
9. Cournand A, Motley HL, Werko L et al. Physiological studies of the effects of intermittent positive pressure breathing on cardiac output in man. Am J Physiol. 1948;152:162–74.
10. Duke JG. Cardiovascular effects of mechanical ventilation. Crit Care Resusc. 1999;1:388–99.
11. Kallet RH, Diaz JV. The physiologic effects of noninvasive ventilation. Respir Care. 2009;54(1):102–14.

Noninvasive Ventilation with Oral Mask: Key Determinants and Clinical Evidence

3

Dilek Ozcengiz and Ersel Gulec

Contents

Abbreviations

ARF	Acute respiratory failure
EPAP	Expiratory positive airway pressure
IPPV	Intermittent positive-pressure ventilation
NIV	Noninvasive ventilation
PEEP	Positive end-expiratory pressure

3.1 Introduction

In 1953, Dr. John Affeldt was the first to use intermittent positive noninvasive ventilation (NIV) via mouthpiece. In 1968, the Bennett lip seal, which fixes the mouthpiece in the mouth for sleep and seals the lips to prevent air leakage out of the mouth, entered the American market [1]. NIV has a considerable impact on the

D. Ozcengiz, MD (✉) • E. Gulec, MD
Department of Anesthesiology, Cukurova University Faculty of Medicine, Adana, Turkey
e-mail: dilekozcendiz@gmail.com; gulecersel@yahoo.com

A.M. Esquinas (ed.), *Noninvasive Mechanical Ventilation: Theory, Equipment, and Clinical Applications*, DOI 10.1007/978-3-319-21653-9_3

treatment of acute respiratory failure (ARF). Proper interface selection is a major determinant in achieving successful NIV because they are associated with adverse events such as air leakage, claustrophobic reaction, facial erythema, acneiform eruptions, and skin or eye injuries [2].

Patients have reported mouthpiece NIV to be easy to use during daily activities such as eating and speaking [1]. However, the use of this technology is not common and it is utilized in only a few centers. Currently, there are no evidence-based guidelines for this application. A small, angled mouthpiece or straw-type mouthpiece with volume-controlled ventilators can be used in patients with neuromuscular disease. An intermittent positive-pressure ventilation (IPPV) technique was used in one study [3]. This study included 257 ventilator users. Mouth IPPV was performed using commercially available mouthpieces for support during daytime and a mouthpiece with lip seal or custom orthodontic interfaces for nocturnal ventilator support. Mouth IPPV alone or other noninvasive ventilatory supports were reviewed for these 257 patients. Mouth IPPV was used during nocturnal support by 163 individuals, 61 of whom had little or no measurable vital capacity or significant ventilator-free breathing time.

In terms of a patient's ability to use the mouthpiece, NIV can be more reliably performed via a Lipseal (Philips-Respironics Inc., Murrysville, PA, USA) or Oracle (Fisher & Paykel Healthcare Inc., Auckland, New Zealand) mouthpiece interface if sedation is required. This kind of oral interface is designed to reduce air leakage. Nose plugs may be required if nasal air leak occurs in the patient (Figs. 3.1 and 3.2).

One study reported that mouthpiece ventilation was used by patients undergoing bronchoscopy [4]. Physiologic parameters consisting of ventilatory parameters, indexes of patients' respiratory effort, gas exchange, leaks and asynchrony, and comfort were evaluated in another study. The study suggested that a mouthpiece is as effective as a full-face mask in reducing inspiratory effort in both hypoxemic ARF and hypercapnic ARF.

A leak is a significant complication during the mouthpiece ventilation. Levels of leaks were relatively moderate and were lower with the largest mask, being present in 36 % of cases with oronasal masks and 60 % with mouthpiece [5]. A mouthpiece is probably more appropriate for patients with chronic conditions than for patients in respiratory failure.

Mouthpiece ventilation increased pH and lowered $paCO_2$ and prevented endotracheal intubation requirements in patients with respiratory failure due to chronic obstructive respiratory diseases and cardiac insufficiency. Mouthpiece ventilation has also been recommended for the treatment of severe sleep-related breathing disorders [1]. A lip seal or custom orthodontic interface has been used for nocturnal mouthpiece noninvasive positive pressure ventilation.

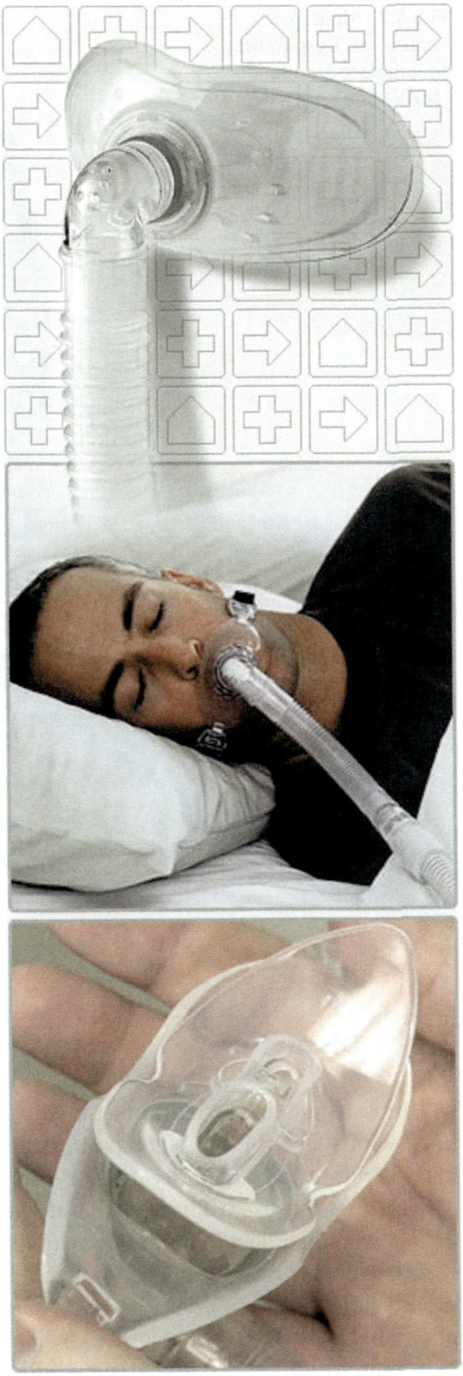

Fig. 3.1 Oracle Fisher oral mask

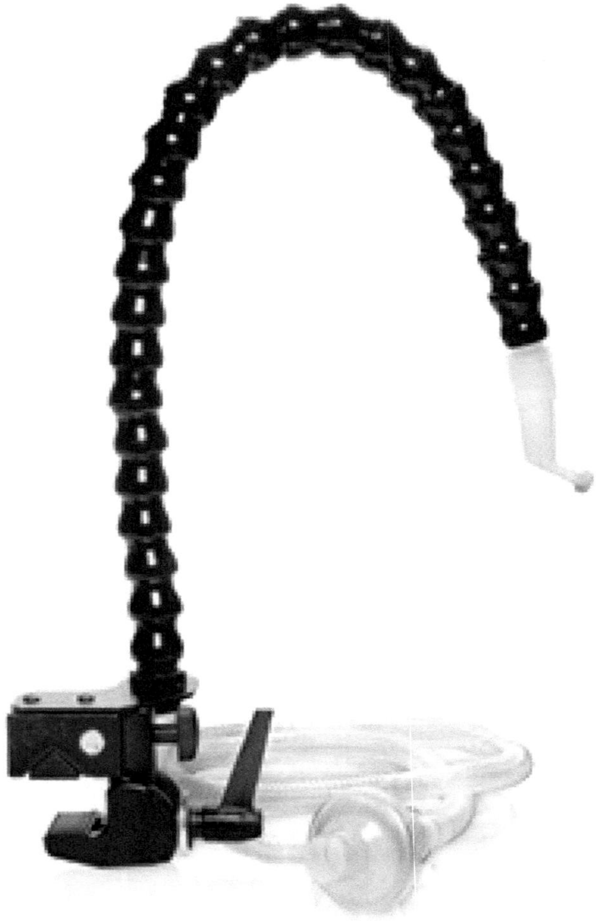

Fig. 3.2 Mouthpiece ventilation. Respironics Mouthpiece Ventilation (MPV) Support System

3.2 Discussion

The most significant benefits of a mouthpiece to support ventilation are less interference with speech, little dead space, better appearance, no necessity of headgear, and, therefore, no possibility of claustrophobia.

The greatest disadvantage is that it is useful predominantly during the daytime except when retained by a lip-covering interface such as Lipseal or Oracle at night [2, 3]. Another disadvantage limiting its use in ARF is nasal leakage, however, mouth air leaks can be controlled with a tight-fitting lip seal and nasal plugs or nose clips can be used to prevent air leak via the nares [3, 6].

Vomit aspiration is a potential complication. In addition, air may be swallowed and cause gastric distention. The advantages and disadvantages of mouthpiece use are summarized in Table 3.1.

Table 3.1 Advantages and disadvantages of mouthpiece use

	Advantages	Disadvantages
Mouthpiece	Lower interference with speech Very little dead space No requirement for headgear Eliminates any possibility of claustrophobia Better appearance	Less effective if patient cannot maintain mouth seal Usually requires nasal or oronasal interface at night Nasal air leakage Mouthpieces can cause gag reflex, salivation, or vomiting Long-term use can cause orthodontic deformities

Mouthpiece ventilation can be obtained with positive expiratory pressure (expiratory positive airway pressure (EPAP) or positive end-expiratory pressure (PEEP)) but it cannot be maintained for patients using open systems of NIV. Obstructive apneas are relieved by sufficient positive inspiratory pressure delivery. Apnea alarms, when present, should be set at the highest threshold to avoid unnecessary activation and nuisance.

The most common ventilator mode used is assist volume-controlled with tidal volume between 0.7 and 1.5 l with no PEEP (EPAP), low pressure alarm set at the minimum, and maximum apnea duration. Although volume cycling permits air stacking, when gastric inflation is severe, volume cycling is discontinued in favor of pressure cycling. A gastrostomy is needed in some patients so that air insufflated into the stomach can be "burped out" during sleep. Mouthpiece NIV is not successful when patients are uncooperative, cannot access the interface, or when a severe bulbar dysfunction causes aspiration of saliva such that the O_2 saturation baseline remains below 95 %. It can cause or exacerbate dry mouth. Heated humidification or switching to oronasal interfaces may beneficial in such patients. Mouthpiece NIV can reduce risk of pneumonias and other respiratory complications. Its use improves cough, speech, and pulmonary compliance. These improvements can obtain high life quality for patients with neuromuscular diseases.

Conclusion

In conclusion, oral masks can delay invasive ventilation and improve the life quality for patients with neuromuscular diseases, sleep apnea, and chronic respiratory failure. The limitation is necessity of high cooperation ability.

Recommendations

- An oral mask can be the first choice for the patient requiring NIV.
- The mask can be helpful for the patient who has a claustrophobia.
- Further study should be recommended to spread use of oral masks.

References

1. Garuti G, Nicolini A, Grecchi B, et al. Open circuit mouthpiece ventilation: concise clinical review. Rev Port Pneumol. 2014;20(4):211–8.
2. Nava S, Navalesi P, Gregoretti C. Interfaces and humidification for noninvasive mechanical ventilation. Respir Care. 2009;54:71–84.
3. Bach JR, Alba AS, Saporito LR. Intermittent positive pressure ventilation via the mouth as an alternative to tracheostomy for 257 ventilator users. Chest. 1993;103:174–82.
4. Tran J, Bach JR, Gonçalves MR. Alternatives to mouthpiece noninvasive ventilatory support to permit dental care. Am J Phys Med Rehabil. 2014;93:182–5.
5. Fraticelli AT, Lellouche F, L'her E, Taillé S, Mancebo J, Brochard L. Physiological effects of different interfaces during noninvasive ventilation for acute respiratory failure. Crit Care Med. 2009;37(3):939–45.
6. Gonzales J, Sharshar T, Hart N, et al. Air leaks during mechanical ventilation as a cause of persistent hypercapnia in neuromuscular disorders. Intensive Care Med. 2003;29:596–602.

Nasal Pillow for Sleep Apnea Syndrome: Key Technical Determinants and Clinical Evidence

4

Yoshinori Matsuoka

Contents

Y. Matsuoka, MD, PhD
Department of Emergency Medicine, Kagoshima Minami Kyushu City, Japan
e-mail: yoshinoriqq216@gmail.com

A.M. Esquinas (ed.), *Noninvasive Mechanical Ventilation: Theory, Equipment, and Clinical Applications*, DOI 10.1007/978-3-319-21653-9_4

4.1 Introduction

4.1.1 Although Nasal Masks Are Effective for the Management of Obstructive Sleep Apnea Syndrome, They Have Many Side Effects

Continuous positive airway pressure (CPAP) therapy is the most effective treatment for patients with obstructive sleep apnea syndrome (OSAS), particularly those with moderate and severe disease [1]. However, the device is cumbersome and compliance rates are only moderately satisfactory [2]. In particular, local side effects directly related to the nasal mask are common, with up to 50 % of patients complaining of pressure sores or ulceration, air leaks, allergic reactions on the face, claustrophobia, or mask dislodgement [3]. Therefore, proper mask fitting and patient education are important for reducing air leaks, ensuring optimal mask adjustment, and improving adherence to treatment [4]. However, despite our best efforts, a significant proportion of patients continue to experience nasal mask-related side effects.

4.1.2 Appearance of Nasal Pillows on the Market

To circumvent nasal mask-related side effects, different interfaces have been introduced to the market. One such interface is the nasal pillow, as developed by Mallinckrodt Corporation [5], Fisher and Paykel, and ResMed. Nasal pillows fit into the nostrils, thereby allowing breathing to be more natural, reducing nasal pressure on the nose, and preventing air leaks. Moreover, the device is less intrusive and can reduce the sense of claustrophobia.

4.2 Discussion and Analysis Main Topic

4.2.1 Clinical Evidence for the Effects of Nasal Pillows

Ryan et al. [6] argue that patients with OSAS find the use of nasal pillows more comfortable than standard nasal masks during CPAP therapy, thereby resulting in improved satisfaction. However, despite these assertions, the compliance rates, objective and subjective effectiveness, and side-effect profile remain unaltered. Although the overall SF-36® quality of life scores were comparable for both devices, the use of nasal pillows resulted in a significant improvement in the "change of health" domain.

4.2.2 Nasal Pillows Can Become a First-Choice Option for CPAP Therapy

In a recent study, the mask type was found to affect adherence to CPAP therapy. Specifically, oronasal masks were found to have a negative impact on CPAP adherence, with the authors suggesting that nasal masks should be the preferred first-choice option [7]. In addition, Ryan et al. [6] confirmed the comparable effectiveness of the nasal pillow to the nasal mask. They observed that both the apnea-hypopnea index and the Epworth sleepiness scale were similarly reduced by both devices, suggesting that the nasal pillow could be the initial choice for CPAP titration in certain patients, particularly when proper mask fitting cannot be achieved with a nasal mask at the initial mask-fitting session.

4.2.3 Nasal Pillows Can Be Used for Patients Requiring High CPAP Pressures

Mask selection is known to affect a patient's experience of CPAP. However, nasal pillows are infrequently used on patients requiring high CPAP pressures, and their performance at these pressures has not been evaluated systematically. Zhu et al. [8] examined the treatment efficacy and user satisfaction of nasal pillows compared with those of nasal masks at CPAP pressures $\geq$12 cm H_2O. They found that nasal pillows were at least as efficacious and subjectively acceptable as nasal masks when treating patients with OSAS at high CPAP pressures. Their study suggests that clinical practice can be amended to allow patients with CPAP the option to choose the most suitable mask type for themselves, regardless of their pressure requirements.

4.2.4 A Weakness Peculiar to Nasal Pillow Use

Belge et al. [9] have reported that the flexibility of nasal pillows can lead them to collapse against the skin, thereby abolishing the therapeutic effect of CPAP. Moreover, because this can occur without inducing leaks that would otherwise awaken patients, it can persist for prolonged periods. This important observation demonstrates that not every nasal pillow type fits every nose. Medical and paramedical personnel working with CPAP machines and interfaces need to be aware of this particular characteristic of soft nasal pillows so that they can remain vigilant for poor therapeutic response and inform patients of the risk.

4.2.5 What Disease Is Most Suitable for Nasal Pillows?

Porszasz et al. [10] evaluated a novel noninvasive open ventilator system that was designed for use by hypoxemic patients with chronic obstructive pulmonary disease (COPD) and intended to be practical to facilitate activities of everyday living. The device was well tolerated by patients in their laboratory study, markedly increasing exercise tolerance and substantially reducing dyspnea. The mechanism of improvement appeared to be through a combination of unloading of the respiratory muscles and improved oxygenation.

Conclusion

The use of a nasal pillow rather than a standard nasal mask for CPAP therapy in patients with OSAS may result in improved comfort and therefore satisfaction. The equivalent effectiveness of the nasal pillow to the nasal mask suggests that nasal pillows can at least be considered a first-choice option for CPAP. Because nasal pillows can be used for patients requiring high CPAP pressures, the adaptation of nasal pillows will be extended to patients with severe OSAS. In addition, nasal pillows have been successfully adapted for patients with COPD and OSAS, effectively facilitating activities of daily living.

Key Major Recommendations

- Nasal pillows should be considered a first-choice option for CPAP.
- Nasal pillows are safe and effective for patients requiring high CPAP pressures.
- Professionals should be vigilant for the risk of collapse peculiar to nasal pillows.
- Nasal pillow appear suitable for patients with comorbid COPD and OSAS.

References

1. Gay P, Weaver T, Loube D, et al. Evaluation of positive airway pressure treatment for sleep related breathing disorders in adults. Sleep. 2006;29:381–401.
2. Reeves-Hoche MK, Meck R, Zwillich CW. Nasal CPAP: an objective evaluation of patient compliance. Am J Respir Crit Care Med. 1994;149:149–54.
3. Pepin JL, Leger P, Veale D, et al. Side effects of nasal continuous positive airway pressure in sleep apnea syndrome. Study of 193 patients in two French sleep centers. Chest. 1995;107:375–81.
4. Weaver TE, Grunstein RR. Adherence to continuous positive airway pressure therapy: the challenge to effective treatment. Proc Am Thorac Soc. 2008;5:173–8.
5. Massie CA, Hart RW. Clinical outcomes related to interface type in patients with obstructive sleep apnea/hypopnea syndrome who are using continuous positive airway pressure. Chest. 2003;123:1112–8.
6. Ryan S, Garvey JF, Swan V, et al. Nasal pillows as an alternative interface in patients with obstructive sleep apnea syndrome initiating continuous positive airway pressure therapy. J Sleep Res. 2011;20:367–73.
7. Borel JC, Tamisier R, Dias-Domingos S, et al. Type of mask may impact on continuous positive airway pressure adherence in apneic patients. PLoS One. 2013;8:e64382.
8. Zhu X, Wimms AJ, Benjafield AV. Assessment of the performance of nasal pillows at high CPAP pressures. J Clin Sleep Med. 2013;9:873–7.
9. Belge C, Delguste P, Mouchart F, et al. Obstructive apneas during continuous positive airway pressure: unexpected finding with nasal pillow interface. Am J Respir Crit Care Med. 2012;185:112–4.
10. Porszasz J, Cao R, Morishige R, et al. Physiologic effects of an ambulatory ventilation system in chronic obstructive pulmonary disease. Am J Respir Crit Care Med. 2013;188:334–42.

ICU Ventilators Versus BiPAP Ventilators in Noninvasive Ventilation

5

Tamer Fahmy and Sameh Salim

Contents

5.1 Introduction

In contrast to the closed-circuit ventilation of invasive ventilation, noninvasive ventilation (NIV) is an open-circuit ventilation where leaks are inherent and, paradoxically, essential to its success. The success of NIV, whether in the acute setting, weaning, or long-term therapy is dependent on all three aspects for its use, appropriate patient selection, suitably fitting interface, and a specifically designed machine. The choice of a ventilator may be crucial for the success of NIV in the acute setting, because intolerance and excessive air leaks are significantly correlated with NIV failure [1].

T. Fahmy, MD, PhD (✉) • S. Salim, MD
Critical Care Medicine, Cairo University Hospitals, Giza, Egypt
e-mail: tfahmy@kasralainy.edu.eg, tamfahmy@gmail.com

A.M. Esquinas (ed.), *Noninvasive Mechanical Ventilation: Theory, Equipment, and Clinical Applications*, DOI 10.1007/978-3-319-21653-9_5

5.2 Leaks and Ventilator Performance

In contrast to unintentional leaks creating difficulties with ventilation, intentional leaks are "venting leaks." They should be created in the system in two instances. The first is to prevent the accumulation of CO_2 and rebreathing due to the dead space present in the interface, which may reach up to 800 ml in total face masks [2]. This accumulated air should be vented via exhalation ports in the interface. In the second instance, single-limb circuits should contain either a port for continuous intentional leaks or an exhalation valve. The intentional leaks are constant and controllable. Other sites of leaks, including that between the interface and the patient's face and mouth leaks with nasal masks, are sudden, variable, and unpredictable.

Leaks are less marked during expiration than during inspiration, because upper airway pressure decreases markedly when mechanical insufflation switches off to permit expiration. However, positive end-expiratory pressure (PEEP) may still promote expiratory leaks, where its level is proportional to the occurrence of leaks. Such leaks interfere with proper ventilation by affecting the trigger, pressurization during insufflations, and cycling off to exhalation. This ultimately leads to poor ventilation, lack of patient compliance, and prolongation or failure of NIV. Expiratory leaks can mimic an inspiratory effort for the ventilator, leading to auto-triggering, and inspiratory leaks can mimic a sustained inspiration, leading to delayed cycling [3].

If leak flow reaches the trigger threshold, auto-triggering occurs. Because of this, the frequency of auto-triggering does not depend on the magnitude of the increase in leak. On the other hand, if the leak is large enough, the ventilator may not detect respiratory efforts, leading to miss-triggering [3]. Vignaux et al. [4] demonstrated that auto-triggering was present in 13 % of patients, and delayed cycling in 23 % of patients during NIV. Auto-triggering per se may also induce miss-triggering if inspiratory time is prolonged, because of auto-triggering overlapping the patient's next inspiratory effort. In other words, cycle asynchrony can produce trigger asynchrony. Additionally, leaks can lead to aerophagia, odynophagia, dry mouth, eye irritation, and nasal symptoms, and noise may result, all of which reduce therapeutic compliance [5].

Ventilators used in NIV must be capable of detecting and properly estimating leaks and compensating for such leaks. Indeed, the response of these ventilators will vary according to the degree of leak, their capability to compensate, ventilation target (pressure vs volume targeted ventilation), and the type of intrinsic lung disease (obstructive vs restrictive pattern).

5.2.1 Leak Estimation and Compensation

The leak volume, as estimated from the difference in inspiratory and expiratory volumes, occurs during both inspiration and expiration. In the past, tidal volume has been estimated from the expiratory volume. However, given the observation that volume is also lost during expiration, tidal volume (Vt) can be underestimated from expiratory volume, and, consequently, crucial inspiratory leakage might be overestimated [6, 7]. Conceivably, the expired-volume method for measuring Vt might underestimate the Vt if leaks occur during expiration and therefore may induce overcompensation.

The simplest way to estimate the patient's Vt during leaks is to measure expiratory Vt and to consider that Vt is underestimated in case of expiratory leakage [7]. Ventilators with an expiratory valve have no expiratory circuit and no pneumotachograph connected to the patient interface. Consequently, these ventilators cannot measure expiratory Vt and, therefore, the patient's real Vt during leaks [7]. By measuring pressure and flow inside the ventilator, while taking into account the ventilator turbine speed throughout the entire respiratory cycle and detecting the beginning and end of inspiration, the ventilators with single-limb circuits with intentional leak are able to rebuild the patient's flow pattern and to establish a "baseline" breathing pattern corresponding to the patient's zero flow [7].

Khairani et al. [7] evaluating the ability of home ventilators to maintain the minimum Vt in volume-targeted pressure support ventilation (VT-PSV) in seven different NIV ventilators using different circuits. They concluded that ventilators that can be used with a single-limb circuit with intentional leak outperform devices that use double circuits or expiratory valves, where the latter could even paradoxically exacerbate the Vt drop during unintentional leak when used in VT-PSV mode. All but one of the studied ventilators with a double-limb circuit and all studied ventilators with an expiratory valve misinterpreted leaks as an increase in Vt and therefore decreased their inspiratory pressure to the minimal preset level, thereby paradoxically exaggerating the fall in Vt.

5.3 Comparison Between Ventilators

Three major types of ventilators have been commonly used for NIV over the past two decades: regular intensive care unit (ICU) ventilator (with no NIV capabilities or algorithm), ICU ventilator with NIV algorithm, and dedicated NIV ventilators. In general, in ICU ventilators without algorithms for leak compensation, a minimal amount of leak can be attained because the ventilator can only minimally compensate for the decline in pressure. If leaks are greater, the ventilator leak alarm will be activated, and the leaks will abort the breath due to disconnection. The failure to operate alarm is activated at higher levels. In the latter case, the system alarm for disconnection may be modified to a higher level, however, this still cannot be compensated for. ICU ventilators are more powerful and have more adjustable features (trigger type and sensitivity, slope of pressurization, cycling criteria) and monitoring capabilities. Their downside is cost, size, and the knowledge required for their safe use.

NIV ventilators, on the other hand, are portable devices with a turbine-type blower capable of delivering a high inspiratory flow rate (>100 l/min), are easier to use, and are less costly [8]. Most of the first generation bi-level ventilators, however, had important technical limitations, including limited pressure-generation ability, poor performance if respiratory-system load increased, risk of CO_2 rebreathing, and lack of ventilatory monitoring, alarms, or battery [1]. Although there have been many updates, NIV ventilators still cannot administer high inspired O_2 concentrations, nor can they reliably provide high (>20 cmH_2O) levels of pressure support. These two factors could prove to be a limitation in patients with hypoxemic respiratory failure, in whom high levels of FiO_2 and PEEP are required. In addition, CO_2 rebreathing can occur with some circuits, and they often lack monitoring capability [8].

Several bench and clinical studies have compared ventilator operability as well as patients' synchrony with different ICU ventilators (with and without leak compensation algorithms) and dedicated NIV ventilators (portable and ICU ventilators). In a randomized, crossover clinical study, Lofaso et al. [8] compared a home device to a device specially designed for intensive care use in seven intubated patients during weaning from mechanical ventilation. The main differences between the two devices were trigger sensitivity and initial flow acceleration. For the same level of pressure support, there were no significant differences in arterial PCO_2, Vt, respiratory rate, or minute ventilation between these two devices. However, the esophageal pressure-time product was 30 % higher with the home device. They concluded that differences exist between devices in terms of occurrence of rebreathing, speed of attainment of stable pressure support level, and expiratory resistance. These differences characterizing the delivery of pressure support may have clinical impact on the inspiratory effort of patients.

Didier et al. (2002) compared an NIV ventilator with three different ICU ventilators in a bench study they found its inspiratory trigger responded as quickly as the ICU ventilators tested, while its speed of pressurization was equal to some ICU ventilators, even at high inspiratory demand, provided the level of pressure support was kept below 20 cmH_2O. At higher levels, the proportional solenoid valve of the ICU machines was clearly at an advantage over the turbine-type blower of the home device [8].

In a bench study, Ferreira et al. (2009) [9] evaluated the ability of nine different ICU ventilators to function in the presence of leaks compared with NIV ventilators. They found that as the leak was sequentially increased, all ventilators, except for one dedicated NIV and another ICU ventilator, needed adjustment of sensitivity and/or inspiratory termination criteria to maintain synchrony, and some ventilators transitioned to backup ventilation. They found that only those two ventilators were able to synchronize with the lung simulator at all leak levels without adjustment. However, the dedicated NIV ventilator outperformed the ICU ventilator.

In a bench and a clinical study, Carteaux et al. (2012) [3] compared 19 different ICU ventilators with dedicated NIV ventilators. They found that in NIV conditions, most dedicated NIV ventilators allowed better patient-ventilator synchronization than ICU ventilators, even when the NIV algorithm was engaged, especially regarding the risk of auto-triggering. Most dedicated NIV ventilators exhibited a synchronization performance in the presence of leaks equivalent to ICU ventilators in the absence of leaks. Moreover, the NIV algorithm usually improved, at least slightly, the triggering and/or cycling synchronization of ICU and transport ventilators in the presence of leaks. The authors suggested that each ICU ventilator should be examined individually regarding its ability to manage NIV conditions. In contrast, dedicated NIV ventilators exhibited more homogeneous behavior during our bench evaluation, with an ability to avoid auto-triggering or delayed cycling while keeping a short triggering delay despite leaks.

Miyoshi et al. (2005) [10] evaluated the effects of gas leak on triggering function during NIV with dedicated NIV and ICU ventilators using a lung simulator. They found that the dedicated NIV ventilators triggered properly at several levels of leak (up to 44.2 l/min at 5 cmH_2O of PEEP) and that triggering was more effective than with the ICU ventilators (but not in NIV mode).

Oto et al. (2013) [11], in a lung model of chronic obstructive pulmonary disease (COPD) and acute respiratory distress syndrome (ARDS) evaluated seven different ICU and NIV ventilators at different levels of leaks up to 36 l/min. They found that ventilators performed better during decreasing than increasing leak, and that ventilators performed better with lower than with higher PEEP. Moreover, miss-triggering occurred more frequently and longer times were required to stabilize Vts in the COPD model than in the ARDS model. On the other hand, auto-triggering occurred more frequently in the ARDS model than in the COPD model. The ventilators may automatically decrease trigger sensitivity according to the level of leak to avoid auto-triggering, but as the leak decreases, the trigger sensitivity increases. This can lead to miss-triggering, particularly if the change is larger than the inspiratory effort. If the change in leak is smaller than the inspiratory effort, miss-triggering is unlikely, though higher patient effort is required to reach this threshold. The authors further added that because all the ventilators measure one or several cycles and adjust trigger/cycling for the subsequent cycles following a leak level change, it is not possible to synchronize on the exact breath that the leak changes. Due to this technical constraint, leak compensation on current acute care ventilators is limited in its ability to provide synchrony.

Nakamura et al. (2014) [2] found that only one of eight tested ICU ventilators was suitable for NIV using a total face mask with large leaks. Four were considered totally nonoperational due to inappropriate turning-off (misinterpretation of disconnection) or auto-triggering, whereas three of the remaining four had problems compensating for the large leaks through the exhalation ports, resulting in inability to keep PEEP and inspiratory pressure, delayed inspiratory triggering, or delayed cycling to expiration.

To increase safety, various manufacturers have limited the leak compensation for ICU ventilators to values equal to or lower than 30 l/min (or 0.5 l/s), values above which the disconnection alarm of the ventilator goes off [13]. However, the authors mentioned in the limitations of their study that some of the failed ICU ventilators upgraded their NIV software to a higher level of leak compensation after the commencement of their study.

To conclude, in different comparative studies:

- There is a wide range of heterogeneity among ICU ventilators in the leak compensation algorithms, while dedicated NIV ventilators are more homogenous. Because the manufacturers have not revealed the exact triggering and cycling algorithms used during system leak, it is difficult to explain the discrepancies among the different studies.

- Dedicated NIV ventilators outperform ICU ventilators in NIV, especially in patient–ventilator synchrony.
- NIV algorithms mostly improve ICU ventilator performance in NIV, however, modifications still have to be carried out to prevent triggering and cycling asynchrony.

5.4 Variation with Different Modes

In addition to the inherent characteristic of the device, the mode and setting also affect the leak compensation mechanisms within the same ventilator. Three different controls are being used in NIV: volume-targeted, pressure-targeted, and volume (average) assured pressure support. The response to different degrees of leak widely differs among these modes/controls.

When a leak is introduced, the peak inspiratory pressure decreases in the system and delivered Vt decreases. In volume-targeted ventilation, compensation is far less effective than in pressure-targeted ventilation [12]. This is expected with most volume-targeted ventilators, where the inspiratory flow is fixed and cannot increase, accounting for its poor leak compensation capabilities [12]. This cannot be overcome by increasing the inspiratory time, as this would also increase the duration of leak at higher pressures. Although increasing the Vt could partially compensate for leaks, this strategy for leak compensation is less effective than using pressure-targeted ventilators. Thus, volume-targeted ventilators would not be the first choice for noninvasive positive-pressure ventilation in patients with substantial air leakage.

On the other hand, when leak occurs in pressure-targeted ventilation, inspiratory flow will increase to maintain system pressurization for an extended time, increasing the inspiratory time. However, this compensatory effect depends on the rate of lung filling and emptying and the absolute inspiratory duration. Prolonging the inspiratory time to the point of inverting the inspiratory-expiratory ratio is counterproductive at higher rates (e.g., 30/min) because of incomplete emptying of the lung, resulting in higher end-expiratory pressure and therefore lower differential pressure [12].

Two counterproductive mechanisms occur. First, increasing pressure also increases leakage further, and the patient may not tolerate it, or it may further lead to aerophagia. Second, increasing the inspiratory time, especially with high rates, leads to expiratory asynchrony, requiring the patient to use the expiratory muscles to cycle off. Hence, this compensatory mechanism leads to increasing the inspiratory time, and at high rates would lead to air trapping, cycling off expiratory asynchrony, and intolerance to NIV [12]. Additionally, if pressure increases, in NIV-dedicated ventilators, inspiratory oxygen fraction obtained in these cases depends on factors such as the mixing of air supplied by the system and the oxygen in the circuit. If greater flow is needed to pressurize the circuit, high oxygen concentrations are harder to reach, even with high flow supplements [5].

This patient response varies among different ventilators and modes. If the patient-ventilator interface develops a large air leak during the attempted delivery of a pressure-targeted, flow-cycled breath, the ventilator will prolong inspiration because it does not sense the drop in flow required to terminate inspiration [13]. The ventilator may not be able to generate enough flow to maintain adequate inspiratory pressure. The patient will then "pull" against the ventilator circuitry, increasing the work of breathing. In contrast, a subset of patients may experience discomfort when exposed to an inspiratory flow exceeding demand [13].

The mechanism of expiratory asynchrony is terminated by a decrease in inspiratory flow up to a maximum duration of 3 s. Therefore, inspiratory time increases during leak because inspiratory flow fails to drop sufficiently to cycle the ventilator [12]. If airway resistance or lung elastance increases, normally Vt can be delivered only in volume targeted ventilation, and decreases in pressure controlled.

5.4.1 Volume (Average Volume) Assured Pressure Support

These devices increase the delivered Vt by increasing inspiratory flow during inspiration. However, when working within a single-circuit configuration without monitoring of the expiratory volume, it may expose to inefficient compensation especially when inspiratory leaks are present [14]. Some have used a proprietary system to adjust their leak compensation, which uses pressure-targeted ventilation to obtain optimal control of both inspiratory positive airway pressure (IPAP) and inspiratory time (Ti) to determine which of these adjustments is most effective for leak compensation [14]. The original feature of their leak compensation mode is that a Ti increase is combined with an IPAP increase to maintain sufficient minute ventilation based on monitoring of the patient's exhaled Vt. The ventilator takes the amount of leakage into account, cycle by cycle, and increases inhaled Vt to obtain an exhaled Vt value as close as possible to the set security Vt [14]. One important limitation of this system is that expiratory leaks may lead to errors by decreasing the exhaled Vt detected by the ventilator. The result may be inappropriately large increases in Ti, inspiratory flow, and IPAP, possibly producing lung overinflation [14]. They concluded that their leak-compensation system is probably less effective in compensating for expiratory leaks than inspiratory leaks and may be ineffective when the entire exhaled Vt leaks around the interface [14, 15].

In the presence of a mild leak during NIV, whether with an ICU ventilator or a dedicated NIV ventilator, either volume-controlled or volume-assured ventilation can be used. However, as the leak increases, pressure-targeted ventilation may be preferred to compensate for the leaks, as long as the pressure still allows (less than 20–25 cmH_2O) and the inspiratory time can still be increased. To best compensate for air leaks, pressure-targeted ventilators should have high and sustained maximal inspiratory flow capabilities.

Conclusion

Because leakage is a prerequisite in the application of NIV, ventilators used for NIV should be specifically designed to overcome this leak. The degree of leak compensation should be enough to build-up the baseline pressure set on the ventilator. ICU ventilators with NIV capabilities or bi-level positive airway pressure units usually have leak compensation between 30 and 60 l/min. Some ICU ventilators may have higher compensation, reaching more than 100 l/min. The set baseline expiratory pressure must not be less than 4 to allow for continuous venting of CO_2 and to prevent rebreathing; therefore, leak compensation must be capable of maintaining that minimum pressure during expiration.

In order for a ventilator to maintain synchrony in the presence of leak, the ventilator must automatically adjust the trigger sensitivity and/or cycling time [11]. Furthermore, in any mode the ventilator should have an algorithm for differentiating the leak from the decrease in base flow for triggering to prevent triggering dyssynchrony (missed efforts and auto-triggering). Similarly, in case of pressure support mode, the ventilator should also be able to discriminate between the leak and the expiratory trigger criteria (cycling) to allow for inspiratory synchrony and the following breath trigger level. In addition, the ventilator should be designed to have a secondary cycling mechanism in case of failure to sense the expiratory trigger level, so that the inspiratory time is not unduly prolonged (i.e., longer than 1.5 s). In such cases, the ventilator will switch from pressure-support mode to pressure control (time cycled). In order for a ventilator to maintain synchrony in the presence of increasing leaks, the ventilator must be able to acclimate by adjustment of both triggering and cycling, ideally automatically [9].

References

1. Scala R, Naldi M. Ventilators for noninvasive ventilation to treat acute respiratory failure. Respir Care. 2008;53(8):1054–80.
2. Nakamura MA, Costa EL, Carvalho CR, Tucci MR. Performance of ICU ventilators during noninvasive ventilation with large leaks in a total face mask: a bench study. J Bras Pneumol. 2014;40(3):294–303.
3. Carteaux G, Lyazidi A, Cordoba-Izquierdo A, Vignaux L, Jolliet P, Thille AW, Richard JC, Brochard L. Patient-ventilator asynchrony during noninvasive ventilation: a bench and clinical study. Chest. 2012;142(2):367–76.
4. Vignaux L, Tassaux D, Carteaux G, Roeseler J, Piquilloud L, Brochard L, Jolliet P. Performance of noninvasive ventilation algorithms on ICU ventilators during pressure support: a clinical study. Intensive Care Med. 2010;36(12):2053–9.
5. Rabec C, Georges M, Kabeya NK, Baudouin N, Massin F, Reybet-Degat O, Camus P. Evaluating noninvasive ventilation using a monitoring system coupled to a ventilator: a bench-to-bedside study. Eur Respir J. 2009;34(4):902–13.
6. Storre JH, Bohm P, Dreher M, Windisch W. Clinical impact of leak compensation during non-invasive ventilation. Respir Med. 2009;103(10):1477–83.
7. Khirani S, Louis B, Leroux K, Delord V, Fauroux B, Lofaso F. Harms of unintentional leaks during volume targeted pressure support ventilation. Respir Med. 2013;107(7):1021–9.
8. Lofaso F1, Brochard L, Hang T, Lorino H, Harf A, Isabey D.Home versus intensive care pressure support devices. Experimental and clinical comparison. Am J Respir Crit Care Med 1996;153(5):1591–9
9. Ferreira JC, Chipman DW, Hill NS, Kacmarek RM. Bilevel vs ICU ventilators providing noninvasive ventilation: effect of system leaks: a COPD lung model comparison. Chest. 2009;136(2):448–56.

10. Miyoshi E, Fujino Y, Uchiyama A, Mashimo T, Nishimura M. Effects of gas leak on triggering function, humidification, and inspiratory oxygen fraction during noninvasive positive pressure ventilation Effects of gas leak on triggering function, humidification, and inspiratory oxygen fraction during noninvasivepositive airway pressure ventilation. Chest. 2005;128(5):3691–8.
11. Oto J, Chenelle CT, Marchese AD, Kacmarek RM. A comparison of leak compensation in acute care ventilators during noninvasive and invasive ventilation: a lungmodel study. Respir Care. 2013;58(12):2027–37.
12. Mehta S, McCool FD, Hill NS Leak compensation in positive pressure ventilators: a lung model study. Eur Respir J. 2001;17(2):259–67.
13. Hotchkiss JR, Marini JJ. Noninvasive ventilation: an emerging supportive technique for the emergency department. Ann Emerg Med. 1998;32(4):470–9.
14. Orlikowski D, Mroue G, Prigent H, Moulin C, Bohic M, Ruquet M, Raphael JC, Annane D, Lofaso F. Automatic air-leak compensation in neuromuscular patients: a feasibility study. Respir Med. 2009;103(2):173–9.
15. Gonzalez J, Sharshar T, Hart N, Chadda K, Raphaël JC, Lofaso F. Air leaks during mechanical ventilation as a cause of persistent hypercapnia in neuromuscular disorders. Intensive Care Med. 2003;29(4):596–602.

Ventilators for Noninvasive Mechanical Ventilation: Theory and Technology

6

Raffaele Scala

Contents

Abbreviations

ARF	Acute respiratory failure
CPAP	Continuous positive airway pressure
CRF	Chronic respiratory failure
EPAP	Expiratory positive airway pressure

R. Scala, MD
Pulmonology and Respiratory Intensive Care Unit,
AUSL8, S. Donato Hospital,
Via Nenni, 20, Arezzo 52100, Italy
e-mail: raffaele_scala@hotmail.com

A.M. Esquinas (ed.), *Noninvasive Mechanical Ventilation: Theory, Equipment, and Clinical Applications*, DOI 10.1007/978-3-319-21653-9_6

f	Respiratory rate
FiO_2	Inspiratory fraction of O_2
IPAP	Inspiratory positive airway pressure
NPPV	Noninvasive positive pressure ventilation
PAV	Proportional assist ventilation
PCV	Pressure-controlled ventilation
PEEP	Positive end-expiratory pressure
PSV	Pressure support ventilation
Ti	Inspiratory time
VAPS	Volume-assured pressure support ventilation
VCV	Volume-controlled ventilation
Vt	Tidal volume

6.1 Introduction

The use of noninvasive positive pressure ventilation (NPPV) to treat both acute respiratory failure (ARF) and chronic respiratory failure (CRF) has been tremendously expanded in the last two decades in terms of spectrum of diseases to be successfully managed, settings of application/adaptation, and achievable goals [1–3]. The choice of a ventilator may be crucial for the outcome of NPPV in the acute and chronic setting as poor tolerance and excessive air leaks are significantly correlated with the failure of this ventilatory technique [3, 4]. Patient-ventilator dyssynchrony and discomfort may occur when the clinician fails to adequately set NPPV in response to the patient's ventilatory demands during acute distress, wakefulness, and sleep [3–5]. Technical properties of the ventilator (i.e., type of circuit, efficiency of trigger and cycling systems, speed of pressurization, air leak compensation, CO_2-rebreathing, blender for O_2, monitoring accuracy, transportability) play a key role in helping NPPV to achieve the goals of mechanical ventilation in ARF (unloading respiratory muscles, improved gas exchange) and CRF (improved gas exchange, sleep quality, quality of life, survival) [3, 4].

With the growing implementation of NPPV, a wide range of ventilators have been produced to deliver noninvasive support, both in randomized controlled trials and in "real-life scenarios." This chapter examines the key points concerning the technology of ventilators for NPPV and their main impact in clinical practice. Because of constraints in length, ventilators for negative pressure ventilation (i.e., iron lung, cuirass, poncho-wrap) are not covered.

6.2 Classification of Ventilators

Even if any ventilator can be theoretically used to start NPPV both in ARF and in CRF, success is more likely if the ventilator is able to (a) adequately compensate for leaks; (b) let clinician continuously monitor patient-ventilator synchrony and ventilatory parameters due to a display of pressure-flow-volume waveforms and a double-limb circuit; (c) adjust the fraction of inspired oxygen (FiO_2) with a blender to assure stable oxygenation; and (d) adjust inspiratory trigger sensitivity and expiratory cycling as an aid to manage patient-ventilator asynchronies [3, 4].

Ventilators may be classified in four categories, whose features are briefly summarized below and in Table 6.1 [3]:

1. *Volume-controlled home ventilators* were the first machines used to deliver NPPV, mostly for a domiciliary care. Even if well equipped with alarms, monitoring system, and inner battery, their usefulness to apply NPPV is largely limited by their inability to compensate for air leaks. Consequently, their NPPV application is today restricted to home-based selected cases of neuromuscular disorders, although they still play a role in the safe invasive support of ventilatory-dependent tracheostomized patients [3].
2. *Bi-level ventilators* are the evolution of home-based continuous positive airway pressure (CPAP) devices and derive their name from their capability of supporting spontaneous breathing with two different pressures: an inspiratory positive airway pressure (IPAP) and a lower expiratory positive airway pressure (EPAP) or positive end-expiratory pressure (PEEP). These machines were specifically designed to deliver NPPV, thanks to their efficiency in compensating air leaks. Because of their easy handling, transportability, lack of alarms and monitoring system, and low costs, the first generation of bi-level ventilators matches the needs for nocturnal NPPV in chronic patients with a large ventilatory autonomy. However, traditional bi-level ventilators showed important technical limitations (risk of CO_2 rebreathing due to their single-limb circuit in non-vented masks; inadequate monitoring; lack of alarms and O_2 blending; limited generating pressures; poor performance to face the increase in respiratory system load, lack of battery), which have been largely overcome by more sophisticated machines. The newer generations of bi-level ventilators have gained popularity in clinical practice to apply acute NPPV, especially in higher levels of care settings, as well as to invasively support ventilatory-dependent chronic patients at home. These new devices are capable of delivering a large extent of more advanced pressometric modalities of ventilation, with the inclusion of "hybrids modes" such as volume-target pressure-preset ventilation (i.e., volume-assured pressure support ventilation, or VAPS), which can dynamically change the level of pressure assistance depending on the measured tidal volume according to different algorithms. Despite their physiological benefits, the real clinical advantages of these "hybrids modes" have yet to be demonstrated compared with the traditional pressometric modalities [3, 4].
3. *ICU ventilators* were initially designed to deliver invasive ventilation via a cuffed endotracheal tube or tracheal cannula to either sick patients in the intensive care unit (ICU) or to allow surgical procedures in the theatre room. Despite good monitoring of ventilatory parameters and of flow-pressure-volume waves, as well as a satisfactory setting of FiO_2 and of ventilation, performance of conventional ICU ventilators in delivering NPPV is poor because they are not able to cope with leaks. Thus, a new generation of ICU ventilators has been developed to efficiently

Table 6.1 Characteristics of the four categories of ventilators for NPPV

	CO_2-rebreathing	Blender O_2	Adjustment of trigger and cycling	Modality of NPPV	Monitoring	Air leak com compensation	Alarms	Battery	Transportability	Costs
Volume-target ventilators	–	No	+	Volumetric	+	–	++	Yes	++	++
Older Bi-level ventilators	+++	No	–	Pressometric	–	+++	–	No	+++	+
Newer Bi-level ventilators	±	No	+++	Pressometric, Volumetric, Hybrids	++	+++	++	Yes	+++	++
Intermediate ventilators	±	Some	++	Pressometric, Volumetric, Hybrids	++	++	+++	Yes	++	++
Conventional ICU ventilators	–	Yes	++	Pressometric and Volumetric	+++	–	+++	Yes	±	+++
New ICU ventilators	–	Yes	+++	Pressometric and Volumetric	+++	+++	+++	Yes	±	+++

assist acute patients with NPPV with to the option of leak compensation (i.e., "NPPV mode"), which allows a partial or total correction of air leak-induced patient-ventilator asynchrony, even with large intermachine variability [5].

4. *Intermediate ventilators* combine some features of bi-level, volume-cycled, and ICU ventilators (dual-limb circuit, sophisticated alarm and monitoring systems, inner battery, both volumetric and pressometric modes, wide setting of inspiratory and expiratory parameters). "Hybrid modes" of ventilation, such as VAPS, are available with the great majority of newer intermediate ventilators. These new machines are designed to meet the patients' needs, both at home and in the hospital, and for the safe transport of critically ill patients [3, 4].

6.3 Technological Issues (Table 6.2)

6.3.1 Source of Gas and Oxygen Supply

ICU ventilators are equipped with high pressure air sources and with a blender in which O_2 from high-pressure sources and room air are variably mixed, making the FiO_2 controlled and stable. Conversely, bi-level and several intermediate ventilators are provided with either a compressor or an electrically supplied turbine pump to pressurize the room air. which may not assure constant stability in the pressurization. Moreover, these machines do not have a blender, so O_2 is delivered from low pressure sources and the FiO_2 during NPPV is not easily predictable because it is dependent on several variables: site of O_2 enrichment, type of exhalation port, ventilator setting, O_2 flow, breathing pattern, and amount of leakage [3]. It was calculated that the highest FiO_2 is achieved with the leak port in the circuit and O_2 added into the mask using low IPAP levels [6]. Assuring a preset precise FiO_2 is a great help in managing acute hospitalized patients suffering from either severe hypoxemia (i.e., requirement of high O_2 inhaled gas) or hypercapnic decompensated CRF (i.e., avoidance of CO_2 rebound due to inappropriately high O_2 delivery).

6.3.2 Circuit

With ventilators having a single-limb circuit there are two possibilities, depending on the type of exhalation system: (1) intentional leak or "vented circuit" and (2) anti-rebreathing expiratory valve or "non-vented circuit" [7]. The original Respironics BiPAP, like most of the first-generation bi-level ventilators, was provided with a vented single-limb circuit. With this device, the exhalation of the expired air occurs through the whisper swivel, a fixed resistance, variable flow, leak port situated either in the circuit proximal to the interface or within the interface itself. According to physiologic bench studies, this type of equipment may theoretically expose the patient to the risk of CO_2 rebreathing, which may be detrimental when treating hypercapnic patients [3]. The CO_2 rebreathing is also influenced by

Table 6.2 Key points of the performance of ventilators for NPPV [3]

Source of gases
Compressed medical gases
Compressor or electrically supplied turbine pump
Oxygen supply
High-pressure sources with a blender
Low-pressure sources with connection at the: ventilator, circuit, mask
Circuit
Single-limb circuit with: non-rebreathing valve, plateau exhalation valve or whisper
Double-limb circuit
Inspiratory trigger with sensitivity changeable or not
Flow, Pressure, Volume, Mixed
Expiratory cycle
Flow-dependent (with threshold changeable or not), *Time-dependent, Auto-function*
Inspiratory flow changeable or not
Back-up respiratory rate
Air leak compensation
Humidification
Heated humidifiers, Heat-moisture exchangers
Battery
Internal, Additional external
Alarms
Lack or minimal
Sophisticated
Monitoring systems
Only some inspiratory parameters
Inspiratory and expiratory parameters
Flow, volume, pressure curves
Mode of ventilation
Only spontaneous modes without (PSV, PAV) or with a guaranteed Vt (VAPS)
Both spontaneous (PSV, PAV) and mandatory modes (VCV, PCV)
Interface
Nasal mask, full-face mask, total-face mask, helmet, mouthpiece

PSV pressure support ventilation, *PAV* proportional assist ventilation, *VAPS* volume-assured pressure support ventilation, *VCV* volume controlled ventilation, *PCV* pressure controlled ventilation

the site of the exhalation port, being significantly lower by using a facial mask with the exhalation port inside compared with a facial mask with the exhalation port in the circuit and a total face mask with the exhalation port inside [8]. The options that the clinician has to prevent this risk are (a) to keep the conventional whisper swivel and apply high EPAP levels, such as 8 cm H_2O, which may be, therefore, poorly tolerated or (b) to use specific devices such as the *plateau exhalation valve*, which has a diaphragm that limits air leaks during inspiration and allows a unidirectional air flow during expiration [3]. However, it should be noted that the clinical impact of the potential risk of CO_2 rebreathing using ventilators equipped with a vented single-limb circuit is probably overestimated.

Ventilators with a non-vented single-limb circuit are provided with a *non-rebreathing valve* (mushroom, diaphragm, or balloon valve), which works a true valve. During inspiration, the diaphragm or its balloon is inflated, with full occlusion of the expiratory circuit limb, whereas during expiration, as the valve is deflated, air is allowed to be exhaled throughout it [7]. According to physiological bench studies, even with large variability, these valves may interfere with resistance and expiratory work and, therefore, may increase lung hyperinflation (i.e., intrinsic PEEP) [3, 4]. However, the clinical significance of these physiological findings is unknown.

With ventilators having a dual-limb circuit in which a complete separation exists between inspiratory and expiratory lines (i.e., ICU, last generation bi-level, and intermediate ventilators) there is no risk of rebreathing. Conversely, dual-limb circuit ventilators are less user friendly and more cumbersome compared with single-limb circuit devices. The latter may be preferable for home-based noninvasive ventilatory treatment of the clinical patterns of CRF patients [3].

6.3.3 Inspiratory Trigger and Expiratory Cycle

The optimization of patient-ventilator interaction during NPPV is essentially based on the technological efficiency of the machine in detecting the patient's minimum inspiratory effort as quickly as possible (i.e., *inspiratory trigger*) and in ending the delivery of mechanical support as close as possible to the beginning of the patient's expiration (i.e., *expiratory cycling*), independent from respiratory system impedance and air leaks [3, 4]. Ideally, the inspiratory trigger should be set at a higher sensitivity capable of reducing the patient's effort required to activate the mechanical support. Bi-level ventilators equipped with flow triggers are associated with lower work of breathing and shorter triggering delay time compared with those equipped with pressure triggers [9]. As a matter of a fact, the chance of patient-ventilator dyssynchrony due to "wasted efforts" for a too "tough trigger" is likely to be lower with the former devices. On the other hand, a too sensitive trigger, especially if flow-based, may induce auto-triggering during NPPV with substantial air leaks, and, consequently, ventilator dyssynchrony due to "unwanted efforts" [5]. Inspiratory trigger function may significantly differ, not only among the different categories of ventilators but also within the same category, because of the structural features of the circuit (i.e., single-limb circuit with high resistive valves, "incomplete dual-limb circuit" and a PEEP valve in the short expiratory limb) and the heterogeneity in their performance (pressure-time and flow-time waveforms, trigger delay, leak-induced auto-triggering during NPPV with flow-triggered ventilators) [3].

The cycling to expiration optimizes the synchrony between the inspiratory time (Ti) of the patient and that of the machine. During pressure support ventilation (PSV), cycling to expiration is flow-dependent and occurs at a threshold, which is the decrease in flow either to a default or changeable percentage (usually 25 %) of inspiratory peak flow or to an absolute flow [3, 4]. Patient-ventilator dyssynchrony with expiratory muscle activation and "wasted efforts" due to incomplete lung emptying may happen under NPPV in the case of excessive air leaks that delay or prevent the inspiratory flow from reaching the threshold (i.e., "inspiratory hang-up") [5]. Successful strategies for preventing inspiratory hang-up that may be applied with some ventilators include (a) setting a suitable threshold and/or a maximum Ti; (b) use of special algorithms (i.e., "auto-track system"); and (c) switching to pressure control ventilation (PCV) mode, in which expiratory cycling is time-dependent [3]. The opportunity to finely set the threshold for expiratory cycling because of the display of mechanics waveforms available in some newer ventilators may be helpful in improving patient-ventilator synchrony during NPPV, as well as comfort and the possibility of success [4, 10].

As observed with the inspiratory trigger, the behavior of different ventilators varies in terms of cycling to expiration, and a marked heterogeneity is reported for a given ventilator in response to various conditions of respiratory mechanics and air leaks. Generally speaking, most of the bi-level ventilators use a cut-off at a higher fraction of inspiratory flow than most of the ICU ventilators to avoid the mask leak-induced deleterious prolongation of Ti. Newer bi-level ventilators tend to prematurely cycle to expiration under normal respiratory system mechanics, and this tendency is exaggerated in restrictive conditions. Conversely, under obstructive conditions, most of the older bi-level ventilators show a delayed cycling, and this behavior is greatly exaggerated by the presence of air leaks. Consequently, at their default setting, bi-level ventilators seem to be better adapted for supporting obstructed patients [3]. Opposite to bi-level ventilators, in the absence of leaks and at their default setting, newer ICU ventilators present some degree of delay in cycling to expiration that is worsened by obstructive conditions, whereas restrictive mechanics lead to premature cycling. The addition of leaks increases the delayed cycling in normal and obstructive conditions and partially corrects premature cycling in restrictive status. This dyssynchrony in expiratory cycling may be prevented by using NPPV modes in normal and obstructive mechanics [3–5].

6.3.4 Inspiratory Flow

It is known that severely dyspneic patients with chronic obstructive pulmonary disease (COPD) cope better with higher inspiratory flow and neuromuscular patients do better with lower inspiratory flow (i.e., pressure rise times of 0.05–0.1 and 0.3–0.4 s, respectively) [3]. In most bi-level ventilators, this parameter is unchangeable; conversely, in more advanced bi-level ventilators, as well as in most intermediate and

ICU ventilators, the rise time may be set with a potential profound effect on unloading of respiratory muscles, tolerance, and leaks. In a physiologic study, the highest pressurization rate was associated with an increased air leakage and poorer NPPV tolerance, even though the diaphragmatic effort was reduced more compared with lower speeds without significant differences in blood gases or breathing pattern. As patient comfort was not different at the lower pressurization speeds, the authors suggested that the individual titration should be targeted to achieve a good tolerance and to minimize air leaks, keeping a relatively high pressurization rate [11].

6.3.5 Back-up Respiratory Rate

Some bi-level ventilators do not have the option of setting a back-up respiratory rate (f), which raises the costs. Conversely, the majority of newer bi-level ventilators and all intermediate and ICU ventilators are equipped with a back-up f. This option is particularly advantageous in sicker patients with instability of their respiratory drive because it prevents the phenomena of apneas and of periodic breathing, such as Cheyne-Stokes in chronic heart failure. Back-up f may also be useful when a cautious sedation is administered to improve patient compliance to NPPV in expert intensive acute care settings [3].

6.3.6 Air Leak Compensation

Because of the kind of interface used, air leak is almost a constant feature of NPPV and may interfere with patient comfort, patient-ventilator synchrony and, eventually, the likelihood of success both in acute and chronic patients [1, 5, 10]. During NPPV delivered by ventilators equipped with a vented single-limb circuit, one must consider both intentional (due to the presence of the exhalation system) and unintentional leaks (throughout the mouth during nasal ventilation and/or between the interface and the face with both nasal and oronasal masks) [7]. Excessive unintentional leaks are strongly correlated with NPPV failure as a consequence of alveolar hypoventilation, discomfort, patient-ventilator asynchronies, and sleep fragmentation. On the other hand, attempting to tightly fit the straps of headgear to reduce air leaks should be avoided, because thus may reduce the patient's tolerance and predispose to skin damage [3, 4]. Consequently, it is important to have a ventilator capable of well compensating air leaks during NPPV. Air leak compensation is greater using bi-level than volume-target home ventilators, with the fall in tidal volume (Vt) >50 % with the latter. Conversely, the fall in Vt is <10 % and in IPAP <8 % with bi-level ventilators in case of leaks because of an adequate increase in the inspiratory flow and in the Ti. However, the effects of air leaks during NPPV are more complex than the simple fall in IPAP and Vt, due to the role played by further variables such as Ti, expiratory cycling and inspiratory trigger sensitivity. Mathematical models that analyze the complex interaction between air leaks and PSV in the obstructive conditions and their potential clinical implications have been recently implemented. Even though all bi-level ventilators and most intermediate and newer ICU ventilators equipped with NPPV modes were able to compensate air leaks, their performance was not uniform [3, 4].

6.3.7 Battery

For both acute and chronic patients with a high level of dependency on NPPV, a battery power source is mandatory in case of electricity supply failure at home and in case of the need to transport the patient within the hospital or to another hospital. However, clinician must be aware that battery duration differs greatly among the different portable ventilators and may be shorter than that reported in the operator's manual. Moreover, portable ventilator battery duration is affected by the setting, the lung impedance characteristics, and the ventilator features [3].

As an alternative or in addition to internal batteries for NPPV ventilators, it is also possible to use external batteries that guarantee a prolonged autonomy of the ventilator in case of loss of electricity. It has to be considered that external batteries may make the ventilator too heavy when it is to be transported.

6.3.8 Alarm and Monitoring System

The need for sophisticated alarms and monitoring systems during NPPV is based on clinical practice because, to date, there is no scientific evidence of their clinical utility. This is especially true for patients on home ventilation. Care must be taken when setting the alarms on the ventilator to ensure that they will only function when a genuine need arises, as frequent, often spurious alarms can significantly disturb the sleep of the patient. The prototype of Respironics BiPAP did not have either alarm or monitoring features, with an advantage in cost and transportability in the home care setting. In the acute setting, the availability of newer bi-level, intermediate, and ICU ventilators with more sophisticated alarms (i.e., low and high pressure, Vt, f, FiO_2, leaks) and monitoring graph (i.e., flow, Vt, and pressure curves) may be useful in terms of safety and in improving patient-ventilator interaction [4, 5]. Conversely, too elaborate alarms may be counter-productive in the clinical practice because they frequently indicate minor air leaks during NPPV [3].

In the context of patient-ventilator interaction, even if some asynchronies may be suspected at bedside by a careful observation of chest and abdomen movements during NPPV, the interpretation of ventilator curves is helpful to noninvasively assess patient-ventilator interaction [7] (Fig. 6.1). The correct identification of the type of asynchrony during NPPV is helpful in choosing the best strategy to improve the degree of patient-ventilator interaction (e.g., choosing a different interface to reduce leaks and/or changing the setting of the ventilator). A randomized controlled trial clearly demonstrated that a curve-driven setting of the ventilator is capable of achieving a correction of acidosis in a shorter time compared with traditional settings in severe COPD exacerbations [10].

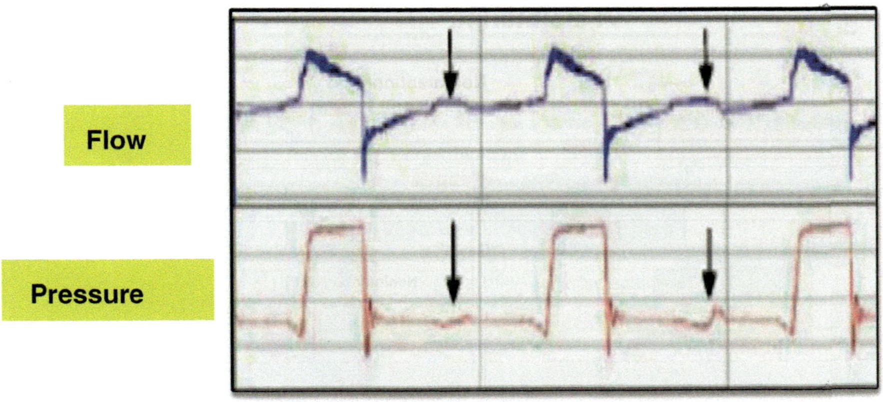

Fig. 6.1 A typical patient-ventilator asynchrony pattern resulting from ineffective efforts during noninvasive ventilation that may be easily suspected by looking at the flow-pressure curves of sophisticated more advanced ventilators

The keys parameters to be monitor during NPPV are expiratory Vt and f, the determinants of the breathing pattern. Concerning the former, the excessive air leaks may cause a significant discrepancy between inspiratory and expiratory Vt. Expiratory Vt assessment is feasible only with ventilators equipped with a dual-limb circuit where expiratory Vt is obtained by subtracting leaks from inspiratory Vt. With these ventilators, monitoring of expiratory Vt is more reliable with machines that take the measurement at the level of the expiratory branch of the Y-tube than with those that take the measurement at the inlet of the expiratory tube into the ventilator [3]. With ventilators having a single-limb circuit there are two possibilities, depending on the type of exhalation system. In presence of a non-vented circuit, the ventilator gives a inspiratory Vt value that is always an actual measurement of volume delivered by the ventilator. The values are computed at the beginning of inspiration, so that, in the presence of leaks, the leaks are considered as part of the delivered inspiratory Vt. In this case, the ventilator is not able to measure and provide an estimation of leaks and of expiratory Vt as well. In presence of a vented circuit, the ventilator provides an estimation (and not a measure) of expiratory Vt that should be the real volume inspired by the patient without the intentional leaks. In this case, the ventilator is able to provide an estimation of leaks. The leak value displayed may be the total value of leak (intentional + unintentional) or only the unintentional leaks according to the algorithm used by the ventilator. Unfortunately, for a very large leak, its estimation, as well as the estimation of expiratory Vt, may become unreliable [7] (Fig. 6.2).

Concerning f assessment during NPPV, there may be a gap between the rate of ventilator-assisted and patient-triggered breaths. Looking at the ventilator-f, ineffective efforts and auto-triggering may cause, respectively, underestimation and overestimation of the effective patient's f [7].

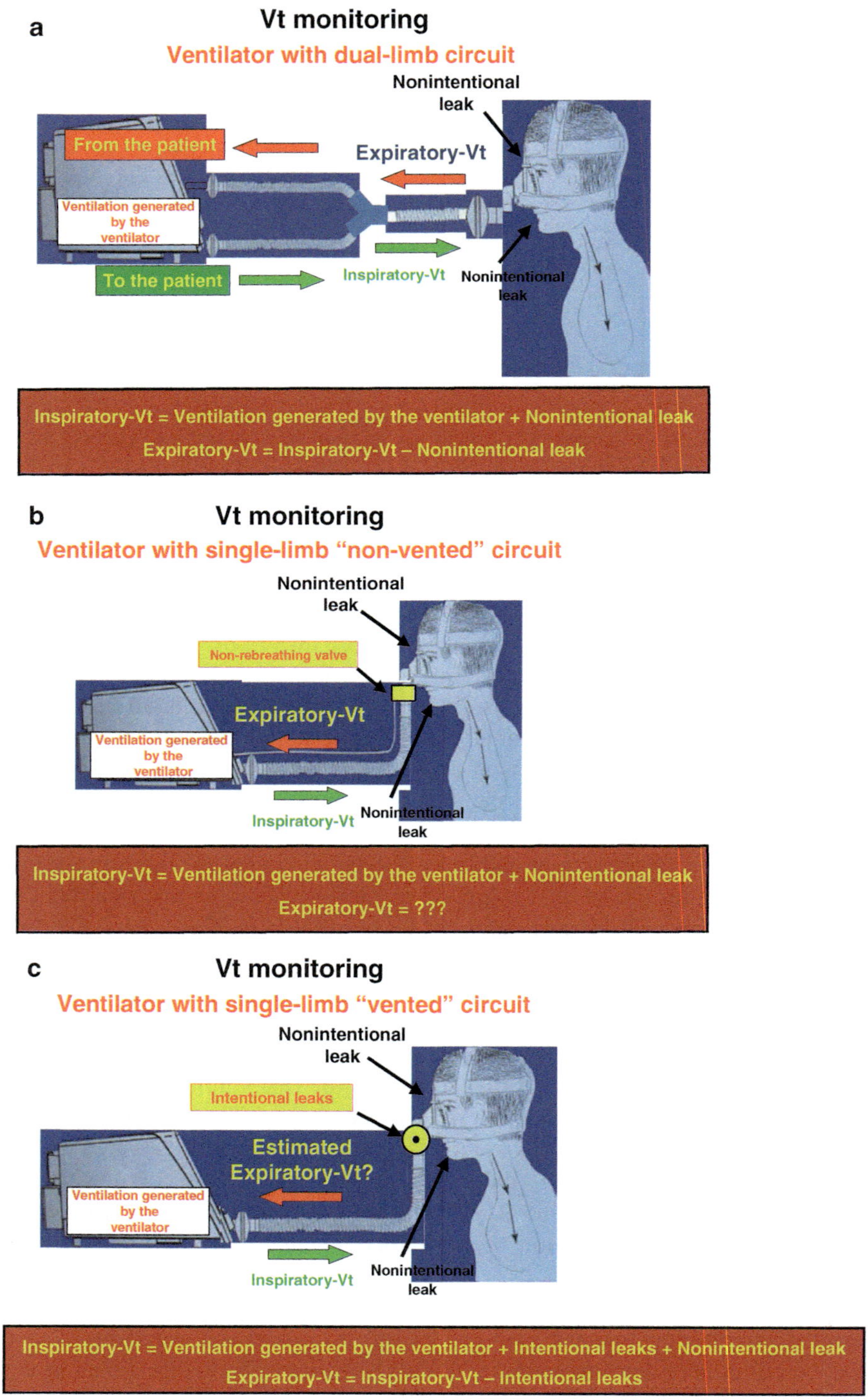

Fig. 6.2 Differences in Vt monitoring during noninvasive ventilation delivered by means of ventilators equipped with double (**a**) or single-limb circuit provided with a non-vented (**b**) or vented (**c**) exhalation system with permission from reference [7]

6.4 Controversial Issues

Because of the huge gap between the increasing number of newer ventilators that are commercially available and their physiologic and clinical careful evaluation, there is no published data about several sophisticated ventilators routinely used in the clinical practice. With few in vivo investigations, the majority of data about the performance of the different available ventilators comes from in vitro studies conducted on lung models. Therefore, some doubts remain about the real clinical significance of the technical differences observed in the bench studies among the vary types of ventilators. Consequently, every extrapolation of these experimental data to the clinical setting must be done cautiously because no lung model can simulate the ventilatory variability observed in patients. This is particularly true when the findings of in vitro studies have to be applied to acute patients under NPPV in the presence of leaks.

Based on the published data of the literature, despite a wide heterogeneity found in each category of machines, several bi-level ventilators demonstrated a better performance than several ICU ventilators [3, 4]. However, no study has shown greater NPPV clinical success for one type of ventilator than another both in the acute and chronic settings. Nevertheless, some points should be clear when the clinician must choose a ventilator [3].

Key Major Recommendations

- As excessive air leaks are correlated with treatment failure, the clinician should choose *ventilators designed for NPPV with leak compensation capability* (i.e., bi-level, some intermediate and new ICU ventilators). Moreover, the capability of *setting several parameters and looking at flow-volume-pressure waveforms* with newer ventilators may be helpful in improving patient-ventilator synchrony, comfort, gas exchange and, hopefully, clinical outcome.
- The choice of ventilator should be tailored to the *pathophysiology and the severity of ARF and CRF*. In the acute setting, for hypoxemic patients, ventilators with an O_2 blender are recommended, whereas in those with hypercapnia, ventilators with a dual-limb circuit have an advantage in lowering $PaCO_2$. In patients with mild COPD exacerbation, the use of home ventilators may be appropriate, particularly if the patient is already on home NPPV. In contrast, patients with life-threatening ARF at risk of intubation should be treated with more sophisticated machines. In the chronic setting, conditions where respiratory drive is good (e.g., COPD) could use a simple ventilator that works in a spontaneous mode, whereas those in whom respiratory drive is impaired must have a mandatory back-up rate. Conversely, in case of fast-progressing neuromuscular diseases, a more sophisticated ventilator with adequate monitoring equipment and an inner battery is recommended. The clinical superiority of new hybrid modes of

NPPV (e.g., VAPS) over the traditional pressometric modes has yet to be demonstrated in both the acute and chronic settings.

- The selection of a ventilator should also take into account *costs and staff experience*. The more sophisticated a ventilator is, the longer the training for clinicians is required. With the tremendous growth of the ventilator market in terms of complexity, some of the new bi-level ventilators are not user-friendly even for trained ICU clinicians. The smaller the variety of devices used, the greater the likelihood that all team members will acquire enough experience in NPPV set-up, with positive repercussions in costs and workload.
- The clinician should be aware of the *multiple interferences of the accessories for NPPV* (interfaces, exhalation systems, pressure settings, and humidification devices) with the performance of the different categories of ventilators. For example, concerning humidification during NPPV, heated humidifiers show great clinical and physiological advantages compared with heat-moisture exchangers, even though the former is more time-consuming.

References

1. Nava S, Hill N. Non-invasive ventilation in acute respiratory failure. Lancet. 2009;374(9685):250–9.
2. Ozsancak A, D'Ambrosio C, Hill NS. Nocturnal noninvasive ventilation. Chest. 2008;133(5):1275–86.
3. Scala R, Naldi M. Ventilators for noninvasive ventilation to treat acute respiratory failure. Respir Care. 2008;53(8):1054–80.
4. Gregoretti C, Navalesi P, Ghannadian S, et al. Choosing a ventilator for home mechanical ventilation. Breathe. 2013;9:394–408.
5. Vignaux L, Vargas F, Roeseler J, et al. Patient-ventilator asynchrony during non-invasive ventilation for acute respiratory failure: a multicenter study. Intensive Care Med. 2009;35(5):840–6.
6. Schwartz AR, Kacmarek RM, Hess DR. Factors affecting oxygen delivery with bi-level positive airway pressure. Respir Care. 2004;49(3):270–5.
7. Scala R. Monitoring choices in acute NIV. In: Simonds AK, ed. ERS Practical Handbook of Noninvasive Ventilation. Sheffield, European Respiratory Society. 2015; pp. 93–101.
8. Schettino GP, Chatmongkolchart S, Hess DR, et al. Position of exhalation port and mask design affect CO_2 rebreathing during noninvasive positive pressure ventilation. Crit Care Med. 2003;31(8):2178–82.
9. Nava S, Ambrosino N, Bruschi C, et al. Physiological effects of flow and pressure triggering during non-invasive mechanical ventilation in patients with chronic obstructive pulmonary disease. Thorax. 1997;52(3):249–54.
10. Di Marco F, Centanni S, Bellone A, et al. Optimization of ventilator setting by flow and pressure waveforms analysis during noninvasive ventilation for acute exacerbations of COPD: a multicentric randomized controlled trial. Crit Care. 2011;15(6):R283.
11. Prinianakis G, Delmastro M, Carlucci A, et al. Effect of varying the pressurisation rate during noninvasive pressure support ventilation. Eur Respir J. 2004;23(2):314–20.

7 Ventilatory Modes and Settings During Noninvasive Ventilation

Claudio Rabec and Daniel Rodenstein

Contents

C. Rabec, MD (✉)
Service de Pneumologie et Réanimation Respiratoire, Centre Hospitalier et Universitaire de Dijon, 2 Bd Maréchal de Lattre de Tassigny, Dijon 21079, France
e-mail: claudio.rabec@chu-dijon.fr

D. Rodenstein, MD, PhD
Service de Pneumologie, Cliniques Universitaires Saint Luc, Université Catholique de Louvain, Bruxelles, Belgium

A.M. Esquinas (ed.), *Noninvasive Mechanical Ventilation: Theory, Equipment, and Clinical Applications*, DOI 10.1007/978-3-319-21653-9_7

Since the early 1980s, when noninvasive ventilation (NIV) showed efficacy in the management of some forms of respiratory failure [1–3], the number of patients receiving this treatment both in the acute setting and at home has steadily increased. This is explained by a growing number of indications in which the effectiveness of NIV has been proven, and also by major technological advances that led to the availability of high-performance portable ventilators and the development of a technical support infrastructure [4]. In the particular case of chronic respiratory failure patients, NIV applications were extended from conventional indications in chest wall and neuromuscular diseases to other more frequent conditions such as obesity hypoventilation and chronic obstructive pulmonary disease (COPD), although, in the latter, the role of NIV is still controversial [5–7].

NIV is predominantly applied at night. Sleep is a unique state that induces profound ventilatory changes, including modifications in ventilatory control, upper airway patency, and respiratory muscle recruitment. These sleep-related physiological changes, although without clinical consequences in healthy subjects, may represent an additional challenge when the respiratory system is in a disease state, exceeding the response capabilities of the system and leading to failure [8]. Furthermore, it has been well demonstrated that sleep-related hypoventilation is the first sign of ventilatory failure preceding daytime chronic respiratory failure [9].

Nocturnal NIV can have sustained effects in correcting arterial blood gases during the day. It has been hypothesized that this improvement is mediated by a number of possible mechanisms: (1) improving ventilatory mechanics, (2) resting fatigued respiratory muscles, or (3) enhancing ventilatory sensitivity to CO_2 [10]. In addition, improvement in sleep stage distribution may increase chemosensitivity and enhance sleep quality [11].

This chapter deals with the equipment and mechanisms for NIV and, in particular, the major ventilator modes and settings.

7.1 NIV: A Short Story

From an historical point of view, negative pressure ventilation (NPV) was the first mode applied to long-term mechanical ventilation. In NPV, a perithoracic subatmospheric pressure is applied to generate inspiration by using body ventilators (e.g., tank or cuirasses). Apart from some specialized centers, this treatment has been almost completely substituted for positive pressure ventilation. The main reasons for this trend were cumbersome NPV devices, the lack of accessibility by the patient, and the danger of inducing upper airway obstruction [12].

The first positive pressure ventilators were powered by a piston chamber, a rotary piston, or a standard compressor. They were large, encumbering, and not versatile and had limited capabilities to modify airflow. Most of them provided only a volume-targeted mode. In the mid-1990s, the development of blower-driven continuous positive airway pressure (CPAP) devices to treat obstructive sleep apnea (OSA) and the growing popularity of NIV influenced the evolution toward the first blower-driven devices providing bi-level positive pressure. These devices were originally conceived to improve the tolerance of patients with OSA and consisted of a CPAP blower modified with a magnetic valve to cycle between two different pressure levels, hence the name bi-level devices [13]. Since then, NIV devices have rapidly evolved with the development of microprocessor-controlled, high-performance, blower-driven micro ventilators. These new technology devices have some advantages, such as flexibility and variability in gas-delivery patterns, high leak compensation capabilities, and "intelligent" inspiratory and expiratory trigger mechanisms. Some of them also have the capability of interfacing with computer systems and built-in monitoring modules that can assess ventilatory parameters and store the data in memory for subsequent analysis.

7.2 Issues of Particular Importance During NIV: Leaks, Upper Airway Resistance, the Type of Exhalation Port, and NIV Ventilators

Compared with invasive ventilation, NIV has two unique characteristics: the non-airtight nature of the system that poses the potential risk of unintentional leaks, and the fact that the ventilator-lung assembly cannot be considered as a single-compartment model because of the presence of a variable resistance represented by the upper airway (UA). Both situations may compromise the delivery of an effective tidal volume. As a consequence, during NIV, increasing the delivered volume or the delivered inspiratory pressure do not necessarily result in increased effective ventilation reaching the lungs [14].

7.2.1 Influence of Unintentional Leaks

Unintentional leaks are very common in NIV [11, 15]. Leakage may be absent or minimal when the patient is awake but may worsen during sleep as a result of the loss of voluntary control and decreased muscle tone. Leaks can take place at the mouth, between the skin and the mask but an amount of air can also be deposited at the oropharyngeal reservoir and even pass to the digestive tract ("internal" leaks) [16]. After having ruled out poor adaptation of the interface, leaks can be classified according to causal factor: as primary or "passive", resulting from hypotonic masseter muscles and/or inability of the soft palate and the oral muscles to counterbalance the high inspiratory pressure insufflated by the ventilator, or secondary to closure of the upper airways occurring at the level of the oropharynx or the glottis [14, 16, 17].

Leaks can impair quality of both ventilation and sleep. They can largely affect ventilator triggering, pressurization, volume delivered, rate of inspiratory pressuring and cycling function and induce sleep fragmentation. A detail of leak-induced abnormalities can be seen in Table 7.1.

Table 7.1 NIV: impact of unintentional leaks (see text for details)

Impact of unintentional leaks depends on:
Ventilatory mode (volume or pressure controlled)
Management of expiration (valve or leak outlet)
Unintentional leaks may affect:
Patient-ventilator synchrony and level of ventilatory assistance by affecting
Inspiratory triggering
Auto-triggering
Ineffective inspiratory efforts
I to E cycling [35, 38]
Rise time
Pressurization
Maintain of desired PEEP level
Tolerance of ventilation
Quality of sleep by inducing frequent arousals and sleep fragmentation
The consequences of leaks on the quality of NIV will depend on:
The ventilatory cycle phase during which the leak occurs
The magnitude of the leak
The continuous or intermittent nature of the leak
The ability of the ventilator to compensate for leaks

7.2.2 Influence of the Upper Airways: A to Component Variable Resistor

During NIV, a variable resistance constituted by the upper airway (UA) is interposed between the ventilator and the lung. This explains why a reduction of airway patency may occur, compromising delivery of an effective tidal volume. Intermittent obstruction of the UA is common during NIV and may be related to two mechanisms. The first corresponds to obstructive events at the oropharyngeal level because of UA collapse, as a result of insufficient expiratory positive airway pressure (EPAP). This mechanism may be present in patients with an unstable UA, such as patients with OSA [7, 18]. Another mechanism corresponds to episodes of intermittent obstruction at the glottal level, reflecting cyclic glottal closure induced by hyperventilation, a type of "ventilation resistance" reflex [19–22].

7.2.3 Influence of Type of Exhalation Device and Connecting Circuits

Whereas intensive care unit (ICU) ventilators classically use a double circuit with an integrated expiratory valve, two different types of circuits can be used to provide

NIV. The first uses a similar assembly to those used in ICU devices and includes either single or double tubing, in which inspiration and expiration are separated and a true expiratory valve is present so that CO_2 rebreathing is not a significant problem (Fig. 7.1a). The other type of ventilators, like the CPAP devices that they were derived from, do not have a true exhalation valve and often use a single-limb circuit with a risk of rebreathing. To avoid rebreathing, this system includes a calibrated leak (called intentional leak) either at the mask level or in the circuit (Fig. 7.1b). Single-circuit pressure-targeted ventilators, provided with a calibrated leak (called bi-level ventilators), are most commonly used for NIV today. These devices cycle between a higher inspiratory positive airway pressure (IPAP) and a lower EPAP that can be independently adjusted. With these devices, a minimum mandatory EPAP level of 4 cm H_2O is needed to ensure an effective washout of CO_2, [23]. The use of specific "anti-rebreathing" valves may also diminish rebreathing, although their clinical relevance remains uncertain. Moreover, some of these devices increase expiratory work of breathing and may potentially lead to dynamic hyperinflation and patient discomfort [23, 24]. Interestingly, one study showed that the exhalation port position influences CO_2 rebreathing with a more efficient CO_2 washout when the leak is positioned within the mask [25].

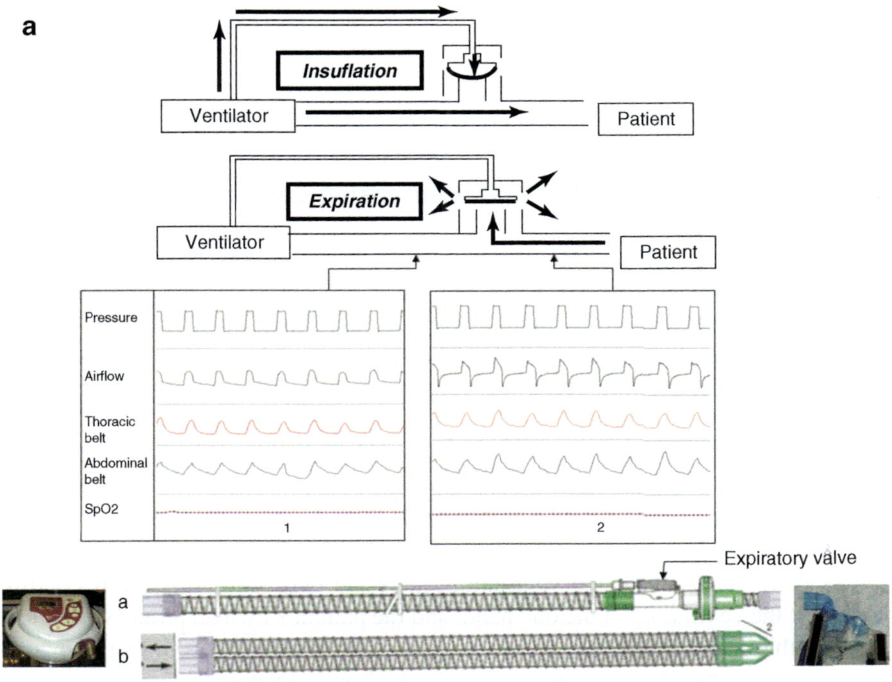

Fig. 7.1 Type of circuits used in non-invasive ventilation (NIV) with (**a**) an expiratory valve and (**b**) intentional leak,Note that when a simple circuit with an intentional leak is used, the leak may be interposed in the circuit or incorporated at the mask

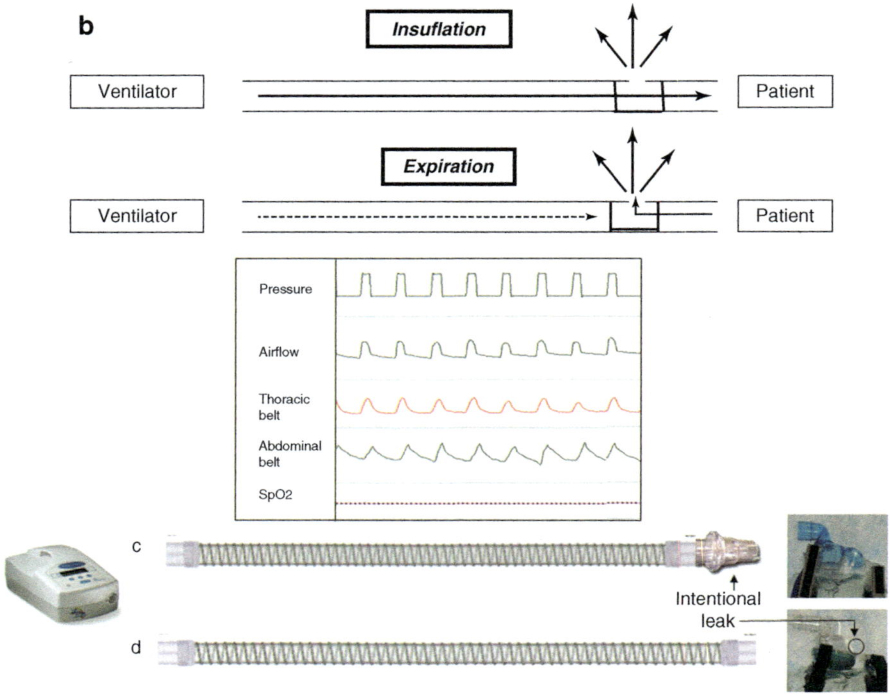

Fig. 7.1 (continued)

7.2.4 Influence of the Ventilator: Intensive-Care (ICU) Versus Home Devices

Both ICU and home ventilators can be used to deliver NIV. The main technical characteristic differentiating them is that, for the former, the driving pressure is supplied by compressed gas, whereas the latter incorporate their own pressure source. Nevertheless, the type of ventilatory support that they provide is similar

7.3 Patient Ventilator Synchrony: One Goal, Two Pumps

When delivering mechanical ventilation, there are two ventilatory pumps acting together: the ventilator, on the one hand, and the patient's own respiratory muscles, on the other hand. These two pumps may work in harmony, but, in fact, they can interact in any number of ways, many of which will create problems rather than solving them. Hence, patient ventilator asynchrony is quite common in patients during NIV [26, 27]. Asynchronies may occur at two levels: during inspiratory triggering, in situations in which there is a mismatch between patient inspiratory effort and ventilator triggering (i.e., ineffective inspiratory effort, double triggering, or auto-triggering) or during cycling from inspiration to expiration, when ventilator cycling does not coincide with the end of patient effort (premature or delayed cycling) [27].

We will begin this section by reviewing the triggering and cycling modes.

7.3.1 How Do Inspiration and Expiration Start and Stop?

The patient can control the initiation (triggering) and the end (cycling) of inspiration or, on the contrary, neither of them, in which case the ventilator controls both the initiation and the end of inspiration.

7.3.1.1 Spontaneous Mode (S)

In this mode, the patient controls the beginning and end of inspiration. Inspiration starts when the ventilator is triggered by the patient. During the low-level expiratory pressure (EPAP), the patient's inspiratory effort modifies the pressure and flow into the circuit, starting the change to the higher inspiratory pressure (IPAP). The pressure is maintained as long as a minimal preset inspiratory flow is occurring. The end of inspiratory assistance (cycling from inspiration to expiration) occurs when the declining inspiratory flow reaches a predetermined percentage of peak inspiratory flow and the pressure in the circuit reverses to EPAP. In this mode, a targeted inspiratory pressure, an inspiratory trigger sensitivity, and a percentage threshold of peak flow for cycling to expiration (see below) must be selected. In some ventilators, these can all be set by the clinician, whereas in others, only the inspiratory pressure can be set. Trigger sensitivity, peak flow, and the level of ventilatory support (IPAP – EPAP) are the main variables that determine the patient's work of breathing Because each cycle is terminated by a flow criterion rather than by volume or time, the patient retains control of cycle length as well as its depth and flow profile. This mode is also called pressure support ventilation (PSV).

7.3.1.2 Assist Mode (A)

In A mode, the patient controls the onset of inspiration but the inspiratory length is regulated by the operator. In this mode, the clinician must select a targeted volume or pressure, an inspiratory-expiratory (I:E) ratio, or an inspiratory time and an inspiratory trigger sensitivity

7.3.1.3 Assist-Control Mode (A/C)

As in assist mode, in A/C mode the patient controls onset of inspiration but end of inspiration is time triggered and determined by the operator. As this mode also allows presetting a backup respiratory rate (RR), if patient RR is lower than the preset ventilator backup RR, the system moves to control mode. Then, this mode allows the patient to trigger the ventilator but also tries to grant a minimum minute ventilation by allowing a backup rate. In this mode, the clinician must select a backup rate, a targeted volume or pressure, an expiratory pressure, an I:E ratio, and inspiratory trigger sensitivity. Trigger sensitivity and peak flow are the main variables that determine the patient's work of breathing.

7.3.1.4 Control Mode (C)

In the control mode, there is a preset automatic cycle based on time. The ventilator controls the beginning and end of inspiration and thus the RR. Therefore, one expects the ventilator to capture and inhibit the patient's respiratory center and the patient to follow the settings imposed by the ventilator. In this mode, the clinician must select a targeted volume or pressure, a fixed RR, and an I:E ratio or inspiratory and expiratory durations. With this mode, the entire work of breathing is supposed to be performed by the ventilator. In some ventilators, this mode is also called timed (T) mode, but it is rarely used.

A particular combination of these modes is available in some NIV ventilators. This mode, called S/T is basically a PSV that provides a backup rate. In this particular mode, cycling from inspiration to expiration is flow limited in patient-triggered cycles and switched to time limited when the patient's spontaneous RR falls below the backup rate. It also happens when, during S cycles, inspiratory time exceeds a predetermined maximal length (see below). A patient-triggered cycle can be seen in curves of ventilation as a negative inspiratory deflection in pressure and flow curves (see trace no 2 in both Fig. 7.2b, c).

7.3.2 How a Ventilator Acts and How Patient Ventilator Synchrony Is Achieved: The Ventilatory Cycle

Inadequate patient cooperation, mask intolerance, and patient selection criteria have been advocated as frequent causes of NIV failure, but little attention has been paid to settings and type of ventilator. However, appropriate settings are essential to obtain optimal patient-ventilator synchrony, a main condition to ensure a good quality of ventilation and a proper tolerance by the patient [28]. The most logical approach to explain how a ventilator acts and how patient ventilator synchrony is achieved is to analyze the different phases of a typical positive pressure ventilatory cycle (Fig. 7.3).

7.3.2.1 Triggering

As described above, the beginning of inspiration can be triggered by time or patient effort. In the A and AC mode, the ventilator must recognize the patients' inspiratory effort. This is called triggering function. Classically, NIV devices propose two types of triggers. The first, called a pressure-based trigger, present in older NIV ventilators, is based on a drop in proximal airway pressure and requires a closed circuit. The amplitude of this drop is a function of preset sensitivity and also of patient respiratory drive. A second, called a flow-based trigger, present in almost all newer NIV devices, is based on detection of an inspiratory flow in the presence of a continuous flow washing out the circuit during expiration.

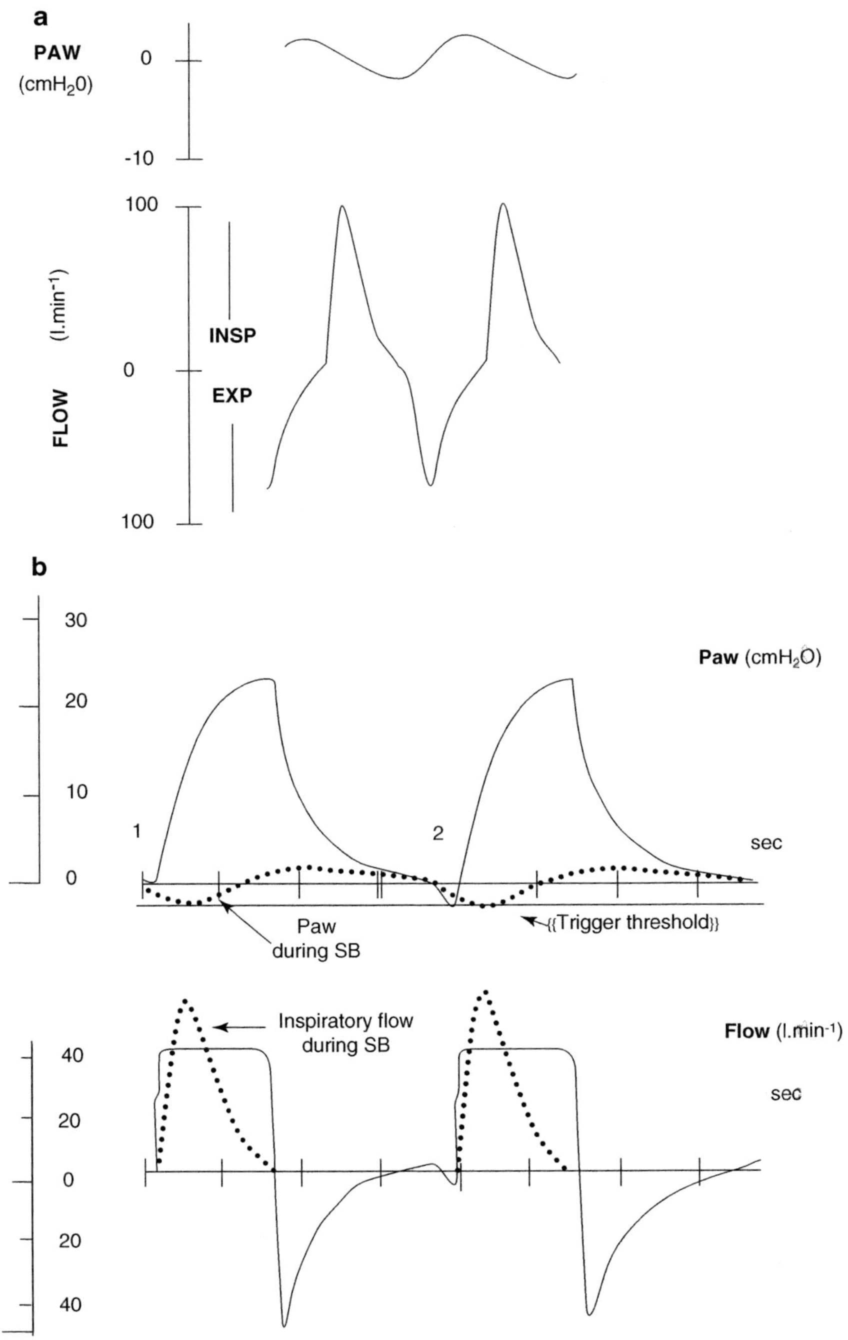

Fig. 7.2 Flow and Paw dynamics during (**a**) spontaneous breathing, (**b**) pressure-targeted ventilation, (**c**) volume-targeted ventilation. *1* Controlled cycle, *2* assisted cycle. *Dashed lines* represent simultaneous theoretical spontaneous breathing kinetics. Note that, during PTM, flow contour remains close to physiological flow dynamics, facilitating a better adaptation to patient ventilatory needs and patient-ventilator synchrony (for details, see text)

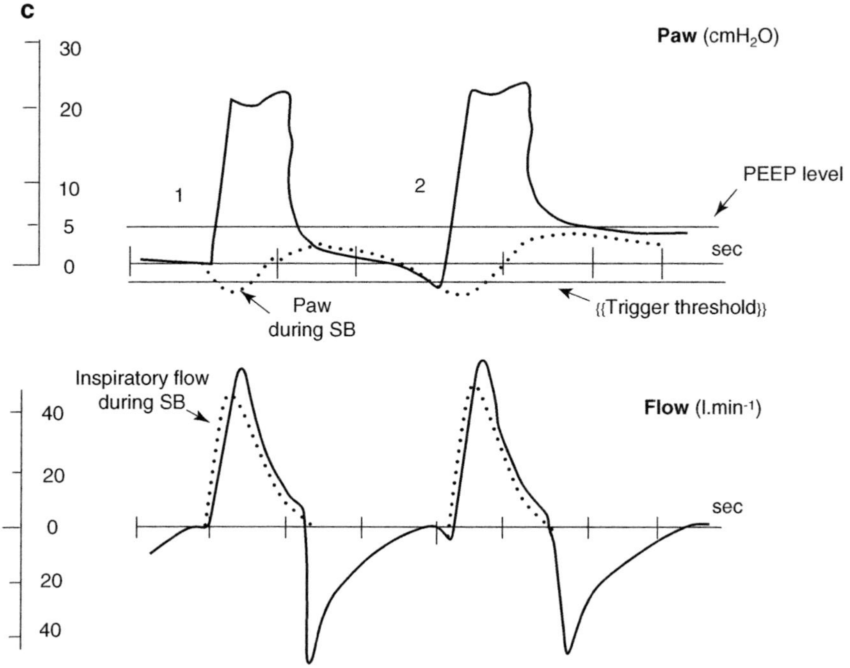

Fig. 7.2 (continued)

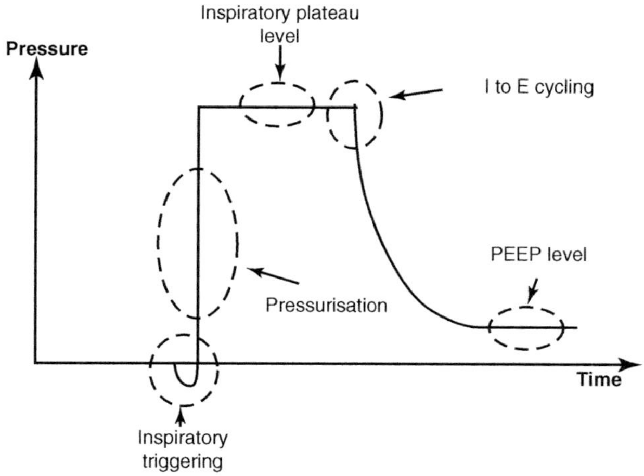

Fig. 7.3 The ventilatory cycle

Patient ventilatory synchrony during the triggering phase needs a match between the three physiological variables characterizing spontaneous breathing (ventilatory drive, ventilatory requirements, and Ti/Tot, which is the ratio of inspiratory time/total time) and the three technological variables characterizing ventilator function (trigger function, gas delivery algorithm, and cycling criteria). Asynchrony during the inspiratory phase is quite common during sleep in patients under NIV, may compromise ventilatory efficacy and sleep quality, and is mainly influenced by the delay duration, trigger sensitivity, and amount of pre-inspiratory effort (which depends itself on respiratory drive and muscle strength) [26]. Therefore, the inspiratory trigger should have a short delay of response (i.e., a short time between onset of inspiratory effort and pressurization) and be sensitive enough to allow the patient to trigger easily without auto-triggering, even in the presence of leaks. It ideally should be <100 ms, inasmuch as higher values can increase work of breathing and lead to asynchrony or discomfort [29]. As opening a demand valve during pressure triggering can impose substantial effort [29], ventilators that use flow triggering have, in general, shorter trigger delays [30]. However, these triggers expose the patient to greater occurrence of auto-triggering [31, 32]. Other than intrinsic performance of the trigger system, triggering depends on type of circuit used (simple or double), the patient profile, the level of auto-positive end expiratory pressure (auto-PEEP), and the presence of leaks [33]. Leaks may greatly affect trigger function, either by precluding detection of patient inspiratory effort (leading to ineffective inspiratory effort) or by mimicking an "inspiratory flow" (when using flow triggering) or dragging EPAP level below trigger threshold (when using pressure triggering), with both of the latter situations possibly leading to autocycling. Finally, other frequent causes of asynchrony during the triggering phase are excessive pressure assistance (as high pressure generates dynamic hyperinflation due to larger tidal volume and shorter expiratory time, contributing to a new inspiratory effort occurring before an incomplete exhalation), additional resistance in the circuit, and dynamic hyperinflation [27, 33].

The newer technologies (microprocessors, servo valves, and fast blowers) have substantially improved trigger response. Moreover, an adjustable inspiratory trigger is an option presently available in most home ventilators. Automated complex trigger algorithms, are available, in which a flow-time waveform is used to trigger the ventilator. With these systems, triggering arises when patient inspiratory effort distorts the expiratory flow waveform and this signal crosses the flow shape signal. This method is said to be more sensitive than classical flow triggering, allows adjusting trigger sensitivity in presence of leaks, and can help to reduce ineffective efforts and autocycling. However, the respective advantages of this sophisticated trigger system have not been assessed in rigorous studies. It should be emphasized that some adjustable-trigger devices are scaled in arbitrary units (1–5 or even 1–10), which makes them difficult to use in real life

7.3.2.2 Pressurization

As the correct pressurization is essential to decrease inspiratory effort and improve synchronization, during this phase, inspiratory flow should be sufficient to match inspiratory demand [34]. Circumstances influencing pressurization are the level of ventilatory support, the amount of time required to reach the target pressure (pressurization slope, also called rise time), compliance and resistance of the respiratory system, and patient inspiratory effort. Studies comparing different ventilators also emphasize the influence of the type of device on pressurization, in particular in situations of high inspiratory demand [35].

A faster rise time has been shown to better unload the respiratory muscles [34]. As the slope becomes flatter, the machine delivers lower flow rates and the patient's work of breathing increases [34]. In these situations, the device acts by creating an increasing hindrance to airflow, simulating a condition in which the patient breathes through a narrow circuit. However, it must be emphasized that if a slow pressurization can increase inspiratory work, an excessive peak flow can also have adverse effects as it may increase the sensation of dyspnea [36], induce double triggering [27], and lead to high peak mask pressure, which favors leaks. Moreover, leaks can themselves impair pressurization [35].

Some new ventilators offer an adjustable rise time, allowing an individual titration that can profoundly affect patient comfort and synchrony. In this context, it must be emphasized that even if the data published show that the steepest pressure ramp slope induced the lowest work of breathing in both obstructed and restricted patients [34], COPD patients tend to prefer relatively rapid rise time (0.05–0.1 s) whereas patients with neuromuscular diseases prefer a slower one (0.3–0.4 s)

Whereas the pressurization capacity of recent bi-level ventilators have shown improvements, NIV blower-powered devices are, in this aspect, clearly at a disadvantage when compared with proportional valve-powered ICU ventilators [35]. Moreover, studies comparing different home ventilators found major differences in terms of pressurization, even when tested at similar rise times, in particular in situations of high inspiratory demand [35]. Regardless, when considering long-term ventilation, this concern is probably not as important as it is in the acute setting because most patients do not have high inspiratory demands

7.3.2.3 Sustainment of Inspiratory Plateau

Inspiratory pressure level is one of the main determinants of efficacy of NIV. Determination of the optimal level can be the result of balancing two opposing aims: the desire to provide effective minute ventilation and the need to minimize leaks and discomfort caused by excessive inspiratory pressure. It must be emphasized that, even if newer ventilatory devices have great capabilities to compensate mild to moderate leaks, greater leaks may compromise the ability of the device to attain a desired level of inspiratory pressure. Because very high IPAP levels may favor leaks and the ability of these devices to compensate for them is limited, these two conditions will determine whether inspiratory pressure level remains stable or decreases. Even if there is no recognized gold standard for the level at which ventilatory support must be set, high IPAP levels must be avoided because, in addition to favoring leaks and discomfort, they can induce central apneas during sleep, leading to arousals and sleep fragmentation [37], and can also cause patient ventilatory asynchrony [27].

7.3.2.4 Cycling from Inspiration to Expiration

Switching from inspiration to expiration can be time cycled or flow cycled. In the time-cycled mode, ventilators use a time criteria chosen by the clinician. In the flow-cycled mode, cycling occurs as inspiratory flow decreases to a preadjusted percentage of the peak inspiratory flow, which is supposed to indicate the end of inspiratory effort. The criteria used to end inspiration may have a clinically relevant impact on quality of ventilation. Ideally, cycling should coincide with the end of patient effort. However, synchronization between end of neural inspiration and ventilator expiratory triggering is mainly determined by respiratory mechanics moving from a premature cycling in restrictive patients to a late cycling in obstructive ones [35, 38]. Moreover, when flow cycling is used, leaks may also delay switching to expiration because flow rate is maintained, in an attempt to maintain pressure, above the level at which cycling into expiration occurs (Fig. 7.4). Both these conditions may lead to patient ventilator expiratory asynchrony, a common condition in patients with COPD [38]. Moreover, this late cycling may aggravate auto-PEEP, also leading to ineffective inspiratory triggering [38]. As with other components of the ventilatory cycle, leaks may profoundly modify I to E cycling, either by advancing or delaying expiratory triggering. In the latter case, increasing the ventilator flow for leak compensation may counterbalance the decrease of inspiratory flow under the preadjusted threshold level, thus impeding recognition of the end of inspiration. This results in abnormal prolongation of inspiratory time that may lead to asynchrony, as patients exhale against the machine (aggravating auto-PEEP, in particular, in obstructive patients) or even inhale without receiving any ventilatory support (inspiratory hang-up) [38].

In older ventilators, expiratory trigger is fixed at 25 % of peak flow, but newer ventilators offer adjustable expiratory triggers. Some of them use arbitrary units, but others allow defining a known percentage of peak flow. These adjustable expiratory triggers may allow tailoring settings to the patient's underlying condition. For instance, Tassaux et al. [39] demonstrate in a COPD population under invasive ventilation that increasing the expiratory trigger from 10 to 70 % of peak flow (this means shortening inspiration to allow a greater expiratory time) was associated with a marked reduction in delayed cycling and intrinsic PEEP. Whether the same is true in patients under NIV remains to be elucidated.

To improve patient ventilator expiratory synchrony, some bi-level ventilators provide intelligent flow-based algorithms that, by "copying" previous ventilatory cycle patterns and by using moving signals, are able to modify cycle thresholds to automatically adjust breath-to-breath inspiratory time. These algorithms are supposed to be useful, in particular to adjust inspiratory time during leaks.

Finally, additional mechanisms proposed by some ventilators can improve cycling to prevent undesired inspiratory time prolongation. Sudden increases in pressure (that can be assumed as secondary to an active expiratory effort) produce, in almost all the devices, early cycling to expiration. Another mechanism is to limit maximal inspiratory time. This maximal inspiratory time (called also Timax) is generally fixed at 3 s but may be adjustable for some devices. The aim of Timax is to switch to a time criterion to terminate the breath to prevent an unsuitable lengthening of inspiratory time (in particular when leaks are present).

7.3.2.5 PEEP Level

PEEP is an above-atmospheric (positive) pressure applied during expiration. When positive pressure is applied during machine breaths, the term PEEP is maintained but when applied during spontaneous breathing the term CPAP is used.

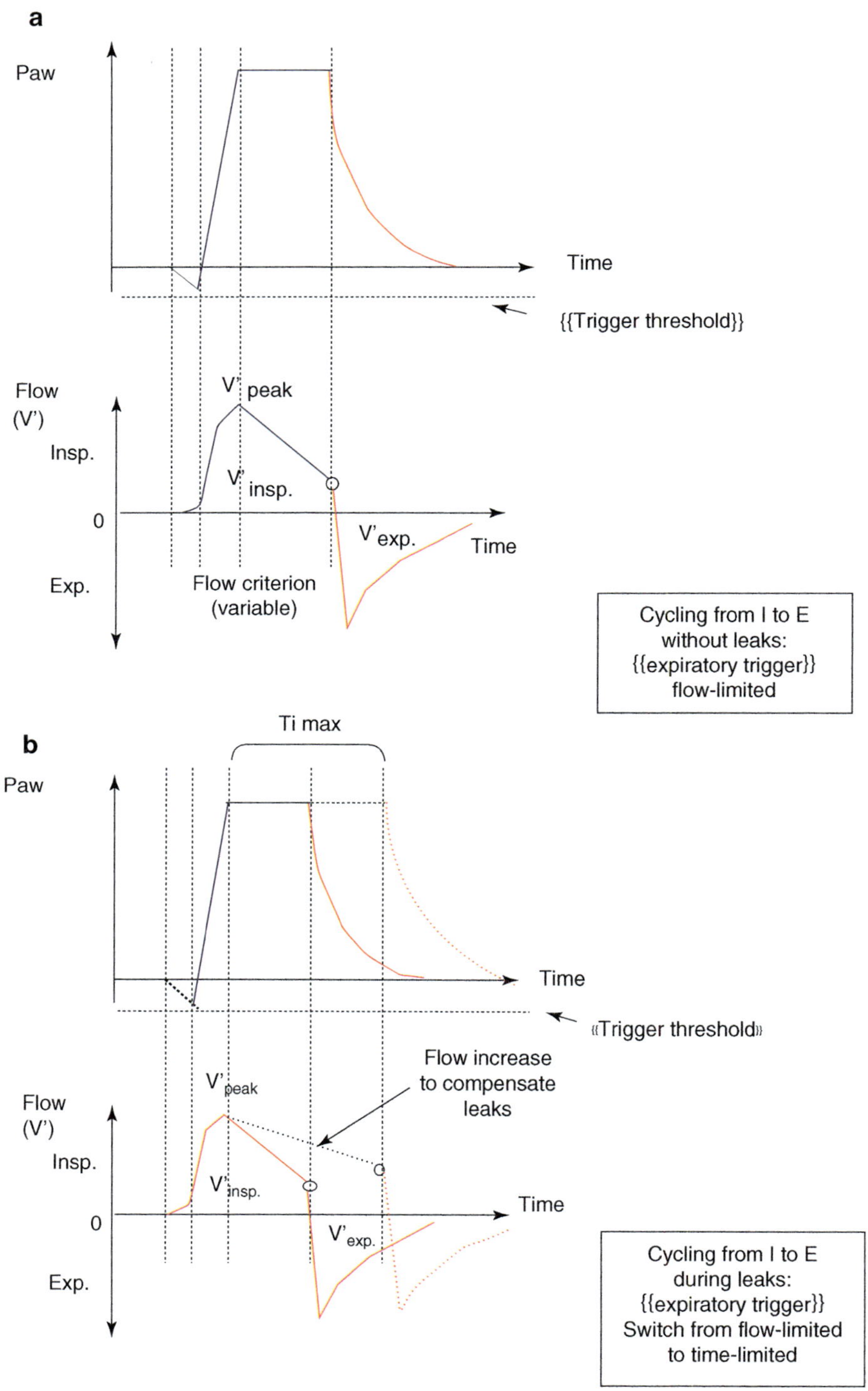

Fig. 7.4 Impact of leaks on I to E cycling during PSV (S in bi-level devices) mode. (**a**) Pressure support ventilation without leaks. (**b**) With leaks. Note that during leaks, the cycle switches to a time mode

With both, the positive pressure is maintained throughout the entire cycle. Providing an external PEEP (called EPAP in bi-level devices) during NIV has many theoretical advantages. Other than flushing dead space CO_2 and preventing rebreathing, EPAP can, in some obstructive patients, reduce dynamic hyperinflation by offsetting intrinsic PEEP [40], thereby reducing inspiratory work required to trigger assisted inspiration. Moreover, an optimal PEEP level can preserve the airway patency in patients with unstable upper airway during sleep. Additional advantages are alveolar recruitment, which increases functional residual capacity and decreases the tendency to microatelectasis. In the three latter situations, higher levels of EPAP (>6 cm) may be needed [41]. Unnecessary increases in EPAP levels should be avoided because inspiratory pressure must be increased in parallel if inspiratory assistance is to be maintained, which can lead to intolerance and favor leaks. As a result and regarding the ventilator category (ICU or home ventilator), the PEEP setting may interfere with either pressure support or IPAP levels. In fact, ICU ventilators propose PEEP and pressure support settings, however, PEEP and IPAP settings are usually associated with home ventilators. Thus, PEEP setting increases IPAP level on ICU ventilators, and PEEP setting decreases pressure support level on home ventilators. Moreover, high EPAP levels may, in some cases, increase work of breathing if lung volume increases to a point where EPAP induces overdistension and increases elastic impedance [42]. A further concern is that the application of a high level of EPAP can result in hemodynamic impairment.

Leaks, if significant, may make it impossible to maintain the set EPAP level. If the device uses a pressure-based inspiratory trigger, this may lead to autocycling because the EPAP levels fall below the trigger threshold.

Measures aimed at improving patient-ventilator synchrony under NIV are detailed in Table 7.2.

7.4 Modes of Ventilation

When NIV was introduced, there were a limited number of modalities and types of ventilators with only a few possible settings. We now have more than 30 brands offering numerous options for settings [43]. Moreover, ventilators are not submitted to stringent medical regulations. This leaves manufacturers free to give different names to the same ventilator modalities and settings and even to "create" new modalities that correspond frequently only to small modifications of a known class. This explains the wide variety of existing terminology describing NIV modalities.

Theoretically, NIV can be delivered using all the modalities used in invasive ventilation. In practice, this is not the case, because the circumstances of ventilation and target population are different but also because available equipment is often limited. Because most ventilators used for NIV deliver either volume- or pressure-targeted modes, and the place of other anecdotally proposed modes for some NIV devices, such as synchronized intermittent mandatory ventilation (SIMV),

Table 7.2 Measures aiming to improve patient-ventilator synchrony under NIV

Component of ventilatory cycle	Measure
Inspiratory trigger	Avoid excessive inspiratory pressure or volume Control unintentional leaks Use device with short response time (ideally <100 ms) Set trigger (if adjustable) sensitive enough to allow easy triggering without auto-triggering, even in the presence of leaks Reduce additional resistance Avoid dynamic hyperinflation Use respiratory backup rate in patients with muscular weakness Use flow-triggered devices (or, better yet, a device with "flow waveform method of triggering") Set EPAP level to counteract intrinsic PEEP (avoiding high EPAP levels)
Pressurization	Control unintentional leaks Use bi-level ventilators offering an adjustable rise time Set "tailored" rise time (faster slope while avoiding excessive peak flow)
Maintain targeted pressure/ volume	Control unintentional leaks Avoid excessive inspiratory pressure or volume Use devices with acceptable capabilities of leak compensation
Cycling from I to E	Control unintentional leaks Reduce IPAP level Tailor flow threshold Set Timax (if available) Avoid high backup RR (in particular in obstructive patients) Use adjustable expiratory triggers or "flow waveform method" of triggering
Sustaining EPAP level	Control unintentional leaks Avoid high EPAP levels

proportional assisted ventilation (PAV) or other "hybrid" modalities, is not yet clear, this chapter focuses only on the former two modes.

7.4.1 Volume-Targeted Mode

In the volume-targeted mode (VTM), also called the flow-limited mode, the ventilator delivers a fixed volume during a given time and with whatever pressure is necessary to achieve this. Pressure in the airways (Paw) results from the interaction between ventilatory settings, compliance and resistance of the respiratory system, and spontaneous inspiratory efforts (Fig. 7.2b). It should be emphasized that any inspiratory effort will not lead to changes in delivered volumes or flows but will only result in a decrease in Paw.

Because each breath is delivered with the same predetermined flow time profile and the area under the flow time curve defines volume, the advantage of this mode is the strict delivery, in the absence of leaks, of the preset volume, whatever the values of C and R. A major disadvantage is, precisely, that delivery of this fixed ventilatory assistance does not allow taking into account the patient's varying requirements. Another inconvenience is that, if there is a leak, there will be no increase in flow rate to compensate and the generated pressure will be lower, so that the effectively delivered volume will be reduced proportionally.

Ventilators that deliver VTM use a simple or double circuit with an integrated expiratory valve. Nevertheless, a new ventilator (Trilogy, Philips, Koninklijken Netherlands) incorporates a volume mode using a simple circuit with intentional leak. To ensure tidal volume, this device includes a complex algorithm to compensate for total leaks. Most older ventilators delivering this mode deliver volumes via a piston or bellows, however, newer devices are blower driven and capable of providing internal PEEP adjustment.

7.4.2 Pressure-Targeted Mode

In the pressure-targeted mode (PTM), also called the pressure-limited mode, the ventilator is set to deliver airflow by generating a predefined positive pressure in the airways for a given time. Therefore, airflow is adjusted so as to establish and maintain a constant Paw according to the preset pressure. Constant analysis of the flow rate and airway pressure determines the flow variations necessary to maintain a flat or "square wave" pressure. Flow is brisk at the beginning of inspiration when the gradient between the circuit pressure and pressure target is large (Fig. 7.2c). As this gradient narrows, flow decelerates until driving flow no longer exists and flow ceases. Thus, for a given patient, the volume delivered is not fixed and will depend on the interaction between the preset pressure, patient inspiratory effort, the physical characteristics of the respiratory system (R and C), and inspiratory time. PTM ventilators can use circuits with or without an expiratory valve. An important advantage of PTM is the ability to compensate for mild to moderate leaks. Simple-circuit PTM ventilators without an expiratory valve (called bi-level ventilators) are used the most for NIV. These devices are provided with a calibrated leak and cycle between IPAP and EPAP. The mathematical difference between both pressures corresponds to a pressure support in S mode or a pressure control in T mode. With these devices, the patient's effort determines flow and, when switching to EPAP, the device delivers a lower positive pressure that splints and maintains a positive alveolar pressure. Therefore, IPAP and EPAP level can be independently adjusted both to augment alveolar ventilation and maintain upper airway patency during sleep. In S mode (and in ST mode above backup RR), the patient can control inspiratory and expiratory time, inspiratory flow, tidal volume, and respiratory rate, with th the ventilator providing only a preset pressure. Therefore, this mode is comfortable and provides a suitable patient ventilator synchrony.

7.4.3 NIV: Volume or Pressure Targeted?

Most of the initial studies concerning NIV used VTM ventilators [1, 44]. However, PTM ventilators were increasingly prescribed and surpassed VTM ventilators at the end of the 1990s. Although studies published showed no significant differences in terms of clinical efficacy or arterial blood gas results [45, 46], a European survey showed that more than 75 % of home-ventilated patients use PTM ventilators and that, in fact, VTM indications were restricted to patients with neuromuscular disease [47]. There are several technological and financial reasons for this trend. Ventilators providing PTM, in particular those of the bi-level type, are smaller, quieter, lighter, more compact, cheaper, and easier to adjust. Moreover, PTM provides better synchronization because this mode (and, in particular, PSV) was primarily designed to facilitate the patient's effort to breathe and flow contour and volume can be varied on a breath-by-breath basis. In addition, as a consequence of the decelerated flow rate, PTM can provide the same delivered tidal volumes by generating lower mean and peak airway pressures [48, 49], allowing less mask tightness and reducing the likelihood of leaks and side effects. An additional benefit of PTM is a better compensation for mild-to-moderate unintentional leaks because the capabilities of these devices to increase inspiratory flow to compensate for a leak-induced pressure drop [50].

A characteristic of NIV is that the magnitude of leaks changes continuously with movement, posture, and sleep stages changes and with the amount of pressure, which may provide a more stable ventilatory support. In fact, some of the modern home PTM devices can achieve peak inspiratory flow rates up to 180 $l \cdot min^{-1}$. A further advantage of small, portable PTV ventilators is the absence of unnecessary alarms, which controls costs and maximizes portability. Finally, a further advantage of PTM concerns the situations in which O_2 must be added. As most of the available portable ventilators do not have an O_2 blender, supplemental O_2 is provided by an additional admission in the ventilator tube. When VTM is used, this flow is added to minute volume delivered to the patient. Therefore, tidal volume needs to be proportionally reduced to impede overventilation. On the contrary, as in PTM, the ventilator targets a preset pressure, the addition of an external flow will not modify tidal volume and then no additional adjustments are needed.

On the other hand, PTM ventilators are less able to compensate for changes in compliance and resistance and the blowers powering most bi-level devices have limited maximal pressure-generation capacities. This may lead to insufficient ventilation. Therefore, PTM ventilators are less reliable than piston-driven volume ventilators when higher insufflation pressures are needed. Moreover, during PTM, delivered tidal volume differs substantially among different pathological entities and also between ventilators, despite similar settings, even in the absence of leaks. This is related to differences in inspiratory flow, rates, inspiratory duration, and even actual pressure delivered [50]. For that, VTM may be preferred in patients with changing respiratory impedance to ensure a given tidal volume and for some situations characterized by reduced thoraco-pulmonary compliance. An additional advantage of VTM is to provide the possibility of air stacking for assisted coughing and increasing the voice volume during NIV. Finally, VTM has been shown to produce more complete offloading of respiratory muscles, but at the expense of comfort [51]. Therefore, as has been suggested, VTM may offer advantages in patients with some conditions, such obesity hypoventilation, chest wall restriction, and neuromuscular disease, who may require high insufflation pressure or in those in whom adequate control is not achieved with PTM [52, 53]. Also, VTM is suitable in more dependent patients needing alarms (as VTM ventilators have better alarm capabilities than simple bi-level ventilators) or built-in battery backup systems (because blower-based technology used by bi-level devices consumes considerably more energy than piston-powered devices, large internal batteries are needed that counterbalance the benefits of light weight and compact size).

A comparative analysis of the two modalities and of corresponding flow and pressure patterns is summarized in Table 7.3.

7.4.4 Volume Targeting Pressure Mode

A limitation of pressure ventilation is that it cannot guarantee a tidal volume delivered to the patient. Volume targeting is a feature available in some bi-level ventilators that can allow overweighting of this limitation. In this hybrid mode, which combines the advantages of the pressure and volume modes, the ventilator estimates the delivered tidal volume and adjusts parameters to achieve a target tidal volume (Vt). Some of them adjust a target volume intracycle (each breath starts as a pressure-limited breath and if the set Vt is not reached, the breath converts to a flow-cycled mode by prolonging the inspiratory time), but most progressively adjust the pressure support level along several cycles within a preset range to provide a Vt as close as possible to the target volume set by the clinician. Whether this feature can improve ventilation effectiveness is not yet clear; as has been demonstrated, a higher level of pressure support is not necessarily associated with a decrease in diaphragmatic energy expenditure because wasted efforts were more common [54]. Interestingly, two studies using of this mode in patients with obesity hypoventilation syndrome (OHS) showed a significant improvement in nocturnal and daytime $PaCO_2$ compared with usual bi-level ventilation, but at the expense of impaired objective quality of sleep [55, 56]. Moreover, there are no differences between the two modes in terms of health-related quality of life.

There are two possible explanations for these findings. One is that pressure variations may induce sleep stages changes and/or arousals. But it is also possible that this altered sleep quality is a consequence of an impairment in patient ventilator synchrony secondary to glottic apneas triggered by increasing inspiratory pressure [21]. Interestingly, one study shows that the respiratory disturbance index was greater when patients were ventilated with volume-targeted mode, supporting the latter hypothesis [56].

Table 7.3 Comparison between pressure- and volume-targeted ventilators

	Volume targeted	Pressure targeted
Type of ventilatory assistance delivered	Fixed volume in spite of changing resistance and compliance	Fixed pressure Tidal volume may vary with changes in C and R
Controlled variable	Maintains a constant inspiratory preset flow	Maintains a constant inspiratory preset pressure
Breath-to-breath adjustments	Not possible. Ventilator delivers a fixed assistance	Possible. Flow and volume can be varied on a breath-to-breath basis.
Possibility to guarantee a fixed tidal volume	Yes (if no leaks)	No
Peak airway pressure	Not limited	Limited (useful in patients at risk of barotraumas or gastric distension)
Size	Tend to be of larger size	Smaller
Powered by	Piston, compressor, blower	Blower
Alarms	Wide range of alarms	Limited alarms (or none)
Breath stacking	Possible	Not possible
Peak airway pressure	Not limited	Limited (useful in patients at risk of barotraumas or gastric distension)
Rebreathing	Minimal	Possible
Leak compensation	Poor, leaks may significantly reduce delivered volume and induce hypoventilation	Good, for mild to moderate leaks
PEEP	Internal PEEP generally not available. External PEEP can be added[a]	Internal PEEP available
Digestive insufflation	Frequent	Infrequent
Comfort	Lower	Higher
Need to adjust settings when oxygen is added	Yes	No

[a]More recent blower-driven volume-targeted ventilation may provide internal PEEP

7.5 Combined or Dual Ventilators

Some manufacturers of home ventilators have developed a category of ventilators that combine some features of bi-level, home VTM, and ICU ventilators. These high-performance micro blower-driven devices, called intermediate ventilators, can provide PTM, VTM, and hybrid modes (such as volume targeting) and have been designed to bridge the gap between bi-level devices, volume-targeted home ventilators, and ICU ventilators. They can guarantee high inspiratory pressures (up to 40 cmH_2O), have adjustable pressure rise time and maximum inspiratory time, and some also have minimal inspiratory time and sophisticated monitoring systems.

Table 7.4 Summary of technical characteristics of NIV ventilators

Ventilatory modes
Pressure targeted
Volume targeted
Hybrids
Circuit type
Single or double limb with expiratory valve
Single limb with calibrated leak
Triggering modes
Assisted
Controlled
Assisted-controlled
Inspiratory trigger function
Timed
Adjustable
Pressure triggered
Flow triggered
Automatic flow-based triggering "flow waveform"
I to E cycling
Timed based
Flow based
Fixed
Adjustable (% of peak flow)
"Intelligent" algorithms
Rise time
Fixed
Adjustable
PEEP
Internal
External
Options
Batteries
Alarms
Oxygen blender
Monitoring modules

Some of these devices offer the possibility to choose between either a single-limb circuit with calibrated leak or a single or double limb with expiratory valve and are able to automatically detect the type of circuit. The role of these hybrid ventilators has not yet been sufficiently explored. Their attraction is the availability of different modes in the same ventilator and the possibility to ensure the best tailored settings for each patient using only one device.

A summary of technical characteristics of NIV ventilators is provided in Table 7.4.

7.6 Choice of Ventilator

In spite of the increasing sophistication and wide difference in available options present in commercial home ventilators, there are, to date, no formal recommendations concerning preference of one particular ventilator. Moreover, technical issues determining the actual quality of devices are neither standardized nor regulated by guidelines. Both ventilator choice and optimal settings are poorly defined and selection is left to the perceptions of the clinician and patient. This underlines the importance of patient-tailored prescription and emphasizes the need for nocturnal monitoring of NIV efficacy. The choice of NIV ventilator should depend on both patient condition and device characteristics, including (1) clinical situation and underlying diagnosis (in particular, the degree of ventilator dependency and mobility); (2) patient comfort; (3) versatility and, if needed, availability of different ventilatory modes; (4) device performance; (5) mechanisms of leak compensation; (6) quality and accuracy of monitoring (asynchronies and unintentional leak detection); and (7) experience of the clinical team. At the same time, as those ventilators can be used regularly and long term at home, devices should be simple and easy to handle. Therefore, the ergonomics of home ventilators must be taken into account as benefits derived from good performance can sometimes be outweighed by a confusing user interface. In a trial evaluating user friendliness of home ventilators frequently used in clinical practice, Gonzalez et al. [57] tested the capacity of physicians experienced in mechanical ventilation to perform a series of standardized usual tasks. They showed major differences in accessibility of settings between the different devices with potentially dangerous delays necessary to accomplish even the simplest maneuver.

In general, patients eligible for home ventilation are in a stable condition. Therefore, in contrast to invasive mechanical ventilation or acute NIV, patients under long-term NIV were not threatened by temporary disruption of ventilation. Consequently, with the exception of patients with little autonomy, home ventilators may not need sophisticated technical systems such as external batteries, supplemental O_2, pressure or volume monitoring, or surveillance devices or alarms that are more of an annoyance than a necessity and must be optional rather than imperative. Moreover, as NIV is generally used at night, these alarms when activated may disrupt sleep quality.

Finally, mechanisms of leak detection and leak compensation capabilities are critical issues that dictate ventilator choice because they determine how well a NIV device performs. Moreover, because knowing the actual Vt is essential to providing the desired ventilatory support, another important aspect is how the device estimates Vt. In a system characterized by leaks, measuring effective ventilation is impossible, thus, Vt can only be estimated from appropriate mathematic algorithms integrating flow and pressure. These algorithms, usually not disclosed by manufacturers, are crucial in determining the quality of a given ventilator as they determine not only the ability of the device to guarantee the prescribed ventilatory support but also because they serve to adjust inspiratory and expiratory triggers. Fortunately, nearly

Table 7.5 The ideal ventilator

User friendly and ergonomic
Portable and quiet
Easy to adjust
Operates in assist and control modes
Pressure targeted (may offer volume-targeted ventilation as an option)
Simple circuit with intentional leak (may offer double circuit with expiratory valve as an option)
May provide high pressure level (up to 40 cm H_2O)
Detects the inspiratory effort as quickly as possible
Sensitive flow-based inspiratory trigger
Not influenced by mild to moderate leaks (preferably of the "flow waveform method" type)
Ending inspiration as close as possible to beginning of patient expiration
Adjustable expiratory trigger
Independent of respiratory impedance
With algorithm compensating for mild to moderate leak
With Timax
Can apply PEEP
Adjustable rise time with possibility of fast pressurization
Basic alarms (may be deactivated)
Low pressure
High pressure
Massive leaks
Power failure
Versatile
Dual voltage
Reliable and robust
Low-cost maintenance
Provides and stores accurate, user-friendly monitoring data
May provide as option
Batteries
Oxygen blender

all newer home ventilators perform as least as well as ICU ventilators and are capable of meeting high ventilatory demands [52]. Conditions to be met by an "ideal" ventilator are listed in Table 7.5

References

1. Leger P, Bedicam J, Cornette A, Reybet-Degat O. Nasal intermittent positive pressure ventilation. Long term follow up in patients with severe chronic respiratory failure. Chest. 1994;105:100–5.
2. Leger P, Jennequin J, Gerard M, Gaussorgues P, Robert D. Nocturnal mechanical ventilation in intermittent positive pressure at home by nasal route in chronic restrictive respiratory insufficiency. An effective substitute for tracheotomy. Presse Med. 1988;17:874.

3. Rideau Y, Gatin G, Bach J, Gines G. Prolongation of life in Duchenne's muscular dystrophy. Acta Neurol (Napoli). 1983;5:118–24.
4. Farre R, Lloyd-Owen SJ, Ambrosino N, Donaldson G, Escarrabill J, Fauroux B, Robert D, Schoenhofer B, Simonds A, Wedzicha JA. Quality control of equipment in home mechanical ventilation: a European survey. Eur Respir J. 2005;26:86–94.
5. Cuvelier A, Molano LC, Muir JF. Domiciliary ventilation in patients with COPD. Rev Mal Respir. 2005;22:615–33.
6. Jounieaux V, Rodenstein DO. Home mechanical ventilation: indications and pathophysiological limitations. Rev Mal Respir. 2004;21:358–66.
7. Rabec C, Merati M, Baudouin N, Foucher P, Ulukavac T, Reybet-Degat O. Management of obesity and respiratory insufficiency. The value of dual-level pressure nasal ventilation. Rev Mal Respir. 1998;15:269–78.
8. Gonzalez MM, Parreira VF, Rodenstein DO. Non-invasive ventilation and sleep. Sleep Med Rev. 2002;6:29–44.
9. Ward S, Chatwin M, Heather S, Simonds AK. Randomised controlled trial of non-invasive ventilation (NIV) for nocturnal hypoventilation in neuromuscular and chest wall disease patients with daytime normocapnia. Thorax. 2005;60:1019–24.
10. Hill NS. Noninvasive ventilation. Does it work, for whom, and how? Am Rev Respir Dis. 1993;147:1050–5.
11. Bach J, Robert D, Leger P, Langevin B. Sleep fragmentation in kiphoscoliotic individuals with alveolar hypoventilation treated by NIPPV. Chest. 1995;107:1552–8.
12. Levy RD, Bradley TD, Newman SL, Macklem PT, Martin JG. Negative pressure ventilation. Effects on ventilation during sleep in normal subjects. Chest. 1989;95:95–9.
13. Sanders MH, Kern N. Obstructive sleep apnea treated by independently adjusted inspiratory and expiratory positive airway pressures via nasal mask. Physiologic and clinical implications. Chest. 1990;98:317–24.
14. Parreira VF, Delguste P, Jounieaux V, Aubert G, Dury M, Rodenstein DO. Glottic aperture and effective minute ventilation during nasal two-level positive pressure ventilation in spontaneous mode. Am J Respir Crit Care Med. 1996;154:1857–63.
15. Rabec C, Georges M, Kabeya NK, Baudouin N, Massin F, Reybet-Degat O, Camus P. Evaluating noninvasive ventilation using a monitoring system coupled to a ventilator: a bench-to-bedside study. Eur Respir J. 2009;34:902–13.
16. Rabec CA, Reybet-Degat O, Bonniaud P, Fanton A, Camus P. Leak monitoring in noninvasive ventilation. Arch Bronconeumol. 2004;40:508–17.
17. Parreira VF, Jounieaux V, Delguste P, Aubert G, Dury M, Rodenstein DO. Determinants of effective ventilation during nasal intermittent positive pressure ventilation. Eur Respir J. 1997;10:1975–82.
18. Pepin JL, Chouri-Pontarollo N, Orliaguet O, Levy P. Alveolar hypoventilation during sleep and domiciliary assisted ventilation. Rev Mal Respir. 2005;22:113–25.
19. Jounieaux V, Aubert G, Dury M, Delguste P, Rodenstein DO. Effects of nasal positive-pressure hyperventilation on the glottis in normal awake subjects. J Appl Physiol. 1995;79:176–85.
20. Jounieaux V, Aubert G, Dury M, Delguste P, Rodenstein DO. Effects of nasal positive-pressure hyperventilation on the glottis in normal sleeping subjects. J Appl Physiol. 1995;79:186–93.
21. Parreira VF, Jounieaux V, Aubert G, Dury M, Delguste PE, Rodenstein DO. Nasal two-level positive-pressure ventilation in normal subjects. Effects of the glottis and ventilation. Am J Respir Crit Care Med. 1996;153:1616–23.
22. Delguste P, Aubert-Tulkens G, Rodenstein DO. Upper airway obstruction during nasal intermittent positive-pressure hyperventilation in sleep. Lancet. 1991;338:1295–7.
23. Lofaso F, Brochard L, Touchard D, Hang T, Harf A, Isabey D. Evaluation of carbon dioxide rebreathing during pressure support ventilation with airway management system (BiPAP) devices. Chest. 1995;108:772–8.
24. Lofaso F, Aslanian P, Richard JC, Isabey D, Hang T, Corriger E, Harf A, Brochard L. Expiratory valves used for home devices: experimental and clinical comparison. Eur Respir J. 1998;11: 1382–8.

25. Schettino GP, Chatmongkolchart S, Hess DR, Kacmarek RM. Position of exhalation port and mask design affect CO2 rebreathing during noninvasive positive pressure ventilation. Crit Care Med. 2003;31:2178–82.
26. Fanfulla F, Taurino AE, Lupo NDA, Trentin R, D'Ambrosio C, Nava S. Effect of sleep on patient/ventilator asynchrony in patients undergoing chronic non-invasive mechanical ventilation. Respir Med. 2007;101:1702–7.
27. Thille AW, Rodriguez P, Cabello B, Lellouche F, Brochard L. Patient-ventilator asynchrony during assisted mechanical ventilation. Intensive Care Med. 2006;32:1515–22.
28. Elliott M. Non invasive ventilation during sleep: time to define new tools in the systematic evaluation of the technique. Thorax. 2011;66(1):82–4.
29. Racca F, Squadrone V, Ranieri VM. Patient-ventilator interaction during the triggering phase. Respir Care Clin N Am. 2005;11:225–45.
30. Aslanian P, El Atrous S, Isabey D, Valente E, Corsi D, Harf A, Lemaire F, Brochard L. Effects of flow triggering on breathing effort during partial ventilatory support. Am J Respir Crit Care Med. 1998;157:135–43.
31. Prinianakis G, Kondili E, Georgopoulos D. Effects of the flow waveform method of triggering and cycling on patient-ventilator interaction during pressure support. Intensive Care Med. 2003;29:1950–9.
32. Vignaux L, Tassaux D, Jolliet P. Performance of noninvasive ventilation modes on ICU ventilators during pressure support: a bench model study. Intensive Care Med. 2007;33:1444–51.
33. Fauroux B, Leroux K, Desmarais G, Isabey D, Clement A, Lofaso F, Louis B. Performance of ventilators for noninvasive positive-pressure ventilation in children. Eur Respir J. 2008;31:1300–7.
34. Bonmarchand G, Chevron V, Menard JF, Girault C, Moritz-Berthelot F, Pasquis P, Leroy J. Effects of pressure ramp slope values on the work of breathing during pressure support ventilation in restrictive patients. Crit Care Med. 1999;27:715–22.
35. Battisti A, Tassaux D, Janssens JP, Michotte JB, Jaber S, Jolliet P. Performance characteristics of 10 home mechanical ventilators in pressure-support mode: a comparative bench study. Chest. 2005;127:1784–92.
36. Manning HL, Molinary EJ, Leiter JC. Effect of inspiratory flow rate on respiratory sensation and pattern of breathing. Am J Respir Crit Care Med. 1995;151:751–7.
37. Meza S, Giannouli E, Younes M. Control of breathing during sleep assessed by proportional assist ventilation. J Appl Physiol. 1998;84:3–12.
38. Calderini E, Confalonieri M, Puccio PG, Francavilla N, Stella L, Gregoretti C. Patient-ventilator asynchrony during noninvasive ventilation: the role of expiratory trigger. Intensive Care Med. 1999;25:662–7.
39. Tassaux D, Gainnier M, Battisti A, Jolliet P. Impact of expiratory trigger setting on delayed cycling and inspiratory muscle workload. Am J Respir Crit Care Med. 2005;172:1283–9.
40. Appendini L, Patessio A, Zanaboni S, Carone M, Gukov B, Donner CF, Rossi A. Physiologic effects of positive end-expiratory pressure and mask pressure support during exacerbations of chronic obstructive pulmonary disease. Am J Respir Crit Care Med. 1994;149:1069–76.
41. Simonds AK. Ventilatory modes. In: Simmonds AK, editors. Non invasive respiratory support. Arnold Publisher. London; 2001.
42. Braun NM, Arora NS, Rochester DF. Force-length relationship of the normal human diaphragm. J Appl Physiol. 1982;53:405–12.
43. Gonzalez-Bermejo J, Laplanche V, Husseini FE, Duguet A, Derenne JP, Similowski T. Evaluation of the user-friendliness of 11 home mechanical ventilators. Eur Respir J. 2006;27:1236–43.
44. Simonds AK, Elliott MW. Outcome of domiciliary nasal intermittent positive pressure ventilation in restrictive and obstructive disorders. Thorax. 1995;50:604–9.
45. Meecham Jones DJ, Wedzicha JA. Comparison of pressure and volume preset nasal ventilator systems in stable chronic respiratory failure. Eur Respir J. 1993;6:1060–4.
46. Restrick LJ, Fox NC, Braid G, Ward EM, Paul EA, Wedzicha JA. Comparison of nasal pressure support ventilation with nasal intermittent positive pressure ventilation in patients with nocturnal hypoventilation. Eur Respir J. 1993;6:364–70.

47. Lloyd-Owen SJ, Donaldson GC, Ambrosino N, Escarabill J, Farre R, Fauroux B, Robert D, Schoenhofer B, Simonds AK, Wedzicha JA. Patterns of home mechanical ventilation use in Europe: results from the Eurovent survey. Eur Respir J. 2005;25:1025–31.
48. Chatburn RL. Which ventilators and modes can be used to deliver noninvasive ventilation? Respir Care. 2009;54:85–101.
49. Nichols D, Haranath S. Pressure control ventilation. Crit Care Clin. 2007;23:183–99.
50. Mehta S, McCool F, Hill N. Leak compensation in positive pressure ventilators: a lung model study. Eur Respir J. 2001;17:259–67.
51. Girault C, Richard JC, Chevron V, Tamion F, Pasquis P, Leroy J, Bonmarchand G. Comparative physiologic effects of noninvasive assist-control and pressure support ventilation in acute hypercapnic respiratory failure. Chest. 1997;111:1639–48.
52. Schonhofer B, Sortor-Leger S. Equipment needs for noninvasive mechanical ventilation. Eur Respir J. 2002;20:1029–36.
53. Simonds A. Equipmente for NIPPV: ventilators, interfaces and accessories. In: Simmonds A, editors. Non-invasive respiratory support. Arnold Publisher. London; 2001.
54. Nava S, Bruschi C, Rubini F, Palo A, Iotti G, Braschi A. Respiratory response and inspiratory effort during pressure support ventilation in COPD patients. Intensive Care Med. 1995;21:871–9.
55. Janssens JP, Metzger M, Sforza E. Impact of volume targeting on efficacy of bi-level non-invasive ventilation and sleep in obesity-hypoventilation. Respir Med. 2009;103:165–72.
56. Storre JH, Seuthe B, Fiechter R, Milioglou S, Dreher M, Sorichter S, Windisch W. Average volume-assured pressure support in obesity hypoventilation: a randomized crossover trial. Chest. 2006;130:815–21.
57. Gonzalez-Bermejo J, Laplanche V, Husseini FE, Duguet A, Derenne JP, Similowski T. Evaluation of the user-friendliness of 11 home mechanical ventilators. Eur Respir J. 2006;27:1236–43.

Software for Home Ventilators and Leak Compensation: Key Technical and Practical Applications

8

Patrick Pasquina, Jean-Paul Janssens, Olivier Contal, and Dan Adler

Contents

Abbreviations

%Trigg	Percentage of respiratory cycles triggered by the patient
ABG	Arterial blood gases
AHI	Apnea-hypopnea index
COPD	Chronic obstructive pulmonary disease
NIV	Noninvasive ventilation
OHS	Obesity hypoventilation syndrome

P. Pasquina • J.-P. Janssens, MD (✉) • D. Adler, MD
Division of Pulmonary Diseases, Geneva University Hospitals,
4-6 rue Gabrielle-Perret-Gentil, Geneva 1211, Switzerland
e-mail: patrick.pasquina@hcuge.ch; jean-paul.janssens@hcuge.ch; dan.adler@hcuge.ch

O. Contal, PhD
University of Health Sciences (HESAV), Lausanne, Switzerland
e-mail: olivier.contal@hesav.ch

A.M. Esquinas (ed.), *Noninvasive Mechanical Ventilation: Theory, Equipment, and Clinical Applications*, DOI 10.1007/978-3-319-21653-9_8

RR Respiratory rate
VE Minute volume
VT Tidal volume

8.1 Introduction

During the past 20 years, long-term noninvasive ventilation (NIV) has become the key treatment for chronic hypercapnic respiratory failure. Technical advances, in particular in bi-level pressure-cycled ventilators, have been tremendous over the years in terms of pressurization, compensation for leaks, size, noise, and improvement of patient-ventilator synchronization through adjustable inspiratory and expiratory triggers. Many newer bi-level ventilators designed for home care are provided with built-in software that supplies detailed information about compliance, tidal volume (VT), minute ventilation (VE), respiratory rate (RR), estimated leaks, respiratory cycles triggered by the patient (%Trigg), and apnea-hypopnea index (AHI) [1, 2]. This chapter discusses the reliability of data recorded by software for home ventilators and highlights their clinical utility based on the published evidence.

8.2 Compliance

Data recorded by ventilator software are extremely useful for assessing compliance and pattern of ventilator use. The pattern of ventilation is an indirect indicator of tolerance of NIV and comfort. For example, multiple interruptions during the night after short periods of NIV or an erratic pattern of use over several days is suggestive of poor adaptation to NIV and patient discomfort (Fig. 8.1). Conversely, a rapid increase in NIV use may suggest imminent exacerbation in patients who are not ventilator dependent (Fig. 8.2). A study by Borel et al. [3] assessed whether data retrieved from a NIV device could be used to predict the risk of exacerbation in patients with chronic obstructive pulmonary disease (COPD) treated by home NIV. In this selected population, some patients increased their adherence to NIV prior to exacerbations (because NIV alleviates dyspnea), whereas other patients reduced its use (reflecting intolerance and/or inadequacy of ventilator settings during exacerbations). As reported by our group, compliance may also be related to the underlying chronic respiratory condition. For instance, neuromuscular patients, especially those suffering from progressive disease, tend to increase their use of NIV over time compared with patients treated for obesity hypoventilation syndrome (OHS) [2]. Monitoring of daily use of NIV may also detect progression of highly dependent patients who need a second ventilator with an internal battery for security reasons.

A detailed report on compliance is important for deciding whether or not to pursue ventilatory support, discussing alternate patterns of daily use of NIV in case of poor tolerance during the night (i.e., daytime sessions), and understanding insufficient impact of NIV on arterial blood gases (ABG) or clinical symptoms.

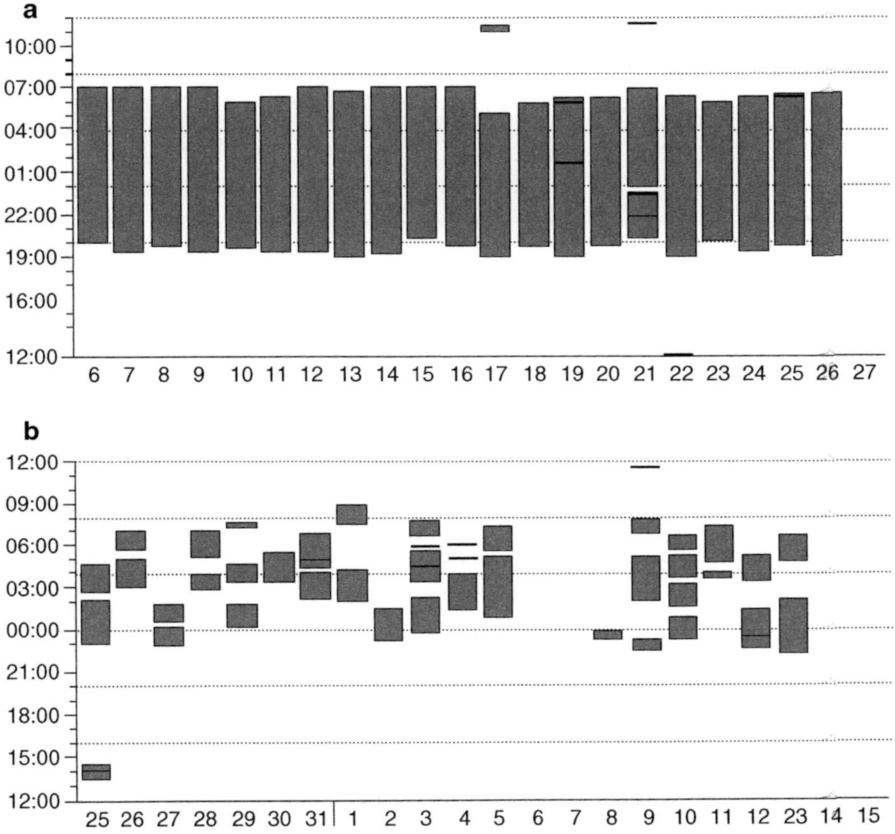

Fig. 8.1 (**a**) Graphic transcription of daily compliance and pattern of use of a ventilator provided by ventilator software in a patient who is well adapted to his ventilator, with excellent compliance. Use of the ventilator during the night is continuous, without interruption, suggesting acceptable quality of sleep. (**b**) Graphic transcription of daily compliance and pattern of use of ventilator provided by ventilator software in a patient who tolerates his treatment poorly, revealing multiple interruptions during the night, and days without ventilator use (Adapted from Ref. [2])

8.3 VT and Minute Ventilation

Although leaks have traditionally been a problem in volume-cycled NIV, pressure cycling and advances in blower technology now allow a certain amount of unintentional leakage without affecting pressurization capabilities and efficient delivery of VT, at least in some ventilators [4]. This is of major importance because unintentional leaks are a clinical reality in unsupervised patients treated by domiciliary NIV.

In single-limb circuits with a vented mask, the built-in flow sensor monitors total gas flow, that is, the sum of respiratory flow and unintentional and intentional leaks (Fig. 8.3). Because there is no direct measurement of expiratory flow in a single-limb

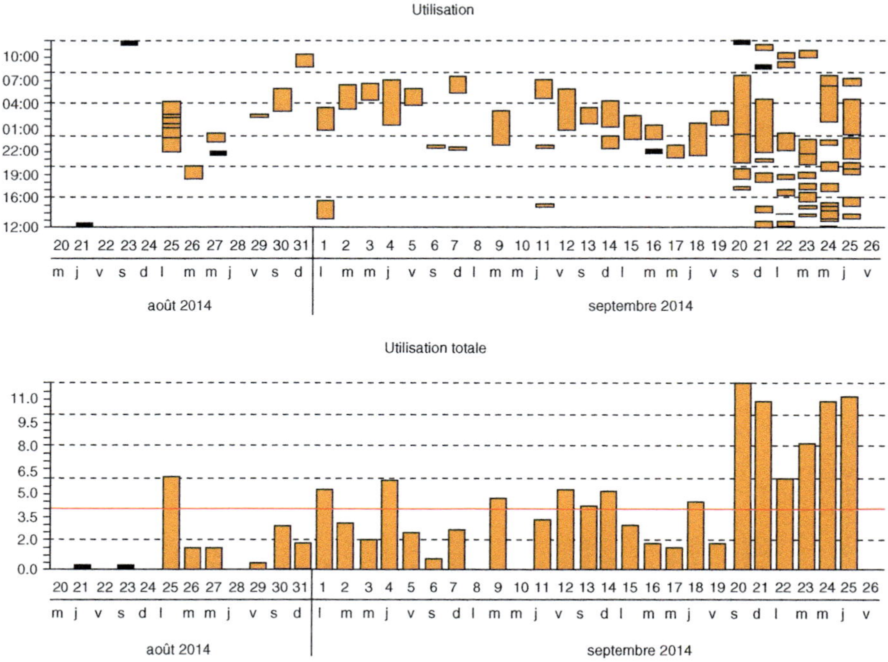

Fig. 8.2 *Upper graph*: pattern of use; *Lower graph*: total daily use. Graphic illustration of pattern of use and total daily use in a COPD patient with poor adaptation to NIV. Note frequent interruption during treatment, days with no treatment, and daily use <4 h. Six days before admission to the respiratory ward for acute exacerbations of COPD, the patient complained of shortness of breath that was alleviated by NIV, as evidenced by a rapid increase in daily use

Fig. 8.3 Flow and leaks during NIV with a bi-level pressure support ventilator (single-tube system and nasal mask vented)

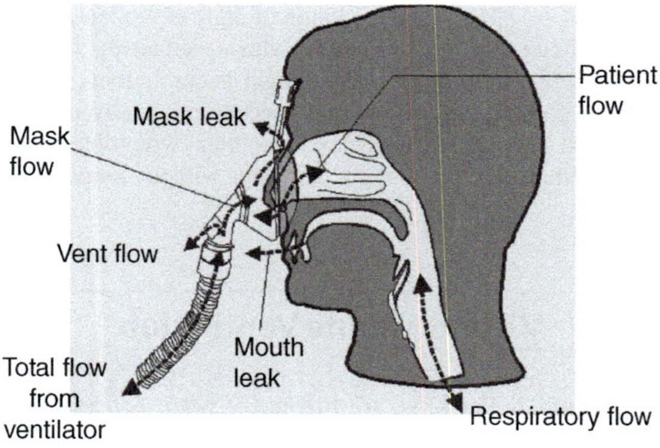

circuit, VT can only be estimated by taking into account changes in flow and unintentional leaks (from the mask or from the mouth), assuming that the intentional leak is known. For most ventilators, built-in software underestimates VT and this underestimation is little affected by leaks. Conversely, higher pressure support increases underestimation of VT [5, 6]. Sogo et al. [7] developed a bench model presented as more representative of clinical leaks by inducing random dynamic leaks during inspiratory or expiratory phases. Unlike previous studies, the authors found that the four ventilators tested significantly overestimated VT (with differences ranging from 18 % ± 7 % to 36 % ± 18 %) suggesting that a portion of the identified leak was erroneously considered by the software as volume delivered to the patient. The inaccuracy in VT estimation has direct clinical implications: commercial software can unpredictably either underestimate or overestimate VT. For these reasons, clinicians should minimize unintentional leaks by adjusting mask fit or changing mask type or ventilator settings. Once leaks have been corrected, clinicians must remain aware of differences in estimation of VT between ventilators and not rely only on information provided by ventilator software to monitor efficacy of NIV.

8.4 Leaks

Unintentional leaks are major contributors to NIV intolerance, patient-ventilator asynchrony, suboptimal correction of ABGs, and nocturnal hypoventilation. Estimation of leaks by the ventilator – if reliable – is a useful contribution to NIV monitoring.

Rabec et al. [8] showed that leaks assessed by built-in software of the VPAP™ III-ResLink™ (ResMed, North Ryde, Australia) ventilators were highly correlated with bench test measurements. These results cannot, however, be extrapolated to all home bi-level ventilators because bench testing of different commercially available home ventilators has demonstrated important discrepancies in leak estimation between devices [5–7]. One important caveat is that devices do not all report estimations of leaks in the same way. For instance, leaks are reported either as an estimation of unintentional leaks or as an estimation of total leaks (i.e., leaks through mask exhalation valves plus unintentional leaks) (Fig. 8.3). Physicians monitoring patients on home NIV should therefore be aware of these differences. Manufacturers have determined an arbitrary threshold for leaks below which pressurization is considered effective. In case of major leaks, the leak compensation may be insufficient and impair efficacy of ventilation, as shown in Fig. 8.4 [8]. Conversely, thresholds reported by manufacturers are not necessarily relevant, inasmuch as recent home ventilators have a high capacity for leak compensation.

8.5 Respiratory Rate and Percentage of Respiratory Cycles Triggered by the Patient

Most ventilator softwares provide information about spontaneous RR and %Trigg. This information must be interpreted with caution according to the clinical scenarios. For instance, a low %Trigg may occur when the patient has a backup RR above his or her spontaneous RR. In this situation, the patient is assumed to be treated with a "controlled ventilation mode." However, in conditions in which inspiratory efforts are potentially not detected by the ventilator (major leaks, patients with severe

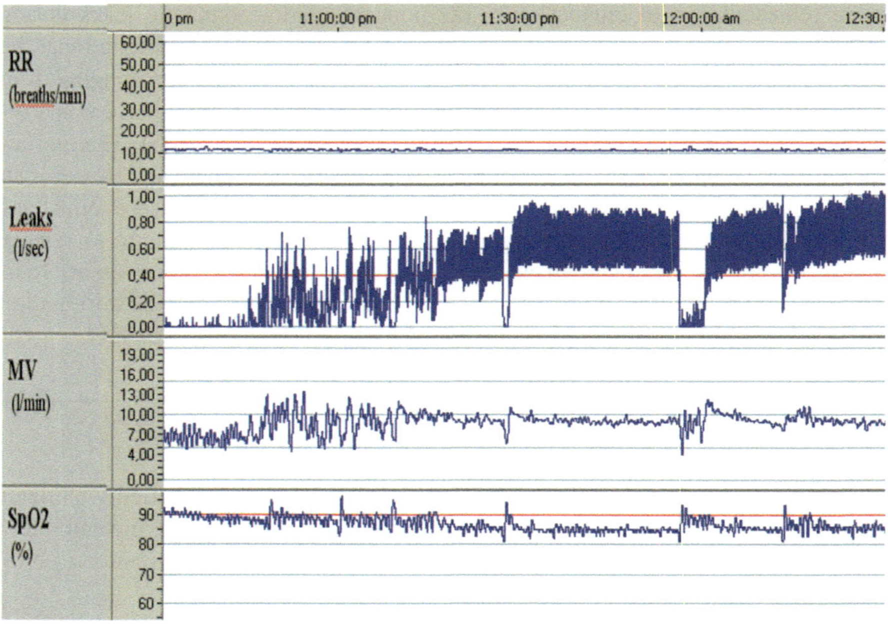

Fig. 8.4 VPAP-Reslink™ characteristic tracing showing – from top to bottom – respiratory rate, leaks (unintentional leaks in liters/second), minute ventilation, and SpO_2. Important unintentional leaks (>0.4 l/s) are associated with a prolonged decrease in SpO_2 directly measured by the device's pulse oximetry module (Adapted from Ref. [8])

neuromuscular disease and low inspiratory muscle strength, intrinsic positive end-expiratory pressure in severe COPD, upper airway closure), a low %Trigg may in fact reflect the inability of the ventilator to respond to the patient's inspiratory efforts, leading to patient-ventilator asynchrony. Conversely, a high value of RR above backup rate and a high %Trigg can represent appropriate detection of triggering efforts in a "spontaneous mode" as well as auto-triggering in case of important unintentional leaks or clinical conditions with low respiratory drive.

Whether it is preferable to use a high or a low backup rate for home NIV is still a matter of debate. It has been a long tradition to "capture" the patient with a backup rate in neuromuscular diseases. In OHS, evidence suggests that using a backup rate may prevent central and obstructive respiratory events [9]. In COPD, evidence as to increasing backup rate is scarce: high-intensity NIV with high inspiratory pressures and a high backup rate improves physiological endpoints [10]; however, a recent randomized controlled trial demonstrated no advantage of associating a high backup rate to high pressure support in night-time ventilator adherence or any of the other measured physiological parameters (including $PaCO_2$) [11]. These data suggest that it is the high-pressure component of the high-intensity NIV approach that plays the therapeutic role in the management of hypercapnic respiratory failure, at least in the COPD population. Using a telemetry approach, Borel et al. [3] recently demonstrated that daily variations in RR and %Trigg are predictors of acute exacerbations in patients with COPD. This "proof of concept" study provides a potentially simple predictive approach through telemonitoring, which requires neither the patient's active involvement nor additional sensors in their environment.

8.6 Apnea-Hypopnea Index

To our knowledge, the validity and accuracy of AHI provided by home ventilators has not been thoroughly studied. The lack of standardized definitions for respiratory events occurring under positive-pressure ventilation and their mode of detection is problematic. In an observational study of OHS patients under NIV, the correlation between AHI provided by the ventilator software and AHI measured simultaneously by polysomnography was high, with a low bias. An arbitrary threshold value of 10 for AHI proved to be sensitive and specific for discriminating between patients appropriately ventilated versus those requiring further adjustment of ventilator settings [12]. This study had, however, a few limitations and should be repeated in other patient groups with different NIV devices before one can determine whether it is possible to rely on AHI indices provided by ventilator software.

Conclusion

Home ventilators with built-in software provide substantial information for monitoring home NIV, such as compliance, pattern of ventilator use, leaks, RR, %Trigg, and AHI. This information may be used to adapt ventilator settings and can have a direct impact on patient management. However, reliability of data is not equivalent between all ventilators. The NIV physician therefore should not completely rely on these data to adapt ventilator settings. Presently, data provided by ventilator software are a useful adjunct to recommended tools for basic monitoring of NIV, such as ABG analysis, nocturnal pulse oximetry, nocturnal capnography, and polygraphy.

Key Points

- A detailed report on compliance is important for deciding whether or not to pursue ventilatory support, discussing alternate patterns of daily use of NIV in case of poor tolerance during the night (i.e., daytime sessions), and understanding insufficient impact of NIV on ABG or clinical symptoms.
- Clinicians monitoring patients on home NIV should be aware of differences in the estimation of leaks between ventilators. They should aim to maintain the 95th percentile of leak values at the lowest possible level by adjusting interface and ventilator settings.
- Home ventilator softwares (see above) does not provide accurate and reliable values of VT and VE. Discrepancies exist between home ventilators and are influenced by leaks. Clinicians should thus not rely only on these data for adjusting ventilator settings.
- RR and %Trigg can help the clinician to better set the backup RR on the home ventilator.

References

1. Janssens JP, Borel JC, Pépin JL. Nocturnal monitoring of home non-invasive ventilation: the contribution of simple tools such as pulse oximetry, capnography, built-in ventilator software and automatic markers of sleep fragmentation. Thorax. 2011;66:438–45.
2. Pasquina P, Adler D, Farr P, Bourqui P, Bridevaux PO, Janssens JP. What does built-in software of home ventilators tell us? An observational study of 150 patients on home ventilation. Respiration. 2012;83:293–9.
3. Borel JC, Pelletier J, Taleux N, Briault A, Arnol N, Pison C, Tamisier R, Timsit JF, Pepin JL. Parameters recorded by software of non-invasive ventilators predict COPD exacerbation: a proof-of-concept study. Thorax. 2015;70:284–5.
4. Battisti A, Tassaux D, Janssens JP, Michotte JB, Jaber S, Jolliet P. Performance characteristics of 10 home mechanical ventilators in pressure-support mode: a comparative bench study. Chest. 2005;127:1784–92.
5. Contal O, Vignaux L, Combescure C, Pepin JL, Jolliet P, Janssens JP. Monitoring of noninvasive ventilation by built-in software of home bilevel ventilators: a bench study. Chest. 2012;141:469–76.
6. Luján M, Sogo A, Pomares X, Monsó E, Sales B, Blanch L. Effect of leak and breathing pattern on the accuracy of tidal volume estimation by commercial home ventilators: a bench study. Respir Care. 2013;58:770–7.
7. Sogo A, Montanyà J, Monsó E, Blanch L, Pomares X, Lujàn M. Effect of dynamic random leaks on the monitoring accuracy of home mechanical ventilators: a bench study. BMC Pulm Med. 2013;13:75.
8. Rabec C, Georges M, Kabeya NK, Baudouin N, Massin F, Reybet-Degat O, Camus P. Evaluating noninvasive ventilation using a monitoring system coupled to a ventilator: a bench-to-bedside study. Eur Respir J. 2009;34:902–13.
9. Contal O, Adler D, Borel JC, Espa F, Perrig S, Rodenstein D, Pépin JL, Janssens JP. Impact of different back up respiratory rates on the efficacy of noninvasive positive pressure ventilation in obesity hypoventilation syndrome: a randomized trial. Chest. 2013;143:37–46.
10. Dreher M, Storre JH, Schmoor C, Windisch W. High-intensity versus low-intensity non-invasive ventilation in patients with stable hypercapnic COPD: a randomised crossover trial. Thorax. 2010;65:303–8.
11. Murphy P, Brignall K, Moxham J, Polkey M, Davidson C, Hart N. High pressure versus high intensity noninvasive ventilation in stable hypercapnic chronic obstructive pulmonary disease: a randomized crossover trial. Int J Chron Obstruct Pulmon Dis. 2012;7:811–8.
12. Georges M, Adler D, Contal O, Espa F, Perrig S, Pépin JL, Janssens JP. Reliability of apnea-hypopnea index measured by a home bi-level pressure support ventilator versus a polysomnographic assessment. Respir Care. 2015;60(7):1051–6.

Maintenance Protocol for Home Ventilation Circuits

9

Michel Toussaint and Gregory Reychler

Contents

Abbreviations

CF	Cystic fibrosis
COPD	Chronic obstructive pulmonary disease
HVC	Home ventilation circuits
MRSA	Methicillin-resistant *Staphylococcus aureus*
PPO	Potentially pathogenic organism

M. Toussaint, PhD (✉)
Centre for Neuromuscular Disease and Centre for Home Mechanical Ventilation UZ-VUB-Inkendaal, Rehabilitation Hospital Inkendaal, Inkendaalstraat, 1, Vlezenbeek 1602, Belgium
e-mail: michel.toussaint@inkendaal.be

G. Reychler, PhD
Pulmonology Unit and the Department of Physical Medicine and Rehabilitation, Cliniques Universitaires Saint-Luc, Université Catholique de Louvain, Avenue Hippocrate 10, Brussels 1200, Belgium
e-mail: Gregory.Reychler@uclouvain.be

A.M. Esquinas (ed.), *Noninvasive Mechanical Ventilation: Theory, Equipment, and Clinical Applications*, DOI 10.1007/978-3-319-21653-9_9

9.1 Introduction

Home mechanical ventilation has become a standard of care to effectively treat chronic respiratory failure, both in patients with restrictive diseases such as neuromuscular and thorax cage disorders and in patients with obstructive diseases such as selected cases of lung and airways disorders. Depending on the group of patients, home ventilation may improve survival and quality of life in the long term and may decrease the rate of lower respiratory tract infections [1].

9.1.1 Equipment for Home Mechanical Ventilation

Home mechanical ventilation requires equipment consisting of a generator of pressure (volume- or pressure-cycled ventilator), a circuit with tubing (with or without expiratory valve), and an interface to deliver air to the patient. In the majority of patients, a nasal mask is the most appropriate interface for nocturnal use. Total face masks may be used in the rare cases where nasal masks are useless. Finally, mouthpieces are preferentially used in waking patients for daytime noninvasive ventilation. Invasive ventilation via tracheostomy may be required when noninvasive ventilation is no longer possible.

9.1.2 Dirtiness and Contamination

Contamination of circuits infers the transient presence of bacteria in the circuits and/or in the airways, whereas colonization infers the multiplication of the germs in the airways of patients that may lead to chronic respiratory infection. In contrast with the hospital setting, transmission of infection by cross contamination is rare in the home setting because patients receiving home mechanical ventilation use their own equipment and have no direct or indirect contact with other patients. The possible causes of contamination are inappropriate maintenance or manipulation of the equipment with contaminated hands. In home use, the question is to what extent home ventilation circuits (HVC) must be disinfected. Is dirtiness of HVC a risk factor for HVC contamination and the patient's self-colonization? What is the best protocol for cleaning? Is disinfection needed and how often is it recommended? The aim of this chapter is to answer these questions and to suggest an adequate protocol for maintenance of HVC.

9.1.3 Maintenance Is Empirically Driven

Although home ventilation is widely used around the world, maintenance of HVC is empirically driven. Instructions given before discharging patients home are mostly taken from the recommended guidelines from other areas such as lung function tests, nebulization techniques, or respiratory monitoring. These instructions are generally based on tradition rather than scientific evidence and vary depending on the country and center. Instructions are often too elaborate and not specifically adapted for patients receiving home ventilation. Current instructions often include the use of a disinfectant solution, vinegar mixed with water or a quaternary ammonium compound, but generally fail to explain how basic maintenance may be achieved by simple cleaning with soap and hot water or with the dishwasher.

9.1.4 A European Survey on Maintenance

In a European survey including more than 20,000 patients receiving home ventilation (two-thirds of patients with restrictive disorders, one-third with obstructive), only 60 % of the participating centers provided written instructions on the cleaning and maintenance of the equipment 2]. There was a significant positive correlation between the size of the center and the proportion of written instructions ($p<0.001$). On average, only 56 % of the centers had protocols for correct cleaning and maintenance of circuits and interfaces. These findings clearly demonstrate that a greater effort is needed to improve communication to patients regarding adequate rules of maintenance before home discharge.

9.1.5 Patients Do Not Clean Their Equipment

In one study, two-thirds patients who were given cleaning instructions prior to discharge did not adequately clean their equipment at home [3]. Tubing and masks were most commonly found as "unacceptably" dirty. It was hypothesized that dirtiness of equipment exposes circuits and masks to a higher risk of contamination. Indeed, the dirtiest circuits were found to be significantly more contaminated than the cleanest ones [3, 4]. Dirtiness and contamination could potentially expose patients to a higher risk of airway colonization, which in turn could cause respiratory infections. However, this relationship has not yet been demonstrated with evidence.

9.1.6 Sensitivity to Infections

Clearly, regular cleaning appears to be the most important instruction that needs to be followed by all patients for the maintenance of HVC. As previously seen, however, there needs to be a considerable effort to target and institute this basic effective cleaning. By contrast with cleaning rules, the instructions for post-cleaning disinfection depend upon the relative sensitivity of patients to respiratory tract infections and the related risks for bacterial colonization of the airways. Two groups of patients need to be considered here: restrictive and obstructive disease patients. Clearly, both groups are not equally sensitive to infections and, as a consequence, should not require a similarly elaborate disinfection level.

9.2 Analysis and Discussion

9.2.1 Restrictive Disorders

By contrast with patients affected by obstructive respiratory diseases, patients affected by restrictive respiratory diseases or hypoventilation syndrome are a priori at low risk for bacterial colonization of airways.

In an uncontrolled study with stable patients receiving written and verbal information on maintenance of HVC (the recommendation was for daily cleaning with soap and water), a Spanish group questioned patients regarding their cleaning habits [3]. They conducted both visual inspection of HVC and sampling of masks (contamination) plus nostrils (colonization) in each patient. As a result, the frequency of cleaning was found as follows: 47 % cleaned their HVC once a week, 23 % cleaned once a month, 15 % cleaned sporadically, and 15 % never cleaned their equipment. In total, 67 % of HVC were deemed as very dirty and a positive relationship between circuit contamination and nostril colonization was highlighted. Bacterial colonization was more important in those patients where HVC were dirtier. The authors could not conclude whether colonization preceded or followed contamination. However, they suggested that adequate cleaning decisively decreased the rate of contamination. However, these authors did not provide a protocol for adequate maintenance of HVC.

In another study, visual and bacterial inspection of HVC was assessed before and after cleaning in a first experiment [4]. In a second experiment, the authors randomly compared cleaning either with a household dishwasher or low-level disinfection with an ammonium-chlorhexidine complex. Their findings were in agreement with the findings of Rodriguez et al. [3]. Prior to cleaning, circuits were found to be dirty in 69 % of the cases. HVC were dirtier in invasive ventilation. There was a significant positive correlation between the level of visual dirtiness and bacteriologic contamination of HVC ($p=0.56$; $p<0.001$). Bacteriologic contamination reached 22 % of noninvasive HVC with little presence of fungi. Nevertheless, by contrast with invasive HVC, contamination of noninvasive HVC did not include potentially pathogenic organisms (PPO) such as *Serratia marcescens*, methicillin-resistant *Staphylococcus aureus* (MRSA), or *Pseudomonas aeruginosa*. In invasive HVC, contamination affected 81 % of HVC and included the important presence of fungi; 19 % of HVC were PPO including *S. marcescens* in two cases, and MRSA in one case, but no *P. aeruginosa* contaminated HVC in this group. In the second experiment of this study, cleaning in the dishwasher was shown to be superior to the chemical compounds for both cleaning and disinfecting HVC. In addition, Gram-negative bacteria and fungi survived in the chemical complex but not in the dishwasher.

In accordance with the findings of Ebner et al. [5], we suggest using either a dishwasher at 65 °C or basic soap and hot water as the best means of cleaning HVC used by restrictive patients (Table 9.1). Nevertheless, a disinfectant agent may be recommended (1) in the very dirty HVC, (2) in circuits from invasive ventilation, and (3) in HVC from patients known for their high sensitivity to respiratory

Table 9.1 Maintenance protocol for home mechanical ventilation circuits

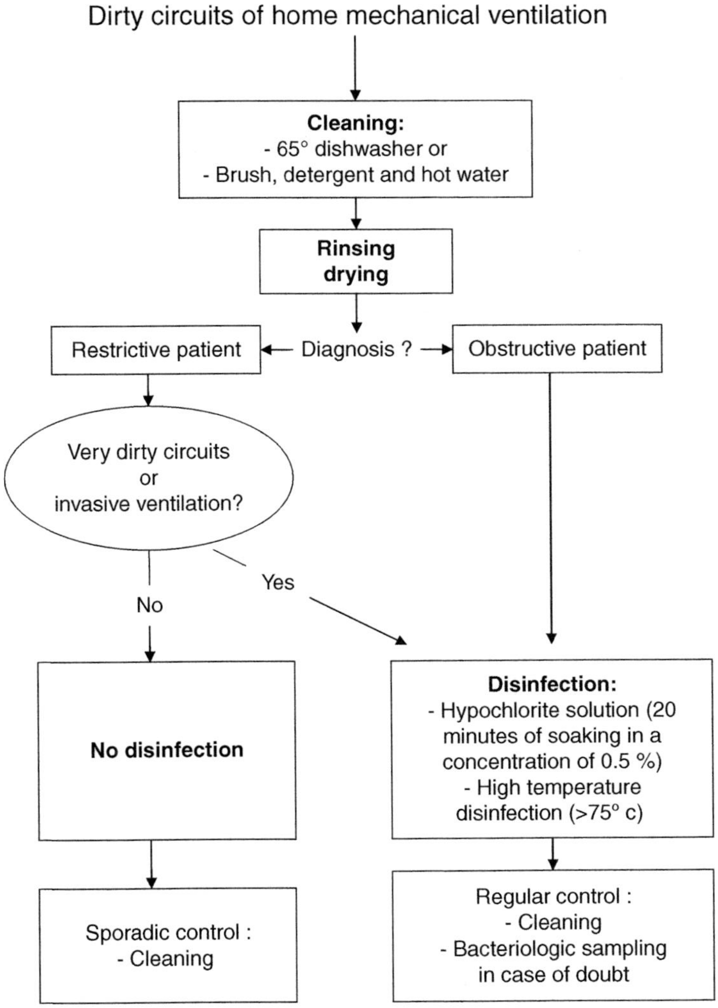

infections, such as obstructive patients. Effective cleaning must always precede any disinfection. It is important to be sure that a thermo-stable HVC is used before cleaning or disinfecting at temperatures >60 °C. Effective disinfection is described below.

9.2.2 Obstructive Disorders

The situation regarding hygiene of HVC is slightly different in obstructive respiratory diseases such as cystic fibrosis (CF) and chronic obstructive pulmonary disease (COPD) compared with restrictive respiratory diseases. The major reason for this difference is a higher sensitivity to bacterial colonization of the airways in these patient populations. The rate of airway colonization often correlates with the severity and/or speed of obstructive disease progression. In addition, there is evidence that the need for noninvasive ventilation becomes more frequent after airway colonization in these patients.

Ventilator-associated pneumonia is well documented. In intensive care units, the use of mechanical ventilation is an important risk factor for the development of nosocomial pneumonia. Moreover, current risk is greater with the use of invasive mechanical ventilation compared with noninvasive ventilation. Unfortunately, the relationship between the use of noninvasive ventilation and an increased risk for nosocomial pneumonia is not demonstrated.

The greater number of manipulations and the presence of an endotracheal tube associated with invasive ventilation contribute to HVC contamination. It can be hypothesized that manipulations related to noninvasive ventilation also represent a potential risk for contamination. This implies a rigorous implementation of classical nonspecific rules of hygiene, including hand washing. Nevertheless, the ventilator, the circuit, and the interface do not represent major risk factors for contamination and colonization, but monitoring potential bacterial contamination of devices and paying attention to the basic rules of hygiene probably remain important challenges.

There is little published research to support the relationship between hygiene and noninvasive ventilation devices in obstructive diseases. In a small study on cystic fibrosis patients (particularly at risk of cross contamination), no evidence was found of pathogenic microbial contamination of NIV devices [6]. However, we can extrapolate findings from therapies such as respiratory physiotherapy devices to patients with obstructive disorders receiving long-term noninvasive ventilation. Indeed, the material involved in noninvasive ventilation is part of the semi-critical devices that are in contact with mucus membranes as defined by the Centers for Disease Control and Prevention. Fortunately, recommendations on hygiene of these devices are available.

In patients affected by CF and other chronic respiratory diseases, nebulizers are considered potential vectors of bacterial infection of airways. Notably, studies showed that nebulizers of CF patients are frequently contaminated [7]. Similarly, it was suggested that nebulizers can lead to nosocomial disease in COPD patients [8]. The bacterial contamination of HVC is related to the duration of its use and the airway colonization of the patient.

Based on this evidence, several recommendations were proposed and could be applied to the pieces of the circuit involved in noninvasive ventilation in obstructive diseases. As shown in Table 9.1, regular cleaning of HVC and masks is mandatory, at least as a basic hygiene procedure and, more specifically, to eliminate the biofilm deposited on the surfaces that further decreases the efficacy of disinfectants [9]. The necessary frequency of cleaning is still being debated. Based on the results of studies on nebulizers, a daily cleaning could theoretically be the recommended timing. However, a less regular cleaning, for instance, once a week, could be acceptable in the practice. The possibility of using tap water for cleaning must be taken into account whether HVC are contaminated by *S. marcescens* and *Stenotrophomonas maltophila*.

When considering disinfection, different methods may be proposed. The choice of the optimal method largely depends on the material chosen to disinfect. A thermal disinfection (e.g., sterilizer, boiling water) may be not suitable for some non-thermo-stable pieces of HVC even though its efficacy is evident with all germs. There are a number of chemical methods and each one has its own characteristics. The duration of soaking and the concentration of the chemical depend on the particular substance used, and the guidelines for each must be followed carefully. Acetic acid is not recommended due to its inefficacy on gram-positive and gram-negative bacteria [10, 11]. In contrast with acid acetic, hypochlorite solution (20 min of soaking in a concentration of 0.5 %) may be the best alternative of those readily available chemical solutions.

After disinfection, rinsing and drying is the last part of the cleaning and disinfection sequence. Drying seems important as a higher contamination rate was related to non-dried nebulizers in CF patients. Because there is a paucity of specific data related to noninvasive ventilation, precise recommendations can not be made. However, it could justify more studies on this topic. Finally, it appears critically important to investigate the relative effectiveness of the different established protocols for cleaning and disinfecting of HVC to maintain their integrity.

Key Major Recommendations

- Cleaning the ventilator, circuits, and interfaces is required 2–4 times per month in all patients receiving mechanical ventilation at home.
- Written instructions on how to clean the equipment for home ventilation are useful. Regular assessment of whether or not circuits and interfaces are correctly cleaned and maintained is mandatory.
- In patients with restrictive disorders, cleaning in the dishwasher is effective and sufficient for thermo-stable circuits and interfaces. Cleaning with soap and hot water may be sufficient for all pieces. Disinfection is not mandatory.
- In patients with obstructive disorders, cleaning must be more frequent than for restrictive disorders. Cleaning always precedes disinfection. After cleaning, rinsing and drying are important. An effective weekly disinfection may be achieved by using a hypochlorite solution (20 min of soaking in a concentration of 0.5 %).
- The expiratory valve must be washed specifically, with care taken so that the balloon is not held underwater.

References

1. Dohna-Schwake C, Podiewski P, Voit T, et al. Non-invasive ventilation reduces respiratory tract infections in children with neuromuscular disorders. Pediatr Pulmonol. 2008;43:67–71.
2. Farre R, Loyd-Owen SJ, Ambrosino N, et al. Quality control of equipment in home mechanical ventilation: a European survey. Eur Respir J. 2005;26:86–94.

3. Rodriguez Gonzalez-Moro JM, Andrade Vivero G, de Miguel Diez J, et al. Bacterial colonization and home mechanical ventilation: prevalence and risk factors. Arch Bronconeumol. 2004;40:392–6.
4. Toussaint M, Steens M, Van Zeebroeck A, et al. Is disinfection of mechanical ventilation needed at home? Int J Hyg Environ Health. 2006;209:183–90.
5. Ebner W, Eitel A, Scherrer M, et al. Can household dishwashers be used to disinfect medical equipment? J Hosp Infect. 2000;45:155–9.
6. Mutagi A, Nash EF, Cameron S, Abbott G, Agostini P, Whitehouse JL, Honeybourne D, Boxall E. Microbial contamination of non-invasive ventilation devices used by adults with cystic fibrosis. J Hosp Infect. 2012;81(2):104–8.
7. Vassal S, Taamma R, Marty N, et al. Microbiologic contamination study of nebulizers after aerosol therapy in patients with cystic fibrosis. Am J Infect Control. 2000;28:347–51.
8. Mastro TD, Fields BS, Breiman RF, et al. Nosocomial Legionnaires' disease and use of medication nebulizers. J Infect Dis. 1991;163:667–71.
9. Merritt K, Hitchins VM, Brown SA, et al. Safety and cleaning of medical materials and devices. J Biomed Mater Res. 2000;53:131–6.
10. Karapinar M, Gonul SA. Effects of sodium bicarbonate, vinegar, acetic and citric acids on growth and survival of *Yersinia enterocolitica*. Int J Food Microbiol. 1992;16:343–7.
11. Reychler G, Aarab K, Van Ossel C, et al. In vitro evaluation of efficacy of 5 methods of disinfection on mouthpieces and facemasks contaminated by strains of cystic fibrosis patients. J Cyst Fibros. 2005;4:183–7.

10 Noninvasive Open Ventilation (NIOV™) Therapy: Clinical Implications

Heidi A. Pelchat, Patrick L. Williams, and Alex H. Gifford

Contents

Abbreviations

COPD	Chronic obstructive pulmonary disease
CF	Cystic fibrosis
EMG	Electromyography
EPAP	Expiratory positive airway pressure

H.A. Pelchat, BS, RRT
Department of Medicine, Section of Cardiology, Cardiac and Pulmonary Rehabilitation, Dartmouth-Hitchcock Medical Center, Lebanon, NH, USA

P.L. Williams, BA, RRT
Department of Respiratory Care, Dartmouth-Hitchcock Medical Center, Lebanon, NH, USA

A.H. Gifford, MD (✉)
Department of Medicine, Section of Pulmonary and Critical Care Medicine, Dartmouth-Hitchcock Medical Center, Lebanon, NH, USA

Section of Pulmonary and Critical Care Medicine, 5C, New Hampshire Cystic Fibrosis Center, Dartmouth-Hitchcock Medical Center, One Medical Center Drive, Lebanon, NH, USA
e-mail: Alex.H.Gifford@hitchcock.org

A.M. Esquinas (ed.), *Noninvasive Mechanical Ventilation: Theory, Equipment, and Clinical Applications*, DOI 10.1007/978-3-319-21653-9_10

FEV_1	Forced expiratory volume in one second
FiO_2	Fraction of inspired oxygen
HFT	High-flow therapy
ILD	Interstitial lung disease
IPAP	Inspiratory positive airway pressure
LPM	Liters per minute
NIPPV	Noninvasive positive pressure ventilation
PEEP	Positive end-expiratory pressure
PTP	Peak-to-peak
V_T	Tidal volume
V_E	Minute ventilation
SpO_2	Oxyhemoglobin saturation

10.1 Introduction

The convention of using trademark only at first mention of product is fine. is a novel portable system for delivering inspiratory positive pressure and supplemental oxygen through a specially designed nasal pillows interface during ambulation. The NIOV system augments tidal volume (V_T), minute ventilation (V_E), and oxyhemoglobin saturation (SpO_2), which in total has beneficial effects on respiratory mechanics, exercise capacity, and symptom burden in chronic obstructive pulmonary disease (COPD), as discussed later in this chapter. Patients and their respiratory care providers can adjust a number of settings on the device to optimize its performance. In this chapter, we describe how NIOV functions, review several studies of its clinical utility, and share some of our experiences with the device in our pulmonary rehabilitation and cystic fibrosis programs.

10.2 Overview of NIOV Technology

The NIOV system consists of a unique nasal pillows interface and a sophisticated microprocessor-controlled ventilator that can be programmed by the clinician to deliver inspiratory pressure in synchrony with the patient's breathing pattern (Fig. 10.1). It requires a compressed gas source for operation. The amount of pressure and volume delivered are determined by the patient's inspiratory effort and respiratory system mechanics. The microprocessor housing is small, lightweight, and designed to be worn at the waist or mounted on a pole. Buttons on the front of the device allow the patient to choose settings that are appropriate for recumbent and sitting positions and ambulation. A large liquid-crystal touch screen display (LCD) depicts the target inspiratory volume, activity setting, current respiratory rate, oxygen flow rate in liters per minute (LPM), and remaining battery life. A speaker for audible alarm output is located in the face of the housing.

Sensing ports located in the nasal pillows interface (Fig. 10.2) detect spontaneous respirations. The system can provide a mean fraction of inspired oxygen (FiO_2)

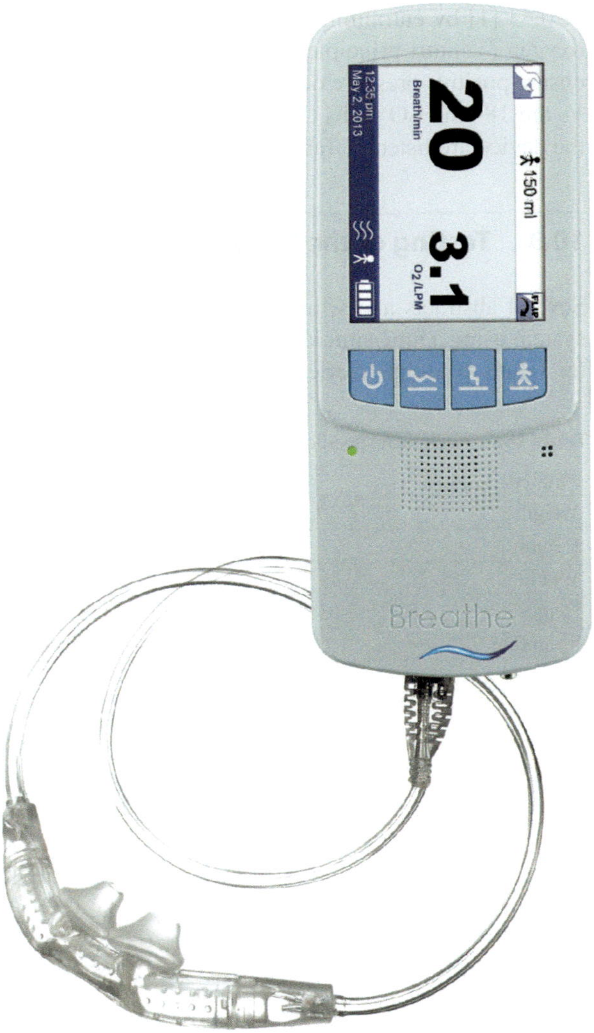

Fig. 10.1 NIOV™ apparatus (compressed oxygen source not shown)

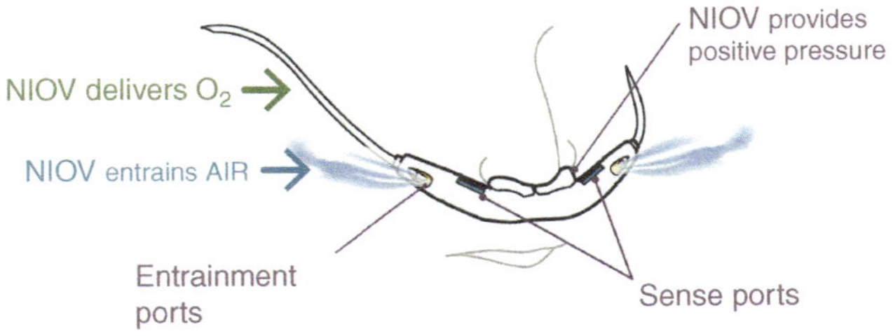

Fig. 10.2 The NIOV™ nasal pillows interface blends oxygen with air entrained through ports in the side of the interface, an application of the Venturi effect. Centrally located sense ports detect patient inspiratory effort, triggering the device to delivery positive pressure through nasal pillows that conform to the patient's nares

of 0.43 [1] by entraining air through two ports and blending it with supplemental oxygen (Venturi principle). Two molded nasal pillows form a seal at the nares to ensure positive pressure delivery. The maximum attainable inspiratory pressure and V_T are 18 cm H_2O and 1150 ml, respectively [1]. Other technical specifications of the device are listed in Table 10.1.

10.3 Testing of the NIOV System Using a Lung Simulator

Several abstracts and white papers have described the performance of the NIOV system using a lung simulator. McCoy and Diesem [2] equipped a breathing simulator (Hans Rudolph, Series 1101, Shawnee, KS, USA) with a simulated nose to

Table 10.1 Technical specifications of the NIOV™ system

Physical	
Weight	1.0 lb (0.5 kg)
Height	3.1 in (7.9 cm)
Width	7.5 in (19.1 cm)
Depth	1.3 in (3.2 cm)
Mounting	Belt clip or pole mount
Features	
Delivered gas	Oxygen with entrained air
Flow delivery	Closed-loop proportional valve
Breath sensing	Proximal in patient interface
Rate (breaths/min)	2–40, based on patient's spontaneous breathing
Internal battery duration	4 h with nominal use
Internal battery charge time	90 % recharged within 2.5 h
Alarm types	Audible and vibrating
User interfaces	Push buttons, LEDs, color LCD touch screen
Patient accessible settings	
Power	On, off
Volume delivery settings	Low, medium, high
Trigger sensitivity	0–9 (−0.01 to −0.34 cm H_2O)
Alarm loudness	1–5
Vibrating alarm	On, off
LCD brightness	1–5
Clinician programmable settings	
Breath timeout	12 breaths/min or 3 LPM
Volume delivery	50–250 ml in 10 ml increments
Inspiratory delivery time	10–40 % of breath period
Clinician programmable alarms	
Breath timeout period	20 or 60 s
High breath rate	5–120 breaths/min
Low breath rate	0–119 breaths/min

accommodate nasal cannulae. They compared NIOV to high-flow therapy (HFT) on the basis of delivered V_T and peak-to-peak (PTP) pressure differentials over a range of values for resistance (5, 10, and 20 cm H_2O/l/s) and compliance (70, 100, and 120 ml/cm H_2O). For all combinations of these parameters, the lung simulator was set to breathe at a rate of 12 breaths per minute with V_T of 500 ml and an inspiratory-to-expiratory time ratio of 1:2. The NIOV was set to 250 ml and 21 % delivery time, defined as the time during which the selected target volume is delivered as a fraction of the patient's spontaneous breath period. HFT was modeled using the AIRVO™ system (Fisher & Paykel Healthcare, Auckland, New Zealand) set to the maximum 45 LPM setting. V_T and PTP pressure differentials were uniformly higher for NIOV than HFT. Importantly, NIOV but not HFT provided inspiratory pressure support, while HFT but not NIOV provided positive end-expiratory pressure (PEEP). This finding highlights different capabilities of the two systems.

In a parallel study using the same lung model and resistance and compliance values, McCoy and Diesem [3] compared NIOV to the LTV® 1100 (CareFusion, San Diego, CA, USA) and VPAP Tx™ (ResMed Corporation, San Diego, CA, USA) on the basis of inspiratory positive airway pressure (IPAP) and expiratory positive airway pressure (EPAP). The NIOV and LTV 1100 devices intrinsically had 0 cm H_2O of EPAP, and the VPAP Tx was set to its minimum EPAP of 3 cm H_2O for testing. Observed mean V_T and pressure support values were statistically similar among all three devices, suggesting that NIOV could generate comparable ventilatory support.

Blakeman and Branson [4] also tested the NIOV apparatus using a bench model of human ventilation. These investigators devised a nasopharynx and trachea in which the resistance to airflow and anatomic dead space were comparable to the human respiratory tract. They employed an ASL 5000 computerized test lung (IngMar Medical, Pittsburgh, PA, USA) to mimic the physiology of a normal human, a human with COPD, and a human with interstitial lung disease (ILD). The NIOV was programmed for V_T of 100, 150, 200, and 250 ml. The device was observed to deliver augmented simulated patient V_T ranging between 362 and 828 ml, increasing the spontaneous V_T by up to 459 ml depending on ventilator settings and type of lung disease the ASL 5000 was supposed to approximate. The delivered FiO_2 was 0.36–0.45, again depending on conditions. Auto-triggering was not observed during any aspect of the study. Using available data, the researchers were able to quantify V_T under normal, COPD, and ILD conditions by a linear regression equation. This important study proved that the NIOV system could theoretically augment V_T and supplement FiO_2 in patients with obstructive and restrictive physiology.

10.4 Clinical Efficacy of the NIOV System

NIOV has mostly been studied in patients with COPD. Porszasz et al. [5] have published the most detailed assessment to date of how the device influences dyspnea, respiratory muscle activation, and pulmonary gas exchange efficiency in COPD patients during constant work rate exercise on the cycle ergometer. The 15 patients were all men with mean percent-predicted forced expiratory volume in 1 s

(FEV_1) = 32.2 ± 12.0 % and exercise-induced oxyhemoglobin desaturation (mean SpO_2 = 86.5 ± 2.9 %) on FiO_2 = 0.21. The mean age of study participants was 65.5 ± 9.1 years, and 53 % of them had class IV disease according to the *G*lobal Initiative for Chronic *O*bstructive *L*ung *D*isease (GOLD) classification system. For each patient, peak work rate was identified by incremental cycle ergometry, and NIOV testing was performed at 80 % of this value.

There were four permutations for exercise testing: unencumbered, NIOV plus air, NIOV plus oxygen, and unencumbered plus oxygen through a nasal cannula. Exercise tolerance was reduced during incremental testing, and patients had ventilatory limitation to exercise by multiple lines of evidence. The authors [5] found that endurance time was significantly longer and Borg dyspnea scores were significantly lower when patients exercised with NIOV plus oxygen compared with all other permutations. Isotime SpO_2 was significantly higher for NIOV plus oxygen, and electromyography (EMG) of respiratory muscles revealed mechanical unloading under these conditions. Moreover, a positive correlation (r = 0.42, p = 0.0053) was identified between isotime Borg dyspnea score reduction and isotime EMG signal reduction. In total, this important study provides a sophisticated mechanistic understanding of the benefits of NIOV to COPD patients.

10.5 Institutional Experience with NIOV at Dartmouth-Hitchcock Medical Center

We have utilized NIOV in our outpatient pulmonary rehabilitation program for individuals who require more than 4 LPM of supplemental oxygen during exercise, those who are unable to maintain SpO_2 ≥90 %, and those who rate their dyspnea severity as ≥3 points on a Borg scale during exercise. The NIOV device has allowed our participants with COPD and ILD to increase exercise workload and duration with decreased dyspnea ratings and improved SpO_2 levels. These individuals have also noted that their portable oxygen tanks were lasting longer because their consumption through the NIOV decreased significantly (i.e., 6–8 LPM continuous flow vs 3–4 LPM via the NIOV). Interestingly, our patients have observed improved SpO_2 levels on their usual supplemental oxygen flow rate after using the NIOV. We have had individuals use the NIOV for exercise training only and others who utilize it as their primary oxygen source during the day. With the increase in V_T, individuals who have significant airway mucus production may note increased mucus clearance and overall improvement in aeration and SpO_2 levels.

Our patients' responses to NIOV have been quite positive. One patient reported, "I can breathe without having to work at it!" Most of these individuals are highly aware of their work of breathing, and the effects of mitigating that perception have been no less than remarkable. Patients have also noticed that their skin tone has gone from dusky to pink, while others have commented on how good they look.

We have also brought the NIOV device to bear on the case of a young woman with advanced cystic fibrosis (CF) during a hospital stay for treatment of acute pulmonary exacerbation. She had a percent-predicted FEV_1 of 36 %, was active on the list for lung transplantation at the time, and required supplemental oxygen by nasal cannula at a flow rate of 6–8 LPM and nocturnal noninvasive positive pressure ventilation (NIPPV). During a 6-min walk test, we observed a reduction in Borg dyspnea score with the introduction of NIOV and reduced work of breathing when she was at rest. Responding to our inquiry a few weeks later about her NIOV experience, she stated that the device reduced air hunger during ambulation and the extent to which she became tachycardic in this setting. She did not sleep well with the NIOV system and instead used her other NIPPV apparatus. Finally, she observed shorter daytime longevity of her compressed oxygen tanks with the NIOV system, but this may have been related to an increased level of physical activity.

Conclusion

NIPPV can clearly improve quality of life and mitigate the distressing symptom of dyspnea in many patients with chronic respiratory insufficiency, including those with COPD and progressive neuromuscular dysfunction. Challenges to the delivery of this important therapy have included unwieldy size and weight of the apparatus and a lack of technical sophistication of the apparatus sufficient enough to allow straightforward and customizable use. The NIOV system appears to have overcome these challenges and, as such, represents an innovative and effective treatment option. Further study is needed, however, in patients with ILD, CF, and partially reversible airflow obstruction.

Key Recommendations

- The NIOV system should be considered as a means of supporting ventilation and oxygenation and mitigating dyspnea in patients with COPD.
- Because the NIOV device allows for customization of numerous parameters, the settings should be defined, adjusted, and monitored for efficacy by specialists in respiratory care.
- Although most of the preclinical and clinical research involving the NIOV system has focused on obstructive lung disease, the system could reasonably be applied to patients with restrictive lung diseases such as ILD.

References

1. Device Technical Specifications: Breathe Technologies, Incorporated, 2013. http://www.breathetechnologies.com/clinician/NIOV/system
2. McCoy R, Diesem R. Bench comparison of non-invasive open ventilation to high flow therapy in various test scenarios. COPD8USA. Chicago; 2013.
3. McCoy R, Diesem R. Bench comparison of non-invasive open ventilation to home and bilevel ventilation in non-invasive conditions. COPD8USA. Chicago; 2013.
4. Blakeman T, Branson R. Evaluation of a volume targeted NIV device: bench evaluation of the breathe technologies Non-Invasive Open Ventilation system (NIOV). COPD. 2014;11:568–74.
5. Porszasz J, Cao R, Morishige R, et al. Physiologic effects of an ambulatory ventilation system in chronic obstructive pulmonary disease. Am J Respir Crit Care Med. 2013;188:334–42.

Transnasal Insufflation: A New Approach in the Treatment of Obstructive Sleep Apnea Syndrome?

11

Giuseppe Fiorentino, Antonio Pisano, and Daniela G. Giordano

Contents

Abbreviations

AHI	Apnea-hypopnea index
CPAP	Continuous positive airway pressure
LV	Left ventricle
OSA	Obstructive sleep apnea
PEEP	Positive end-expiratory pressure
RDI	Respiratory disturbance index
REM	Rapid eye movement

G. Fiorentino, MD (✉)
Division of Respiratory Physiopathology and Rehabilitation, A.O.R.N. "Dei Colli" – Monaldi Hospital, Naples, Italy
e-mail: giuseppefiorentino1@gmail.com

A. Pisano, MD • D.G. Giordano, MD
Cardiac Anesthesia and Intensive Care Unit, A.O.R.N. "Dei Colli" – Monaldi Hospital, Naples, Italy
e-mail: antoniopisanoMD@libero.it; danielagiordano04@libero.it

A.M. Esquinas (ed.), *Noninvasive Mechanical Ventilation: Theory, Equipment, and Clinical Applications*, DOI 10.1007/978-3-319-21653-9_11

SDB Sleep-disordered breathing
TNI Transnasal insufflation
WOB Work of breathing

11.1 Introduction

Obstructive sleep apnea (OSA) is a condition of cyclic or repetitive obstruction of the upper airway during sleep, with micro-arousals occurring at the end of a respiratory event. OSA is thought to affect 2 % of female and 4 % of male adults, whereas its prevalence is higher than 8 % among men aged 40–59 years [1]. Continuous positive airway pressure (CPAP), usually applied nasally, is the established treatment for moderate-to-severe OSA. However, although CPAP is an effective treatment for OSA, it is widely acknowledged that significant limitations to its actual use by patients exist. In fact, adherence to nasal CPAP is substantially low. It has been shown that only 46 % of patients used nasal CPAP for at least 4 h during 70 % of the observed nights [1]. Nonadherence to CPAP generally occurs early during the first week of therapy, usually by the second to fourth day, primarily because of the mask and head gear required for maintaining positive pressure during sleep [2]. Transnasal insufflation (TNI) has been introduced as an alternative method for improving respiration during sleep.

11.2 Discussion and Analysis

11.2.1 Mechanisms of OSA

During wakefulness, tonic and phasic output to the respiratory muscles of the upper airway is similar (and proportional) to that of the thoracic pump: throughout each breath, the upper airway is stiffened, thus preventing lumen closure during the generation of a subatmospheric intraluminal pressure. During sleep, however, the uniformity of motor output is lost and the airway becomes more compliant and vulnerable to collapse. If the stiffness of the soft tissues in the narrowest segments of the passive airway is inadequate to counteract the negative intraluminal pressure that is generated during inspiration, airway obstruction occurs. As a result, the central nervous system adjusts sleep to a lighter level to increase muscle tone and, thus, allow opening of the airway and resumption of the breathing cycle. In patients with OSA, there is a reduction in the expansion forces of the pharyngeal dilator muscles, as in the case of genioglossus muscle dysfunction, and a lack of coordination between the inspiratory activity of this muscle and respiratory effort. Additional factors that may contribute to OSA are excessive or elongated tissues of the soft palate, macroglossia, tonsillar hypertrophy, and a redundant pharyngeal mucosa [3].

The therapeutic mechanism of ventilatory treatment of OSA involves the creation of a "pneumatic splint" by an effective positive pressure applied to the pharynx, which provides immediate relief from obstruction, thus allowing sleep continuity and preservation of sleep architecture.

11.2.2 Effect of TNI

The use of TNI, consisting of high flow rates of room air or room air/oxygen mixtures delivered to the patient via a nasal cannula (Fig. 11.1), has been suggested for the treatment of respiratory diseases such as OSA and for respiratory failure. These high flow rates (ranging from 16 to 40 l/min) are tolerable because the air is warmed and humidified and because nasal cannulas are designed not to create a jet directed to mucosal surfaces.

Several studies have shown that TNI improves oxygenation, increases end-inspiratory lung volume, reduces airway resistance, increases functional residual capacity, and flushes nasopharyngeal dead space (thus reducing CO_2 rebreathing) [4].

The nasopharynx facilitates the humidification and warming of inspired gases through contact with its large surface, but this generates an appreciable resistance to the gas flow. However, TNI minimizes the inspiratory resistance of the nasopharynx by providing a nasopharyngeal gas flow that matches or exceeds the patient's peak inspiratory flow. The resulting change in resistance translates into a decrease in resistive work of breathing (WOB) [4].

Parke et al. [5] measured airway pressure during TNI at 30, 40, and 50 l/min in healthy individuals with both open and closed mouth. They found a positive linear relationship between the flow imposed and airway pressure. In patients recovering

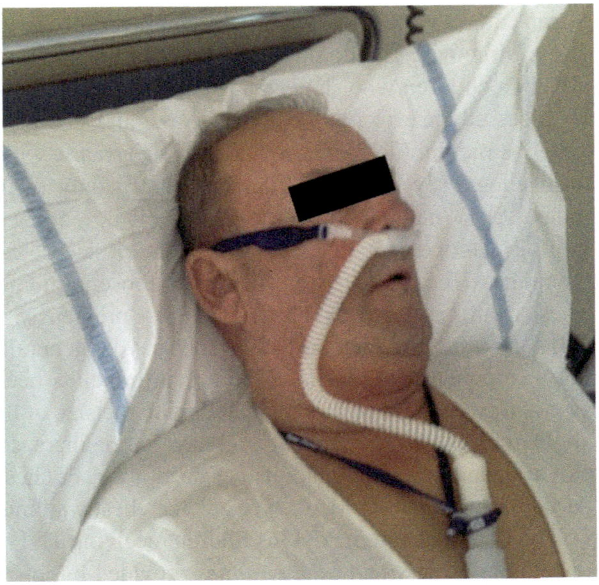

Fig. 11.1 A patient treated with transnasal insufflation (TNI)

from cardiac surgery, a mean positive airway pressure of 2.7 cmH_2O was measured with a flow of 35 l/min with the mouth closed. In healthy individuals, TNI generated a flow-dependent median positive expiratory pressure of 7.4 cmH_2O at 60 l/min with the mouth closed [6]. However, a large interpatient variability was reported, probably due to differences in air leak around the outer part of the nasal cannula and the wide variability in the size of the nostrils. A smaller leak may create an increased resistance to expiration, resulting in higher nasopharyngeal pressure and, therefore, in an increased positive end-expiratory pressure (PEEP) effect [5]. Although this mechanism is particularly effective in neonates, it could also be potentially useful in adult patients.

Moreover, by delivering humidified air, TNI may prevent drying of the airway, thus avoiding the consequent inflammatory response and improving mucociliary function, and could facilitate the clearance of secretions and reduce the formation of atelectasis. Finally, conditioning (warming) of the gas mixture administered can also minimize airway constriction, resulting in a reduction of WOB, which may help to maintain effective delivery of oxygen to the lungs [4].

11.2.3 TNI in Children with OSA

CPAP is the most effective treatment option for children with OSA who are not eligible for surgical interventions (adenotonsillectomy is the treatment of choice when there is adenoid or tonsil hypertrophy), whose parents refuse adenotonsillectomy, or who have residual OSA after surgery. However, as mentioned, adherence to CPAP is relatively low. Accordingly, a large number of children remain untreated [4].

The use of TNI in children with OSA may offer several advantages. First, the patient interface is a nasal cannula, which is less bulky than a nasal mask and avoids facial compression. Accordingly, it might be better tolerated by children during sleep. Moreover, TNI could represent a therapeutic option even more effective than CPAP in children who showed a suboptimal response to the latter. McGinley et al. [7] assessed the effect of TNI (20 l/min of air), compared with CPAP, on upper airway obstruction in 12 children, aged 10 ± 1 years, with mild to severe OSA (2–36 events/hour), by measuring the inspiratory duty cycle and the apnea-hypopnea index (AHI) (namely, the rate of obstructive events per hour of sleep) during both rapid eye movement (REM) and non-REM sleep. They found that the improvements in AHI with TNI were similar to those with CPAP in most of the children. These results appear to be better than those previously shown in adult OSA patients [5]. A possible explanation is that TNI may be generally more effective in increasing pharyngeal pressure in children than in adults because of the relatively larger size of the nasal cannula as compared with the size of the nostrils. Alternatively, the slight increase in pharyngeal pressure might increase lung volume to a greater extent in children than in adults because of higher chest wall and lung compliance, particularly during REM sleep (when the chest wall musculature is hypotonic).

The improvement in AHI in children receiving TNI suggests that the increases in inspiratory airflow and tidal volumes provided by this technique may be sufficient to prevent hypoxia and/or arousals. If these data are confirmed by larger investigations, the implications for the management of sleep-disordered breathing in children could be significant.

11.2.4 TNI in Adults with OSA

TNI has also been used in adult patients with OSA (see Fig. 11.1). McGinley et al. [8] assessed its efficacy in 11 patients with mild-to-severe obstructive apnea–hypopnea syndrome. TNI reduced the overall AHI by 63.2 % (from 28 ± 5 to 10 ± 3 per hour, $p < 0.01$), and some improvement in the AHI was observed in each subject. In a larger study, TNI was shown to reduce the respiratory disturbance index (RDI), namely the mean number of episodes of apnea, hypopnea, and respiratory event-related arousal per hour of sleep, below a clinically acceptable threshold (10 events/hour) in approximately one-quarter of the 56 patients who required CPAP. Overall, RDI decreased by 31 % (from 22.6 ± 15.6 to 17.2 ± 13.2 events/hour, $p < 0.01$) [3].

Nilius and colleagues [3] also investigated the predictors for treatment responses with TNI and found that they were independent from the severity of the sleep apnea disease and the level of prescribed CPAP. Also, anthropometric characteristics did not predict treatment responses. However, the success rate was markedly increased in patients who predominantly had hypopneas and in patients with mild upper airway obstruction. Conversely, the presence of >10 % central apneas predicted poor response to TNI. In other words, TNI therapeutic responses probably depend on the severity of upper airway obstruction but not on its frequency (i.e., the severity of the OSA disease). It is possible that insufflation of air into the nose, by washing out the anatomic dead space, leads to a reduction in CO_2 rebreathing, thereby contributing to the occurrence of central apneas.

As highlighted in the aforementioned investigation, the main mechanism by which TNI reduces the RDI seems to be the increase in pharyngeal pressure that is associated with a rise in the inspiratory airflow. At a rate of 20 l/min, in fact, TNI increases nasal pressure by about 2 cmH_2O and inspiratory airflow by about 100 ml/s. Because the mean peak inspiratory airflow for hypopneas and flow-limited breaths ranges from approximately 150 to 200 ml/s, the additional flow provided by TNI will develop an inspiratory airflow of 250–300 ml/s, a level previously associated with stabilization of breathing patterns [8].

Finally, the results of the study by Nilius et al. [3] also suggest that response rates to TNI would be higher in adults with a predominance of REM-sleep-disordered breathing events, as compared with non-REM sleep associated events.

11.2.5 TNI in Adults with OSA and Stroke

In a 10-year follow-up study on stroke patients, the presence of OSA (with AHI >15 events/hour) was shown to increase the risk of death by 75 %, mostly due to cardiac complications [9]. In fact, futile inspiratory effort against a closed glottis, as occurs in OSA, leads to the generation of negative intrathoracic pressure and increases venous return to the right heart. As a result, right ventricle distention and diastolic leftward shift of the interventricular septum occur. This adversely affects left ventricle (LV) filling and causes reduced stroke volume and delayed LV relaxation. Haba-Rubio et al. [10] examined both tolerability and efficacy of treatment with TNI in patients with acute stroke and sleep-disordered breathing (SDB). To ensure maximum comfort, they used a slightly lower flow rate (18 l/min) compared with the above-mentioned studies (20 l/min). TNI was shown to be well accepted, and no significant side effects were reported. Globally, TNI significantly lowered both the AHI (by 23.8 %) and the oxygen desaturation index (ODI, i.e., the number of times per hour of sleep that arterial oxygen saturation drops by 3 % or more from baseline). TNI also improved sleep stage distribution, with an increase in slow-wave sleep. However, the magnitude of such improvement was rather modest. Moreover, the response to TNI was heterogeneous, with only modest effects on respiratory events in most patients. Indeed, it is likely that nasal CPAP is more effective than TNI in reducing AHI in these patients. Nevertheless, as CPAP is often poorly tolerated, especially in the acute phase of stroke, TNI offers a simplified nasal interface for delivering relatively low levels of pharyngeal pressure and it does not require titration. Accordingly, it could be an alternative option for the treatment of SDB when CPAP is not feasible.

Conclusions

In children, the effects of TNI on SDB suggest that it might provide an alternative to surgery and, compared with CPAP, might be a more readily accepted treatment option. The minimally intrusive nasal interface of TNI may improve adherence to treatment in children and, ultimately, may prove to be more effective in managing the long-term morbidity and mortality of OSA. In adults, TNI offers an alternative to the standard CPAP therapy, especially in patients who predominantly have obstructive hypopnea.

Key Major Recommendations

- TNI could be an alternative treatment for OSA in patients who are poorly adherent to CPAP.
- In adults, TNI seems to be as effective as CPAP in only some subgroups of OSA patients (prevailing hypopneas, mild upper airway obstruction), whereas it is poorly successful in others (e.g., frequent central apneas).
- TNI seems to be particularly effective in children with OSA and may represent a valid alternative to surgery and, compared with CPAP, a more readily accepted treatment option.
- In stroke patients with SDB, TNI should be considered only when nasal CPAP is unfeasible.

References

1. Lee W, Nagubadi S, Kryger MH, et al. Epidemiology of obstructive sleep apnea: a population-based perspective. Expert Rev Respir Med. 2008;2(3):349–64.
2. Weawer TE, Grustein RR. Adherence to continuous positive airway pressure therapy: the challenge to effective treatment. Proc Am Thorac Soc. 2008;5:173–8.
3. Nilius G, Wessendorf T, Maurer J, et al. Predictors for treating obstructive sleep apnea with an open nasal cannula system (transnasal insufflation). Chest. 2010;137:521–8.
4. Dysart K, Miller TL, Wolfson MR, et al. Research in high flow therapy: mechanisms of action. Respir Med. 2009;103:1400–5.
5. Parke RL, McGuinness SP. Pressures delivered by nasal high flow oxygen during all phases of the respiratory cycle. Respir Care. 2013;58(10):1621–4.
6. Groves N, Tobin A. High flow nasal oxygen generates positive airway pressure in adult volunteers. Aust Crit Care. 2007;20:126–31.
7. McGinley B, Halbower A, Schwartz AR, et al. Effect of a high-flow open nasal cannula system on obstructive sleep apnea in children. Pediatrics. 2009;124:179–88.
8. McGinley BM, Patil SP, Kirkness JP, et al. A nasal cannula can be used to treat obstructive sleep apnea. Am J Respir Crit Care Med. 2007;176:194–200.
9. Sahlin C, Sandberg O, Gustafson Y, et al. Obstructive sleep apnea is a risk factor for death in patients with stroke: a 10-year follow-up. Arch Intern Med. 2008;168(3):297–301.
10. Haba-Rubio J, Andries D, Rey-Bataillard V, et al. Effect of transnasal insufflation on sleep-disordered breathing in acute stroke: a preliminary study. Sleep Breath. 2012;16(3):759–64.

Exhalation Ports and Interface: Key Technical Determinants and Clinical Implications

12

Henry K.H. Kwok

Contents

Abbreviations

CO_2	Carbon dioxide
COPD	Chronic obstructive pulmonary disease
EPAP	Expiratory positive airway pressure
ICU	Intensive care unit
NIV	Noninvasive positive pressure ventilation
PEEP	Positive end-expiratory pressure
RVEA	Resident volume of expired air
SARS	Severe Acute Respiratory Syndrome

H.K.H. Kwok, MBBS(HK), MPH, MRCP(UK), FCCP, FHKAM
Respiratory Medicine, Private Practice, Hong Kong, SAR, China
e-mail: hkwok@hkoccmed.com

A.M. Esquinas (ed.), *Noninvasive Mechanical Ventilation: Theory, Equipment, and Clinical Applications*, DOI 10.1007/978-3-319-21653-9_12

12.1 Introduction

Noninvasive positive pressure ventilation (NIV) is the delivery of mechanical ventilation without endotracheal intubation and has been established as the treatment of choice for various causes of respiratory failure, one of which is hypercapnic respiratory failure [1]. Although traditional intensive care unit (ICU)-type ventilators can be used, NIV is more commonly delivered through the more portable NIV or so-called "bi-level" devices, which are able to alternate between a high inspiratory and a low expiratory pressure. In contrast with the ICU types of ventilators, which usually have separate inhalation and exhalation arms of a circle system design, the usual NIV setup involves a single ventilator tube, an exhalation device for the escape of carbon dioxide (CO_2), and the user interface, which can be any type of nasal, oronasal, or full face mask. The single ventilator tube is a concern because of the possibility of CO_2 rebreathing [2].

Because of the setup of the breathing circuit, CO_2 can escape from the breathing system either through the exhalation device or other leaks from the mask–patient interface. Such exhalation devices that facilitate the escape of CO_2 are theoretically important in the determination of the overall performance of a NIV breathing circuit and, therefore, the overall success of the NIV therapy. It should be noted that other ways of CO_2 escape are inevitably present, such as through the leaks from the incomplete seal between the face and the mask. Such leaks are usually minimized to allow the delivery of a desired pressure support to the patient.

Several issues arise that could affect the performance of the NIV breathing circuits. These include (1) whether different types of exhalation devices would make a difference in the CO_2 elimination, (2) effects of different position of exhalation devices on the removal of CO_2, and (3) effects of different types of exhalation devices on the dispersion of aerosols into the surroundings.

12.2 Different Types of Exhalation Devices on the Effects of CO_2 Elimination

Various types of exhalation devices are available for use in the NIV circuit. These devices can either be (1) *built in* on the air hose or on the mask or (2) *separate and connectable devices* on the circuit. The built-in devices usually take the form of a series of small holes, either in the mask itself or on the elbow connector on the mask. For those separate devices not built in on the mask, various forms are available, ranging from a single hole on the connector (Disposable Exhalation Port, Respironics Inc., Murrysville, PA, USA), a fixed valve connector with several narrow slits (Whisper Swivel, Respironics Inc., Murrysville, PA, USA), a connector with a circumferential leak design that allows the gas to escape along the direction of the air hose (Whisper Swivel II, Respironics Inc., Murrysville, PA, USA), or to a specially designed valve with a variable resistor that minimizes rebreathing (Plateau Valve, Respironics Inc., Murrysville, PA, USA) (Fig. 12.1).

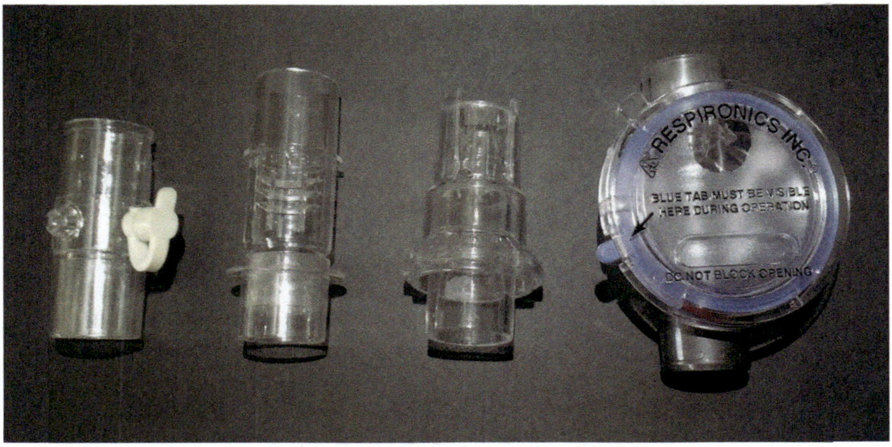

Fig. 12.1 Different types of connectable exhalation ports. *From left to right*: Disposable Exhalation Port, Whisper Swivel, Whisper Swivel II, and Plateau Valve (Respironics Inc., Murrysville, PA, USA)

The built-in exhalation ports have the advantage of being a built-in device without the need to worry about an additional connector on the circuit, whereas the connectable devices have the advantage of being a separate piece of equipment that can be replaced more easily and also allow easier disinfection after use. The question is whether there are any differences in the performance of these different devices in CO_2 exhalation. Additional factors, such as the size of the dead space in using the different types of built-in or connectable devices that could affect the performance of CO_2 exhalation, will not be addressed in this chapter.

12.2.1 Product Information from the Manufacturer

Laboratory studies have been performed to compare the CO_2 elimination of these different types of exhalation devices. The product specification leaflet from the manufacturer of the masks or exhalation ports provides information about the leak rate at different pressure levels used in treatment, an example of which is found from Philips Respironics Inc. [3]. It appears that the newly designed masks commonly have built-in exhalation ports rather than using the conventional detachable exhalation ports. As listed by the manufacturer, the intentional leak is increased with increasing level of applied pressure, and the leaks are usually similar between the different masks and are within a narrow range for different types of masks with different exhalation devices, except for a specific model (Small Child Profile Lite), which has a higher levels of leaks compared with other models (Table 12.1).

Table 12.1 Intentional leak rates for masks and exhalation ports

	Mask	Whisper Swivel 2	ComfortGel Blue EasyLife	ComfortGel ComfortFusion ComfortSelect ComfortClassic ProfileLite	ComfortGel Full ComfortFull 2	FullLife	FitLife	OptiLife all cushions	Small Child Profile Lite	ComfortLite 2 Simple cushion	ComfortLite2 Pillows cushion Direct seal Cushion	Simplicity with 15 mm elbow
Pressure (cmH_2)	2.5	11	12	13	12	13	8	11	20	13	14	11
	5	17	18	18	19	19	13	16	31	19	20	16
	10	26	26	26	28	26	20	23	45	27	29	22
	15	33	32	31	34	32	26	29	57	33	35	28
	20	40	37	37	40	37	31	34	68	38	41	32
	25	45	42	41	44	42	35	38	74	43	46	36
	30	50	46	45	48	46	40	42	82	47	51	39
	35	55	50	49	52	50	43	45	89	51	55	42
	40	59	54	52	56	53	47	49	96	55	59	45

Adapted from Respironics [3]

12.2.2 Laboratory and Clinical Investigations on CO_2 Elimination Performance

Clinical investigators have also performed studies on the performance of different exhalation devices. In a lung model study, Lofaso et al. [4] demonstrated that when the usual type of exhalation port (Whisper Swivel) was used, significant CO_2 rebreathing occurred with resident volume of expired air (RVEA) of up to 55 % of tidal volume detected at a positive end-expiratory pressure (PEEP) level of 1.3 cmH_2O and an inspiratory pressure of 9.4 cmH_2O. When a non-rebreathing valve (Sanders NRV-2 Non-Rebreathing Valve, Respironics Inc., Murrysville, PA, USA) was used to replace the usual type of exhalation port, an auto-PEEP effect was noted, raising the level of PEEP to 2.4 cmH_2O, and at the same time, the RVEA was eliminated.

In a small-scale clinical study of seven critical care patients, Lofaso et al. [4] compared the effect in blood gas and ventilator changes when using conventional intensive care ventilators, NIV with usual type of exhalation port (Whisper Swivel), and NIV with a non-rebreathing exhalation port (Sanders NRV-2 Non-Rebreathing Valve). The authors found that there were no significant effect on $PaCO_2$ and respiratory rate, although a small nonsignificant rise in PaO_2 for the NIV with usual type of exhalation port was observed.

In another clinical study of chronic stable chronic obstructive pulmonary disease (COPD) and normal volunteers, Ferguson and Gilmartin [5] evaluated the effects of different exhalation devices on the $PaCO_2$ levels, CO_2 rebreathing, and other respiratory parameters under different NIV pressure settings. The authors found that significant CO_2 rebreathing could occur at low expiratory pressure levels ($\leq$4 cmH_2O), and they also found that CO_2 rebreathing could be eliminated at an expiratory positive airway pressure (EPAP) of 8 cmH_2O. Such CO_2 rebreathing could be effectively eliminated by the use of the Plateau Valve, which was designed to minimize rebreathing by a variable resistor that permits more air to escape at low expiratory pressures than the traditional type of exhalation devices.

On the other hand, Hill et al. [6] directly compared the effectiveness of the traditional exhalation valve with a three-slit design (Whisper Swivel) to the Plateau Valve in the blood gas and respiratory outcomes among patients receiving long-term nocturnal nasal ventilation for various causes and using low expiratory pressure of $\leq$4 cmH_2O. The authors found that the use of the Plateau Valve did not improve daytime or nocturnal gas exchange or symptoms in patients receiving long-term nasal NIV. The authors attributed the lack of differences to the presence of air leakage from other routes (e.g., through the mouth or under the mask) during nocturnal ventilation.

In summary, exhalation ports are usually built in on the masks, or the ports can be available in the form of a detachable device. Most of the masks with built-in exhalation ports have similar performance in leaks when compared with the commonly used detachable exhalation port, with very few exceptions. Laboratory studies have shown that different detachable exhalation devices have different CO_2 elimination efficacy, with the non-rebreathing valve being more effective in CO_2

elimination. In small-scale clinical studies, however, studies on different patient groups have shown different performance of various exhalation devices. Specific types of exhalation valves, such as the Plateau Valve, have shown different results when assessed in different studies, with a favorable result in the study by Ferguson and Gilmartin [5] and a neutral result in the study by Hill et al. [6]. Other factors, such as the level of PEEP or the dead space of the mask, might have a role in influencing the efficiency of the CO_2 elimination.

12.3 Position of the Exhalation Port on the Removal of CO_2 from the Breathing Circuit

As the exhalation port serves to eliminate CO_2 from the breathing circuit, its position should be placed as near the patient as possible to more effectively capture the CO_2 exhaled by the patient and to decrease the chance of CO_2 being washed up into the breathing circuit. With reference to the different designs of the interface and the circuits, the position of the exhalation port can either be placed on the ventilator tubing or on the mask itself. Studies have been conducted to evaluate whether there are any differences in the CO_2 efficacy if the exhalation port is positioned differently.

Lofaso et al. [7], in a bench study of different types of NIV ventilators, tried placing side holes in the inspiratory circuit of a NIV device to allow venting of expiratory gas to the atmosphere, but found that these side holes on the circuit were not effective.

In a laboratory study, Schettino et al. [8] evaluated CO_2 rebreathing in three different types of interface setting: (1) the full face mask with a exhalation port on the mask over the nasal bridge, (2) a facial mask using the Whisper Swivel exhalation port on the circuit connected to the mask, and (3) the Total Face Mask (Respironics Inc., Murrysville, PA, USA) with the exhalation port within the mask. The authors found that the facial mask with built-in exhalation port could more effectively clear CO_2 from the mask and circuit, whereas the facial mask with an in-circuit Whisper Swivel exhalation port performed similarly to the Total Face Mask, which had a much larger dead space. The authors also found that increasing the EPAP level from 4 cmH_2O to 8 cmH_2O had only a small effect in decreasing the CO_2 rebreathing when masks with exhalation ports within the mask were tested.

In a study by Chen et al. [10], seven patients with COPD were treated with NIV with the path of exhalation connected to the side hole on the mask. The authors found that CO_2 rebreathing could be minimized with such a setup modification when compared with the usual setup of placing the exhalation port on the circuit [9]. This study led some investigators to suggest that exhalation ports over the nasal bridge should become the "standard" in NIV.

In summary, position of the exhalation port may impact the performance of the CO_2 elimination, as shown in different laboratory and small-scale human studies, with some suggestion that CO_2 elimination is most favorable when the exhalation port is placed on the top of the mask near the nasal bridge. Because of the small number of studies having been conducted, and also because of the involvement of other factors such as air pressures, types of patients, and the size of the dead space of different masks, further studies are needed to confirm such observations.

12.4 Effects of Different Types of Exhalation Devices on the Dispersion of Aerosols to the Surroundings

A more contemporary issue related to exhalation is the dispersion of bioaerosols from the port. This issue stems from the epidemic of the severe acute respiratory syndrome (SARS) in 2003, when 8,098 patients were infected, resulting in the death of 774 people, with a case fatality rate of 9.6 % [11], including a significant proportion of health-care workers [12]. The question of whether NIV could cause dispersion of infectious bioaerosols become a heated debate, and many pulmonologists and professional societies have issued precautionary statements and guidelines on the use of NIV for patients with pulmonary infections [13]. Since then, studies have been conducted on the dispersion of bioaerosols from NIV both in laboratory settings and in human studies.

In a laboratory study by Hui et al. [14], oil-based smoke particulates were used to assess the dispersion distances of bioaerosols from two different combinations of mask and exhalation device (Respironics Inc. ComfortFull 2 full face mask with built-in exhalation diffusers vs Image 3 full face mask with an external Whisper Swivel exhalation port). It was found that the Image 3–Whisper Swivel exhalation port had a higher maximal dispersion distance at all the tested IPAP pressures: 0.95 m at IPAP 10 cmH_2O, >0.95 m at IPAP 14 and 18 cmH_2O. This was compared with dispersion distances of 0.65, 0.65, and 0.85 m at IPAP 10, 14, and 18 cmH_2O for the ComfortFull 2 mask. The diffusion from the Image 3-Whisper Swivel combination was also more diffuse and extensive. The difference in dispersion distance could be related to the design of the mask and the exhalation port.

In another setting using human subjects, Simmonds et al. [15] recruited three groups of participants (normal subjects, subjects with coryzal symptoms, and subjects with chronic lung disease exacerbations) and gave them a series of respiratory therapies, including chest physiotherapy, oxygen therapy, neubilized medications, and NIV. NIV was delivered either through a vented full face mask or using a modified circuit with a non-vented full face mask coupled with a viral/bacterial filter placed between the mask and the expiratory leak. Measurements of aerosol sizes and number were made at two positions, one immediately adjacent to the participants (D1) and from a second position at 1 m from the participants (D2). The authors found that, after treatment with NIV using standard circuits with vented full face mask, a significant increase in amount of aerosols larger than 10 μm was found at position D1 for subjects with chronic lung diseases and for coryzal subjects. At position D2, coryzal subjects were also found to generate significantly more aerosols of sizes 3–5 μm and 5–10 μm and a borderline significant increase in aerosols at >10 μm size range. Although this study has not compared the propensity for different exhalation ports to generate bioaerosols, it illustrates that in a real-life situation, bioaerosols generated from NIV through the exhalation port can be minimized by the installation of a bacterial/viral filter placed between the patient interface and the exhalation port.

Conclusion

Different types of exhalation devices are available for use in NIV, from the conventional detachable types of exhalation ports to the built-in exhalation ports on the NIV mask, which are increasingly popular. Performance in CO_2 elimination among the different exhalation devices varies, but the difference tends to be small, with some advantages in certain non-rebreathing devices. It appears from a few small-scale studies that the position of the exhalation port is best placed near the top of the NIV mask near the nasal bridge for the most efficient CO_2 elimination performance. That being said, confounding variables such as the level of EPAP and the dead space of the mask itself should be noted in the overall evaluation of the exhalation port effectiveness. A more contemporary issue relates to the dispersion of bioaerosols through the exhalation port, highlighting the importance of infection control when using NIV for patients with pulmonary infections.

References

1. Mehta S, Hill NS. Noninvasive ventilation. Am J Respir Crit Care Med. 2001;163(2):540–77 [Research Support, U.S. Gov't, P.H.S. Review].
2. Szkulmowski Z, Belkhouja K, Le QH, Robert D, Argaud L. Bilevel positive airway pressure ventilation: factors influencing carbon dioxide rebreathing. Intensive Care Med. 2010;36(4):688–91.
3. Respironics P. Intentional leak rates for masks and exhalation ports. Philips Res. [Cited 2015, 20 April 2015]. Available from: http://medtoyou.com/files/Product_Resources/KnowledgeCenter/1036867_MaskLeakRates_Poster.pdf.
4. Lofaso F, Brochard L, Touchard D, Hang T, Harf A, Isabey D. Evaluation of carbon dioxide rebreathing during pressure support ventilation with airway management system (BiPAP) devices. Chest. 1995;108(3):772–8 [Clinical Trial Comparative Study Randomized Controlled Trial Research Support, Non-U.S. Gov't].
5. Ferguson GT, Gilmartin M. CO_2 rebreathing during BiPAP ventilatory assistance. Am J Respir Crit Care Med. 1995;151(4):1126–35 [Clinical Trial Randomized Controlled Trial].
6. Hill NS, Carlisle C, Kramer NR. Effect of a nonrebreathing exhalation valve on long-term nasal ventilation using a bilevel device. Chest. 2002;122(1):84–91 [Clinical Trial Research Support, Non-U.S. Gov't].
7. Lofaso F, Brochard L, Hang T, Lorino H, Harf A, Isabey D. Home versus intensive care pressure support devices. Experimental and clinical comparison. Am J Respir Crit Care Med. 1996;153(5):1591–9 [Clinical Trial Comparative Study Randomized Controlled Trial Research Support, Non-U.S. Gov't].
8. Schettino GP, Chatmongkolchart S, Hess DR, Kacmarek RM. Position of exhalation port and mask design affect CO2 rebreathing during noninvasive positive pressure ventilation. Crit Care Med. 2003;31(8):2178–82 [Research Support, Non-U.S. Gov't].
9. Chen R, Zhang X, He G. Modification of facial mask on the dead space effect in non-invasive mask ventilation. Zhonghua jie he he hu xi za zhi = Zhonghua jiehe he huxi zazhi = Chin J Tuberculosis Respir Dis. 2000;23(12):734–6 [Clinical Trial Randomized Controlled Trial].

10. Elliott MW. The interface: crucial for successful noninvasive ventilation. Eur Respir J. 2004;23(1):7–8 [Comment Editorial].
11. Hui DS, Chan PK. Severe acute respiratory syndrome and coronavirus. Infect Dis Clin North Am. 2010;24(3):619–38 [Case Reports Review].
12. McDonald LC, Simor AE, Su IJ, Maloney S, Ofner M, Chen KT, et al. SARS in healthcare facilities, Toronto and Taiwan. Emerg Infect Dis. 2004;10(5):777–81 [Review].
13. Hong_Kong_Lung_Foundation. Practice Standards of Respiratory Procedures: Post SARS Era. Noninvasive Positive Pressure Ventilation. Hong Kong Lung Foundation; 2005.
14. Hui DS, Chow BK, Ng SS, Chu LC, Hall SD, Gin T, et al. Exhaled air dispersion distances during noninvasive ventilation via different Respironics face masks. Chest. 2009;136(4):998–1005 [Research Support, Non-U.S. Gov't].
15. Simonds AK, Hanak A, Chatwin M, Morrell M, Hall A, Parker KH, et al. Evaluation of droplet dispersion during non-invasive ventilation, oxygen therapy, nebuliser treatment and chest physiotherapy in clinical practice: implications for management of pandemic influenza and other airborne infections. Health Technol Assess. 2010;14(46):131–72 [Research Support, Non-U.S. Gov't].

Technological Aspects and Safe Use of Noninvasive Mechanical Ventilation Devices: Key Technical and Practical Recommendations

13

Sven Stieglitz

Contents

Abbreviations

CO_2	Carbon dioxide
FFM	Full face mask
ICU	Intensive care unit
NIV	Noninvasive ventilation
NM	Nasal mask

S. Stieglitz, MD
Department of Pneumology and Cardiology,
Petrus Hospital Wuppertal, Academic Teaching Hospital of the University of Duesseldorf,
Carnaper Str. 48, 42283 Wuppertal, Germany
e-mail: sven.stieglitz@cellitinnen.de

A.M. Esquinas (ed.), *Noninvasive Mechanical Ventilation: Theory, Equipment, and Clinical Applications*, DOI 10.1007/978-3-319-21653-9_13

13.1 Introduction

The first patients to be ventilated were patients in Denmark with poliomyelitis. Before the 1950s, the iron lung (negative pressure tank) was the only available ventilator and, from some points of view, these ventilators may be regarded as noninvasive. Negative pressure tanks were able to treat hypercapnic failure but were not a good solution for treating severe hypoxemic failure.

The next stage in the development of ventilators was the introduction of positive-pressure ventilators, which worked by a simple push-pull bellows pump that ventilated patients via an endotracheal tube and a breathing circuit. The smaller proportions of these ventilators led to a worldwide distribution of ventilators in intensive care units (ICUs), which now is considered a key technology in the ICU [1]. The main technical features of ICU ventilators are the different modes and a variety of ventilator settings, the use of a breathing circuit with low or even very low leakage, a reliable oxygen supply, a high level of safety with a maximum of alarming, some tools for ventilator settings (e.g., for determining upper and lower inflection points), and a large display indicating parameters and curves. There are two different pneumatic principles of ICU ventilators. The one drive system operates with compressed gas sources that are dispensed and mixed by high-precision valves. The other drive system works independently of a central compressed air supply by sucking in ambient air via a turbine and mixing additional oxygen from a gas source. Most modern ICU ventilators operate by high-precision valves that require central gas sources. Because they are dependent on a gas source, this type of ventilator is immobile. Compared with invasive ventilation, the distinguishing features of noninvasive ventilation (NIV) are the non-hermetic nature of the system, with intended and unintended leaks, and the presence of variable resistance resulting from the upper airway [2]. This explains a major disadvantages of ICU ventilators driven by a central gas source: they are not suitable for handling leakage. This makes them inappropriate for NIV, despite the fact that an increasing number of ICU ventilators offer a NIV mode.

The history of NIV ventilators is exciting because the development was driven in two different ways. Some ventilators were engineered as portable ventilators with a bellows pump. The first ventilators specifically designed for long-term home mechanical ventilation were the volume-controlled PLV 100 (Philips Respironics, Amsterdam, Netherlands), followed by the pressure-controlled PV 401 (Breas Medical, Herrsching, Germany). These portable ventilators were lightweight and economical compared with ICU ventilators. At the time, NIV was also applied as volume-controlled ventilation, like the ventilators that operated only in this mode. Other ventilators were developed from continuous positive airway pressure (CPAP) machines that were designed to pump a flow of air into the nasal passages to keep the airway open in sleep apnea. These devices, used in sleep medicine, were driven by a turbine. Modification of these devices led to ventilators that had an inspiratory pressure of 20 mbar and a simple S-mode (spontaneous), which corresponds to the pressure support ventilation (PSV) of ICU ventilators. Later, ST and T (timed) modes were developed. Today, both types of ventilators are turbine driven. Most NIV ventilators operate as pressure-controlled ventilators and are turbine driven. An increasing number of features of ICU ventilators, such as configuring the inspiratory trigger-threshold or displaying ventilator curves are transferred to portable NIV ventilators. This brief history of the development of ventilators explains the confusing diversity of nomenclature of modes in NIV. Nevertheless, one may recognize the different types of NIV ventilators. One type works with a breathing circuit with an integrated expiratory valve (either active or passive) and the other requires a mask with a pre-defined leakage that works as a passive expiratory "valve" (vented mask).

Three different types of ventilators can be found in a hospital or even within a single ICU:

1. Dedicated ICU ventilators working with gas sources and high-precision valves
2. Dedicated NIV ventilators that are turbine-driven and approved for NIV only
3. Portable turbine-driven ventilators that are approved for invasive (either for breathing support or for life-sustaining ventilation) as well for noninvasive ventilation

13.2 Discussion and Analysis

13.2.1 Choice of Ventilator

Dedicated ICU ventilators that operate with compressed gas sources are limited regarding the maximum of possible flow that they might deliver by the central gas source. They usually achieve a maximum of flow about 120 l/min, although some manufacturers find technical solutions by a built-in tank working as a reservoir that allows generation of flows of about 180 l/min. Turbine-driven portable ventilators are able to achieve flow rates above >200 l/min. Today, the highest possible flow is generated by turbine-driven ICU ventilators with flow rates of 260–300 l/min. When ventilating patients noninvasively, it is important to employ ventilators that generate high flow rates. The flow is necessary to compensate for the leakage at the mask, to avoid CO_2 rebreathing (especially in single circuits and passive expiratory valves), and to handle the high flow that may be generated by spontaneously breathing patients, especially in case of acute respiratory failure. As shown above, for technical reasons the small portable turbine-driven ventilators are superior in NIV compared with dedicated ICU ventilators that operate with valves and central gas sources. The latter are not recommended in NIV, even when the manufacturers of the ventilator offer a "NIV" mode.

13.2.2 Oxygenation

ICU ventilators are able to ensure an adequate oxygen delivery, which is sometimes less well balanced in dedicated NIV ventilators. In NIV, the oxygen is usually delivered by a constant flow. Nevertheless, the delivery of oxygen varies because the concentration of oxygen that reaches the patient depends on the pressure (which is generated by the flow of the turbine), the flow of the spontaneously breathing patient, and the leakage within the breathing circuit or mask (which again will increase the flow to compensate for the leakage). Particularly large leakage may reduce the concentration of inspired oxygen. There is another observation that can be made: patients sometimes require a higher oxygen delivery when they are ventilated with NIV compared with spontaneous breathing. This happen when the flow of the spontaneous breathing is lower than the flow generated by NIV. In this case, the oxygen is diluted by the ambient air, which may reduce the hemoglobin oxygen saturation and require an increase of the oxygen flow during NIV. Therefore, patients with severe hypoxemia who are ventilated with NIV require an optimal medical surveillance.

When NIV is started, it is important to begin the ventilation first and to connect the oxygen afterwards. This prevents the oxygen from getting into the ventilator, which generates a fire hazard. Many manufacturers also require the use of a pressure valve to avoid oxygen intrusion into the ventilator.

There are only few ventilators approved for NIV that have a separate input for oxygen. In general, the oxygen may be introduced either near the mask or near the ventilator. These two possibilities seem to be equal with regard to the oxygenation of the patient.

13.2.3 Misconnections of Invasive and Noninvasive Ventilation

Whereas mechanical ventilation in the ICU is performed within a limited area by a defined team that is well trained and ventilates patients only in the ICU, performing NIV in conventional medical wards not only extends the location where NIV is performed but also increases the group of people faced with NIV and the problems of the patients who use NIV. Performing NIV out-of-hospital further increases this group and adds the patients themselves (and their relatives) who must utilize the NIV correctly and the employees of the home-care provider. As shown above, the situation is complicated by the three categories of ventilators: dedicated ICU ventilators, dedicated NIV ventilators, and portable turbine-driven ventilators that are approved for invasive and noninvasive ventilation.

NIV is usually used with a single-circuit ventilation system. The advantage of single circuits is their lower weight compared with double-circuit systems of invasive ventilation, which is important considering the fitting of the mask. The handling is simpler, which is particularly important in the use of NIV outside of the hospital.

The situation is further complicated by two competing systems: one using a breathing circuit with an integrated expiratory valve (active or passive), which requires a non-vented mask, and the other using a breathing circuit without an expiratory valve but requiring a vented mask. The most common misconnections in NIV seems to be the misconnection of a breathing circuit with an expiratory valve integrated with a vented mask, leading to an abnormal leakage that impairs an adequate increase of the pressure, and the misconnection of a breathing system without an expiratory valve with a non-vented mask, which leads to a failure of CO_2

elimination. This is especially dangerous because it might be overlooked in the clinical routine. Even marked hypercapnia can be associated with normal oxygen saturation when additional oxygen is administered. In fact, hemoglobin oxygen saturation is only a marker for ventilation when patients are breathing room air. Therefore, we recommend routine measurement of CO_2 by blood gas analysis or by transcutaneous measurement (end-tidal measurement of CO_2 works only in invasive ventilation). Regrettably, there is no solution for this problem, although the connection between the mask and tubing (the elbow piece) of vented and non-vented masks is sometimes designed in different colors. Because the elbow piece fits both types of masks, the error still has the potential to occur, especially after removing this piece to clean the mask [3].

Another type of misconnection applies to the use of ventilators that offer both invasive and noninvasive modes. Although these ventilators are approved for both modes, the setting of the mode is done manually. It is possible to connect a ventilator that operates with a simple single circuit (without expiratory valve) in a NIV mode to a breathing tube, leading to severe hypercapnia. There is no technical solution to avoid this. Therefore, we recommend a clear separation between invasive and noninvasive ventilators and, in our clinical routine, ventilators that are approved for both modes are used exclusively for either invasive or noninvasive ventilation.

The incorrect use of the ventilator equipment and, therefore, the human factor are the main reasons for critical incidents in respiratory medicine. Thus, continued training of doctors, nursing staff, respiratory therapists, and caregivers is required. One should always also take into account that misuse occurs by the patients, their relatives, and employees of home-care provider.

13.2.4 Pressure Constancy

The pressure constancy of portable turbine-driven ventilators varies ±2.5 mbar (sometimes even higher) for most portable ventilators. This explains the observation that many patients remark on a difference after exchange of the ventilator even if the ventilator settings remain unchanged. Therefore, an exchange of the ventilator always requires a clinical control (e.g., blood gas analysis). This is especially important in home mechanical ventilation and chronic hypercapnic failure.

13.2.5 Manipulation of Interfaces

NIV is often underestimated with regard to its effectiveness and its complexity. Additionally, as mentioned above, the group of people helping to provide NIV is larger than the small, specialized teams who care for invasive ventilation in an ICU. This might explain why manipulation of the NIV may sometimes be observed, with the potential risk of harm to the patient. We recommend appointing one nurse (or a team) or respiratory therapist who controls the NIV in daily routine and checks the ventilator equipment.

13.2.6 Rapid Eye Movement Rebound

Rapid eye movement (REM) rebound occurs after initiation of CPAP and may also play a role in NIV. In clinical studies, the increase of REM after one night of CPAP amounts to 20 % [4], but in single cases REM may increase to more than 70 % after initiation of CPAP [5]. In REM, the CO_2- and O_2-threshold for ventilation are changed and the stimulation of breathing due to hypoxemia or hypercapnia is markedly reduced. Additionally, the threshold for awakening is reduced in REM. This all together contributes to a challenging situation that requires clinical care of the patient and an optimal control of the ventilator equipment in the first few nights after initiation of NIV. Special attention should be given to the displacement of the mask and disconnection of the breathing tube in this situation.

13.2.7 Importance of the Interface

The most commonly used interfaces in NIV are the full face (FFM) and the nasal mask (NM) [6]. There seems to be a trend toward the FFM, especially when high-pressure (>25 cmH_2O) NIV is performed [7]. In this regard, it is important to recognize that NIV failure may occur not only because of the chosen ventilation strategy (invasive vs noninvasive) or the ventilator setting (pressure difference, frequency, triggering, ramp, etc.) [2] but also as a result of the chosen interface. Furthermore, also sedation affects the effectiveness of NIV and the interaction of interface and ventilation [8]. The study of Oto et al. [8] showed that the NM is superior to the FFM in unconscious patients. For these reasons, changing of the interface (e.g., from NM to FFM) requires a medical control of the ventilation.

Conclusion

The use of turbine-driven NIV ventilators allows ventilation of patients outside the ICU and even at home. However, a specialized team is required to care for the NIV equipment and for the patients. The presence of vented and non-vented systems is a pitfall that requires good care of all the equipment used. The flow of the NIV ventilator reduces the hemoglobin oxygen saturation in the case of additional oxygen supply. REM rebound may occur after initiation of NIV, which may potentially harm patients because of the reduced hypercapnic and hypoxemic stimulation of ventilation in REM. Therefore, good medical care is required after initiation of NIV.

Key Major Recommendations

- Turbine-driven ventilators are recommended for NIV.
- Because a higher oxygen delivery may be necessary with NIV compared with spontaneous breathing due to dilution with ambient air, optimal medical surveillance is necessary when patients are hypoxemic.

- To avoid misconnections of vented and non-vented systems and any manipulation of the interfaces, the foundation of a specialized "NIV team" who cares for all ventilator equipment is strongly recommended.
- Clinical care of the patient and optimal control of the ventilator equipment in the first few nights after initiation of NIV are required to avoid critical incidents resulting from REM rebound, with special attention paid to the displacement of the mask and disconnection of the breathing tube in this situation.

References

1. Marini J. Mechanical ventilation: past lessons and near future. Crit Care. 2013;17 Suppl 1:51.
2. Rabec C, Rodenstein D, Leger P, et al. Ventilator modes and settings during non-invasive ventilation: effects on respiratory events and implications for their identification. Thorax. 2011;66(2):170–8.
3. Stieglitz S, George S, Priegnitz C, et al. Life-threatening events in respiratory medicine: misconnections of invasive and non-invasive ventilators and interfaces. Pneumologie. 2013;67(4):228–32.
4. Brillante R, Cossa G, Liu PY, et al. Rapid eye movement and slow-wave sleep rebound after one night of continuous positive airway pressure for obstructive sleep apnea. Respirology. 2012;17:547–53.
5. Bue AL, Salvaggio A, Insalaco G, et al. Extreme REM rebound during continuous positive airway pressure titration for obstructive sleep apnea in a depressed patient. Case Rep Med. 2014;2014:292181.
6. Silva RM, Timenetsky KT, Neves RC, et al. Adaptation to different noninvasive ventilation masks in critically ill patients. J Bras Pneumol. 2013;39(4):469–75.
7. Murphy PB, Brignall K, Moxham J, et al. High pressure versus high intensity noninvasive ventilation in stable hypercapnic chronic obstructive pulmonary disease: a randomized crossover trial. Int J Chron Obstruct Pulmon Dis. 2012;7:811–8.
8. Oto J, Li Q, Kimball WR, et al. Continuous positive airway pressure and ventilation are more effective with a nasal mask than a full face mask in unconscious subjects: a randomized controlled trial. Crit Care. 2013;17:R300.

CPAP Device Therapy for Noninvasive Mechanical Ventilation in Hypoxemic Respiratory Failure: Key Technical Topics and Clinical Implications

14

Rodolfo Ferrari

Contents

Abbreviations

AA	Acute asthma
ABG	Arterial blood gas analysis
ACPE	Acute cardiogenic pulmonary edema
AHRF	Acute hypoxemic respiratory failure
ARDS	Acute respiratory distress syndrome
ARF	Acute respiratory failure
CHF	Chronic heart failure
COPD	Chronic obstructive pulmonary disease
CPAP	Continuous positive airway pressure
DNI	Do not intubate
ED	Emergency department

R. Ferrari, MD
Medicina d'Urgenza e Pronto Soccorso, Policlinico Sant'Orsola – Malpighi, Dipartimento dell'Emergenza – Urgenza, Azienda Ospedaliero – Universitaria di Bologna, Via Albertoni, 10, Bologna 40138, Italy
e-mail: dr.rofer@gmail.com; rodolfo.ferrari@aosp.bo.it

A.M. Esquinas (ed.), *Noninvasive Mechanical Ventilation: Theory, Equipment, and Clinical Applications*, DOI 10.1007/978-3-319-21653-9_14

FEV_1	Forced expiratory volume in 1 second
FiO_2	Fraction of inspired oxygen
FRC	Functional residual capacity
HMDU	High medical dependency unit
ICU	Intensive care unit
IMV	Invasive mechanical ventilation
NCPAP	Noninvasive continuous positive airway pressure
NIMV	Noninvasive mechanical ventilation
NPPV	Noninvasive double-level positive pressure ventilation
OOH	Out of hospital
OSAS	Obstructive sleep apnea syndrome
PaO_2	Arterial oxygen pressure
PEEP	Positive end-expiratory pressure
RCCT	Randomized controlled clinical trial
RR	Respiratory rate
SO_2T	Standard oxygen therapy
SpO_2	Oxygen saturation
TI	Tracheal intubation
VPM	Ventilation / perfusion mismatch
WB	Work of breathing

14.1 Introduction

Continuous positive airway pressure (CPAP) entails delivering to the opening of the airways, by an external interface or an endotracheal tube, a positive (over-atmospheric) pressure, continuously, during both expiration and inspiration. Although CPAP cannot literally be defined as a noninvasive mechanical ventilation (NIMV) technique: it is often, but not always, noninvasive; it is sometimes mechanically generated, but there are many simpler ways to perform it; and it cannot strictly be considered "ventilation," because, even if in specific cases CPAP is able to increase alveolar ventilation, it cannot perform any work of breathing (WB).

Today, CPAP is universally accepted and included in the field of NIMV, because, as opposed to the "mandatory controlled" way of ventilating, it represents the "spontaneous" way: the patient is in charge of the whole WB and must be able to individually manage each period of the inhalation phase (triggering, limiting, and cycling). In the last two decades, NIMV demonstrated its main role in the treatment of acute respiratory failure (ARF). It is safe and effective when delivered early to carefully selected patients who do not meet the criteria for tracheal intubation (TI), because of its ability to reduce morbidity and mortality related to invasive mechanical ventilation (IMV) [1].

The use of noninvasive CPAP (NCPAP) in treating acute hypoxemic respiratory failure (AHRF) has spread in the everyday real world of clinical practice in emergency care, coming out of the intensive care units (ICUs) to reach the high-dependency medical units (HMDUs), the emergency department (ED), and the out-of-hospital

(OOH) setting. NCPAP is also the cornerstone for treating, even at home, such chronic condition as chronic heart failure (CHF) and obstructive sleep apnea syndrome (OSAS). With the spread of NCPAP, today, even in the scientific medical literature, the term CPAP has become synonymous with NCPAP. Similarly, the acronym PEEP (positive end-expiratory pressure) is often used with the same meaning as CPAP.

Nevertheless, we can never forget that NIMV and NCPAP are not actually a real "therapy," as they are not able to resolve by themselves the cause of the ARF. They are a "bridge" we use to support the WB while therapy is ongoing to confront and resolve the acutely decompensated basic pathological condition. Drugs remain the mainstay of medical etiopathogenetic treatment.

14.2 Background

NCPAP, versus standard oxygen therapy (SO_2T), has proven its efficacy in reducing the rate of TI and hospital mortality in ARF resulting from acute cardiogenic pulmonary edema (ACPE) [2]. Its success is mainly due to the increase in intrathoracic pressure and its subsequent hemodynamic cardiovascular and respiratory effects. In many other clinical conditions, unresponsive to SO_2T alone, NCPAP showed lower levels of evidence and strength of recommendation [3]. The pathophysiological rationale is often in the increased ventilation/perfusion mismatch (VPM) complicated by AHRF, and the capability of interfering with atelectasis and the shunt effect.

Key determinants for the success of the technique include the right selection of patients, an early intervention, the choice of a comfortable and well-fitting interface, careful monitoring, and a skilled team [4, 5]. Once NCPAP is established as part of the treatment for ARF in a particular patient, some further choices are then pivotal:

- Which positive pressure level must be set (usually expressed as cmH_2O), depending on the underlying clinical condition and the hemodynamic state of the patient?
- Which fraction of inspired oxygen (FiO_2, expressed as a percentage) to start with, depending on the ideal target in oxygen saturation (SpO_2)?
- Which interface to choose?
- Where to perform the treatment, and which kind of monitoring is needed?
- How to prepare in case of NIMV failure?

One must always keep in mind that any unnecessary delay in recognizing the need for IMV, and its dramatic consequences, should be avoided.

14.3 Technical Topics: Devices and Interfaces

CPAP can be provided in many different ways, by many different devices and systems. For the treatment of ARF in the acute care setting, NCPAP is usually provided by simple high-flow generators needing only an oxygen source (standalone systems,

Table 14.1 NCPAP: high-flow generators versus ventilators

High-flow generators	Ventilators
Pros	*Pros*
Simpler, less parameters needed to set	No limits in high flow versus high FiO_2
Cheaper	Leak compensation, more stable pressure
No triggering system	Waveforms, alarms, monitoring
Easier and lighter for transport or OOH use	Known FiO_2
Cons	*Cons*
Compromise between high flow and/or high FiO_2	More complex, more parameters to set
Less stable positive pressure	Expensive
No alarms, no monitoring	Need for synchronization and triggering
Inaccurate FiO_2	Need for batteries or electricity
Lower performances	Need for specific NIV module

Venturi-like, Boussignac®-like, etc.) or by turbine- or piston-driven ventilators (with a NIMV module). The main pros and cons are listed in Table 14.1.

Today there is no reason to strongly recommend a specific device over another. A pivotal factor in the approach and the choice is the need to provide a high flow, high enough to meet the needs of a patient with ARF, mainly in the very early phase of inhalation. Some other simpler devices, with or without oxygen supply, are particularly tailored for home treatment of chronic conditions. On the other hand, patient comfort and tolerance of the interface are probably the crucial factors for successful NIMV [6]. Oro-nasal masks, full or total face masks, and helmets can be used to provide NCPAP in treating ARF. The pros and cons are listed in Table 14.2. Nasal masks, nasal prongs, and mouthpieces are used outside of the acute care setting; interfaces covering both the mouth and the nose are the first choice for acute NIMV. The ideal mask does not exist and cannot be expected a priori for an individual patient.

In an ideal situation, even in the emergency setting, it is useful to be able to change the size or rotate different interfaces to reduce the rate of complications (Table 14.3) and increase patient comfort during NCPAP. The most common complications associated with interfaces for NCPAP can be, at least in part, prevented, treated, and resolved [3, 7]. The contribution provided by the nursing staff in the management of the interface can make the difference in the success of the treatment. Training, experience, skills, and motivation are vital factors, primarily in the early phases of treating ARF by NIMV, for a successful outcome [4].

14.4 Main Clinical Indications

The efficacy of NIMV on patient outcome predominantly depends on the underlying pathology. ACPE provides the best evidence for efficacy of NCPAP in ARF [8]. By reducing WB and improving gas exchanges, lung and thorax mechanics (compliance, functional residual capacity (FRC)), right ventricular preload, and left

Table 14.2 NCPAP interface characteristics

Oro-nasal Mask	Full/total face mask	Helmet
Pros	*Pros*	*Pros*
Few air leaks	Scarce air leaks	Minimum air leaks
Stable airway pressure	Easy fitting	Neither nasal nor facial skin damage
Easy application	Stable airway pressure	No problem in facial trauma, burns, edentulism
Less cooperation required	No nasal bridge skin lesions	Less flow resistance
Cheaper	Less noisy	Easier speaking
		Panoramic view
		Possible drinking
		Enteral nutrition allowed
		Easier coughing and expectoration
		More suitable for long-lasting treatments
Cons	*Cons*	*Cons*
Nasal skin decubitus	Facial skin lesions	Very high gas flow required
Vomiting	Vomiting	Noisy
Claustrophobia	Claustrophobia	High dead space
Eyes irritation	Eyes irritation	Risk for CO_2 rebreathing
Difficult seeing	Difficult speaking	Less stable airway pressure
Difficult speaking	Ophthalmopathies	Axillae or neck skin lesions
Neither eating nor drinking	Expensive	Longer time for application
		Difficult humidification
		Expensive

ventricular afterload, it demonstrates the power to reduce mortality and rate of TI versus SO_2T.

In 2008, a famous randomized controlled clinical trial (RCCT), which confirmed how NIMV can induce a quicker improvement in respiratory distress and metabolic disturbances versus SO_2T, raised uncertainty about the ability of NIMV to reduce the rate of TI and mortality [9]. The paper was widely and harshly criticized for its methods and the structure of the study protocol [10, 11], but, even today, its consequences, when defining the grade of recommendation for NIMV in ACPE, endure [2].

In the field of NIMV, there is no recommendation to date that favors NCPAP over noninvasive double-level positive pressure ventilation (NPPV) for treating ACPE, even though the published data are slightly stronger for NCPAP [8]. Because it is easier and cheaper, NCPAP is considered by many authors as the first-line treatment in ACPE. Moreover, the presence of hypercapnia during an episode of ARF due to ACPE does not represent an indication to prefer NPPV over NCPAP; they are comparable in efficacy, even in this subgroup of cases. This confirms (and is a consequence of the fact) that hypercarbia, in the context of ACPE, is not mainly due to pump failure but has a multidimensional pathophysiological explanation [12].

Table 14.3 Most common complications due to NCPAP interfaces

Leaks
Pressure sores and ulcers
Discomfort
Soft skin tissue damage
Claustrophobia
Aspiration
Mucous plugging
Conjunctivitis
Keratitis
Eye irritation
Oral and nasal dryness
Nasal congestion
Vomiting
Gastric distention
Aerophagia
Difficult speaking
Difficult eating
Difficult hearing
Noise
Allergy

NCPAP has demonstrated different, lower levels of evidence versus SO_2T in the early treatment of other different causes of AHRF in the acute care setting. The pathophysiological background for NCPAP in these conditions is, most likely, one of the following reasons:

- To reduce atelectasis
- To regain and recover ("recruit") flooded alveoli to ventilation (to open and keep open)
- To increase compliance and FRC
- To decrease WB
- To unload respiratory muscles
- To increase tidal volume
- To decrease VPM
- To improve oxygenation and correct gas exchange abnormalities

Many promising experiences have been reported in the literature regarding NCPAP for the treatment of AHRF resulting from blunt chest trauma, pneumonia (with or without chronic obstructive pulmonary disease (COPD)), peri- and postoperatively (for both prevention and treatment), mild acute respiratory distress syndrome (ARDS), pandemics, aspiration, pleural effusion, restrictive conditions, facilitation of weaning/extubation, and prevention of extubation failure [1, 3, 13, 14].

Acute asthma (AA) is worthy of special mention. Currently, in the field of chronic obstructive pulmonary diseases, AA is a peculiar entity and one of the most common reasons for NIMV application in EDs in the United States [15]. For AA, NCPAP showed positive results in early prevention of AHRF, and less strong data in the treatment of AHRF itself, even with a convincing pathophysiological background (Table 14.4).

NCPAP also has pathophysiological significance for ARF resulting from acute exacerbations of COPD, overcoming intrinsic PEEP and acting as a kind of mechanical bronchodilator, and reducing both dyspnea and WB. In this area, the efficacy of NPPV versus SO_2T, and also versus CPAP, is evident [16].

NCPAP is used to treat AHRF in chronic conditions such as OSAS [17] and CHF, and also in some carefully selected patients, often overlapping, with neuromuscular diseases, obesity hypoventilation syndrome, restrictive pulmonary diseases, thoracic cage deformities, partial upper airway obstruction, sleep disorders, idiopathic pulmonary fibrosis, and so on. In these chronic conditions, the purpose for NCPAP is to achieve physiologic benefits, palliate symptoms, improve quality of life, decrease pulmonary morbidity, reverse reversible superimposed conditions responsible for acute deterioration, prevent hospitalizations, and, in some cases, extend survival.

Regardless of the specific causes of AHRF, there is a high grade of recommendation for NIMV and NCPAP in immunocompromised patients [3]. This is mainly due to the high rate of infectious complications during IMV and its consequences in terms of hospital mortality. The subgroup of immunosuppressed patients features one of the most striking and strong indications for NIMV and NCPAP, in terms of efficacy and outcome, for the treatment of various forms of ARF [18, 19].

In summary, each unusual or off-label application of NCPAP for AHRF has lights and shadows, and, even in cases of promising preliminary results, remains controversial. Large, prospective, multicenter RCCTs are needed. Out of shared indications, NCPAP should be provided early, cautiously, safely and carefully, during the proper "window of opportunity," by an experienced team, in an appropriate setting (ICU or HMDU), with a quick access to facilities for TI and IMV [1, 3, 4].

Table 14.4 Pathophysiological rationale for NCPAP in AA

Increased bronchodilation (mechanically, equal pressure point, alveolar patency at end expiration), decreased airway resistance, re-expanded atelectasis (collateral reinflation), promoted removal of secretions, enhanced bronchial clearance, influencing medical treatment
Increased functional residual capacity, raised minimal pleural pressure, decreased swing in transdiaphragmatic pressure, decreased adverse hemodynamic effects
Reduction of respiratory muscles load, accessory recruitment and work: reduced transdiaphragmatic pressure, pressure time product for the inspiratory muscles and diaphragm, and fractional inspiratory time (endurance); reduction of elastic work (due to intrinsic PEEP); offset intrinsic PEEP and rest respiratory muscles;
Reduction of dyspnea, respiratory rate, pulse rate
Improvement in arterial blood gas exchanges, reduced inspiratory work (improved efficiency and decreased energy cost), increased FEV_1
Need of lower inspiratory pressures versus IMV
Reduced side effects and avoided complications versus TI, reduced need for sedation versus TI; decreased adverse hemodynamic effects of large negative peak and mean inspiratory pleural pressures; reduced need/frequency/duration of hospital admission

14.5 Indications and Contraindications, Criteria for Inclusion or Exclusion

A proper selection process to identify the right candidates to NCPAP for AHRF is the mainstay of the clinical management for critical cases. In the acute care setting characterized by AHRF, it is not easy to fix strict criteria for beginning NCPAP, particularly in the ED. The first decision is based exclusively on clinical grounds, when deeper diagnostic assessment is yet to be started, and only a little help from limited "point of care" imaging data or laboratory information is available. In this situation, the good candidate for NCPAP is the patient, suffering from severe acute respiratory distress, who we clinically consider will not be able to resolve AHRF by SO_2T and, at the same time, is not showing indications for TI and IMV.

In the early clinical decision phase, the first point to set, and the first question to answer, in an emergency situation is, is the patient really able to "spontaneously" breath and perform the needed amount of WB by him or herself, protecting his or her airways? The main indications to start NCPAP are listed in Table 14.5.

Special attention must be paid to cooperation and sensorium disturbances. Even though, in conditions such as ACPE, a neurologic status score such as a Kelly-Matthay grade 4 [20] can be considered a "relative" contraindication for NCPAP, in different situations (such as AA) any slight worsening in alertness should be considered, evaluated and treated as a "red flag" to move toward IMV. Contraindications for NCPAP are described in Table 14.6.

Many conditions previously considered as absolute contraindications have become relative contraindications or are no longer contraindications:

- NCPAP use after thoracic or major abdominal surgery (also facial, upper airway, or gastroesophageal tract) showed a good outcome both in preventing and treating ARF.
- New interfaces have overcome problems related to peculiar craniofacial shapes or skin damage such as burns or decubitus.
- The presence of a pneumothorax, if narrow or after drainage, does not adversely condition noninvasive treatment of blunt chest trauma.
- The use of light sedation or analgesia showed some benefit for reducing intolerance to the interface in properly selected cases.

In the recent past, when approaching ARF, the failure of a SO_2T "trial" was considered an indication for NIMV. Today, when identifying early indications for

Table 14.5 Criteria to start NCPAP in AHRF

Moderate to severe respiratory distress
RR >30 breaths per minute
Increased WB
Ventilatory accessory muscles recruited
Impaired sensorium
PaO_2/FiO_2 <200 mmHg

Table 14.6 Contraindications for NCPAP in AHRF

Cardiac arrest
Respiratory arrest
Gasping
Coma (Kelly-Matthay grade ≥4)
Multiorgan failure
Shock
Upper gastrointestinal bleeding
Respiratory fatigue
Ventilatory muscle pump exhaustion
Inability to protect the airway
High aspiration risk
Inability to clear secretions
Inability to fit the noninvasive interface
Swallowing impairment
Major tachyarrhythmias
Bradycardia < 50 pulse per minute
Systolic blood pressure <70 mmHg
Agitation, confusion, encephalopathy
Inability to cooperate
Seizures
pH <7.10

NCPAP, any delay in starting NIMV has to be considered as deleterious as a delay in TI and IMV [21] and, similarly, must be avoided. NIMV and NCPAP should no longer be considered as merely "alternatives" to IMV or SO_2T; NIMV has gained its own significant role with its own specific indications.

14.6 Predictors for Success or Failure

Once an indication to start NCPAP in a patient with AHRF has been assessed, it is necessary to perform an early risk stratification to identify cases that are likely to fail or succeed. This decision-making process has an impact on clinical outcome. It is necessary to recognize predictive signs of failure early, choosing the right setting for the right patient, primarily concerning monitoring, access and availability of TI and IMV, and also of NPPV, especially in off-label cases [4, 22]. The most significant predictors of outcome are listed in Tables 14.7 and 14.8.

14.7 New Perspectives and Future Development

Many promising improvements in NCPAP for AHRF are possible. RCCTs in the acute care setting are needed to define and enlighten efficacy in applications such as AA, mild ARDS, pneumonia, and blunt chest trauma. Studies of NCPAP are needed,

Table 14.7 NCPAP in AHRF: predictors for success

Preserved sensorium, better neurologic score
Airways protection
Good tolerance to the interface
Few air leaking
Low acuity of illness, low physiologic score
ACPO
Mild hypoxaemia
Mild pH abnormality
Few secretions
Younger age (<45 years old)
Intact dentition
Improvement in RR and ABG after 1 and 2 h

Table 14.8 NCPAP in AHRF: predictors of failure

Poor nutritional status
Multiple comorbidities
Diabetes
Obesity
Severe hypoxemia (PaO_2/FiO_2 <60 mmHg)
RR >38 breaths per minute
Sensorium disturbances (Kelly-Matthay grade ≥4)
Impaired mental status
Agitation
Uncooperative
Inability to correctly protect the airway
Inability to control the entire inhalation phase
Excessive secretions
Nasal breathing
Edentulism
Inability to fit the interface
Inability to tolerate the interface
High physiologic status
ARF "de novo"
ARDS
Clinical worsening
Worsening symptoms
New complications
Failure to improve RR, heart rate, blood pressure, ABG after 1 and 2 h

focusing on "special" cohorts of patients (more than specific diseases) with AHRF, patients with DNI (do-not-intubate) orders, and those for whom NCPAP can be considered a ceiling treatment or palliation, near the end of life, for symptomatic or ethical reasons, to treat acute and reversible causes of ARF and respiratory distress, with no impact on medium-term survival. RCCTs are not easy to carry out [23] in

Table 14.9 Criteria to stop NCPAP in case of success

RR <25 breaths per minute during NCPAP
SpO_2 >94 % during NCPAP with FiO_2 <40 %
PaO_2 >75 mmHg in SO_2T with FiO_2 <50 %

these cases (DNI most of all) [24], which are often managed in the ED without subsequent admission to ICUs [25].

New devices and systems for NCPAP need to be developed to ensure high flows, stable pressures, and known precise FiO_2, even in difficult settings such as OOH or during transport. It is not clear how to noninvasively set the proper pressure level from the start. We know that 7.5–10 cmH_2O is usually needed to offset atelectasis; it is also commonly accepted to set lower PEEP in COPD patients (to avoid undue expiratory resistances and subsequent air trapping) or in hypotensive or hypovolemic cases (due to the reduction in gradient of systemic venous return and then in right ventricular preload). In some other conditions (ARDS, restrictive disorders, etc.), a higher PEEP may be advisable. To date, arterial blood gas analysis (ABG) and hemodynamic parameters have been the mainstay of the decision-making process to set PEEP. Point of care ultrasound has shown promises in this field [26]. FiO_2 is usually set referring to a target SpO_2 (≥94 % in critical patients with AHRF, SpO_2 between 88 and 92 % in COPD cases) [27], but these criteria are not universally specifically validated for NIMV and NCPAP patients.

Even the best way to deliver inhalation therapy is under debate [28, 29]. Are nebulizers or pressurized metered dose inhalers better? And is it better to treat during NCPAP or during intervals? The use of NIMV for treating ARF, since the last decades, has grown continuously and spread outside the ICUs.

In the future for NCPAP, location, setting, environment, and welfare will be important topics in ARF patient care [1]. Adequate staffing, 24 h a day and 7 days a week, is mandatory. After pioneering trials, HMDUs and step-down units, mainly inside the ED, strictly linked to the emergency room, were shown to have every necessary characteristic to successfully deliver NIMV [12, 30]. Some general ward, OOH, and even long-term acute care facilities show promise in delivering NCPAP in AHRF [30]. Culture, education, training, technical and nontechnical skills, and enthusiasm always make the difference in terms of efficacy, efficiency, and outcome [4, 31, 32].

It is unlikely that shared criteria will be defined or that a consensus will be reached regarding strong recommendations, but studies are needed to try to standardize a "weaning" strategy from NCPAP to SO_2T, referring, for example, to ABG (improvement in pH and gas exchange), severity of respiratory distress, trends of RR and SpO_2, and so on (Table 14.9). Different hypotheses and trials have been described toward the discontinuance of NCPAP for AHRF. Some authors have suggested a gradational decrease of PEEP, others in FiO_2, and still others a reduction in time length of NCPAP, always with careful monitoring during intervals. At present, there is no consensus about the way to end NCPAP, and, even in the real-life world of emergency medicine, most frequently, the

Table 14.10 Criteria to stop NCPAP in case of failure

Inability to correctly protect the airway
Excessive secretions
Coma
Agitation
Sensorium worsening
Seizures
Hemodynamic instability
Electrocardiographic instability
Hypotension not responding in 1 h to fluid resuscitation
Inability to tolerate the interface
Inability to control leaks
Worsening (or inability to improve) dyspnea
Worsening (or inability to improve) respiratory distress
Signs of fatigue
PaO_2 <65 mmHg with FiO_2 ≥60 %

right time is often recognized by patients who independently decide to stop [1]. On the other hand, it is much clearer when to stop NCPAP in case of failure, switching to IMV (Table 14.10).

References

1. British Thoracic Society Standards of Care Committee. Non invasive ventilation in acute respiratory failure. Thorax. 2002;57:192–211.
2. Vital FM, Ladeira MT, Atallah AN. Non-invasive positive pressure ventilation (CPAP or bilevel NPPV) for cardiogenic pulmonary oedema. Cochrane Database Syst Rev. 2013;(5):CD005351.
3. Nava S, Hill N. Non-invasive ventilation in acute respiratory failure. Lancet. 2009;374:250–9.
4. Antonelli M, Conti G, Moro ML, et al. Predictors of failure of noninvasive positive pressure ventilation in patients with acute hypoxemic respiratory failure: a multi-centre study. Intensive Care Med. 2001;27:1718–28.
5. Nava S, Navalesi P, Conti G. Time of non-invasive ventilation. Intensive Care Med. 2006;32:361–70.
6. Mehta S, Hill NS. Noninvasive ventilation. Am J Respir Crit Care Med. 2001;163:540–77.
7. Carron M, Freo U, BaHammam AS, et al. Complications of non-invasive ventilation techniques: a comprehensive qualitative review of randomized trials. Br J Anaesth. 2013;110:896–914.
8. Masip J, Roque M, Sànchez B, et al. Noninvasive ventilation in acute cardiogenic pulmonary edema: systematic review and meta-analysis. JAMA. 2005;294:3124–30.
9. Gray A, Goodacre S, Newby DE, et al. Noninvasive ventilation in acute cardiogenic pulmonary edema. New Engl J Med. 2008;359:142–51.
10. McDermid RC, Bagshaw SM. Noninvasive ventilation in acute cardiogenic pulmonary edema. New Engl J Med. 2008;359:2068–9.
11. Masip J, Mebazaa A, Filippatos GS. Noninvasive ventilation in acute cardiogenic pulmonary edema. New Engl J Med. 2008;359:268–9.
12. Purro A. Questa o quella per me pari sono … due diverse scelte, stessa efficacia: CPAP vs NPPV nell'ACPE. Ital J Emerg Med. 2012;2:15–9 (article in Italian).

13. Ambrosino N, Vagheggini G. Noninvasive positive pressure ventilation in the acute care setting: where are we? Eur Respir J. 2008;31:874–86.
14. Ambrosino N, Guarracino F. Unusual applications of noninvasive ventilation. Eur Respir J. 2011;38:440–9.
15. Hess DR, Pang JM, Camargo JA. A survey of the use of noninvasive ventilation in academic emergency departments in the United States. Respir Care. 2009;54:1306–12.
16. Appendini L, Patessio A, Zanaboni S, et al. Physiologic effects of positive end-expiratory pressure and mask pressure support during exacerbations of chronic obstructive pulmonary disease. Am J Respir Crit Care Med. 1994;149:1069–76.
17. Basner RC. Continuous positive airway pressure for obstructive sleep apnea. New Engl J Med. 2007;356:1751–8.
18. Squadrone V, Massaia M, Bruno B, et al. Early CPAP prevents evolution of acute lung injury in patients with haematologic malignancy. Intensive Care Med. 2010;36:1666–74.
19. Bello G, De Pascale G, Antonelli M. Noninvasive ventilation for the immunocompromised patient: always appropriate? Curr Opin Crit Care. 2012;18:54–60.
20. Kelly BJ, Matthay MA. Prevalence and severity of neurologic dysfunction in critically ill patients. Influence on need for continued mechanical ventilation. Chest. 1993;104:1818–24.
21. Cabrini L, Landoni G, Oriani A, et al. Noninvasive ventilation and survival in acute care settings: a comprehensive systematic review and meta analysis of randomized controlled trials. Crit Care Med. 2015;43:880–8.
22. Hess DR. Noninvasive ventilation for acute respiratory failure. Respir Care. 2013;58:950–72.
23. Nava S, Ferrer M, Esquinas A, et al. Palliative use of non-invasive ventilation in end-of-life patients with solid tumours: a randomised feasibility trial. Lancet Oncol. 2013;14:219–27.
24. Curtis JR, et al. Noninvasive positive pressure ventilation in critical and palliative care settings: Understanding the goals of therapy. Crit Care Med. 2007;35:932–9.
25. Antro C, Merico F, Urbino R, et al. Non-invasive ventilation as a first-line treatment for acute respiratory failure: "real life" experience in the emergency department. Emerg Med J. 2005;22:772–7.
26. Bouhemad B, Brisson H, Le-Guen M, et al. Bedside ultrasound assessment of positive end-expiratory pressure–induced lung recruitment. Am J Respir Crit Care Med. 2011;183:341–7.
27. O'Driscoll BR, Howard LS, Davison AG, et al. BTS guideline for emergency oxygen use in adult patients. Thorax. 2008;63 Suppl 6:vi1–68.
28. Parkes SN, Bersten AD. Aerosol kinetics and bronchodilator efficacy during continuous positive airway pressure delivered by face mask. Thorax. 1997;52:171–5.
29. Dhand R, Tobin M. Inhaled bronchodilator therapy in mechanically ventilated patients. Am J Respir Crit Care Med. 1997;156:3–10.
30. Hill NS. Where should noninvasive ventilation be delivered? Respir Care. 2009;54:62–70.
31. Elliott MV, Confalonieri M, Nava S. Where to perform noninvasive ventilation? Eur Respir J. 2002;19:1159–66.
32. Liesching T, Kwok H, Hill NS. Acute application of noninvasive positive pressure ventilation. Chest. 2003;124:699–713.

Noninvasive Neurally Adjusted Ventilatory Assist (NIV-NAVA) in Children and Adults

15

Jennifer Beck, Yun Liu, and Christer Sinderby

Contents

J. Beck, PhD (✉)
Department of Pediatrics, University of Toronto, Toronto, ON, Canada

Keenan Research Centre for Biomedical Science, St. Michael's Hospital, Toronto, ON, Canada
e-mail: jennifer.beck@rogers.com

Y. Liu, MD
Department of Critical Care Medicine, Jiangsu Province Hospital, Nanjing Medical University, Nanjing, Jiangsu Province, China
e-mail: lyjz.2007@163.com

C. Sinderby, PhD
Keenan Research Centre for Biomedical Science, St. Michael's Hospital, Toronto, ON, Canada

Department of Critical Care Medicine, St. Michael's Hospital, Toronto, ON, Canada
e-mail: sinderby@rogers.com

A.M. Esquinas (ed.), *Noninvasive Mechanical Ventilation: Theory, Equipment, and Clinical Applications*, DOI 10.1007/978-3-319-21653-9_15

Abbreviations

Edi	Electrical activity of the diaphragm
FRC	Functional residual capacity
NAVA	Neurally Adjusted Ventilatory Assist
NIV-NAVA	Noninvasive Neurally Adjusted Ventilatory Assist
PEEP	Positive end-expiratory pressure

15.1 Introduction

Neurally Adjusted Ventilatory Assist (NAVA) is a mode of ventilation controlled by the electrical activity of the diaphragm (Edi) and can be delivered invasively (NAVA) or noninvasively with different interfaces (NIV-NAVA). NAVA was US Food and Drug Administration approved and has been commercially available since 2007. More than 28 peer-reviewed studies in adults and infants ($n=376$ patients) have demonstrated unequivocally that, compared with conventional (pneumatically controlled) modes of ventilation, patient-ventilator interaction – both in terms of timing and proportionality – is much improved with NAVA and NIV-NAVA. For those studies ($n=261$ patients) reporting an Asynchrony Index (AI), NAVA has a significantly lower AI (4.7 %) compared with pneumatically controlled mechanical ventilation (25.6 %).

The improvement in synchrony observed with NAVA and NIV-NAVA is achieved by the use of a neural signal (the Edi), which is independent of pneumatics for the purpose of controlling the ventilator. Often neglected, but equally important in the evaluation of respiratory effort and respiratory metrics, is the additional benefit of using the Edi signal as a monitoring tool. The Edi signal represents the final output of the respiratory centers, after receiving multiple afferent inputs about lung stretch, diaphragm force, arterial blood gases, and voluntary influences (Fig. 15.1). Furthermore, the natural coordination of the upper airway (dilator) muscles with the neural activation of the diaphragm allows efficient delivery of assist during NIV-NAVA, without opposition from the upper airway constrictor muscles. The interested reader is referred to several detailed descriptions about NAVA, NIV-NAVA, and the Edi signal [1–3]. This chapter provides an update of the clinical and experimental findings of the use of NIV-NAVA since the 2013 Minerva publication [2].

15.2 Discussion and Analysis of NIV-NAVA

15.2.1 Equipment and Theory

The most important feature when using NIV-NAVA pertains to the Edi catheter (a routinely used naso- or orogastric feeding tube with miniaturized sensors embedded to record Edi), available in sizes suitable for adults and children (Fig. 15.2). The

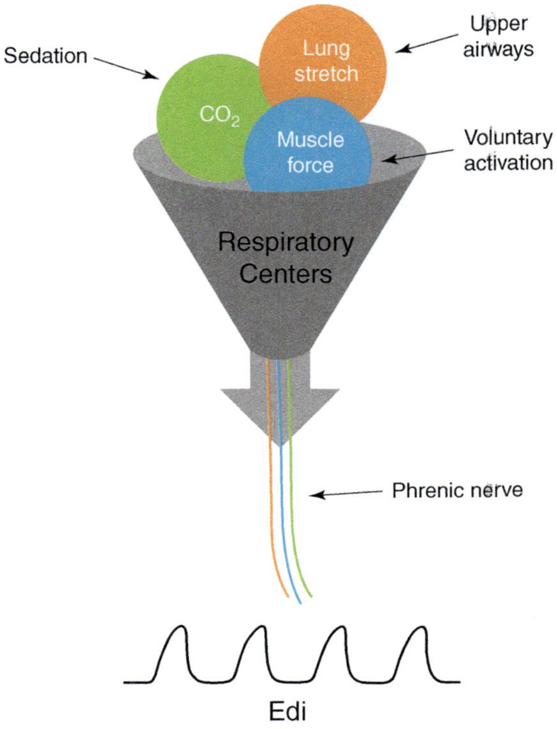

Fig. 15.1 Multiple afferent signals continuously meet and integrate in the respiratory centers. The electrical activity of the diaphragm (Edi) is the final neural output from the respiratory centers (efferent stimulation of the diaphragm) but contains the afferent information about lung stretch, $PaCO_2$, and muscle force

Edi catheter is connected to a SERVO-i or SERVO-U or SERVO-n ventilator (Maquet Critical Care, AB, Solna, Sweden). The catheter is well tolerated and easy to place, as described in the literature. During NIV-NAVA, any interface can be used (e.g., face mask, helmet, nasal prongs) with maintained synchrony, because the control of the ventilator is not affected by leaks.

15.2.2 Ventilator Control

To initiate a ventilator breath, the Edi signal triggers inspiration once a threshold change in Edi has been exceeded. The pressure delivered after triggering increases during inspiration in proportion to the Edi, until neural exhalation begins, and the ventilator cycles off (70 % of the peak Edi). The NIV-NAVA level determines the proportionality between the Edi and the ventilator pressure. After cycling off, the assist returns to a user-defined positive end-expiratory pressure (PEEP) level. In this fashion, the patient is in control of their own ventilator rate and level of assist, which can vary on a breath-by-breath basis. Figure 15.3 demonstrates Edi and ventilator pressure tracings for an infant patient breathing on NIV-NAVA, and demonstrates the synchrony between the Edi (patient) and airway pressure (ventilator), both in terms of timing and proportionality. As in any another mode of mechanical

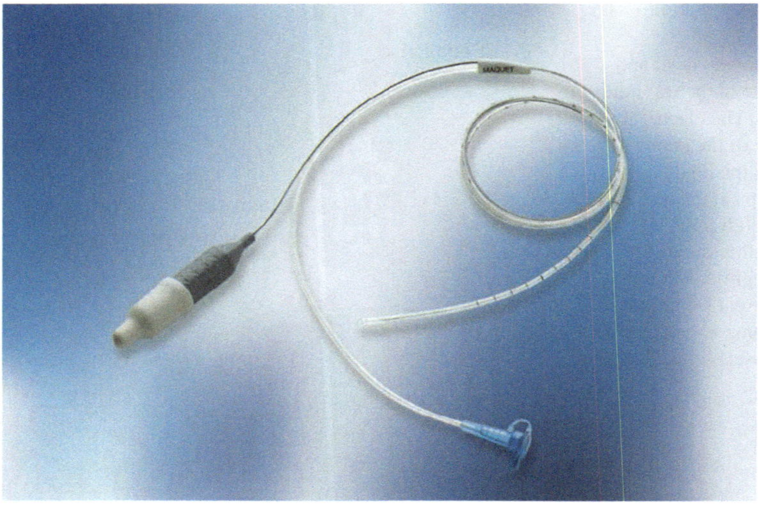

Fig. 15.2 Example of an Edi catheter (8 F size shown), used for feeding and measuring of diaphragm electrical activity (Maquet, Solna, Sweden)

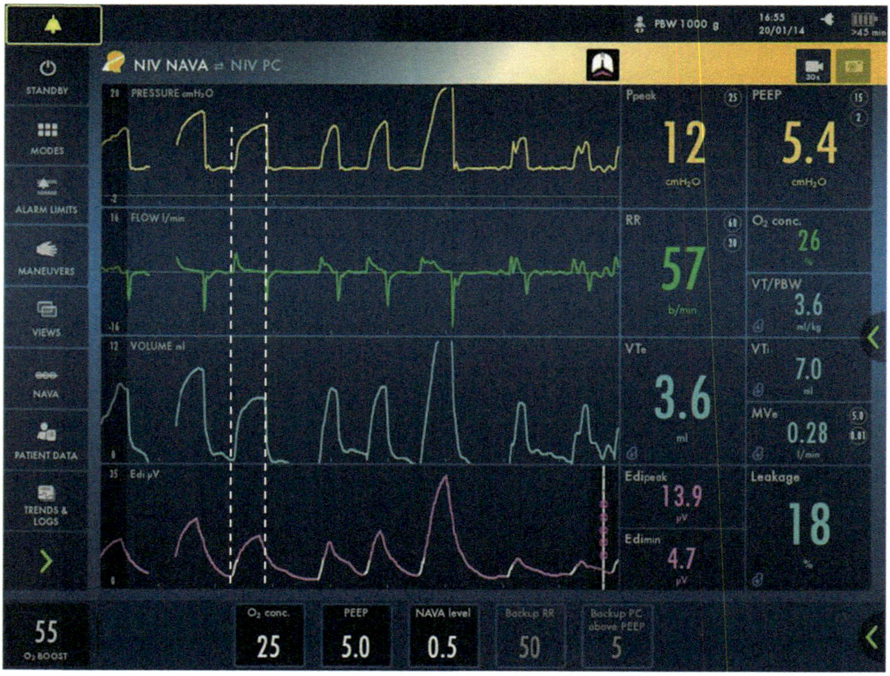

Fig. 15.3 Example of time tracings for ventilator pressure (*top*, *yellow*), flow (*green*), volume (*blue*), and Edi (*bottom*, *magenta*). Note the synchrony and proportionality between Edi and ventilator pressure, despite a leak (18 %)

ventilation, upper pressure limits can be set. Backup ventilation is provided in the case of apnea or accidental catheter removal.

15.2.3 Neural Integration with Respiratory Reflexes

The neural drive to breathe during NIV-NAVA is controlled by multiple afferent inputs originating in the lungs (stretch receptors), the central and peripheral chemoreceptors (CO_2 and pH sensitive), the respiratory muscles (muscle tension receptors), and the upper airway muscles (chemical and pressure receptors). Depending on clinical practice, a further influence on respiratory drive is sedation and analgesia. These multiple afferent inputs are continuously being "centralized" and "integrated" in the respiratory centers of the brainstem, with the resultant package of respiratory-related information being sent out via the phrenic nerves to electrically activate the diaphragm (i.e., the Edi) and other respiratory muscles (Fig. 15.1). Therefore, the physiological responses driving the patient's diaphragm are also simultaneously driving the ventilator throughout each breath during NIV-NAVA.

15.2.4 Recent Publications About NIV-NAVA

A total of 21 papers appear on PUBMED with the topic of NIV-NAVA since its release in 2008. Since the update in Minerva in 2013 [3], five clinical NIV-NAVA studies and one experimental study have been published [4–9]. Three of these articles were accompanied by editorials [10–12].

In 12 adult patients with COPD, Doorduin et al. [4] performed automated patient-ventilator interaction analysis during NIV-pressure support ventilation (PSV) (delivered with two separate ventilators, Maquet's SERVO-i and Respironics' Vision) and NIV-NAVA. Synchrony was superior (the Neurosync index was low, 5 %) during NIV-NAVA compared with NIV-PSV (24 % Vision, 21 % SERVO-i). The improvement in synchrony was mainly due to reduced triggering and cycling-off delays. The authors also found that there was a progressive number of wasted efforts as the triggering and cycling-off delays got worse.

In pediatrics, three studies have all shown feasibility and tolerance of NIV-NAVA, as well as insertion of the Edi catheter [5–8].

Vignaux et al. [5] demonstrated in six children (interquartile range 5–27 months) requiring NIV for respiratory failure after surgery, that NIV-NAVA improved patient-ventilator interaction (asynchrony index 2.3 %) compared to NIV-PSV (asynchrony index 40 %), even with optimization of expiratory trigger setting in PSV with Edi feedback. The improvement in synchrony was mainly due to reduced trigger delays and a reduction in ineffective efforts.

In younger children receiving NIV for respiratory support following cardiac surgery, Houtekie et al. [6] performed a cross-over study by randomizing babies (age range 1–22 weeks and weight <5 kg) to either nasal continuous positive airway pressure (CPAP) or NIV-NAVA immediately after extubation. The peak Edi values during NIV-NAVA were significantly lower, indicating more diaphragm unloading compared with nasal CPAP. Synchrony analysis was reported for NIV-NAVA and showed (despite average leakage of 70 %) 99 % neural triggering (compared with 95 % in the Vignaux et al. [5] study), with a low inspiratory trigger delay.

More recently, in another physiological cross-over study, NIV-NAVA was compared with conventional NIV in 13 children admitted to the pediatric intensive care unit for respiratory failure (interquartile age range 2–109 months), 8 of whom had pneumonia or bronchiolitis [7]. The authors found that during conventional NIV, patients spent between 27 and 32 % of the time in asynchrony, whereas it was only 8 % of the time in NIV-NAVA. This was mainly a result of reduced trigger delay, cycling-off delay, and ineffective efforts. These same authors also described the clinical importance of monitoring the Edi signal during all NIV modes after extubation in a recent review [13].

In 11 children with viral bronchiolitis who were failing nasal CPAP (aged on average 35 days), Baudin et al. [8] studied patient-ventilator interaction during nasal pressure assist control (settings determined clinically) versus NIV-NAVA (2 h each). With matching peak pressures in both modes, breath-by-breath analysis revealed a lower asynchrony index during NIV-NAVA, mainly due to less trigger delays. Ineffective efforts were extremely prevalent during nasal pressure assist control (~22 events per minute), and did not occur during NIV-NAVA. The number of auto-triggering events was higher in assist control (8 per minute) compared with NIV-NAVA. The neural respiratory rate and ventilator rate were comparable for NIV-NAVA; however, in pressure assist control, neural respiratory rate was higher than the ventilator rate.

In animals with early experimental injury, Mirabella et al. [9] examined lung injury markers after 6 h of volume control ventilation with a lung protective strategy (6 ml/kg with PEEP), compared with 6 h of NIV-NAVA and spontaneous breathing and no PEEP, and found a lower lung injury score and plasma interleukin (IL)-8 for the NIV-NAVA group. Interestingly, despite no PEEP being applied during NIV-NAVA, the upper airways were able to aid in the maintenance of functional residual capacity (FRC).

Conclusion

NAVA is a promising technique for NIV because it is able to provide synchronized and proportional assist, even in the presence of large leakage. In light of studies demonstrating the role of asynchrony on intensive care unit length of stay, duration of mechanical ventilation, and mortality [14], it would seem that improving synchrony should be a priority. NIV-NAVA allows the patient the freedom to choose their own breathing pattern, and to recruit the lung when needed with large inspirations (sighs) or maintenance of FRC with tonic activation of the diaphragm. The upper airway dilator muscles are coordinated with the onset of diaphragm activation, and therefore, the risk of gastric insufflation may be reduced with NIV-NAVA. We acknowledge that, in the presence of large leaks, pressure delivery may be underestimated, and it is possible that the NAVA level should be increased to compensate. The Edi signal offers the tool for this evaluation, as increasing the NAVA level – if resulting in unloading of the diaphragm – could be monitored. In addition, if respiratory rate is an important clinical metric, the neural frequency (which is unaffected by leaks) offers a reliable measurement, restoring confidence in decision support.

Key Major Recommendations

- Use NIV-NAVA to improve synchrony.
- Use Edi during NIV to obtain a reliable measure of neural respiratory drive.
- Use Edi during NIV to obtain a reliable measure of respiratory rate.

Disclosure Drs. Beck and Sinderby have made inventions related to neural control of mechanical ventilation that are patented. The patents are assigned to the academic institution(s) where the inventions were made. The license for these patents belongs to Maquet Critical Care. Future commercial uses of this technology may provide financial benefit to Drs. Beck and Sinderby through royalties. Dr. Beck and Dr. Sinderby each own 50 % of Neurovent Research Inc. (NVR). NVR is a research and development company that builds the equipment and catheters for research studies. NVR has a consulting agreement with Maquet Critical Care.

References

1. Sinderby C, Beck J. Neurally adjusted ventilatory assist. In: Tobin MJ, editor. Principles and practice of mechanical ventilation. 3rd ed. New York: McGraw Hill; 2012.
2. Sinderby C, Beck J. Neurally adjusted ventilatory assist in non-invasive ventilation. Minerva Anestesiol. 2013;79(8):915–25.
3. Oppersma E, Doorduin J, van der Heijden EH, et al. Noninvasive ventilation and the upper airway: should we pay more attention? Crit Care. 2013;17(6):245.
4. Doorduin J, Sinderby CA, Beck J, et al. Automated patient-ventilator interaction analysis during neurally adjusted non-invasive ventilation and pressure support ventilation in chronic obstructive pulmonary disease. Crit Care. 2014;18(5):550.
5. Vignaux L, Grazioli S, Piquilloud L, et al. Patient-ventilator asynchrony during noninvasive pressure support ventilation and neurally adjusted ventilatory assist in infants and children. Pediatr Crit Care Med. 2013;14(8):e357–64.
6. Houtekie L, Moerman D, Bourleau A, et al. Feasibility study on neurally adjusted ventilatory assist in noninvasive ventilation after cardiac surgery in infants. Respir Care. 2015;60(7):1007–14.
7. Ducharme-Crevier L, Beck J, Essouri S, et al. Neurally adjusted ventilatory assist (NAVA) allows patient-ventilator synchrony during pediatric noninvasive ventilation: a crossover physiological study. Crit Care. 2015;19:44.
8. Baudin F, Pouyau R, Cour-Andlauer F, et al. Neurally adjusted ventilator assist (NAVA) reduces asynchrony during non-invasive ventilation for severe bronchiolitis. Pediatr Pulmonol. 2014. doi:10.1002/ppul.23139.
9. Mirabella L, Grasselli G, Haitsma JJ, et al. Lung protection during non-invasive synchronized assist versus volume control in rabbits. Crit Care. 2014;18(1):R22.
10. Quintel M, Moerer O. Another brick in the wall of needs for invasive ventilation? Crit Care. 2014;18(2):122.
11. Ramet J, De Dooy J. Patient-ventilator asynchrony during noninvasive pressure support ventilation and neurally adjusted ventilatory assist in infants and children. Pediatr Crit Care Med. 2013;14(7):728–9.

12. Nava S, Pisani L. Neurally adjusted non-invasive ventilation in patients with chronic obstructive pulmonary disease: does patient-ventilator synchrony matter? Crit Care. 2014;18(6):670.
13. Ducharme-Crevier L, Du Pont-Thibodeau G, Emeriaud G. Interest of monitoring diaphragmatic electrical activity in the pediatric intensive care unit. Crit Care Res Pract. 2013;2013: 384210.
14. Blanch L, Villagra A, Sales B, et al. Asynchronies during mechanical ventilation are associated with mortality. Intensive Care Med. 2015;41(4):633–41.

Off-Cycling During NIV in Chronic Obstructive Pulmonary Disease: Clinical Implications

16

Lars-Olav Harnisch and Onnen Moerer

Contents

16.1 Introduction

Noninvasive mechanical ventilation (NIV) has evolved to be part of the current standard therapy for patients suffering from acute exacerbation of chronic obstructive pulmonary disease (aeCOPD) [1]. Using noninvasive ventilation in this condition helps to avoid the common complications of invasive ventilation, such as ventilator-associated pneumonia, and has been shown to substantially improve the course of the disease and decrease length of hospital stay [2].

Although NIV is widely used with great benefit in aeCOPD, there are patients for whom and situations where NIV does not provide satisfactory support or even adds further stress and increases the patient's work of breathing. A main cause is poor patient-ventilator interaction attributed to patient-ventilator asynchrony, which is reported to be common in NIV [3]. Additionally, the characteristics of the chosen

L.-O. Harnisch • O. Moerer (✉)
Department of Anesthesiology, Emergency- and Intensive Care Medicine, University of Goettingen Medical School, Robert-Koch-Str. 40, Goettingen 37099, Germany
e-mail: lars-olav.harnisch@med.uni-goettingen.de; omoerer@med.uni-goettingen.de

A.M. Esquinas (ed.), *Noninvasive Mechanical Ventilation: Theory, Equipment, and Clinical Applications*, DOI 10.1007/978-3-319-21653-9_16

interface, individual patient characteristics, and suboptimal ventilator settings have been found to be a major source of this asynchrony. During pressure support ventilation (PSV) - the ventilator mode of assisted mechanical ventilation mainly used for NIV at present - patient ventilator interaction is of major importance.

Delayed recognition of the patient's inspiratory effort (inspiratory trigger delay) by the ventilator at the beginning of the inspiration, and especially a prolonged inspiratory phase at the end of the patient's inspiratory phase (expiratory trigger delay or off-cycling delay), lead to considerable asynchrony between the patient's and the ventilator's inspiratory and expiratory phases. The transition from inspiration to expiration, known as ventilator (off-)cycling, occurs when inspiratory flow provided by the ventilator decreases to a predetermined fraction of peak inspiratory flow [4]. Prolonged pressurization by the machine into the patient's expiratory phase can lead to expiratory asynchrony and increased work of breathing [2].

Ideally, cycling should coincide with the end of the patient's inspiratory effort and no delay or premature termination should be observed. However, clinically, untimely off-cycling is always present but can be small or large in value and, therefore, varies in relevance for the individual patient.

Delayed off-cycling is a crucial determinant for patient-ventilator synchrony and most likely occurs in the presence of COPD [4, 5] if a low and fixed value for expiratory triggering and off-cycling is used, as is the case with many mechanical ventilators. Adjusting the off-cycling criterion should improve patient-ventilator synchrony (Moerer O et al., unpublished data). To reduce asynchrony, fitting the ventilator well to the patient, lung mechanics in COPD, pressure and flow curves, ventilator performance, and patient-ventilator interaction have to be thoroughly understood.

16.2 Discussion and Analysis

16.2.1 Lung Mechanics in COPD

In comparison with respiration in a healthy person, COPD is characterized by a profound change in respiratory mechanics and respiratory muscle function [6]. The pathophysiological hallmark of COPD is an expiratory flow limitation. In flow-limited patients, expiratory time is often too short to allow lung volume to decline to its physiological functional residual capacity. Dynamic hyperinflation occurs in flow-limited patients when the inspired tidal volume increases and/or the expiratory time decreases, resulting in variable increases of end-expiratory lung volume. Acute exacerbations of COPD are marked by an abrupt increase in airway resistance, worsening expiratory flow limitation and consequently increasing end-expiratory lung volume. Because of the failure of the muscle pump, patients are not able to maintain a sufficient tidal volume and often adopt a rapid, shallow breathing pattern that further limits expiratory time [7].

Viewed from a pressure point of view, dynamic hyperinflation can be defined as intrinsic positive end-expiratory pressure ($PEEP_i$). The additional remaining volume in the lung increases airway pressure at the end of expiration. This pressure has to be overcome at the beginning of the next inspiration, which takes more work than without PEEPi because the compliance curve of the lung is sigmoid and more pressure is therefore needed to inflate the lung sufficiently.

16.2.2 Flow and Pressure Curves and Ventilator Performance

A normal breath starts with contractions of the diaphragm, creating a negative pressure in the respiration system that can be measured at mouth level. This value is known as $p_{0.1}$, and it is measured by a short inspiratory occlusion maneuver and depictures strength of inspiration force. In unassisted spontaneous breathing, inspiration goes on as long as there is a pressure difference between the pressures inside the lung and the surrounding atmosphere, that is, until they are equaled. At the end of inspiration, the diaphragm relaxes and expiration is said to happen passively, meaning that there is normally no active contraction of muscles involved. Nevertheless, there is an active recoil of stretched elastic structures such as thorax and lung tissue. In flow-limited patients, the active recoil of elastic structures often lacks force to overcome the increased airway resistance, and these patients additionally use muscles (intercostal and abdominal) that reduce the size of the thoracic cavity to increase expiration force. Because of the increased airway resistance, it takes longer for these patients to exhale their tidal volume, which can clinically be seen as a prolonged expiration time.

PSV is mainly used for NIV at present. In this ventilation mode, start and stop of the patient's inspiration are marked by pressure changes in the ventilation system (patient, ventilator, connecting tubes, etc.) detected by the ventilator. Modern ventilators use either a pressure or a flow trigger for cycling; in some machines, the trigger can be chosen.

If a pressure trigger is used, the ventilator measures $p_{0.1}$ directly and cycles when a certain (preset) value appears. In flow triggering, the ventilator tries to hold the pressure in the ventilation system steady. When the patient initiates inspiration, a flow directed away from the ventilator occurs that is measured as pressure drop within the ventilator or deflection of a membrane in the breathing stream. This is what causes the ventilator to cycle when, again, a preset value is reached. Knowing this, a pressure curve of noninvasive ventilation can be viewed as follows: Starting at PEEP-level, first a pressure drop appears. When the ventilator starts pressure support, this pressure drop is equaled to PEEP-level and then turned into a positive pressure with preset variables. This pressure will be held until the off-cycling criterion is reached; after this point, expiration is "allowed" by the ventilator. During expiration, airway pressure decreases back to PEEP-level with its own time constant. A flow curve of noninvasive ventilation might be described like this: From a constant (bias-) flow, flow increases up to a maximum (F_{MAX}) and decreases a little, but continuously, from that point on. This decreasing flow goes on up to the off-cycling criterion where flow is stopped, returns to bias flow, and expiration is therefore facilitated.

The majority of modern ventilators allow for an individual adjustment of off-cycling criteria. The main challenge is, by and large, the decision of when and how to sufficiently adjust this parameter.

16.2.3 Patient-Ventilator Interaction

The impaired lung mechanics in COPD and knowledge of ventilator performance and its limits are the basis for optimizing patient-ventilator interaction. Although the latter is usually the case with COPD patients, impaired off-cycling of the ventilator to herald the expiratory phase can either be too early or too late.

16.2.4 Premature Off-Cycling

Having set the off-cycling criterion to high values of about 60 and 70 % peak flow, double triggering can be observed regularly as a specificity of asynchrony. At these high off-cycling values, pressure support appears only for a short duration of time in the breathing cycle. In these cases, pressure support stops when the patient has not yet stopped the inspirational effort. As a consequence, problems occur when the ventilator is ready for on-cycling again while inspiration effort is still going on. In these cases, the ventilator misinterprets ongoing inspiration as another inspiration and will administer pressure support. This extra pressure support leads to overinflation of the lungs; it adds expiratory pressure load and, therefore, even more expirational work of breathing to the already impaired expirational flow, and, last but not least, $PEEP_i$ is increased. All of these are unfavorable effects. As a side note, these effects seem to be less frequent when using a ventilation helmet compared with a nose-and-mouth-ventilation mask because flow and pressure transmissions from patient to ventilator are somewhat impaired due to the internal volume of the helmet [8].

16.2.5 Delayed Off-Cycling

Setting the off-cycling criterion to very low values of about 10 and 20 %, nonsupported inspirational effort is likely to appear. With the ventilator "waiting" for flow to decrease to 10 % or even 20 % of peak inspiratory flow, pressure support often goes on into the next breathing cycle, and sometimes flow does not even reach these low flow values. In these cases, the ventilator still facilitates expiration while the patient already wants to have another inspiration. Therefore, obviously, no inspirational pressure support can be given and work of breathing or tidal hyperinflation increases for that breath. Again, these effects seem to be related to the ventilation device used. Nonsupported inspirational effort seems to be more likely to occur using a nose-and-mouth ventilation mask than using a ventilation helmet. Once again, impaired transmissions resulting from internal helmet volume seems to be liable.

Taking a stepwise approach to understanding the effects of adjustment of the off-cycling criterion, a mode result would most likely look like this: Setting the off-cycling criterion to low values about every second inspirational effort will not be supported by the ventilator. Raising the off-cycling criterion nonsupported inspirational effort will disappear, but the $PEEP_i$ measured by the ventilator will still be large. Raising off-cycling further, $PEEP_i$ will diminish further. Raising off-cycling further still, suddenly double triggering will be present in high off-cycling criteria. Because this model seems to be common in COPD, the off-cycling criterion that allows the best synchrony was found to be 50 % peak inspiratory flow on average (Moerer O et al., 2014, unpublished data) (Figs. 16.1 and 16.2). However, this value should not be set blindly. There are a large variety of influencing and biasing factors that have an impact on synchrony and asynchrony. As mentioned before, the connecting ventilation device has its specific characteristic influence, but there are other factors such as respiration frequency, height of pressure support, and, of course, the ventilator itself with its specific mechanical and software characteristics. The prime influencing factor, however, is the patient him or herself. Lung mechanics such as compliance, resistance, mucus production, and airway smooth muscle tone, just to mention a few, change on a breath-to-breath basis, throughout an exacerbation and throughout the course of the disease as a whole. This makes it pretty clear that no single off-cycling criterion can be recommended generally. Rather, finding the perfect off-cycling criterion for the aeCOPD patient is an ongoing trial-and-error bedside process that needs to be reviewed and adjusted over and over again, throughout the day if needed, that is, when asynchrony is present.

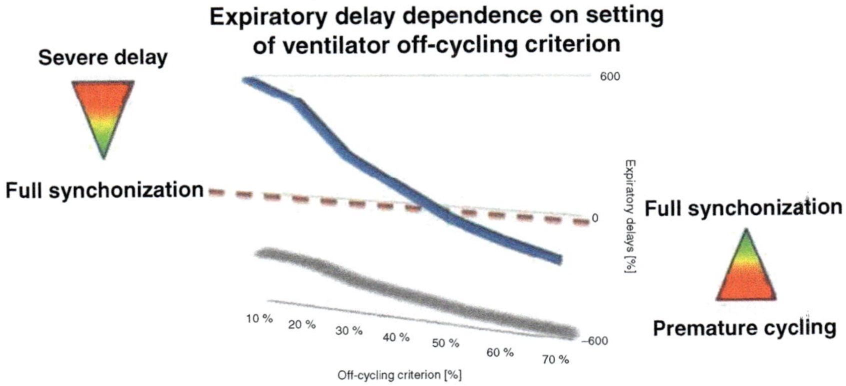

Fig. 16.1 Influence of ventilator off-cycling on patient-ventilator synchronization in COPD. Symbolized presentation of the findings from several studies and data from the authors' own investigations [3, 4] (Moerer O et al., 2014, unpublished)

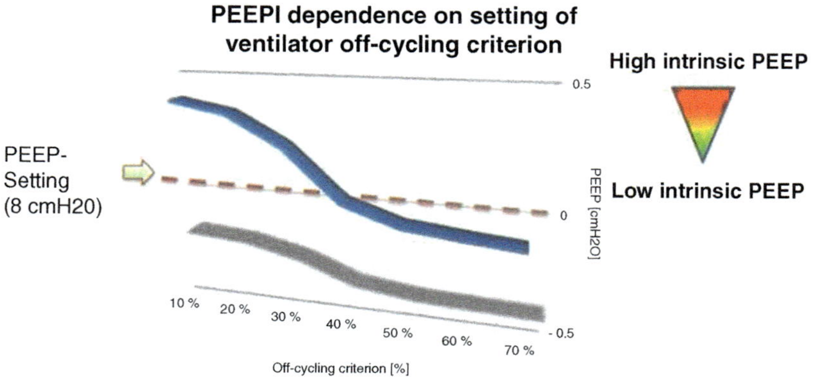

Fig. 16.2 Influence of set ventilator off-cycling on the development of intrinsic $PEEP_i$ (symbolized presentation of the findings from several studies and data from the authors' own investigations [4, 5] (Moerer O et al., 2014, unpublished). Obviously, the lowest $PEEP_i$ values appear at an off-cycling criterion of 40–50 %. Negative values are very small and therefore negligible; they are due to the inability of many ventilators to maintain PEEP in the face of leakage. Because the default value in ventilators is often 25 % peak flow, this setting needs to be adjusted in COPD patients

Conclusion

The off-cycling criterion needs to be adjusted very precisely, but there is not one single value that can be recommended. Nevertheless, some assistance can be granted as to how to find the optimal setting for the individual patient.

The existence of high $PEEP_i$, prolonged inspiratory plateau phase and mechanical inspiration time, an end-inspiratory increase in pressure, or nonsupported inspirational effort suggest a belated off-cycling. In their presence, off-cycling criteria should be raised as long as the measured values are not satisfactory or until nonsupported inspirational effort disappears. As an indicator of accuracy of the off-cycling criterion setting, the value may very well be larger than 30 % peak flow in COPD patients.

On the other hand, when double triggering or decreased tidal volume are present, which can be detected easily in clinical practice, they are likely to depicture premature off-cycling. Here, off-cycling criteria should be decreased until double triggering disappears and tidal volume increases to a maximum. Furthermore, curve-tracings can be easily done inasmuch as any ventilator displays the ventilation curves. In doing so, dissenting characteristics, such as convexity in an expiratory flow curve or concavity of an expiratory pressure curve, depicturing expiratory flow limitation may be found.

As has been said before, setting the off-cycling criterion cannot be done in a "drive-by" mode, but one has to take the time to assess the parameters and curves described to adjust the ventilator to the patient. Once the optimal setting has been found, one has to go over the process just described again and again to readjust the off-cycling criterion because lung mechanics as well as human afflictions are dynamic processes.

After all, to be honest, good patient-ventilator synchrony has not been shown to be of benefit. But bad synchrony has been shown to produce bad comfort for the patient [3], can be responsible for prolonged mechanical ventilation and NIV failure [9], and is clearly associated with increased morbidity and mortality [10]. Thus, finding the optimal setting regarding off-cycling seems not to be an auxiliary task but rather a *conditio sine qua non!*

Recommendations

- Reevaluation and adjustments of off-cycling criteria must not be viewed as auxiliary but rather mandatory, especially in patients suffering from COPD, and should be part of the daily routine.
- Detect patient-ventilator asynchrony by clinical events or tracing of flow- and pressure curves and values measured by the ventilator.
- *Raise* the off-cycling criterion as long as nonsupported inspiratory effort, prolonged inspiratory time, or high $PEEP_i$ persists.
- *Decrease* the off-cycling criterion as long as double triggering or low tidal volumes due to asynchrony persist.

References

1. Crimi C, Noto A, Princi P, et al. A European survey of noninvasive ventilation practices. Eur Respir J. 2010;36:362–9.
2. Burns KE, Adhikari NK, Meade MO. A meta-analysis of noninvasive weaning to facilitate liberation from mechanical ventilation. Can J Anaesth. 2006;53:305–15.
3. Vignaux L, Vargas F, Roeseler J, et al. Patient-ventilator asynchrony during non-invasive ventilation for acute respiratory failure: a multicenter study. Intensive Care Med. 2009;35:840–6.
4. Gentile MA. Cycling of the mechanical ventilator breath. Respir Care. 2011;56:52–60.
5. Jubran A, Van de Graaff WB, Tobin MJ. Variability of patient-ventilator interaction with pressure support ventilation in patients with chronic obstructive pulmonary disease. Am J Respir Crit Care Med. 1995;152:129–36.
6. Bergmann N. Intrapulmonary gas trapping during mechanical ventilation at rapid frequencies. Anesthesiology. 1972;37:626–33.
7. O'Donnell DE, Parker CM. COPD exacerbations. 3: pathophysiology. Thorax. 2006;61:354–61.
8. Moerer O, Fischer S, Hartelt M, et al. Influence of two different interfaces for noninvasive ventilation compared to invasive ventilation on the mechanical properties and performance of a respiratory system: a lung model study. Chest. 2006;129:1424–31.
9. Thille AW, Rodriguez P, Cabello B, et al. Patient-ventilator asynchrony during assisted mechanical ventilation. Intensive Care Med. 2006;32:1515–22.
10. Chao DC, Scheinhorn DJ, Stearn-Hassenpflug M. Patient-ventilator trigger asynchrony in prolonged mechanical ventilation. Chest. 1997;112:1592–9.

Part II

Monitoring Respiratory Care, Phisiotherapy and Rehabilitation

17 Monitoring Patients During Noninvasive Ventilation: The Clinical Point of View

G. Caironi, G. Gadda, R. Rossi, and Andrea Bellone

Contents

G. Caironi, RN
Emergency Department, A.O. Sant'Anna (Presidio di Como), Como 22100, Italy
e-mail: caironiguido@gmail.com

G. Gadda, LN
Emergency Unit, A.O. Guido Salvini (Presidio di Rho), Como 22100, Italy
e-mail: gadda.giorgio@gmail.com

R. Rossi, LN
Emergency Unit, A.O. Sant'Anna (Presidio di Cantù), Como 22100, Italy
e-mail: roberto.rossi73@hsacomo.org

A. Bellone, MD (✉)
Emergency Department, UOC di PS-OSA, Via Ravona 1, San Fermo della Battaglia, Como 22100, Italy

Emergency Department, A.O. Sant'Anna (Presidio di Como), Como 22100, Italy
e-mail: andreabellone@libero.it

A.M. Esquinas (ed.), *Noninvasive Mechanical Ventilation: Theory, Equipment, and Clinical Applications*, DOI 10.1007/978-3-319-21653-9_17

17.1 Introduction

Noninvasive ventilation (NIV) has proved to be an excellent technique in selected critical patients with acute respiratory failure due to different causes. Careful patient selection is imperative for successful outcomes, and a number of predictors have been identified to maximize success on NIV [1, 2].

Equally important, however, is the monitoring, because only careful and continuous patient care may prematurely detect improvements or worsening of the clinical condition. Monitoring is the set of actions that confirms the correct choice of ventilation, analyzes the patient's condition, guides all adjustments of the ventilator settings, and assesses the patient-ventilator interaction. Monitoring includes five different levels: (1) information about the patient and positioning; (2) choice of interface and reduction of the main adverse effects (leaks, patient-ventilator missed interaction); (3) patient observation, assessment of vital signs, evaluation of clinical condition (state of consciousness, anxiety level, and characteristics of breathing); (4) evaluation of laboratory data (arterial blood gas); and (5) continuous checking of ventilation parameters on the basis of clinical response. The combination of these different aspects, integrated in a continuous development of events, comprises monitoring.

Finally, the objective is to assess the patient-ventilator interaction, making sure that the ventilator "has to adapt" to the patient, and not patient to ventilator, improving patient outcome. Clinical observations provide measures for objective progress evaluation and assessing the opportunity for weaning.

17.2 Discussion

17.2.1 Time: Start – Patient Positioning, Information, and First Care

Nurses must communicate care, composure, and competence, as dyspneic patients are distressed, often fearing the worst. Confident and professional care may ease the patient's distress, gaining cooperation and motivating the patient to adapt to NIV [3].

Generally, the sitting position is preferred by patients with respiratory distress. In case of an overweight patient with a protuberant abdomen, the semi-sitting or supine position for ventilating is sometimes preferable, if possible. Sitting upright with the head well supported, or in a more advanced position with upper body forward and elbows resting on a support, promotes better recruitment of respiratory muscles and better diaphragmatic excursion. The patient should be placed in stable, comfortable, and convenient position, using supports and pillows to maintain the correct position.

Assess the patient's consciousness level with the Glasgow Coma Scale or, better, the Kelly scale. Assess that the patient's airways are not obstructed and that patient is able to cough and expectorate. Examine the abdomen for distension, air swallowing, and nausea as possible immediate complications in NIV. These inspections must be ensured at the beginning and also throughout the entire ventilation treatment [4].

Before treatment begins, it is appropriate to provide information about and explain the purpose and potential benefits of NIV, obtaining verbal consent and screening the bed to protect patient privacy and dignity.

Encouraging patients to hold the mask to their face while the ventilator is on and asking them to breathe is a good way for begin. Patients can also be shown how to release the mask quickly so they feel they have some control over the system [3].

17.2.2 Time: First 15 Min – Selection and Management of Interface Device, Patient-Ventilator Interaction, and Reduction of Major Adverse Effects

17.2.2.1 Interface Device

Choice of interface is an important determinant of NIV success or failure and the goal is to maximize patient comfort, minimizing leaks and allowing patient-ventilator synchrony [5]. This chapter will not discuss whether it is preferable to use a facial mask or a helmet. Many studies show the effectiveness of both devices, identifying their advantages and disadvantages. A helmet ensures better tolerability but allows CO_2 rebreathing and potential patient asynchrony. Masks are sometimes poorly tolerated and may result in skin lesions.

Recently, preliminary data showed that an optimized setup for helmet bi-level positive airway pressure (PAP), which limits device compliance and ventilator circuit resistance as much as possible, might be highly effective in improving pressure support delivery and patient-ventilator interaction [7]. Simultaneously, it is widely accepted that a helmet is the best interface with a very high tolerability when prolonged and continuous assistance is needed, for instance, in an intensive care unit or during pre-hospital treatment. On the other hand, in the emergency department, where the ventilation time is short and patients are often older with high comorbidities, including chronic obstructive pulmonary disease (COPD), the best interface for delivering bi-level PAP seems to be the face mask. However, as for the comparison between continuous positive airway pressure (CPAP) and bi-level PAP modalities of NIV, the choice of ventilator interfaces should be based on factors such as staff experience, habit, and individual patient's choice [3, 4].

In choosing a mask, the appropriate mask size, the correct size of headgear, the presence of a mask cushion, and the size of the dead space (to minimize CO_2 rebreathing) are important [6]. A full face mask is recommended for the initial 24 h and is better for patients with COPD, who tend to mouth breathe [7].

It is important to have a different kind of interfaces available (helmet, oro-nasal mask, total face mask) with different sizes because a variety of interfaces for NIV can be used in the acute care setting. Prevention and monitoring of side effects related to interfaces and evaluation of patient tolerance are crucial to avoiding NIV failure as protocols shared by the whole team [3].

Table 17.1 Causes of leaks

Descriptor	% of nonadaptation
Face format	30.5
Discomfort	28.8
Air leaking	27.7
Claustrophobia	18.6
Uncooperative patient	10.1
Patient agitation	6.7
Other causes	

17.2.2.2 Leaks and Adjusting Interface Devices

The first step in monitoring is to observe and assess the leaks of air around the interface device. The primary cause of leaks is a poor fit between mask and skin caused by several factors (Table 17.1) [8]. Position the interface device comfortably, avoiding making it too tight. Keep the device adherent to the patient's face manually for some minutes, allowing the patient to become familiar with the chosen interface device. This procedure also allows checking to see whether the device choice is the correct shape and size and if it fits the patient's face. Then, the mask should be secured in place with straps and/or headgear and reassessed after few minutes.

There are many possible side effects and adverse events. If the mask causes discomfort, it is possible to check the fit, adjust the straps, or choose another mask type. Masks can cause erythema or nasal bridge ulceration and it is appropriate to apply artificial skin (hydrocolloid dressing) to prevent this. In prolonged treatment, nasal or oral dryness may occur and the recommendation is to use nasal saline/emollient. To prevent leaks, an oro-nasal mask is sometimes preferred or pressures can be reduced slightly. Check for air leaks into the eyes (which can lead to conjunctivitis), around the nose, and at the side of the interface.

High-performing ventilators show leaks through a numerical estimate expressed as a percentage and compensate for them. In the first 10–15 min of treatment, the percentage of acceptable leaks is not more than 20 %. A successful patient adaptation and a patient-ventilator interaction should then progress to a reduction in the percentage of leaks from the system.

The effectiveness of treatment is achieved by obtaining the right balance between high leaks and excessive intolerance of the interface device. Remember that when positive pressure (inspiratory positive airway pressure, or IPAP) reaches more than 20 cmH_2O, it may cause a marked increase in leaks.

17.2.2.3 Patient-Ventilator Interaction and Pressure-Flow Graph Interpretation

Especially in the first 10–15 min of ventilation, it is crucial to monitor the adaptation of the patient to the ventilator and whether the ventilator is really assisting with the patient's respiratory efforts. One hand should be positioned on the abdomen of the patient, feeling breaths and then comparing them with those reported in the graphs of flow and pressure (Fig. 17.1). Each inspiration by the patient should match

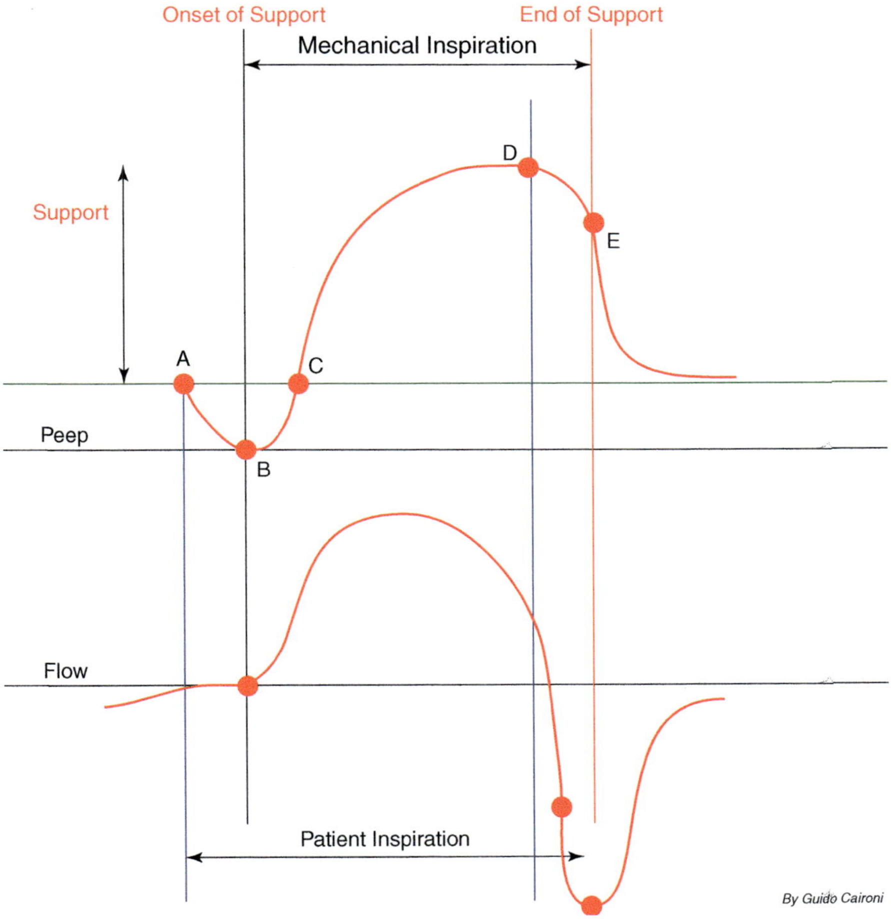

Fig. 17.1 Matching patient effort and ventilator assistance

the curve of respiratory support delivered by the ventilator and shown on the graph. The assessment of inspiratory function includes evaluation of synchronization between inspiratory effort and the onset of ventilation assistance and trigger sensitivity. Synchronization is evaluated by assessing the time lag between the onset of effort and the initial delivery of flow.

In Fig. 17.1, the interval A-B on the *x*-axis (time) represents the trigger delay, corresponding to trigger sensitivity. Inadequate matching between ventilator and patient could be to the result of a delay of ventilation assistance exceeding 360 ms [9] (too hard a trigger, inadequate circuit connections).

Ineffective efforts (muscle contractions not able to trigger the ventilator) are the most frequent problems in patients with obstruction and ventilated with high inspiratory pressures and high tidal volumes that avoid complete exhalation of the accumulated air. Therefore, the patient tries to start a new breath (Fig. 17.2, part a) when

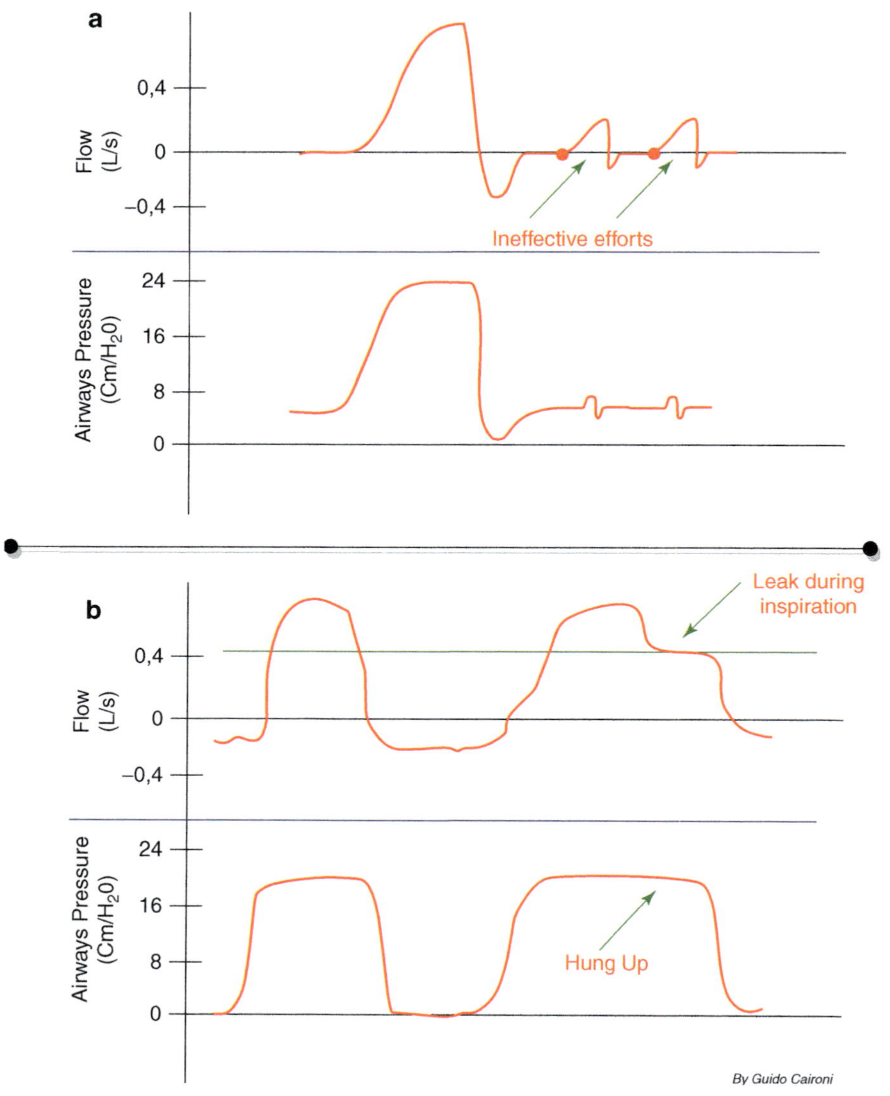

Fig. 17.2 Ineffective efforts (part **a**) and "hung up" phenomenon (part **b**)

the degree of hyperinflation is too high to allow him or her to return to the equilibrium point of the respiratory system and then to trigger the ventilator. The analysis of the parameters of flow and airway pressure shows a few small " bumps" that are not followed, or are contemporaneous, to an inspiratory support by the ventilator. The patient is unsuccessfully attempting to trigger the machine.

An assisted inspiration followed quickly by another one (or three, in "triple triggering") is another problem. It can be explained by setting a flow too high, or a too sensitive expiratory trigger, that requires a modest flow fall to switch from the inspiratory phase to the expiratory phase. Figure 17.2 part b shows a prolonged inspiratory act, and the graph of flow shows a fall, followed by a plateau; this is the "hung up" phenomenon. The patient does not appear to reach a predetermined dropping flow level to switch to the expiratory phase. The problem is usually caused by circuit or interface device leaks that interfere with the ventilator algorithm, increasing the inspiratory time over the maximum established [9]. If the patient is not able to adapt, it is appropriate to ensure that he or she is not muscularly exhausted, that there is no airway obstruction, and that the circuit does not suffer from leaks or disconnections.

17.2.3 Time: After the First 15 Min – Monitoring Vital Signs and Blood Gas Analysis

17.2.3.1 Vital Signs and Clinical Status

The patient treated with NIV should be located in a special area, with an available cohort of staff with adequate experience, equipped with a multi-parameter monitor and devices for emergency management. Primarily, and in the first minutes, it is necessary to assess the work of breathing through the observation of accessory muscle recruitment (such as sternocleidomastoid muscle activity) and respiratory rate. Lack of reduction in respiratory frequency indicates that alveolar ventilation is not obtained because of a wasted ventilation. Causes include inappropriate ventilation setting leading to patient intolerance, leaks, and missed coordination with the ventilator [3, 10].

Improvement in dyspnea is usually seen within 15 min to 1 or 2 h and is usually accompanied by an improvement of the neurological state [3]. Therefore, the evaluation of tidal volume is crucial, expecting a value of 8 ml/kg (better the *expiratory tidal volume*, shown by the ventilator monitor, because it is less influenced by leaks).

In the published papers about NIV ventilation, there are few data on oxygen saturation or transcutaneous CO_2. However, several studies have shown that oxygen levels improve early with NIV: SpO_2 monitoring is likely helpful, although does not replace the need for measurements of arterial blood gas tensions in the early stages of treatment. Oxygen saturation should be monitored continuously for at least 24 h after beginning NIV and supplementary oxygen administered to maintain saturation between 85 and 90 %. Transcutaneous CO_2 monitoring can also be used when it is available because it provides a more complete picture of alveolar ventilation as an integration of arterial blood gas analysis.

Monitoring of the vital signs must be done through a multi-parametric monitor, which is capable of showing the electrocardiographic trace, heart rate, and hemoglobin saturation. Our purpose is a standard protocol, with clinical observation and collection of vital signs at fixed times: every 15 min in the first hour; every 30 min in the next 3 h; then hourly for the next 8 h. Clinical observation should include comfort, mental status, verbal and nonverbal cues, airway patency, nasal congestion, dryness, gastric insufflation, conjunctiva irritations, inability to sleep and, importantly, patient-ventilator synchrony. Vital signs should include respiratory rate (observing chest-wall movement and use of accessory respiratory muscles), saturation, pulse rate, rhythm, blood pressure (noninvasive), evaluation of skin, and diuresis characteristics. Obviously, observation and collection of vital signs can be repeated as needed regardless of proposed standards.

17.2.3.2 Arterial Blood Gas Analysis

Arterial or arterialized capillary blood gas analysis of pH, $PaCO_2$, PaO_2, and relationship between PaO_2 and fraction of inspired oxygen (P/F) are important in the assessment of patients on NIV. Timing of arterial blood gas measurement will depend on the patient's condition, but we propose to consider fixed intervals (Table 17.2), and to carry out these measurements rather than relying on the duty doctor. During the first 24 h, the use of an indwelling arterial line should be considered to reduce patient's discomfort and pain [3, 4].

Frequency will depend on the patient's progress and the different etiologies of respiratory failure. Where the patient's condition is rapidly improved, blood samples should not be taken frequently as these patients are often sleep deprived and need to sleep and relax. When there is no improvement or it is very slow, assessments should be more frequent to guide ventilator setting or interface adjustments, or to consider invasive ventilation. We propose a standard, based on fixed times, for taking samples of arterial blood: after 30 min, then at 120 and 240 min.

It is important to realize that failure of improvement in arterial blood gas tensions is not a criterion for simply increasing the FiO_2 but for clinical re-evaluation. Any changes in oxygenation cannot be assessed in the absence of inspired oxygen concentration information; the metered flow rate and the mode of supplementation should always be clearly recorded.

Table 17.2 Vital signs and arterial blood gases monitoring

Hour	Time	Vital signs, comfort, and clinical observation	Arterial blood gas analysis
1	0	Yes	Yes
	15	Yes	Not routinely
	30	Yes	Yes
	45	Yes	Not routinely
	60	Yes	Yes
2	90	Yes	Not routinely
	120	Yes	Yes
3	150	Yes	Not routinely
	180	Yes	Not routinely
4	240	Yes	Yes
5	300	Yes	If necessary
Etc.	Etc.	–	–

17.2.3.3 Alarms

Alarms are based on flow, pressure, or volume. A low-pressure alarm detects disconnection or excessive leakage, but alarms based on flow are more informative and can warn of changing leakage, worsening airflow obstruction, or partially occluded tubing. By measuring flow and leaks, some ventilators compute tidal volume and, hence, minute volume, with greater monitoring potential with settings such as a larger or smaller tidal volume or low or too high respiratory rate. Alarms for a multi-parametric monitor should be set to warn about a too high heart rate or hypotension.

Conclusions

Patients undergoing NIV require a complex service and high-quality and global care. In many cases, the patient can be ventilated for 24 consecutive hours. Remember that breaks in NIV should be made for drugs, physiotherapy, and meals. It is important to ensure the most appropriate nursing care and the correct clinical and instrumental observation for these patients. Monitoring and continuous care are the key to success of the treatment and to guarantee a good outcome.

Here, we have divided the monitoring actions into sections: observing clinical conditions and care, control of laboratory tests, and examination of flow and pressure charts. However, monitoring is a set of coordinated and continuing actions, divided into distinct phases to make it easier.

Using a standard assessment as well as the one proposed here may help professionals in the management of these complex patients. It allows a rational use of resources, avoiding abuse of diagnostic procedures that are often painful and unnecessary for the patient. Finally, a high level of professionalism is expressed through continuous updating and training of the team caring for these patients, mainly in an emergency department.

Key Major Recommendation

- Give information to the patients about NIV and ensure the correct patient position and comfort.
- Select an interface device. If it is a mask (oro-nasal or total face), hold it in place for the first few minutes to help familiarize the patient with it, then secure with straps, checking for leaks.
- Set up the ventilator and use a multi-parametric monitor and pulse oximeter.
- Check the patient-ventilator interaction.
- Observe clinical status, arterial blood samples, and vital signs as indicated at fixed times or when needed.

References

1. Vital FMR, Ladeira MT, Atallah AN. Non-invasive positive pressure ventilation (CPAP or bilevel NPPV) for cardiogenic pulmonary edema. Cochrane Database Syst Rev. 2013;5:CD005351.
2. Hess DR. The evidence for noninvasive positive-pressure ventilation in the care of patients in acute respiratory failure: a systematic review of the literature. Respir Care. 2004;49(7):810–29.
3. BTS Standards of Care Committee. Non-invasive ventilation in acute respiratory failure. Thorax. 2002;57(3):192–211.
4. Keenan SP, et al. Clinical practice guidelines for the use of noninvasive positive-pressure ventilation and noninvasive continuous positive airway pressure in the acute care setting. Can Med Assoc J. 2011;183(3):195–214.
5. Nava S, Navalesi P, Gregoretti C. Interfaces humidification for noninvasive mechanical ventilation. Respir Care. 2009;54(1):71–84.
6. Mojoli F, Iotti GA, Currò I, et al. An optimized set-up for helmet noninvasive ventilation improves pressure support delivery and patient-ventilator interaction. Intensive Care Med. 2013;39:38–44.
7. Elliott MW. The interface: crucial for successful noninvasive ventilation. Eur Respir J. 2004;23:7–8.
8. Silva RMD, et al. Adaptation analysis of different noninvasive ventilation interfaces in critically ill patients. Crit Care. 2011;15 Suppl 2:1.
9. Nava S, Fanfulla F. Ventilazione meccanica non invasiva. Milan: Springer; 2010.
10. Hill NS. Noninvasive ventilation for chronic obstructive pulmonary disease. Respir Care. 2004;49(1):72–87.

Monitoring Accuracy of Home Mechanical Ventilators: Key Technical Elements and Clinical Implications

18

Manel Luján, Xavier Pomares, and Ana Sogo

Contents

Abbreviations

CPAP Continuous positive airway pressure
ICU Intensive care unit
IPAP Inspiratory positive airway pressure
NIV Noninvasive ventilation.

18.1 Introduction

The interest in monitoring home noninvasive ventilation (NIV) has increased in the last 10 years. In this setting, NIV manufacturers have introduced some improvements in their ventilators that allow the clinician to obtain information about

M. Luján, MD, PhD (✉) • X. Pomares, MD • A. Sogo, MD
Pneumology Service, Hospital de Sabadell Corporació Parc Taulí,
Universtat Autònoma de Barcelona, Sabadell, Spain
e-mail: mlujan@tauli.cat; jpomares@tauli.cat; asogo@hotmail.com

A.M. Esquinas (ed.), *Noninvasive Mechanical Ventilation: Theory, Equipment, and Clinical Applications*, DOI 10.1007/978-3-319-21653-9_18

patient-ventilator interactions during the use of the device. This information is sometimes available in real time, but also it can be downloaded from the internal memory of the ventilators and displayed, often breath to breath, by means of the pressure-time and flow-time graphics through specific software (the so-called *built-in software*). Then, in the daily practice, the clinician has, at least in theory, two devices (ventilator and monitor) in a single machine.

However, one of the main drawbacks of the "monitorization" of home mechanical ventilators is the important differences found in comparative bench studies in the estimated leak and delivered tidal volume values by built-in software of ventilators from different manufacturers (in pressure-limited modes) [1]. The differences in estimated delivered tidal volume ranged from −50 to + 450 ml when the ventilators were submitted to different levels of external controlled continuous leakage in a bench design with single limb and leak port. One of the consequences of these deviations is that a European expert committee in NIV (the Somno-NIV group), although recognizing some clinical value, attributed to the built-in software a low level of evidence in their recommendations for monitoring and titrating NIV home ventilators [2].

The main function of the built-in software should be to display accurately in the device screen the amount of gas entering into the patient's upper respiratory airway. This simple point, easy to understand, can certainly be complicated to apply in the practice, because the ventilator monitors the pressure and flow inside the device and there are several physical phenomena, for example, related to the controlled leak port or to the presence of unintentional leaks by a poorly fitted interface, that might occur between the ventilator's exit and the patient's upper respiratory airway. In this setting, the signal obtained inside the ventilator should be modified through mathematical algorithms, trying to reflect the true gas entering into the patient. In our opinion, one of the most important conclusions of the above-mentioned study that can explain their findings is that manufacturers apply different modifying algorithms of the native signal in their built-in software [1].

In this chapter, we review the basis for monitorization of NIV and how the external factors usually present in its clinical application can interfere with the reliability of this monitorization. Nearly all concepts are based on the findings in pressure-limited modes (the most used in clinical practice), but the conclusions can be also easily applied to volume-limited modes.

18.2 Discussion and Analysis

18.2.1 Morphology and Characteristic of the Native Graphics

The use of mechanical ventilators at home has resulted in a simplification, not only of the ventilators (smaller, portable) but also of the tubing used for delivering the gas into the patient's airway. The use of a double-limb system, however (as in intensive care units (ICUs) or anesthesia), can add a significant complication for the management at home, and systems with single limb are preferred for home

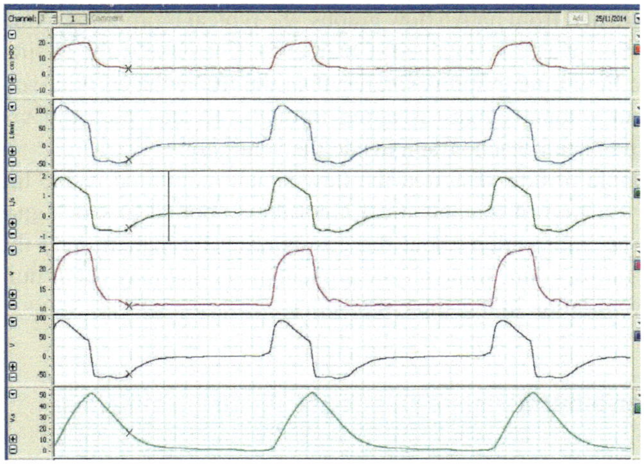

Fig. 18.1 Reproduction of the correction for the intentional estimated leaks in native flow-time graphics (see text for more details) in the laboratory with the help of a simulator. The abrupt "drop" in the uncorrected volume-time graphic (Channel 3) is related to the reset in the integral of the flow-time graphic (in the transition negative-positive of the flow-time graphic – Channel 2-). Usually, built-in software displaying volume-time graphics can present this drop in the presence of leaks

ventilation today. But the use of single-limb systems is also associated with the mandatory use of an alternative expiratory system (intentional leak port or active valve). In both systems, there are important differences in the flow and pressure graphics monitored inside the ventilator compared with those at the patient's airway.

From a generic point of view, it can be considered that the total gas exiting the ventilator should be considered as a sum of the gas entering the patient (tidal volume) plus the intentional (if a system with leak port and single limb is used) and unintentional (attributable to a suboptimal fitting of the mask) leaks. Finally, the compressible volume (CV) remaining in the limb(s) should also be considered (Eq. 18.1):

$$\text{Total gas Flow} = \text{VT} + V(\text{IL}) + V(\text{NIL}) + \text{CV} \tag{18.1}$$

where VT = tidal volume, V (IL) corresponds to the flow or volume exiting through the leak port, V (NIL) is the flow/volume of unintentional leaks, and CV is the compressible volume.

In the laboratory environment, and with the help of a simulator, the morphology of the native graphics can be reproduced, placing a pneumotachograph at the exit of the ventilator. For example, in a system with single limb and leak port, and without unintentional leaks, the morphology can be similar to that represented in Fig. 18.1.

In fact, the native flow-time graphic contains, in the inspiratory phase (Fig. 18.1, Channel 2) the amount of gas delivered to the patient plus the gas escaping through the valve (calculated from the pressure-leak equation in Channel 4). When the estimated leaks are subtracted from native flow graphs, the typical morphology with equal positive and negative phases is obtained (Channel 5). Conversely, the expiratory phase in the native flow-time graph is smaller than the true exhaled tidal volume because there is an amount of gas escaping through the leak port and not directly monitored by the pneumotachograph inside the ventilator.

This is only an example of how distorted the flow signal monitored inside the ventilator can be. The function of mathematical algorithms applied to this signal should be to provide true information about the gas entering the patient, and the algorithms should take into account some physical phenomena that may occur during noninvasive home ventilation in the clinical practice.

18.2.2 Physical Phenomena

18.2.2.1 The Expiratory System

Today, due to its simplicity, not only for the patient but also for caregivers, the single limb with an expiratory leak port embedded in the mask or as an independent piece between the mask and the tubing is probably the preferred configuration in home noninvasive ventilation. This expiratory leak port acts as a continuous leak, with a higher resistance than the tubing itself. The behavior of this continuous leak can be easily determined in the laboratory by means of the so-called "leak test": with the distal end of the mask or tubing occluded, the system is submitted to increasing pressure levels (e.g., in continuous positive airway pressure (CPAP) mode) and a pneumotachograph inside the ventilator captures only the flow leaks. Finally, the data are plotted on an *X-Y* graph and a second-degree equation can approximate with reasonable accuracy the amount of intentional leak for each level of pressure. These values can be subtracted from the native graphics to obtain the true gas flow entering and exiting from the patient.

This approach has two drawbacks, however. First, it is not always easy to perform a leak test when the port is built into the mask because the seal of the distal end might be incomplete. The second drawback appears in the presence of leaks. In this setting, and explained by Poiseuille's law regarding the flow of fluids, with a higher flow exiting from the ventilator, the pressure difference between the true monitoring point (inside the ventilator) and the expiratory leak port also increases. This phenomenon can lead to an overestimation of leaks and progressive underestimation of tidal volume at increasing leak values [3]. The latter phenomenon, however, can be overcome by the introduction of a correction factor based on the resistance of the tubing and following Poiseuille's law. This factor attempts to calculate the distal (in the leak port) pressure as a function of exiting flow, resistance, and proximal pressure values.

On the other hand, if an active valve is used, there are also some drawbacks associated with the monitoring. The most important is that, although there is not an intentional leakage during the inspiratory phase, the built-in software "misses" the signal corresponding to the expiratory phase because the expired gas is exhaled through the valve. In this setting, the only technical solution is to place a pneumotachograph between the valve and the interface.

18.2.2.2 The Unintentional Leak

Classically, the influence of the leaks in monitoring in the laboratory has been performed with models of continuous leakage. Even in a review focused on bench studies, leaks are "standardized" as holes of different diameter [4]. However, the behavior of leaks in clinical practice might not correspond to this pattern. In fact, a poorly fitted mask can generate leaks only during inspiration, or inversely, a patient wearing a nasal mask can theoretically exhale through the mouth. In both cases, the relationship of proportionality between inspiratory and expiratory phases of the respiratory cycle disappears.

For these reasons, the unintentional leak should be considered in a different way, with a "nonlinear "or "dynamic random" approach [5]. In fact, in one study, four home ventilators from different companies were tested in a bench environment in conditions of random or nonlinear leak. The results obtained in this study (overestimation of tidal volume in a model of inspiratory leaks and underestimation in expiratory leaks) reinforced the hypothesis that the approach of considering unintentional leaks as a linear parameter can lead to significant misestimation of tidal volume. In the same study, an algorithm based on the assumption of lack of proportionality between inspiratory and expiratory phases showed minimal deviations in the estimation of tidal volume and unintentional leaks.

But the drawbacks of this misestimation can go beyond wrong information for the clinician. It should be highlighted that, in some new modes of noninvasive ventilation (the dual-control or volume-targeted pressure support modes), the ventilator makes its own decisions based on target tidal volume estimation. If random leaks appear, as demonstrated in a recent study, the ventilator can modify its pressure support level in a different way than expected [6]. In this setting, it seems reasonable to recommend setting in the ventilator a safety lower level of pressure support.

18.2.2.3 The Compressible Volume

The compressible volume refers to the excess of volume contained in the tubing between both phases of the respiratory cycle. From a mathematical perspective, it can be quantified as follows:

$$\mathrm{VC} = \mathrm{PIP} - \mathrm{PEEP} / C$$

where VC is the compressible volume, PIP is the peak inspiratory pressure (in pressure support modes it can be considered as an equivalent of IPAP), and C is the compliance of the tubing (ml/cmH_2O/m).

Being that the compressible volume is a parameter directly related to the length of the tubing, it is easy to understand that, in the configuration with double tubing, the amount of compressible gas can be twice that in comparison with single tubing. In the same way, the use of extremely compliant tubing can increase the compressible volume.

The effects of compressible volume depend on the use of pressure- or volume-limited modes. In fact, if pressure-limited modes are used, the monitored tidal volume can be overestimated in the presence of compressible volume. When volume-limited modes are used, the delivered tidal volume can be less than that set in the ventilator. Under normal circumstances, the compressible volume is not higher than 10 % of the delivered gas, and many companies introduced in their ventilators a compensation factor for this phenomenon [7].

18.3 Conclusions and Clinical Implications

The built-in software for different ventilators shows important variability, suggesting that each manufacturer has its own algorithm in the management of native graphics. An effort should be made to standardize the treatment of pressure and flow native graphics, considering all the physical phenomena and clinical scenarios that may distort the native graphics.

Key Major Recommendations

- The clinician should consider that the graphics displayed by the built-in software of the ventilators are usually treated by mathematical algorithms.
- Manufacturers can use different algorithms to treat native graphics. This fact can explain some differences between the devices from different companies.
- Configuration of the limbs (single or double) and expiratory system (leak port, active valve) plays an important role in the monitoring of home ventilators.

References

1. Contal O, Vignaux L, Combescure C, Pepin JL, Jolliet P, Janssens JP. Monitoring of noninvasive ventilation by built-in software of home bi-level ventilators: a bench study. Chest. 2012;141:469–76.
2. Janssens JP, Borel JC, Pepin JL, SomnoNIV Group. Nocturnal monitoring of home noninvasive ventilation: the contribution of simple tools such as pulse oximetry, capnography, built-in ventilator software and autonomic markers of sleep fragmentation. Thorax. 2011;66:438–45.
3. Luján M, Sogo A, Pomares X, Monsó E, Sales B, Blanch L. Effect of leak and breathing pattern on the accuracy of tidal volume estimation. Respir Care. 2013;58(5):770–7.
4. Oliveri C, Costa R, Conti G, Navalesi P. Bench studies evaluating devices for non-invasive ventilation: critical analysis and future perspectives. Intensive Care Med. 2012;38:160–7.
5. Sogo A, Montanyà J, Monsó E, Blanch L, Pomares X, Lujàn M. Effect of dynamic random leaks on the monitoring accuracy of home mechanical ventilators: a bench study. BMC Pulm Med. 2013;13:75.
6. Luján M, Sogo A, Grimau C, Pomares X, Blanch L, Monsó E. Influence of dynamic leaks in volume-targeted pressure support noninvasive ventilation: a bench study. Respir Care. 2015;60(2):191–200.
7. Bachiller PR, McDonough JM, Feldman JM. Do new anesthesia ventilators deliver small tidal volumes accurately during volume-controlled ventilation? Anesth Analg. 2008;106:1392–400.

Capnography as a Tool to Improve Noninvasive Ventilation: Technical Key Topics and Clinical Implications

19

Eren Fatma Akcil, Ozlem Korkmaz Dilmen, and Yusuf Tunali

Contents

19.1 Introduction

Noninvasive ventilation (NIV) is a mechanical ventilation method frequently used in the treatment of acute and chronic respiratory failure. As it is a noninvasive method, it prevents complications related to intubation and invasive mechanical ventilation and thus decreases morbidity and mortality. The clinical conditions that benefit most from NIV are acute exacerbation of chronic obstructive pulmonary disease (COPD) and cardiogenic pulmonary edema. Its application in pneumonia and acute respiratory distress syndrome (ARDS) is limited; however, it is beneficial in thoracic trauma and postoperative mild hypoxic respiratory failure [1]. Monitoring of respiration during NIV enables the evaluation of its effectiveness and prevents delays in the initiation of invasive mechanical ventilation and also prevents complications. For this purpose, respiratory rate, pulse oximetry, arterial blood gas analysis (ABG), and capnography are frequently used. This section provides an overview of the importance and contributions of capnography in NIV.

E.F. Akcil, MD (✉) • O.K. Dilmen, MD • Y. Tunali, MD
Department of Anaesthesiology and Intensive Care Medicine,
Istanbul University Cerrahpasa School of Medicine, Istanbul, Turkey
e-mail: erenfat@yahoo.com; ozlemkorkmaz1978@mynet.com; ytunali@yahoo.com

A.M. Esquinas (ed.), *Noninvasive Mechanical Ventilation: Theory, Equipment, and Clinical Applications*, DOI 10.1007/978-3-319-21653-9_19

19.2 Discussion

Capnography was first used in the Central Military Hospital in Holland in 1962 by Professor Bob Smalhout. Since 1988, it has been used in operating rooms as a part of routine clinical practice. Accompanied by technological developments, capnography has been recommended in many practice fields for patient safety, not only in intubated patients, but also in nonintubated patients (Table 19.1) [2]. The primary goal of anesthesiologists is to prevent hypoxia, and capnography helps identify situations that can lead to hypoxia, such as disconnection of the circuit and hypoventilation. It also prevents undesirable results of hypoxia, among which irreversible brain damage is the most important. Because of these advantages, the utility of capnography has recently been extended outside the operating room to emergency rooms, endoscopic suites, X-ray rooms, and even on-site emergency and trauma fields.

Although there is an opportunity for end-tidal CO_2 ($etCO_2$) monitoring in nonintubated patients with the developing technology in mainstream and sidestream capnographies, false results can be obtained as a result of obstruction due to water and secretion. Microstream (MST) is a new method developed for CO_2 measurement, based on molecular correlation spectroscopy. In this method, a specific infrared radiation wavelength is used to detect CO_2, which is not affected by the other gases (i.e., O_2, N_2O, He, inhaled anesthetics). In the MST procedure, a low sample flow rate (50 ml/min) is adequate, which makes the procedure useful in different types of patients, such as neonates. MST can be used in intubated and nonintubated patients, and it is widely available for monitoring $etCO_2$ during NIV [3].

In nonintubated patients, capnography provides information about the respiratory rate, airway obstruction (bronchospasm), apnea, hypoventilation/hyperventilation, and dead space ventilation. During NIV, these features of capnography are employed. While capnography is used in the evaluation of the effectiveness of NIV on ventilation and CO_2 elimination, it also provides information about CO_2 rebreathing [4]. In the monitoring of end-tidal CO_2 pressure ($PetCO_2$) during NIV, the type and size of the mask, the sampling site, and the localization of the exhalation port are important. Nuccio et al. [4] applied continuous positive airway pressure (CPAP) and bi-level positive airway pressure (BIPAP) at two different pressure levels in three groups and obtained $etCO_2$ samples from three locations, including

Table 19.1 Recommendations for capnography

	OR	ICU	Recovery	Sedation	CPR	ED
NAP4	2011	2011	2011			2011
ASA	1987			2011		
AAGBI	1988	2009	2009	2009	2009	2009
Resusc. Council					2010	
ICS		2011				

NAP4 National Audit Project 4, *ASA* American Society of Anesthesiologists, *AAGBI* The Association of Anesthetists of Great Britain and Ireland, *Resusc. Council* Resuscitation Council, *ICS* Intensive Care Society, *OR* operating room, *ICU* intensive care unit, *CPR* cardiopulmonary resuscitation, *ED* emergency department

the nasal/oral cannula, mask sample port, and ventilator circuit connector. They found that the best measurement could be obtained with different minute ventilations and different amounts of leakage in nasal/oral cannula applications. It has been demonstrated that in sampling from the nasal/oral cannula, $etCO_2$ levels are not affected by the mask type but are correlated with baseline values in different ventilation parameters, and the wave form in the capnogram is not disturbed. Therefore, nasal/oral cannulas are preferred for $etCO_2$ monitoring in NIV.

CO_2 rebreathing in NIV is an important problem, as it decreases CO_2 elimination and increases work of breathing. Increasing positive end-expiratory pressure (PEEP) and CPAP levels and the addition of non rebreathing valves to the breathing circuits decrease rebreathing [5]. However, in NIV applications in which the exhalation port is located in the breathing circuit instead of the mask, and in which high volume masks are used, increasing PEEP and CPAP does not sufficiently decrease rebreathing. It has been demonstrated that the systems in which the exhalation port is present in the mask and in which low volume masks are used decrease rebreathing [6].

Another problem that influences capnography in NIV is leakage. In most of the ventilators used in NIV, there is leakage compensation, and a small amount of leakage is tolerated to prevent the firm placement of the mask on the face of the patients. Increasing this amount causes a disruption in ventilation, a decrease in CO_2 elimination, and a decrease in $etCO_2$ levels in capnography.

Conclusions

Capnography is essential for monitoring of the respiration system. MST is a new technique of capnography. NIV and MST are both noninvasive methods, and their synergy provides for the safe management of respiratory failure.

Key Recommendations

- Nasal/oral cannula should be the preferred tool for capnography during NIV.
- Leaks must be minimized for accurate measurement.
- More experience is required with MST and NIV.

References

1. Ferrer M, Torres A. Noninvasive ventilation for acute respiratory failure. Curr Opin Crit Care. 2015;21:1–6.
2. Whitaker DK. Time for capnography - everywhere. Anaesthesia. 2011;66:539–49.
3. www.capnography.com/new/technology/microstream. Bhavani-Shankar Kodali copyright©2013.
4. Nuccio P, Hochstetler G, Jackson M. End-tidal CO_2 measurements with noninvasive ventilation. Anesth Analg. 2007;105(S 6):111.
5. Lofaso F, Brochard L, Touchard D, et al. Evaluation of carbon dioxide rebreathing during pressure support ventilation with airway management system (BIPAP) devices. Chest. 1995;108:772–8.
6. Schettino G, Chatmongkolchart S, Hess D, et al. Position of exhalation port and mask design affect CO_2 rebreathing during noninvasive positive pressure ventilation. Crit Care Med. 2003; 31:2178–82.

20 Humidification for Noninvasive Ventilation: Key Technical Determinants and Clinical Evidence

Aylin Ugurlu Ozsancak and Antonio M. Esquinas

Contents

Abbreviations

AH	Absolute humidity
ARF	Acute respiratory failure
CPAP	Continuous positive airway pressure
FiO_2	Fractional inspired oxygen
HH	Heated humidifiers
HME	Heat-and-moisture exchangers
IMV	Invasive mechanical ventilation
IPAP	Inspiratory positive airway pressure

A.U. Ozsancak, MD (✉)
Department of Pulmonary Medicine, Baskent University Hospital, Istanbul, Turkey
e-mail: aozsancak@hotmail.com

A.M. Esquinas, MD, PhD, FCCP
Intensive Care and Non Invasive Ventilatory Unit, Hospital Morales Meseguer, Murcia, Spain
e-mail: antmesquinas@gmail.com

A.M. Esquinas (ed.), *Noninvasive Mechanical Ventilation: Theory, Equipment, and Clinical Applications*, DOI 10.1007/978-3-319-21653-9_20

NAWR	Nasal airway resistance
NIV	Noninvasive ventilation
SRBD	Sleep-related breathing disorders
WOB	Work of breathing

20.1 Introduction

During spontaneous breathing, inhaled air conditioning (i.e., heating and humidification of air) is provided by the upper airways. Artificial humidification is recommended when the upper airway is bypassed, such as during invasive mechanical ventilation (IMV), to prevent hypothermia, disruption of the airway epithelium, bronchospasm, atelectasis, and airway obstruction [1].

Noninvasive ventilation (NIV) has been increasingly used at hospitals for acute respiratory failure (ARF) [2]. It is also used at home for chronic respiratory failure and sleep-related breathing disorders (SRBD). Unfortunately, it might lead to complications, including nasal congestion and/or upper airway dryness (especially when there is air leakage), which might in turn result in intolerance or decrease in patient's compliance and subsequently in NIV failure. Gas conditioning can prevent these adverse effects. It can be either done actively by heated humidifiers (HH) or passively by heat-and-moisture exchangers (HME). Currently, active humidification by HH is suggested for NIV by the American Association of Respiratory Care, as it may improve adherence and comfort [1].

In this chapter, we summarize the effects of inefficient gas conditioning during NIV, factors worsening these effects, types of humidifiers and their properties, and current recommendations for humidification.

20.2 Discussion and Analysis

20.2.1 Effects of Inefficient Gas Conditioning During NIV and Contributing Factors

During normal breathing, the upper airway heats and humidifies inhaled air so that the gas entering the alveoli reaches body temperature and is fully saturated with water vapor [3]. The upper airway recovers added inspiratory heat and moisture partially during exhalation. During IMV, when the upper airway is bypassed by an endotracheal tube or tracheostomy, inadequately humidified dry gases were shown to cause changes of respiratory tract structure and function (including inflammation, necrosis, and squamous metaplasia), deterioration in lung function, and increase in tenacity of sputum leading to airway/endotracheal tube occlusion [4].

During NIV, the inspired gas is conditioned by the upper airways. However it can be overwhelmed in case of inhalation of cool, dry gas with high flow, especially during utilization of intensive care ventilators (using anhydrous wall air or oxygen)

Table 20.1 Effects of inadequate humidification during NIV and factors affecting humidification

Effects of inadequate humidification	Factors affecting humidification
Anatomical and functional changes of nasal mucosa	Presence of leak
Nasal dryness and/or congestion	Type of mask
Increased NAWR and WOB	Type of ventilator
Mucus plugs, secretion retention, atelectasis, airway obstruction, difficult intubation in case of NIV failure	Level of FiO_2 and airflow Level of IPAP
Symptoms (mouth dryness, discomfort) leading to decrease in tolerance or compliance	Temperature of the environment and inhaled gas

Abbreviations: *FiO2* fraction of inspired oxygen, *IPAP* inspiratory positive airway pressure, *NAWR* nasal airway resistance, *NIV* noninvasive ventilation, *WOB* work of breathing

or during leak compensation. A clinical review examined the effects of inappropriate gas conditioning during NIV [5] (Table 20.1). *Structural and functional deterioration of nasal mucosa* was reported, including metaplastic changes and keratinization of the nasal epithelium and submucosa, both for acute and chronic NIV use, and change in ciliary activity, mucus secretion, and local blood flow. Unidirectional inspiratory nasal airflow, worsened by mouth air-leaks, can lead to nasal dryness, which would decrease the capacity of gas conditioning of upper airways and stimulate release of inflammatory mediators leading to *nasal congestion*, *increased nasal airway resistance* (*NAWR*), and *work of breathing* (*WOB*). The secretions can become tenacious and result in *mucus plugs*, *atelectasis*, and life-threatening *airway obstruction*. Additionally, *difficult intubation* can be another consequence of non-humidified dry air during NIV use. Up to 50–60 % of patients using continuous positive airway pressure (CPAP) (especially with nasal mask) for management of ARF or SRBD experience nasal dryness or congestion. Because of nasal or mouth dryness, dry/sore throat, cough, reduced sense of smell, or discomfort, *compliance* with NIV or *tolerance* can be adversely affected for chronic or acute use of NIV, leading to NIV failure.

Some conditions can worsen gas conditioning during NIV (Table 20.1). *Presence of leaks, type of interface and ventilator, level of fractional inspired oxygen (FiO2), and inspiratory positive airway pressure (IPAP)* are the major contributors. *Unintentional leaks* through mouth or at the periphery of the mask can cause unidirectional airflow, resulting in continuous decrease in absolute humidity (AH) (i.e., the total water present in the gas) of air in airways with increased nasal airway resistance, as explained above [5]. This risk is increased with use of *nasal masks* rather than *oro-nasal masks*. Some physicians prefer a helmet, especially for ARF. When *inspiratory flow* is medium or low (FiO_2 of 0.21), humidification during delivery by *helmet* may be less necessary than during other modes, because of mixture of inspired ambient air with expired humidified gas in a relatively larger inner space [6]. However, with higher FiO_2 ($\geq$0.50), AH drops by half to an unacceptable level (9.7 mg H_2O/l), because of the greater proportion of anhydrous dry medical gas in inspired air. *Increased IPAP* as well as *high flow rates* (up to 90 l/min) can lead to inadequate humidification even with humidifiers. *Ventilator type* is another crucial factor, as intensive care unit (ICU) ventilators, obtaining dry medical gas from pipes, provide lower levels of humidity than home ventilators, using compressed room air. Therefore, the clinician should carefully adjust humidification level taking these factors into account.

20.2.2 Effects of Humidifiers During NIV Use

Humidification through artificial humidifiers can prevent these adverse effects of inadequately humidified air inhalation during NIV. Decrease in WOB, nasal airway resistance, and symptoms (such as dry throat) with improved comfort have been shown by utilization of humidifiers in short-term users [5, 7, 8]. In long-term NIV use, especially for SRBD, although there is an improvement in nasopharyngeal symptoms (such as dryness) with humidification during NIV, there are conflicting data that humidification increases patient adherence to and tolerance of CPAP [5].

20.2.3 Recommendations About Humidifier Use for NIV

There are actually no large epidemiological studies to determine whether or not humidification is routinely required for every patient for short- or long-term use. However, the guideline by the American Association of Respiratory Care published in 2012 suggested use of humidification for NIV with possibility of improvement in adherence and comfort [1]. However, in real life, the surveys of physicians manifest that a quarter to nearly half of physicians did not employ humidification during NIV use in acute settings [9, 10]. On the other hand, the American Association of Sleep Medicine also recommended its use as a practice parameter in 2006 to improve CPAP utilization in management of SRBD in adults [11]. Accordingly, some insurance companies (along with the Medicare and Medicaid programs in the United States) pay for it [3]. Unfortunately, this is not possible in every country (such as in Turkey), possibly due to socioeconomic restrictions.

20.2.4 Types of Humidifiers

There are two main types of humidification devices: HH and HME, used for both short- and long-term NIV [4]. By use of HH, gases may be actively warmed and moistened by passing air over the surface of a heated water reservoir attached to the ventilator. The system may have a heated wire in the inspiratory limb of the ventilator circuit to prevent cooling and condensation of the air. On the other hand, HME, usually placed between the Y-piece and the interface, passively humidifies air by recovering patient's expired heat and moisture and returning them to the patient during inhalation.

Both types of humidifiers can result in some complications [1, 4]. HH may lead to electrical shock, thermal injury, hypo/hyperthermia, inadvertent overfilling or pooled condensate with risk of improper ventilator performance and nosocomial

Table 20.2 Pros and cons of humidification systems during NIV

	Pros	Cons
HH	Smaller or no addition of dead space with less CO_2 retention[a] Less WOB[a] Provides effective humidification for clinical use in hypercapnic ARF	More expensive More difficult to use "Condensation fog" formation, fever and discomfort with increasing heat (helmet) Needs electricity
HME	Easier to use Cheaper No need for electricity Extensively used during IMV Condensation prevention Better preservation of humidity during low ambient temperature and at high flow	Bigger internal volume Increased dead space CO_2 retention[a] Increased NAWR (especially with leaks) Increased WOB[a] Decreased performance in case of leaks

Abbreviations: *ARF* acute respiratory failure, *CO2* carbon dioxide, *IMV* invasive mechanical ventilation, *NAWR* nasal airway resistance, *NIV* noninvasive ventilation, *WOB* work of breathing
[a]Recent studies reported no difference for work of breathing with similar CO_2 elimination by using positive end-expiratory pressure or HME with smaller dead space

infection, and patient-ventilator asynchrony. HME can increase dead space, leading to hypoventilation due to hypercapnia. There is also a potential increased risk for airway occlusion with HME due to impaction of mucus secretions compared with HH. Both can cause under-hydration and mucus plugs (<26 mg H_2O/l) with hypoventilation and/or alveolar gas trapping.

Although humidifiers have demonstrated beneficial therapeutic effects during NIV, there is still controversy over the selection of the best humidifier to obtain the best outcomes, such as improved compliance and/or gas exchange, or decreased intubation [5]. Both humidifiers have some pros and cons (Table 20.2). In a long-term (12-month) randomized crossover pilot study, HH were found to result in no differences for NIV compliance, tolerance, rate of hospitalization, or for most of the complications related to dry gases (except for dry throat) when compared with HME during NIV use for chronic respiratory failure [8]. However, at the end of the study, a higher number of patients (10/14) preferred to continue with HH for home use.

In short-term studies, HH were reported to deliver gases with higher water content than HME during NIV, especially in case of leaks [7]. This is probably because of the inability of HME to recover heat and moisture due to unidirectional flow during leaks. Therefore, it is crucial to consider the presence of mouth or mask leaks when choosing the humidifier type. HH were also shown to improve alveolar ventilation and CO_2 elimination and decreased WOB at zero end-expiratory pressure when compared with HME [12], which could be related to substantial dead space added to the ventilator circuit by HME. The lack of improvement in gas exchange with CO_2 retention is an important factor predisposing NIV failure. Therefore, based on these data, the current recommendations were made by the American Association of Respiratory Care favoring the use of HH over HME during NIV [1].

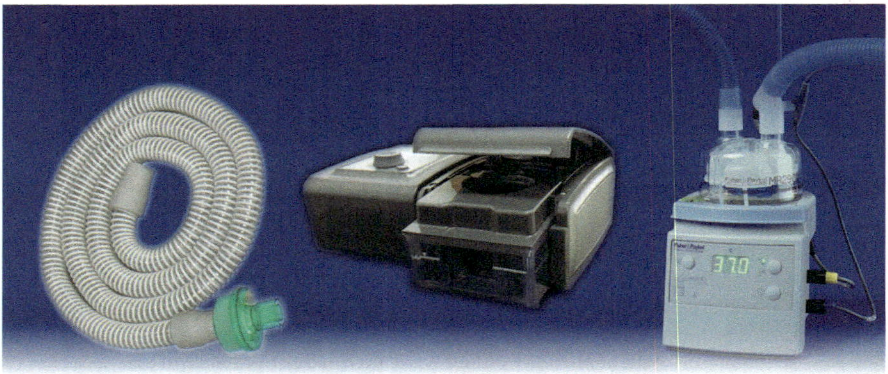

Fig. 20.1 Types of humidifiers: (*from left to right*) Heat-and-moisture exchanger (HME electrostatic filter, Covidien Inc., Boulder, CO, USA), a built-in heated humidifier in A-flex Auto CPAP (Philips Respironics, Murrysville, PA, USA), and heated humidifier (MR 850; Fisher & Paykel Healthcare Limited, Panmure, Auckland)

However, HME with small dead space were recently reported to have similar effects on respiratory parameters (such as respiratory rate, minute ventilation, end-tidal CO_2, oxygen saturation, etc.) and comfort perception as HH [13]. Additionally, a multicenter randomized controlled study declared that the short-term physiologic benefits of HH in comparison with HME during NIV with ICU ventilators were not observed [14]. The authors explained that this lack of difference could be the result of use of positive end-expiratory pressure during real-life NIV application, reducing the impact of the difference in dead space between humidification systems. Intubation rate and long-term outcomes (including NIV duration, length of stay, and mortality) were also reported to be similar. Based on these results, the recommendation of HH as a first-line treatment in all patients with ARF should be revisited (Fig. 20.1).

20.2.5 Humidifier Settings

Humidifiers can be used in critical care, acute care in-patient, operating room, home care, extended nursing facilities, and transport settings [1]. There is no clear recommendation regarding its settings. Exposure to humidity below 25 mg H_2O/l for 1 h or 30 mg H_2O/l for $\geq$24 h was shown to be associated with mucosal dysfunction [1]. Lellouche et al. [7] measured water content during NIV without humidification or with HME or HH (10 min of each period) in healthy subjects and reported these results based on type of ventilator used (turbine or ICU ventilator) and level of FiO_2. There was a dramatic decrease in AH, down to 5 mg H_2O/l, during NIV when an ICU ventilator was used; but gas humidity was equivalent to ambient air hygrometry with a turbine ventilator at minimal FiO_2 (12.5 H_2O/l). Humidifiers (HME and HH) had comparable performances (25–30 mg H_2O/l), which is adequate for the physiologic functioning of the upper airway. Based on ratings of respiratory discomfort, it was suggested that the *minimal level of AH required during NIV* was *15 mg H2O/l*. Gas temperatures during NIV were also suggested to be set based on patient comfort/tolerance, adherence, and underlying pulmonary condition [1]. Comfort measures can vary, especially in patients with ARF using a longer duration of NIV; however, this is the only available data at this time.

Conclusion

The utilization of NIV can lead to detrimental effects on airway mucosa, especially in patients with mouth leaks, receiving dry gases by ICU ventilators, high FiO_2, or high inspiratory flows. Although there is no recommendation for routine use of supplemental humidification in all patients receiving NIV, its use in symptomatic patients (such as nasal congestion or thick or tenacious secretions) with the above risk factors may be helpful to prevent deleterious effects of NIV and improve compliance and adherence. The choice of humidifier type will depend on ventilator and mask type, humidifier availability, and patient's clinical condition. Heated humidifiers are recommended over HME by current guidelines, inasmuch as HME may increase WOB and circuit dead space leading to hypercapnia. However, based on latest literature, the use of HME (ideally with a low dead space) seems to be acceptable.

Key Major Recommendations

- Humidification during NIV can be helpful in preventing symptoms such as dryness of upper airways due to dry gas inhalation, and therefore may improve tolerance and adherence.
- Supplemental humidification would better be applied in symptomatic patients with risk factors for increased moisture loss (e.g., dry gas inhalation by ICU ventilators, nasal mask use, mouth leaks, high IPAP or FiO_2)
- The type of humidifier should be chosen based on properties of ventilator and mask, availability of the humidifier, and the patient's clinical condition.
- Although current guidelines recommend use of HH over HME due to increased WOB and circuit dead space with HME, the latest literature manifested no differences between the two.

References

1. Restrepo RD, Walsh BK, AARC Practice Guideline. Humidification during invasive and noninvasive mechanical ventilation: 2012. Respir Care. 2012;57(5):782–8.
2. Schnell D, Timsit JF, Darmon M, et al. Noninvasive mechanical ventilation in acute respiratory failure: trends in use and outcomes. Intensive Care Med. 2014;40(4):582–91.
3. Branson RD, Gentile MA. Is humidification always necessary during noninvasive ventilation in the hospital? Respir Care. 2010;55(2):209–16.

4. Kelly M, Gillies D, Todd DA, et al. Heated humidification versus heat and moisture exchangers for ventilated adults and children. Cochrane Database Syst Rev. 2010;4:CD004711.
5. Esquinas AM, Scala R, Soroksky A, et al. Clinical review: humidifiers during non-invasive ventilation - key topics and practical implications. Crit Care. 2012;16:203–9.
6. Ueta K, Tomita T, Uchiyama A, et al. Influence of humidification on comfort during noninvasive ventilation with a helmet. Respir Care. 2013;58(5):798–804.
7. Lellouche F, Maggiore SM, Lyazidi A, et al. Water content of delivered gases during non-invasive ventilation in healthy subjects. Intensive Care Med. 2009;35:987–95.
8. Nava S, Cirio S, Fanfulla F, et al. Comparison of two humidification systems for long-term noninvasive mechanical ventilation. Eur Respir J. 2008;32:460–4.
9. Chanques G, Jaber S, Delay JM, et al. Phoning study about postoperative practice and application of noninvasive ventilation. Ann Fr Anesth Reanim. 2003;22:879–85.
10. Crimi C, Noto A, Princi P, et al. A European survey of noninvasive ventilation practices. Eur Respir J. 2010;36:362–9.
11. Kushida CA, Littner MR, Hirschkowitz M, et al. American Academy of Sleep Medicine: practice parameters for the use of continuous and bilevel positive airway pressure devices to treat adult patients with sleep-related breathing disorders. Sleep. 2006;29:375–80.
12. Lellouche F, Maggiore SM, Deye N, et al. Effect of humidification device on the work of breathing during noninvasive ventilation. Intensive Care Med. 2002;28:1582–9.
13. Boyer A, Vargas F, Hilbert G, et al. Small dead space heat and moisture exchangers do not impede gas exchange during noninvasive ventilation: a comparison with heated humidifier. Intensive Care Med. 2010;36:1348–54.
14. Lelouche F, L'Her E, Abroug F, et al. Impact of humidification device on intubation rate during noninvasive ventilation with ICU ventilators: results of a multicenter randomized controlled trial. Intensive Care Med. 2014;40:211–9.

NIV Aerosol Therapy: Key Technical Determinants and Clinical Evidence

21

Serpil Ocal and Arzu Topeli

Contents

Abbreviations

BIPAP	Bi-level positive airway pressure
CPAP	Continue positive airway pressure
DPI	Dry powder inhaler
EPAP	Expiratory positive airway pressure
IMV	Invasive mechanical ventilation
IPAP	Inspiratory positive airway pressure
MV	Mechanical ventilation
NIV	Noninvasive mechanical ventilation
pMDI	Pressurized metered-dose inhaler

S. Ocal, MD (✉) • A. Topeli, MD
Medical Intensive Care Unit, Hacettepe University, Faculty of Medicine,
Sihhiye, Ankara 06100, Turkey
e-mail: drserpilgocmen@yahoo.com

A.M. Esquinas (ed.), *Noninvasive Mechanical Ventilation: Theory, Equipment, and Clinical Applications*, DOI 10.1007/978-3-319-21653-9_21

21.1 Introduction

Aerosol therapy during noninvasive mechanical ventilation (NIV) is commonly used in critically ill patients. Bronchodilators, steroids, prostanoids, surfactants, mucolytics, and antibiotics are the best major aerosol drugs and can be administered to mechanically ventilated patients by the inhalation route. Interestingly, the use of drugs such as atropine, furosemide, heparin, terlipressin, and milrinone by the inhalation route has also been reported [1]. Treatment of pulmonary diseases such as chronic obstructive pulmonary disease, asthma, cystic fibrosis, and pneumonia with aerosol drugs offers advantages over oral and parenteral drugs. The use of aerosol drugs allows selective treatment of the lungs, directly achieving more rapid onset of action and high drug concentrations while using lower doses and, therefore, reducing systemic adverse effects by minimizing systemic drug levels. Inhaled β_2 agonist bronchodilators especially produce a more rapid onset of action through the inhalation route than through oral delivery. Some drugs are only active with aerosol delivery, such as cromolyn and ciclesonide for patients with asthma and dornase alfa for patients with cystic fibrosis. Bronchodilators and steroids are the most frequently used aerosol drugs during NIV [2]. Some studies have been carried out on inhaled bronchodilator therapy in NIV, but issues related to optimum aerosol delivery during NIV are unexplored [3–7].

Moreover, the physiology of aerosol delivery during NIV is not same as the physiology of aerosol delivery during invasive mechanical ventilation (IMV). Patients undergoing NIV can receive aerosol drugs in two different ways: (1) If the patient can tolerate brief periods of discontinuation, NIV can be removed and aerosol drugs can be administered by a nebulizer or a pressurized metered-dose inhaler (pMDI) in the standard manner. (2) In patients for whom NIV should be applied without interruption due to severe hypoxemia or dyspnea, aerosol drugs should then be administered by pMDI with a spacer or nebulizer. Aerosol delivery has been shown to be better when applied during NIV in the emergency department or the intensive care unit. Pollack et al. [3] found that albuterol delivery by a nebulizer during bi-level positive airway pressure (BIPAP) applied with a nasal interface resulted in a greater increase in peak expiratory flow in patients with acute asthma compared with when it is applied with a nebulizer alone. Furthermore, Fauroux et al. [4] reported better aerosol deposition in children with cystic fibrosis when a nebulizer was used with pressure support ventilation of 8–10 cm H_2O with positive end-expiratory pressure. Salbutamol delivery by pMDI with a spacer during NIV is feasible and has been shown to result in significant bronchodilation [5].

Successful aerosol therapy depends on adequate drug deposition and penetration at the intended site of action in the lung. Both in vitro and in vivo studies have contributed to our understanding of the complex factors governing aerosol delivery during mechanical ventilation. The heterogeneity between the in vivo and in vitro data might have been caused by several factors such as the circuit or the humidity, and aerosol losses during exhalation were not taken into account in vitro studies.

Hence, in vitro data should be confirmed clinically. Factors related to pulmonary deposition of aerosol in patients with IMV also differ from those in spontaneously breathing patients.

21.2 Discussion and Analysis

Factors influencing aerosol delivery during NIV are not completely understood. Multiple factors, including the mechanical effect of the applied pressure itself, independent of the drug delivered, as well as penetration, positive pressure applied to recruit collapsed alveoli, increase in tidal volume and functional residual capacity, and decrease in respiratory rate and inspiratory flow rate might have roles in improving ventilation-perfusion mismatch and therefore aerosol delivery. Unfortunately, aerosol drug losses in the ventilator circuit, interfaces, and upper airways reduce the efficiency of drug delivery during NIV. Moreover, outflow of aerosol to the environment due to mask leak creates health risks to patients and health-care providers. Aerosol delivery during NIV depends on several factors.

21.2.1 Ventilator-Related Factors

Critical care ventilators, bi-level ventilators, and home care ventilators can be used to provide NIV. The characteristics of these ventilators may significantly influence the aerosol delivery into the lungs during NIV. Critical care ventilators have the advantages of capability of precise control of fraction of inspired oxygen, presence of various modes and inspiratory flow patterns, and capability of separating inspiratory and expiratory flow to limit rebreathing. Bi-level ventilators are available specifically to provide NIV. Unlike critical care ventilators, they use a single-limb circuit and function well in the presence of leaks. However, aerosol delivery with a bi-level ventilator is more complex because of single-circuit design and the presence of a leak port.

Ventilator mode significantly influences aerosol delivery into the lung. Fink et al. [6] showed that continuous positive airway pressure (CPAP) increased albuterol delivery from a pMDI with a spacer compared with controlled mechanical ventilation, assist-control ventilation, and pressure support ventilation at similar tidal volumes. CPAP delivers positive airway pressure at a level that remains constant through the respiratory cycle (inspiration and expiration). This keeps the upper airway open, thus preventing upper airway collapse or narrowing during sleep. Additionally, increased functional residual capacity and improvement in lung compliance allow a higher volume change per unit of pressure change and, therefore, lead to potentially better aerosol distribution.

BIPAP with a higher inspiratory positive airway pressure (IPAP) and lower expiratory positive airway pressure (EPAP) settings produces better tidal volume, resulting in more retrograde flow into the ventilator circuit. Therefore, the aerosol concentrations in the circuit at the end of the expiratory phase and the aerosol delivery in the next inspiratory phase with a jet nebulizer placed between the patient and leak port during NIV with single limb circuit increase [7]. Moreover, higher IPAP is also associated with longer inspiratory time, which allows more time for the aerosol to reach to the circuit outlet. On the other hand, with higher EPAP, increased flow during the expiratory phase results in increased clearance of the aerosol from the BIPAP device circuit through the leak port and, hence, a decreased aerosol delivery.

Inspiratory flow rate significantly influences aerosol delivery into the lung. High inspiratory flow rates increase turbulent flow and produce stronger inertial forces, leading to impaction of particles in the oropharynx and proximal airways [8]. Lower inspiratory flow rates may be used to improve drug delivery during NIV as long as this is tolerated by the patient. Aerosol delivery can be influenced by the respiratory rate, pressure settings, and breath-triggering mechanism.

21.2.2 Circuit-Related Factors

The gas in the ventilator circuit is heated and humidified to prevent drying of the airway mucosa, but humidification increases loss of aerosol drugs in the ventilator circuit [6]. During NIV, unlike IMV, air is heated and humidified during its passage through the nose. The humidification capacity of the nose may be overwhelmed by the sustained high airflow rates employed during NIV. Although the optimum method of humidification for patients with acute respiratory failure has not been established, the intensivist may prefer heated humidification for patients with acute respiratory failure as it decreases the work of breathing and increases CO_2 clearance. A heat and moisture exchanger is not recommended for NIV.

The dual-limb circuit is the most common circuit used with general-purpose critical care ventilators. However, home-care and BIPAP ventilators can be used with single-limb circuits. There are two types of single-limb circuits: (1) those with built-in expiratory valves and (2) those with a leakage-type exhaust valve. Branconier and Hess [9] evaluated different positions of the leak port in BIPAP devices with a single-limb circuit and detected higher aerosol delivery when the leak port was in the circuit rather than the mask.

21.2.3 Type of Interface

The most commonly used interface for NIV in the intensive care unit is an oronasal mask. Other interfaces include nasal, total face masks, helmets, mouthpieces, and nasal pillows. A variety of sizes and designs are commercially available. Unsuccessful aerosol therapy can occur more often in the nasal mask or poorly fitted oronasal mask at particularly setting higher positive pressure due to major leaks. Anisocoria can develop in patients undergoing NIV who receive ipratropium via a poorly fitting oronasal mask. Total face masks and helmets should not be used for aerosol delivery.

21.2.4 Type of Aerosol-Generating Device and Its Configuration

Bronchodilators are among the most commonly used aerosol drugs in the intensive care unit. These drugs are available in the three principal types of inhaler devices, which include pMDI, dry powder inhaler (DPI), and nebulizers. Only pMDIs and nebulizers have been adapted for clinical use during NIV. The efficiency of aerosol delivery with a DPI in this setting is likely to be low because of the known effect of humidity in reducing aerosol delivery from such devices. Nebulizers or pMDIs with in-line spacers are used to administer inhaled medications during NIV.

Nebulizers: The three basic types of nebulizer devices are jet, ultrasonic, and mesh nebulizers. Nebulizers are connected in the single-limb circuit between the leak port and interface [10], but the optimum position of nebulizer in the dual-limb circuit is yet to be determined. Nebulizer performance is affected by both technical and patient-related factors. Mesh nebulizers are lighter and more portable than jet and ultrasonic nebulizers. Moreover, mesh nebulizers usually deliver the medication dose more quickly and lead to higher aerosol delivery than jet nebulizers. To avoid infection, nebulizers should be cared for appropriately because of the risk of contamination. Additionally, when jet and ultrasonic nebulizers are used, aerosol deposition occurs in the nebulizer cup, which causes ineffective aerosol therapy.

pMDIs: The pMDI is the most commonly used aerosol device for inhalation therapy worldwide. The drug is released from the canister through a metering valve and stem that fits into an actuator boot designed and extensively tested by the manufacturer to work with that specific formulation. A spacer is needed to adapt the pMDI into the ventilator circuit, and a variety of spacers are used for aerosol drug delivery in mechanically ventilated patients. Types of spacers include inline devices (unidirectional and bidirectional) and chamber. These are placed in the inspiratory limb of the dual-limb circuit. The spacer type influences the efficiency of aerosol delivery during mechanical ventilation. Whereas a bidirectional spacer is superior to a unidirectional spacer in dose delivery, a chamber spacer with pMDI is more efficient for aerosol drug delivery compared with a bidirectional or a unidirectional spacer. With a chamber spacer, the aerosol particle has an opportunity to slow and propellant evaporation decreases the size of aerosol particles. Both of these phenomena reduce aerosol drug losses caused by particle impaction on the walls of the ventilator circuits and interface. The aerosolized bronchodilator delivery is also significantly reduced when the pMDI is actuated during the expiratory phase, hence it is important that it is actuated at the initiation of the inspiratory phase.

If a dose counter is not used with a pMDI, it becomes difficult to determine the dose left in the pMDI. The dose counters, which are attached to the top or boot of the pMDI, are manufactured by different companies. Several commercially adapters or actuators are used to connect the pMDI canister to the ventilator circuit.

21.2.5 Drug-Related Factors

Ideally, the majority of the drug particles in pMDI and nebulizer aerosols should be in the range 1–5 μm. While smaller aerosol particles will likely be quickly exhaled before reaching the lung tissue, larger aerosol particles are trapped in the ventilator circuit and on the interface and deposited in the proximal airways during NIV. Additionally, aerosol delivery could be influenced by the drug dose and formulation and duration of action.

21.2.6 Patient-Related Factors

During NIV, tidal volume is variable depending on the compliance of the lung and the chest wall and the resistance of the airways. Accordingly, higher lung compliance and lower airway resistance provide better distal deposition of aerosol drug. Successful therapy is influenced by several additional variables, such as the presence and severity of airway diseases, presence of mucus, counter-regulatory effects of inflammation and other drugs, and patient's response. The best way to deliver aerosol drugs to a patient is in the sitting position. However, if the patient cannot sit in the bed during inhalation therapy, the head of the bed should be elevated at least 20–30° above for better aerosol administration during NIV.

21.3 Administration Techniques

Successful aerosol therapy for inhaled bronchodilator drugs in patients undergoing NIV requires careful attention to the administration technique. When these techniques are employed, adequate pulmonary drug deposition is achieved and a significant response to bronchodilators is observed (Tables 21.1 and 21.2).

Table 21.1 Optimal technique for drug delivery by pMDI in patients undergoing NIV

1. Review order, identify patient, and asses the need for bronchodilator therapy
2. Minimize leaks in the mask and/or circuit
3. Shake pMDI and warm it to hand temperature
4. Be sure that the dose counter is attached to the pMDI
5. Place the pMDI with chamber spacer
(a) Near the "Y" adapter in inspiratory limb for dual-limb circuit
(b) Between the leak port and mask for single-limb circuit
6. Coordinate pMDI action with beginning of inspiration
7. Wait at least 15 s between actuations, and administer the total dose
8. Remove pMDI with spacer from circuit
9. Monitor for adverse effects

Table 21.2 Optimal technique for drug delivery by a nebulizer in patients undergoing NIV

1. Review order, identify patient, and asses the need for a bronchodilator therapy
2. Minimize leaks in the mask and/or circuit
3. Place mesh/jet nebulizer
(a) Between the leak port and mask in a single-limb circuit
(b) Near the "Y" adapter in the inspiratory limb of a dual-limb circuit
4. Pour the recommended drug volume into the nebulizer
5. Set the gas flow to nebulizer at 2–10 l/min, based on the manufacturer label
6. Run until the nebulizer begins to sputter
7. Remove the nebulizer from the circuit, rinse with sterile water, run dry
8. Monitor for adverse effects

Conclusion

Despite the common use of aerosol drugs during NIV, it is still unclear which technique should be used for aerosol delivery. In recent decades, a number of bench model studies during NIV and in vitro studies during IMV have defined some settings allowing successful aerosol therapy. Unfortunately, only a few investigators have studied aerosol delivery in patients undergoing NIV. Aerosolized bronchodilator therapy is effective albeit complex during NIV and more studies are needed for optimum aerosol delivery.

Key Major Recommendations

- Both the nebulizer and the pMDI with spacer are appropriate for delivery of bronchodilators during NIV.
- Proper technique when using a pMDI with spacer, or nebulizer during NIV should be applied.
- Precautions to decrease contamination and to avoid aerosol particles depositions should be in place.

References

1. Ehrmann S, Roche-Campo F, Sferrazza Papa GF, et al. Aerosol therapy during mechanical ventilation: an international survey. Intensive Care Med. 2013;39(6):1048–56.
2. Dolovich MB, Ahrens RC, Hess DR, et al. Device selection and outcomes of aerosol therapy: evidence-based guidelines: American College of Chest Physicians/American College of Asthma, Allergy, and Immunology. Chest. 2005;127(1):335–71.

3. Pollack Jr CV, Fleisch KB, Dowsey K. Treatment of acute bronchospasm with beta-adrenergic agonist aerosols delivered by a nasal bilevel positive airway pressure circuit. Ann Emerg Med. 1995;26(5):552–7.
4. Fauroux B, Itti E, Pigeot J, Isabey D, et al. Optimization of aerosol deposition by pressure support in children with cystic fibrosis: an experimental and clinical study. Am J Respir Crit Care Med. 2000;162(6):2265–71.
5. Nava S, Karakurt S, Rampulla C, et al. Salbutamol delivery during non-invasive mechanical ventilation in patients with chronic obstructive pulmonary disease: a randomized, controlled study. Intensive Care Med. 2001;27:1627–35.
6. Fink JB, Dhand R, Duarte AG, et al. Aerosol delivery from a metered-dose inhaler during mechanical ventilation. An in vitro model. Am J Respir Crit Care Med. 1996;154:382–7.
7. Calvert LD, Jackson JM, White JM, et al. Enhanced delivery of nebulized salbutamol during non-invasive ventilation. J Pharm Pharmacol. 2006;58(11):1553–7.
8. Dolovich M. Influence of inspiratory flow rate, particle size, and airway caliber on aerosolized drug delivery to the lung. Respir Care. 2000;45:597–608.
9. Branconier MP, Hess DR. Albuterol delivery during noninvasive ventilation. Respir Care. 2005;50(12):1649–53.
10. Chatmongkolchart S, Schettino GP, Dilman C, et al. In vitro evaluation of aerosol bronchodilator delivery during noninvasive positive pressure ventilation: effect of ventilator settings and nebulizer position. Crit Care Med. 2002;30:2515–9.

22 Skin Breakdown in Patients with Acute Respiratory Failure Undergoing Noninvasive Ventilation: Key Topics

Samantha Torres Grams and Wellington Pereira Yamaguti

Contents

Abbreviations

ARF Acute respiratory failure
NIV Noninvasive ventilation
SB Skin breakdown

22.1 Introduction

Noninvasive ventilation (NIV) has been recognized as an effective treatment to avoid the need for invasive mechanical ventilation and its associated complications in patients with acute respiratory failure (ARF). Compared with invasive mechanical ventilation, the use of NIV has the advantage of decreasing the risk of ventilator-associated pneumonia, as well as a reduction in the hospital stay and mortality.

NIV has particularly been indicated to treat patients with chronic obstructive pulmonary disease exacerbation, acute cardiogenic pulmonary edema, hypercapnic

S.T. Grams, MSc • W.P. Yamaguti, PhD (✉)
Rehabilitation Service, Hospital Sírio-Libanês, Centro de Reabilitação, São Paulo, SP, Brazil
e-mail: samanthagrams@gmail.com; wellington.psyamaguti@hsl.org.br

A.M. Esquinas (ed.), *Noninvasive Mechanical Ventilation: Theory, Equipment, and Clinical Applications*, DOI 10.1007/978-3-319-21653-9_22

respiratory failure secondary to chest wall deformity or neuromuscular diseases, pulmonary infection in immunosuppressed subjects, acute pancreatitis, and in weaning from tracheal intubation. However, some complications and injurious effects with the use of NIV have also been identified, such as aerophagia, inefficiency to handle copious secretions, bronchoaspiration, hemodynamic instability, and patient-ventilator asynchrony. Other factors that may limit the use of NIV are interface-related problems such as air leaks and mask intolerance due to claustrophobia and anxiety. The development of facial skin breakdown (SB) in the zones of greatest contact pressure between the mask and the patient's skin has also been recognized as one of the most serious complications related to the use of an interface in patients with ARF because it can increase the discomfort reported by the patient, resulting in interface intolerance and, consequently, in NIV failure [1]. Therefore, this chapter reviews the classification, frequency, and potential treatment-related risk factors for SB. Early identification of these factors is fundamental to preventing the development of SB, thus providing the best quality of care to patients.

22.2 SB Classification

Constant pressure during a critical 1–2-h interval increases the risk of SB development due to the production of microscopic pathologic tissue changes [2]. According to the European Pressure Ulcer Advisory Panel and the American National Pressure Ulcer Advisory Panel [3], SB may be classified as:

- Stage I: when intact skin has non-blanchable redness of a localized area, usually over a bony prominence (may indicate "at risk" persons);
- Stage II: when there is partial thickness loss of dermis presented as a shallow open ulcer with a red-pink wound bed;
- Stage III: when there is full thickness tissue loss;
- Stage IV: when there is exposed bone, tendon, or muscle. Serious complications such as osteomyelitis (infection of the bone) or sepsis (infection carried through the blood) can occur.

22.3 Frequency of SB

Few studies have investigated the frequency of SB in patients undergoing NIV. In a multicenter randomized study, the frequency of SB was evaluated when comparing a prototype oronasal mask and a conventional oronasal mask in adult patients with ARF [4]. The results showed that the patients who used the prototype oronasal mask, specifically designed to allow a more comfortable patient-mask interface, had significantly lower frequency of SB (43 %) compared with the conventional oronasal mask (100 %). In a more recent study [5], the frequency of SB was lower in a similar population after the use of NIV with oronasal mask (14.4 %). It was demonstrated that 13.1 % of patients showed SB at Stage I, 1.3 % had SB at Stage II, and no patient developed skin necrosis (Stage III). The authors explained that these differences in results, among other factors, may be due to the use of a protective dermal sheet applied over the nasal bridge during NIV. This study also evaluated the frequency of SB in patients who used NIV with total face mask, and the results showed that the use of this type of interface avoided SB development (only 1.6 % of patients had SB).

In children, the frequency of SB was observed in 48 % of the patients with obstructive sleep apnea, neuromuscular disorders, and cystic fibrosis undergoing NIV via nasal mask [6]. Among the patients, 18 % showed transient erythema (Stage I), 23 % had prolonged erythema (Stage II), and 8 % developed skin necrosis (Stage III).

22.4 Treatment-Related Risk Factors for SB

It has been demonstrated that the total duration of NIV and the use of oronasal mask were considered independent risk factors for the development of SB in patients with ARF:

- Total duration of NIV use: 24–26 h of NIV use is associated with increased risk of skin injury [4, 5]. Longer periods of NIV use are associated with a higher risk of SB: in a previous study, 70 % of patients who continuously used NIV for 48 h presented skin injury [7]. These findings reinforce the hypothesis that the risk of development of SB in subjects undergoing NIV is time dependent. Although longer periods of NIV are more associated with SB, it is important to note that constant pressure for 1–2 h is sufficient to cause tissue damage and cell death [2] and, therefore, even short periods of NIV deserve attention.
- Type of interface: previous studies showed that an oronasal mask may also be considered an independent risk factor for the development of SB in adult patients [4, 5]. The use of other types of interface that produce less pressure against the face, such as total face mask and helmet, has been proposed as an alternative to treat ARF, with better tolerance, comfort, and less risk of SB than oronasal mask [5, 8, 9]. Another recommendation to prevent SB in patients who need prolonged NIV is to use different types of mask periodically, changing the zones of pressure on the face [10].

Higher levels of respiratory pressures and the ventilatory modes could be considered other treatment-related risk factors for the development of SB. During NIV with high levels of respiratory pressures, the interface is usually tightly sealed to the skin to reduce possible air leaks. If this mask pressure against the face exceeds the skin capillary pressure, the tissue perfusion is impaired and, consequently, the risk of SB development could be higher in this condition [9]. During the application of CPAP, air leaks are less problematic because the pressure is constant and does not require a very tight-fitting mask adjustment. On the other hand, as bi-level positive airway pressure ventilation involves oscillation of high level to lower level pressures, the mask adjustment should be tighter. For these reasons, it could be expected that ventilatory modes and higher levels of respiratory pressures would be associated with greater risk of developing skin lesions. However, this relation was not found in a previous study [5]. The authors explained that the ventilatory mode and its level of pressure applied did not seem to influence the occurrence of SB in their population because the mask was properly fitted.

Key Recommendations

- Total face mask and helmet may be considered in patients who need prolonged NIV to prevent SB.
- Different types of masks could be used periodically, changing the zones of pressure on the face.

References

1. American Thoracic Society, European Respiratory Society, European Society of Intensive Care Medicine, Société de Réanimation de Langue Française. International Consensus Conferences in Intensive Care Medicine: noninvasive positive pressure ventilation in acute respiratory failure. Am J Respir Crit Care Med. 2001;163(1):283–91.
2. Breuls RG, Bouten CV, Oomens CW, et al. Compression induced cell damage in engineered muscle tissue: an in vitro model to study pressure ulcer aetiology. Ann Biomed Eng. 2003;31(11):1357–64.
3. European Pressure Ulcer Advisory Panel, National Pressure Ulcer Advisory Panel. Prevention and treatment of pressure ulcers: quick reference guide. 2009. http://www.epuap.org/guidelines/Final_Quick_Prevention.pdf. Accessed 08 Mar 2015.
4. Gregoretti C, Confalonieri M, Navalesi P, et al. Evaluation of patient skin breakdown and comfort with a new face mask for non-invasive ventilation: a multi-center study. Intensive Care Med. 2002;28(3):278–84.
5. Yamaguti WP, Moderno EV, Yamashita SY, et al. Treatment-related risk factors for development of skin breakdown in subjects with acute respiratory failure undergoing noninvasive ventilation or CPAP. Respir Care. 2014;59(10):1530–6.
6. Fauroux B, Lavis JF, Nicot F, et al. Facial side effects during noninvasive positive pressure ventilation in children. Intensive Care Med. 2005;31(7):965–9.
7. Beltrame F, Lucangelo U, Gregori D, et al. Noninvasive positive pressure ventilation in trauma subjects with acute respiratory failure. Monaldi Arch Chest Dis. 1999;54(2):109–14.
8. Chacur FH, Vilella Felipe LM, Fernandes CG, et al. The total face mask is more comfortable than the oronasal mask in noninvasive ventilation but is not associated with improved outcome. Respiration. 2011;82(5):426–30.
9. Nava S, Navalesi P, Gregoretti C. Interfaces and humidification for noninvasive mechanical ventilation. Respir Care. 2009;54(1):71–84.
10. Fraticelli AT, Lellouche F, L'her E, et al. Physiological effects of different interfaces during noninvasive ventilation for acute respiratory failure. Crit Care Med. 2009;37(3):939–45.

Nutrition During Noninvasive Ventilation: Clinical Determinants and Key Practical Recommendations

23

Anneli Reeves, Khoa Tran, and Peter Collins

Contents

Abbreviations

COPD	Chronic obstructive pulmonary disease
ETF	Enteral tube feeding
NIV	Noninvasive ventilation
ONS	Oral nutrition support

A. Reeves, BSc Grad Dip Nut & Diet, Adv APD (✉)
Nutrition Services Department, Logan Hospital, Meadowbrook, QLD, 4131, Australia
e-mail: annelireeves@gmail.com; anneli.reeves@health.qld.gov.au

K. Tran, MBBS, FRACP, FCICM
Respiratory Medicine, Logan Hospital, Meadowbrook, QLD, 4131, Australia
e-mail: khoa.tran@health.qld.gov.au

P. Collins, PhD, APD
Nutrition and Dietetics, School of Exercise and Nutrition Sciences, Faculty of Health, Queensland University of Technology, Kelvin Grove, QLD, 4059, Australia
e-mail: pf.collins@qut.edu.au

A.M. Esquinas (ed.), *Noninvasive Mechanical Ventilation: Theory, Equipment, and Clinical Applications*, DOI 10.1007/978-3-319-21653-9_23

23.1 Introduction

Malnutrition is a common problem affecting between 25 and 40 % of individuals with advanced chronic obstructive pulmonary disease (COPD) [1]. As COPD patients have some of the highest incidences of repeat hospital admissions [2] and with malnutrition in COPD associated with a prolonged length of hospital stay, the optimization of nutritional intake during these periods is important. Despite malnutrition being highly prevalent and associated with poor clinical outcomes, recent systematic reviews and meta-analyses have shown that, if it is identified, it is treatable [3, 4]. Nutritional support was found to not only significantly improve nutritional intake and nutritional status [3] but also to translate to improvements in respiratory muscle strength, functional capacity, and quality of life [4]. However, only two studies included in the reviews targeted inpatients, and these were in non-acute, stable COPD patients with no reported use of noninvasive ventilation (NIV) [3].

23.2 Nutritional Depletion and Respiratory Disease

The association between nutritional depletion and chronic respiratory disease is well known. During exacerbations of respiratory disease, pulmonary function can be impaired to a level that negatively impacts an individual's ability to achieve their nutritional requirements [5]. The etiology of nutritional depletion in this instance is multifactorial and a combination of an inability to achieve altered nutritional requirements against a background of elevated systemic inflammation, impaired functional capacity, and medication side effects [5]. Although medical interventions such as NIV can serve as an additional physical barrier to the intake of food, NIV has been shown to be associated with an improvement in nutritional status in those previously identified as at nutritional risk [6]. Budweiser and colleagues [6] acknowledged the complexity of weight loss in COPD and speculated that NIV could assist in producing a positive nutritional balance required for weight gain through reducing the work associated with breathing. Similar improvements in body weight have also been reported following lung volume reduction surgery [5, 6]. It is also feasible that NIV results in improved nutritional status through other mechanisms such as improvement of hypercapnia and acidosis, which are known to negatively impact protein synthesis [6]. Elevated systemic inflammation, particularly during acute episodes of the disease, is known to negatively impact on appetite, nutrition intake, and protein synthesis and breakdown [5, 6]. As NIV assists in reducing episodes of respiratory failure, hypoxia, and elevated inflammation, this may reduce periods of negative energy balance and catabolism [6]. Acute exacerbations that did not involve the use of NIV have been associated with reduced nutritional intake and increased energy expenditure in COPD patients [7]. There is limited research describing nutritional intake of hospitalized patients receiving NIV, with no protocols currently available to guide health-care professionals in the nutritional management of this patient group. One prospective study of 36 hospitalized patients receiving NIV showed that more than 75 % of the patients had inadequate intake [8]. Intake was lower with increasing time on NIV, and earlier during their hospital admission. Patients who were enterally fed received significantly more energy and protein than those who were receiving oral nutrition only [8].

23.3 Nutritional Intervention in Respiratory Disease

As malnutrition in respiratory disease is a significant clinical problem leading to increased mortality risk, patients at risk of malnutrition need to be identified and to receive prompt appropriate nutrition support. This requires routine nutritional screening followed by appropriate nutritional intervention (such as nutritional supplements or enteral feeds) for patients identified as malnourished or at risk of malnutrition. Malnutrition assessment includes consideration of low body mass index (<20 %), low fat free mass (<17 % for males and <15 % for females), and involuntary weight loss of 5 % or more during the last 6 months [5]. Oral nutritional support is the preferred method of management of malnutrition with high-energy, high-protein foods offered. Texture-modified foods or minced and moist foods might be used as they require less chewing in a breathless patient and are easily swallowed. High-energy, high-protein, liquid multi-nutrient oral nutritional supplements (ONS) are also used and can be divided into doses throughout the day to assist with tolerance [9]. Where patients are unable to achieve 75 % of their estimated nutritional requirements despite these oral nutritional support strategies, a period of enteral tube feeding (ETF) is indicated [10]. Although there is robust evidence for the clinical effectiveness of ONS in stable COPD [3, 4], only one randomized placebo-controlled trial to date has used nocturnal ETF in a small sample of stable, malnourished COPD patients [10]. Despite ETF only being provided for 16 days, the intervention group gained a significant amount of weight (3 kg) and experienced significant improvements in respiratory muscle function.

23.4 Composition of Nutritional Support

It has long been known that nutrition and ventilation are linked with oxygen needed for energy production, and it was thought that a lower carbohydrate and higher fat intake in patients requiring ventilation would be beneficial in optimizing oxygen utilization while minimizing carbon dioxide production [1]. Clinical evidence supporting this practice is limited and, more recently, it has been recognized that avoiding overfeeding and providing excessive substrate that needs to be oxidized is more critical [1]. In addition, the delayed gastric emptying with aggressive feeding and the potential negative impact on breathing mechanics will further increase the burden on the respiratory system [1]. In fact, there is data showing patients experience less dyspnea after a carbohydrate-rich liquid ONS than after an isocaloric fat-rich ONS that would have a longer gastric transit time [7]. However, oral nutrition support achieves best results not by manipulating macronutrient composition but by being given in small, frequent doses, thereby avoiding complications and improving compliance [1, 9]. There remains interest in how nutrition can be manipulated to provide better care for respiratory patients, and one such study investigated the effect of ETF enriched with eicosapentaenoic and gamma-linoleic acid versus a high-fat ETF in ventilated patients [11]. Those ventilated patients who received the omega-3 fatty acid–enriched ETF had significantly improved oxygenation by day 4, a shorter requirement for ventilation, and significantly reduced mortality at 28 days [11]. These extremely promising results demonstrating the benefits of nutritional support and its potential immunomodulatory effects indicate further exploration in other respiratory groups is warranted. This is particularly the case in patient groups where malnutrition and elevated systemic inflammatory markers are hallmarks.

Conclusion

The etiology of malnutrition in respiratory disease and those requiring NIV is complex, but the result is poor clinical and economic outcomes and poorer quality of life for the patient. However, in conditions such as stable COPD, malnutrition is treatable and can be prevented. This results in improvements in nutritional status, functional capacity, and quality of life. To maximize the effectiveness of nutritional support, the nutritional management of patients requires a coordinated approach and consideration of care in the acute and stable phases of the disease. Routine nutritional screening and assessment are needed to promptly identify malnourished individuals and those at risk of malnutrition, with the initiation of nutritional support ideally overseen by a dietitian.

Key Points

- COPD patients receiving NIV should be routinely screened for malnutrition, and nutritional intake should be monitored for adequacy.
- Early referral to a dietitian and/or commencement of nutrition support is recommended for patients identified as at nutritional risk.
- Ventilated patients have a great variation in nutritional needs depending on whether they are hypometabolic, normometabolic, or hypermetabolic. Regular nutritional assessment of ventilated patients is required.
- Although there are some promising results around the manipulation of nutrition and the use of specialist enteral feeds in critically ill patients, more evidence is needed before they can be recommended over standard enteral formulas.
- Current evidence recommends use of high-energy, high-protein, and low-volume oral nutritional supplements in addition to maximizing oral intake. If nutrition support cannot be managed orally, enteral tube feeding is indicated and should be considered.

References

1. Anker SD, John M, Pedersen PU, Raguso C, Cicoira M, Dardai E, Laviano A, Ponikowski P, Schols AM, DGEM (German Society for Nutritional Medicine), Becker HF, Böhm M, Brunkhorst FM, Vogelmeier C, ESPEN (European Society for Parenteral and Enteral Nutrition). ESPEN guidelines on enteral nutrition: cardiology and pulmonology. Clin Nutr. 2006;25(2):311–8.
2. Porter J, Herring J, Lacroix J, Levinton C. CIHI survey: avoidable admissions and repeat admissions: what do they tell us? Healthc Q. 2007;10(1):26–8.
3. Collins P, Stratton R, Elia M. Nutritional support in chronic obstructive pulmonary disease: a systematic review and meta-analysis. Am J Clin Nutr. 2012;95:1385–95.
4. Collins P, Elia M, Stratton R. Nutritional support and functional capacity in chronic obstructive pulmonary disease: a systematic review and meta-analysis. Respirology. 2013;18(4):616–29.
5. Schols A, Ferreira I, Franssen F, Gosker H, Janssens W, Muscaritoli M, Pison C, Rutten-van M, Slinde F, Steiner M, Tkacova R, Singh S. Nutritional assessment and therapy in COPD: Metabolism and nutrition: shifting paradigms in COPD management. http://ow.ly/AsOxh 201 from http://www.ciro-horn.nl/en/publications-2014/An official systematic review of the European Respiratory Society. European Respiratory Society statement from ERS Publications Taskforce Report.
6. Budweiser S, Heinemann F, Meyer K, Wild P, Pfeifer M. Weight gain in cachectic COPD patients receiving noninvasive positive-pressure ventilation. Respir Care. 2006;51(2):126–32.
7. Vermeeren MA, Wouters EF, Nelissen LH, van Lier A, Hofman Z, Schols AM. Acute effects of different nutritional supplements on symptoms and functional capacity in patients with chronic obstructive pulmonary disease. Am J Clin Nutr. 2001;73(2):295–301.
8. Reeves A, White H, Sosnowski K, Tran K, Jones M, Palmer M. Energy and protein intakes of hospitalised patients with acute respiratory failure receiving non-invasive ventilation. Clin Nutr. 2014;33(6):1068–73.
9. Broekhuizen R, Creutzberg EC, Weling-Scheepers CA, Wouters EFM, Schols AMWJ. Optimizing oral nutritional drink supplementation in patients with chronic obstructive pulmonary disease. Br J Nutr. 2005;93(6):965–71.
10. Whittaker JS, Ryan CF, Buckley PA, Road JD. The effects of refeeding on peripheral and respiratory muscle function in malnourished chronic obstructive pulmonary disease patients. Am Rev Respir Dis. 1990;142:283–8.
11. Singer P, Theilla M, Fisher M, Gibstein L, Grozovski E, Cohen J. Benefit of an enteral diet enriched with eicosapentaenoic acid and gamma-linoleic acid in ventilated patients with acute lung injury. Crit Care Med. 2006;34(4):1033–8.

24 Mechanical Insufflation-Exsufflation as Adjunctive Therapy During Noninvasive Ventilation with Airways Encumbrance: Key Technical Topics and Clinical Indications in Critical Care

Andrea Vianello, Oreste Marrone, and Grazia Crescimanno

Contents

24.1 Introduction

Patients undergoing noninvasive positive pressure ventilation (NPPV) for acute respiratory failure (ARF) may experience retained secretions from several causes, including reduced mucociliary clearance, increased mucus volume and consistency, and an inability to cough effectively as a result of weakened respiratory and/or bulbar muscles. A noninvasive approach to the management of tracheobronchial secretions, based on the combination of NPPV and expiratory muscle aid, may result in a reduced need of nasal suctioning and conventional endotracheal intubation (ETI) and/or tracheostomy. In addition, preventive application of assisted coughing techniques after extubation may provide a clinically important advantage to patients with neuromuscular disorders (NMDs) by averting the need for reintubation and shortening their stay in the intensive care unit (ICU).

A. Vianello, MD (✉)
Respiratory Pathophyisology Division, University-City Hospital of Padova, Padova, Italy
e-mail: andrea.vianello@sanita.padova.it

O. Marrone, MD • G. Crescimanno, MD
Institute of Biomedicine and Molecular Immunology, CNR, Palermo, Italy
e-mail: oreste.marrone@ibim.cnr.it; grazia.crescimanno@ibim.cnr.it

A.M. Esquinas (ed.), *Noninvasive Mechanical Ventilation: Theory, Equipment, and Clinical Applications*, DOI 10.1007/978-3-319-21653-9_24

24.2 Mechanically Assisted Coughing in the Critical Care Setting

Airway clearance techniques have the potential to improve mucociliary clearance during NPPV therapy or immediately after extubation by reducing mucus plugging and enhancing the removal of secretions. It is important to distinguish between secretion mobilization techniques (clearance of peripheral airways), including postural drainage, chest wall vibration, positive expiratory pressure therapy, high-frequency chest compression, and high-frequency chest wall oscillation, and cough augmentation techniques (clearance of central and upper airways), including manually and mechanically assisted coughing. Among cough augmentation aids, mechanically assisted coughing (MAC) can be delivered by a device consisting of a two-stage axial compressor that provides positive pressure to the airway, then rapidly shifts to negative pressure, thereby generating a forced expiration. It is usually applied via a facemask. It commonly produces a decrease in pressure by approximately 80 cm H_2O in 0.2 s; the insufflation and exsufflation pressure and time are independently adjustable. The device can deliver maximum positive and negative pressures of about 60 cm H_2O.

The use of mechanical insufflation-exsufflation (MI-E) devices for MAC has been proposed as a complement to NPPV in patients with NMD with an inability to generate an effective cough who develop an intercurrent respiratory tract infection, with the goal to expel secretions, allay secretion-associated dyspnea, and increase oxyhemoglobin saturation and pulmonary parameters.

Ability to effectively cough can be evaluated by measuring peak cough flow (PCF), the maximum airflow generated by the patient during cough, which is dependent on lung volume, airway caliber, compliance of the respiratory system, and inspiratory and expiratory muscle strength. Normal individuals may produce a PCF as great as 720 l/min (occasionally higher in healthy individuals). The minimum effective PCF was inferred from patients who were being weaned from mechanical ventilation, showing that successful extubation requires at least 160 l/min (2.7 l/s). Bach and Saporito [1], in fact, conducted a mixed-population study in 49 patients that found that those with PCF below 160 l/min, irrespective of the ability to breathe, failed extubation or decannulation. On this basis, indications for the use of MI-E in the acute setting have been considered as the following:

- An established diagnosis of paralytic/restrictive disorder
- Patient unable to cough or clear secretions effectively with a PCF less than 160 l/min using lung volume recruitment (LVR) with bag or volume ventilator
- Patient overly fatigued when performing LVR with the resuscitation bag or volume ventilator [2]

The following contraindications should be carefully considered before using MI-E:

- A patient with a history of bullous emphysema
- Susceptibility to pneumothorax or pnuemomediastinum
- Recent barotraumas

Because MI-E releases positive pressure, the following precautions should also be considered before its use: facial fractures; recent esophageal, pulmonary, or anti-reflux surgery; gastric distention; cardiovascular system instability (hypotension and arrhythmias); raised intracranial pressure; pain; nausea; bronchospasm; pulmonary edema; extreme tachypnea; large airway carcinoma; and unexplained hemoptysis [3].

Physiologically, MI-E has been shown to increase PCF in patients with NMD [3, 4]; an increase in PCF is thought to improve the efficacy of cough and thus assist in secretion removal. A study performed in individuals with amyotrophic lateral sclerosis demonstrated significant increases in PCF from baseline unassisted coughs, in patients both with and without bulbar muscle weakness, when using either exsufflation alone, or MI-E. In those without bulbar muscle involvement, the weakest patients (Vital Capacity < 50 %) demonstrated the largest increases in PCF [4].

In the acute setting, MAC has been utilized in combination with NPPV to avoid ETI and tracheotomy, to facilitate extubation and decannulation, and to prevent post-extubation failure in patients with NMD [5–9]. Servera et al. [5] conducted a prospective cohort study in the respiratory medicine ward of a university hospital to study the success rate of the use of continuous NPPV and manually and mechanically assisted coughing to avert ETI in 24 consecutive episodes of ARF for 17 patients with NMD. NPPV and coughing aids were used to reverse decreases in oxyhemoglobin saturation and relieve respiratory distress that occurred despite oxygen therapy and appropriate medication. Noninvasive management was successful in averting death and ETI in 79.2 % of the acute episodes, with bulbar dysfunction resulting the only independent risk factor for failure of the noninvasive approach.

In our experience, we compared 11 NMD patients who received a mean ± SD 2.7 ± 0.9 MI-E sessions per day to 16 historical matched controls who were treated with postural drainage, and suction when required. The results of the retrospective study showed that patients who received MI-E had a lower treatment failure rate (defined by the need to insert a mini-tracheostomy or the need to intubate; 2/11 vs 10/16; $p = 0.047$). There was no significant difference between the groups in the duration of NPPV ($p = 0.93$) or in the proportion of patients requiring bronchoscopy ($p = 0.71$). In addition, MI-E did not produce serious side effects and was well tolerated by all subjects [6]. On this basis, MI-E in combination with NPPV can be suggested as an effective alternative to ETI in managing ARF in NMD patients with mucous encumbrance.

Extubation failure is an outcome to be avoided because it is independently associated with increased hospital mortality, prolonged ICU and hospital stay, higher costs, and greater need for tracheotomy [10]; therefore, strategies preventing this occurrence are required. To avert extubation failure in patients at high risk, recent studies have evaluated the effectiveness of NPPV as a preventive strategy, concluding that its application can reduce the need for reintubation and mortality rate in the ICU in individuals with chronic respiratory disorders (including chronic obstructive pulmonary disease, obesity hypoventilation, sequelae of tuberculosis, chest wall deformity, and chronic persistent asthma), congestive heart failure, and/or hypercapnia of different etiologies [11, 12]. Unfortunately, poor cough strength and inability of patients to protect their upper airway, with the need for airway suctioning and an increased risk of aspiration and pneumonia, are a common occurrence among patients with NMD, leading to extubation intolerance and, finally, failure, regardless of the use of inspiratory aids. As a consequence, the combination of NPPV and cough assistance may become essential to prevent extubation failure in neuromyopathic patients. Bach et al. [8] reported data collected on 152 consecutive unweanable patients who could not pass a spontaneous breathing trial (SBT) before or after extubation. They were administered a protocol including extubation once SpO_2 was maintained ≥95 % in ambient air to full NPPV support and aggressive manually assisted coughing. Extubation success was defined as not requiring reintubation during the hospitalization. The first attempt protocol extubation success rate was 95 % (144 patients). All 96 extubation attempts on patients with assisted PCF ≥ 160 l/m were successful. Six of 7 patients who initially failed extubation succeeded on subsequent attempts, so only one with no measurable assisted PCF underwent tracheotomy. The author concluded that the standardized use of NPPV and cough assist can lead to effective extubation of almost all "unweanable" patients with NMD who could not pass an SBT, supporting the argument that timely provision of inspiratory and expiratory aids allows for virtual elimination of post-extubation failure in patients with NMD.

In our experience, we reported the prospective analysis of the short-term outcomes of 10 patients with NMD who were treated by NPPV and assisted coughing immediately after extubation, comparing them with the outcomes of a population of 10 historical control patients who received standard medical therapy (SMT) alone [13]. Need for reintubation despite treatment was evaluated. Significantly fewer patients who received the treatment protocol required reintubation and tracheostomy compared with those who received SMT (reintubation, 3 vs 10; tracheostomy, 3 vs 9; $p = .002$ and .01, respectively). Mortality did not differ significantly between the two groups. Patients undergoing the weaning protocol remained for a shorter time in the respiratory ICU compared with historical controls (7.8 ± 3.9 vs 23.8 ± 15.8 days; $p = .006$).

Finally, MI-E has also been successfully used in the acute setting in the treatment of postoperative sputum retention following major surgery in patients with NMD, permitting quick extubation of subjects with profuse airway secretions. In particular, a case has been reported demonstrating the successful postoperative management of a child with spinal muscular atrophy undergoing a single-stage posterior spinal fusion procedure. An MI-E device was used to successfully treat bronchial mucous encumbrance and avoid a tracheotomy [14].

According to these results, we conclude that MI-E combined with NPPV provides greater success in weaning patients with NMDs from invasive mechanical ventilation than do conventional methods.

Key Major Recommendations

- Ineffective cough with mucous encumbrance is a major cause of mortality and morbidity in patients with NMD who develop ARF.
- A normal cough requires the ability to generate transient PCFs of at least 160 l/min.

- The use of MI-E in combination with NPPV should be considered in the management of mucous retention in patients with NMD developing ARF.
- Preventive application of assisted coughing techniques combined with NPPV after extubation may avert the need for reintubation or tracheostomy.

References

1. Bach JR, Saporito LR. Criteria for extubation and tracheostomy tube removal for patients with ventilatory failure. A different approach to weaning. Chest. 1996;110:1566–71.
2. Toussaint M, Boitano LJ, Gathot V, et al. Limits of effective cough-augmentation techniques in patients with neuromuscular disease. Respir Care. 2009;54:359–66.
3. Chatwin M, Ross E, Hart N, Nickol AH, Polkey MI, Simonds AK. Cough augmentation with mechanical insufflation/exsufflation in patients with neuromuscular weakness. Eur Respir J. 2003;21:502–8.
4. Mustfa N, Aiello M, Lyall RA, et al. Cough augmentation in amyotrophic lateral sclerosis. Neurology. 2003;61:1285–7.
5. Servera E, Sancho J, Zafra MJ, et al. Alternatives to endotracheal intubation for patients with neuromuscular diseases. Am J Phys Med Rehabil. 2005;84:851–7.
6. Vianello A, Corrado A, Arcaro G, et al. Mechanical insufflation-exsufflation improves outcomes for neuromuscular disease patients with respiratory tract infections. Am J Phys Med Rehabil. 2005;84:83–8.
7. Bach JR, Gonçalves M. Ventilator weaning by lung expansion and decannulation. Am J Phys Med Rehabil. 2004;83:560–8.
8. Bach JR, Gonçalves MR, Hamdani I, Winck JC. Extubation of patients with neuromuscular weakness: a new management paradigm. Chest. 2010;137:1033–9.
9. Gonçalves MR, Honrado T, Winck JC, Paiva JA. Effects of mechanical insufflation-exsufflation in preventing respiratory failure after extubation: a randomized controlled trial. Crit Care. 2012;16(2):R48.
10. Epstein SK. Extubation failure: an outcome to be avoided. Crit Care. 2004;8:310–2.
11. Ferrer M, Valencia M, Nicolas JM, et al. Early noninvasive ventilation averts extubation failure in patients at high risk: a randomized trial. Am J Respir Crit Care Med. 2006;173:164–70.
12. Ferrer M, Sellarés J, Valencia M, et al. Non-invasive ventilation after extubation in hypercapnic patients with chronic respiratory disorders: randomised controlled trial. Lancet. 2009;374:1082–8.
13. Vianello A, Arcaro G, Braccioni F, Gallan F, et al. Prevention of extubation failure in high-risk patients with neuromuscular disease. J Crit Care. 2011;26:517–24.
14. Marchant WA, Fox R. Postoperative use of a cough-assist device in avoiding prolonged intubation. Br J Anaesth. 2002;89:644–7.

Role of Complementary Chest Physiotherapy Techniques: Strategies to Prevent Failure During Noninvasive Mechanical Ventilation

25

Sergio R.M. Mateus

Contents

Abbreviations

IPPB Intermittent positive pressure breathing
IPV Intrapulmonary percussive ventilation

25.1 Introduction

Use of noninvasive ventilation in many clinical scenarios, including those with a strong evidence such as in the exacerbation of chronic obstructive pulmonary disease and in cardiogenic pulmonary edemas is agreed upon [1]. However, results noninvasive ventilation can be optimized through the identification of the cause and, consequently, type of respiratory failure, the patient's state of consciousness,

S.R.M. Mateus, PT, MSc, PhD
Assistant Professor, Physical Therapy, Post Graduate Program in Biomedical Engineering, University of Brasília – UnB, Brasília, Brazil
e-mail: sergiomateus@unb.br

A.M. Esquinas (ed.), *Noninvasive Mechanical Ventilation: Theory, Equipment, and Clinical Applications*, DOI 10.1007/978-3-319-21653-9_25

collaboration, and understanding of the procedure, and the adaptation of the interface and the ventilator equipment [2]. Respiratory monitoring during noninvasive ventilatory assistance, along with early identification of the clinical alterations that may occur, can result in an immediate therapeutic intervention.

There are two types of respiratory failure. Type I is characterized by a deficit of oxygenation, that is, hypoxemia, caused by a reduction of regional ventilation and of airway clearance, ineffective coughing, disturbance of the patient's diffusion capacity, and change in ventilation and perfusion. Such alterations take place due to pulmonary parenchyma dysfunction. Type II appears as the ventilatory pump failure allowing ventilation and respiratory disorders, that is, hypercapnia and hypoxemia, to be observed. Alterations in the respiratory drive or respiratory mechanics and neuromuscular disorders can also be noted. It is important to identify the type and cause of the respiratory failure so that the correct physiotherapy technique can be prescribed and the results of the noninvasive ventilation optimized [3]. Independent of the type of respiratory failure, there is frequently an increase in bronchial secretions, either due to an increase in production, as occurs in an infectious process, or to the patient's inability to cough [4]. Such a condition constitutes a risk factor for failure of the noninvasive ventilation [5], and chest physiotherapy techniques may constitute a strategy that can be used in this case [6].

The failure of noninvasive ventilation can be divided into three periods: immediate (<1 h), early (1–48 h), and late (>48 h) [5]. Fifteen percent of failures occur in the immediate period, 68 % in the early period, and 17 % in the late period. The clinical condition that contributes most to failure during the immediate period is a weak cough reflex and/or excessive secretions [5]. Nevertheless, chest physiotherapy measures can effectively contribute to the success of noninvasive ventilation [6]. For a chest physiotherapy technique to be selected, it is necessary to consider the patient's age, severity of disease, the viability of the procedure in terms of practicality and ease of use, patient comfort [4], execution time, and the patient's level of dependency on noninvasive ventilation. The aims of physiotherapy in respiratory dysfunction are to improve global and/or regional ventilation and lung compliance, reduce airway resistance and the work of breathing, and clear airway secretions, consequently oxygenation is optimize by improving ventilation possible to optimize oxygenation by improving ventilation.

25.2 Airway Clearance Techniques

25.2.1 Manual Techniques

25.2.1.1 Percussion, Vibration, and Shaking

Despite the lack of evidence of the effectiveness of manual techniques, we emphasize that these maneuvers depend on the operator, whose must reach a specific frequency and rhythm necessary for the secretion to be dislocated toward a more central airway [7].

Percussion involves rhythmical beating, at a frequency of 3–6 Hz, with properly shaped hands on the chest wall over specific regions of the lungs to remove the mucus. Manual vibration of the chest wall can be performed by placing both hands firmly on the chest wall over the treated region of the lungs and making fast and continuous pressing movements during both inspiration and expiration. Shaking of the chest wall is performed by pressing the sides of the chest wall with flatly placed hands [7]. We suggest that it begin after inspiration. It can be associated with postural drainage for the improvement of the dislocation of secretions. Both percussion and vibration cause air oscillations inside the airway, facilitating mucus transport [7]. These techniques should take into consideration the time of execution in the individual with noninvasive ventilation, due to the risk that the reduction of oxygen may lead to discomfort. Furthermore, to be considered efficient, it must be finished with measures to induce spontaneous coughing, manually assisted coughing, huffing, or aspiration. The technique is contraindicated in cases where the patient has coagulation disorders. With respect to the lack of evidence, it is possible that the clinical outcomes investigated in the studies were not sensitive enough for any clinical difference to be detected [8]. After the performance of manual techniques, assisted or voluntary coughing, huffing, or tracheal aspiration should be induced for the elimination of bronchial secretions.

25.2.2 Cough

25.2.2.1 Cough Evaluation

Coughing has three phases. In the inspiratory phase, it is necessary to maintain the integrity of the inspiratory musculature, pulmonary and thoracic complacency, and the maximum inspiratory effort, which increases the pulmonary volume until it draws near the total pulmonary capacity. The second phase is characterized by the closure of the glottis and a rise in the intrathoracic pressure, which occurs due to the action of bulbar muscles, following the reopening of the glottis in 0.2 s. Finally, there is the expulsion phase, which consists of the liberation of the respiratory flow through the contraction of the expiratory muscles, especially the abdominal muscles [9]. If the patient presents any alterations in any of these phases, it will directly affect the peak flow of the cough. Thus, the peak flow of the cough should be evaluated considering that, below 160 l/min, the cough is ineffective and may predict the failure of noninvasive ventilation; between 160 and 270 l/min, it represents a moderate risk of complication. However, cough assistance measures are effective in the latter context [10]. At this point, strategies for bronchial hygiene can be defined.

25.2.2.2 Cough Assistance

There are three kinds of cough assistance: manual, mechanical, and functional electrical stimulation. In patients receiving noninvasive ventilation, only the manual and mechanical options are used.

25.2.2.3 Manual Assistance

The manually assisted cough consists of the manual compression of the abdomen's epigastric region, which must be synchronized with the moment in which the glottis is opened. It can be performed by the placement of both hands on the abdomen or with one hand on the thoracic region and the other on the abdomen. This technique increases the cough's peak flow [11]; however, it depends on the integrity of the inspiratory musculature or on techniques of maximum insufflation capacity, which ensures the first phase of the cough, inspiratory volume. In addition, the integrity of the bulbar musculature is also required, because it is responsible for glottal control and, consequently, compression of gas. The abdominal compression increases the intra-abdominal pressure, which is transmitted to the thoracic pressure with the dislocation of the diaphragm and the rise in the expiratory flow.

25.2.2.4 Mechanical Assistance or Cough Machine

Cough assist equipment promotes positive pressure during inspiration, assisting the first phase of cough. With the increase in the inspiratory volume, a thoracic expansion can be observed, and, after a few seconds (2–3), the patient is asked to cough. With the glottis open, a negative pressure is applied to promote a suction of the secretion. This system is also known as mechanical insufflation-exsufflation, and the pressure is applied by a mask or mouthpiece. It is important to always begin and end with the inspiratory pressure, thus expanding the lungs before moving to the suction phase of negative pressure. It is also relevant to repeat some of the phases only with inspiration, which is similar to the technique of intermittent positive pressure breathing (IPPB). After the patient is fully adapted and understands the process, the complete cycle may be utilized, that is, positive pressure, insufflation, and negative pressure. Although there is no consensus on the subject, we suggest that the pressure to be applied is around +40 cmH_2O to –60 cmH_2O. It is important to adjust this pressure to the thoracic and pulmonary complacency so that the expansion is adequate to enhance the inspiratory volume and, consequently, the efficiency of the cough. This technique is able to ensure the inspiratory pulmonary volume. In addition, it can be executed quickly and efficiently to eliminate bronchial secretions. The method is applicable to patients using noninvasive ventilation assistance and contributes to the success of the treatment.

Complications such as pneumothorax due to barotrauma, aerophagia, and abdominal distension can occur.

25.2.3 Intrapulmonary Percussive Ventilation

Intrapulmonary percussive ventilation (IPV) equipment provides a pulsatile air flow during inspiration. Based on a method modified from IPPB, IPV generates mini bursts of air with frequencies ranging from 100 to 300 cycles per minute, oscillations from 1.7 to 5 Hz, and pressures from 5 to 35 cm H_2O. The system produces a shock wave from the airways, then the vibration dislocates the secretions, which are conducted by the airflow to the central region. The equipment may be associated with postural drainage [12]. Presenting evidence of level 1, it has also proven to be effective when used in patients with exacerbated chronic obstructive pulmonary diseases, acute respiratory failure, atelectasis [13], and cystic fibrosis [12]. The cooperation of the patient is essential, and during the performance of this technique, the individual will be disconnected from noninvasive ventilation. IPV is also used in cases of noninvasive ventilation though a helmet [14].

25.2.4 Orotracheal and Nasotracheal Aspiration

Aspiration must be carried out when secretions cannot be eliminated. This procedure is, thus, an option for bronchial hygiene. It is executed by the introduction of a suction catheter in the trachea, either orally (orotracheal suctioning) or nasally (nasotracheal suctioning). This technique is not always easy to execute because it is performed blindly, that is, the operator does not have sight of the end of the catheter. We suggest lubricating the nostrils with gel and careful introducing the aspiration catheter, because, when it approaches the epiglottis, the patient's coughing reflex is frequently activated, usually followed by inspiration. At this moment, the catheter is introduced and aims at the trachea, where the suctioning of the secretion is carried out. To optimize the technique and direct the catheter toward the trachea, an oropharyngeal (Fig. 25.1) or a nasopharyngeal (Fig. 25.2) tube may be used. The nasopharyngeal

Fig. 25.1 Position of an oropharyngeal tube in the airway

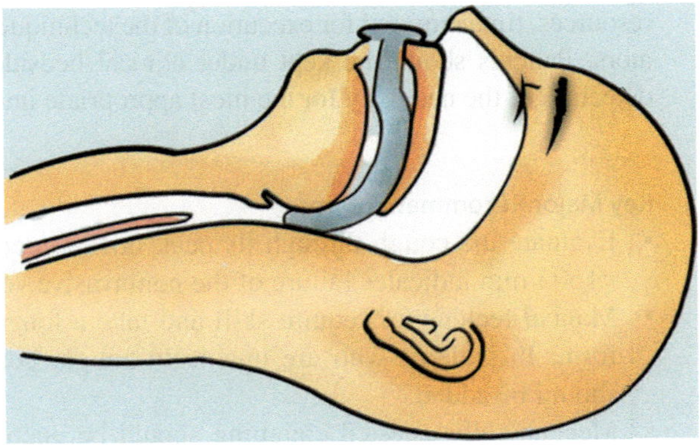

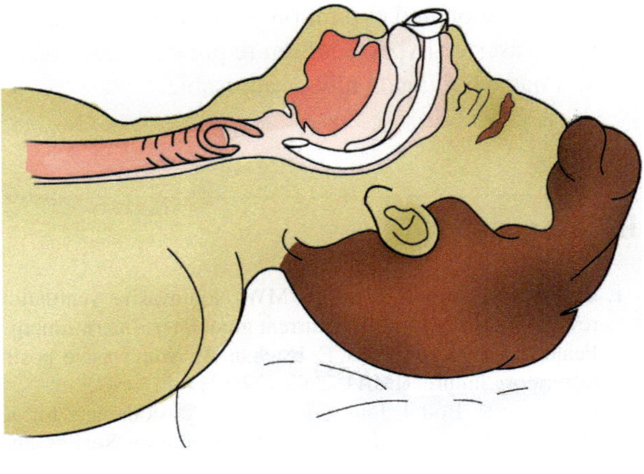

Fig. 25.2 Position of a nasopharyngeal tube in the airway

tube is indicated for hypersecretion, due to the necessity of a higher frequency of aspiration, reducing traumas on the nasal mucosa and on the superior airway. Some measures must be taken before initiating this procedure, including raising the inspired fraction of oxygen. During the performance of suctioning, the patient's oxygenation, cardiovascular function, and perfusion should be monitored [15]. There are many complications associated with this procedure, including bleeding, vomiting, arrhythmia, tachycardia, bradycardia, and cardiac arrest due to vagal stimulation [15]. Hence, this technique should only be utilized as a last resort for bronchial clearance.

Conclusion

An objective of chest physiotherapy techniques is to promote bronchial hygiene to make sure that the patient's airways remain pervious. Therefore, the methods described here contribute to decreasing resistance in the airways and, consequently, respiratory effort, preventing atelectasis and other respiratory complications. In the case of the noninvasive ventilation, tracheal intubation is avoided, leading to more favorable prognoses. There are numerous chest physiotherapy measures that can contribute to the success of noninvasive ventilation. Decisions to undertake such measures are based on scientific evidence, clinical scenario, available material resources, time required for execution of the technique, and experience of the operators. Patients should be kept under clinical bedside monitoring to allow early detection of the necessity for the most appropriate intervention.

Key Major Recommendations

- Evaluate the cough through its peak flow, remembering that an index of <160 l/min indicates failure of the noninvasive ventilation.
- Manual techniques require skill and take a longer period of time to perform. In patients who are unable to cough, cough assistance measures should be added.
- Mechanically assisted coughing should be encouraged as a measure for bronchial clearance because it is useful in two important phases of cough – inspiration and expiration – and can be quickly executed.
- In cases of hypersecretion requiring nasotracheal suctioning, the usage of a nasopharyngeal tube is advisable.

References

1. Berg KM, Clardy P, Donnino MW. Noninvasive ventilation for acute respiratory failure: a review of the literature and current guidelines. Intern Emerg Med. 2012;7:539–45.
2. Penuelas O, Frutos-Vivar F, Esteban A. Noninvasive positive-pressure ventilation in acute respiratory failure. CMAJ. 2007;177:1211–8.
3. Gosselink R, Bott J, Johnson M, et al. Physiotherapy for adult patients with critical illness: recommendations of the European Respiratory Society and European Society of Intensive

Care Medicine Task Force on Physiotherapy for Critically Ill Patients. Intensive Care Med. 2008;34:1188–99.
4. Volsko TA. Airway clearance therapy: finding the evidence. Respir Care. 2013;58:1669–78.
5. Ozyilmaz E, Ugurlu AO, Nava S. Timing of noninvasive ventilation failure: causes, risk factors, and potential remedies. BMC Pulm Med. 2014;14:19.
6. British Thoracic Society Standards of Care C. Non-invasive ventilation in acute respiratory failure. Thorax. 2002;57:192–211.
7. van der Schans CP, Postma DS, Koeter GH, Rubin BK. Physiotherapy and bronchial mucus transport. Eur Respir J. 1999;13:1477–86.
8. Rubin BK. Designing clinical trials to evaluate mucus clearance therapy. Respir Care. 2007;52:1348–58; discussion 58–61.
9. Flume PA. Airway clearance techniques. Semin Respir Crit Care Med. 2003;24:727–36.
10. Kang SW, Bach JR. Maximum insufflation capacity: vital capacity and cough flows in neuromuscular disease. Am J Phys Med Rehabil. 2000;79:222–7.
11. Bach JR. Mechanical insufflation-exsufflation. Comparison of peak expiratory flows with manually assisted and unassisted coughing techniques. Chest. 1993;104:1553–62.
12. Bott J, Blumenthal S, Buxton M, et al. Guidelines for the physiotherapy management of the adult, medical, spontaneously breathing patient. Thorax. 2009;64 Suppl 1:i1–51.
13. Deakins K, Chatburn RL. A comparison of intrapulmonary percussive ventilation and conventional chest physiotherapy for the treatment of atelectasis in the pediatric patient. Respir Care. 2002;47:1162–7.
14. Antonaglia V, Lucangelo U, Zin WA, et al. Intrapulmonary percussive ventilation improves the outcome of patients with acute exacerbation of chronic obstructive pulmonary disease using a helmet. Crit Care Med. 2006;34:2940–5.
15. AARC Clinical Practice Guideline. Nasotracheal suctioning—2004 revision & update. Respir Care. 2004;49:1080–4.

Noninvasive Ventilation in Cardiovascular Rehabilitation

26

Vinicius Zacarias Maldaner da Silva, Gerson Cipriano Jr., and Graziela Franca Bernadelli Cipriano

Contents

Abbreviations

BPAP	Bi-level positive airway pressure
COPD	Chronic obstructive pulmonary disease
CPAP	Continuous positive airway pressure
DH	Dynamic hyperinflation
EPAP	End positive airway pressure
HF	Heart failure
LV	Left ventricular

V.Z.M. da Silva, PT, PhD (✉)
Hospital de Base do Distrito Federal, Brasilia, Brazil

Division of Physical Therapy, University of Brasilia, SQS 215 Bloco A apto 305 ASA SUL, 70294–010, Brasília, DF, Brazil
e-mail: viniciusmaldaner@gmail.com

G. Cipriano Jr., PT, PhD • G.F.B. Cipriano
Division of Physical Therapy, University of Brasilia, SQS 215 Bloco A apto 305 ASA SUL, 70294–010, Brasília, DF, Brazil

A.M. Esquinas (ed.), *Noninvasive Mechanical Ventilation: Theory, Equipment, and Clinical Applications*, DOI 10.1007/978-3-319-21653-9_26

NIV	Noninvasive ventilation
PT	Peak torque
Pw	Peak work
TW	Total work

26.1 Introduction

Patients with heart failure (HF) are often prematurely functionally limited as a result of excessive fatigue, dyspnea, or a combination of both, independent of etiology. Pathophysiological abnormalities specific to HF, such as metabolic derangements in skeletal muscle, peripheral blood flow reduction, and excessive ventilator requirements (leading to inspiratory muscle fatigue and increased muscle metaboreflex) have been documented [1–4] and are related to exercise intolerance and respiratory muscle weakness. These abnormalities may limit these patients in performing at moderate-to-high intensity or for an adequate time during an exercise training rehabilitation protocol, which can reduce the beneficial physiological effects [5]. The use of noninvasive ventilation (NIV) support during rehabilitation sessions has been proposed as an alternative to improve exercise tolerance and cardiopulmonary performance. This chapter discusses the major concepts regarding use of NIV during cardiopulmonary rehabilitation and its level of evidence.

26.2 Discussion and Analysis

26.2.1 Effect of NIV on Hemodynamic Parameters

Positive airway pressure appears to enhance cardiac function in patients with HF [6]. During a regular cardiac rehabilitation program, acute cardiovascular adjustments are required to maintain an adequate blood flow supply to activated muscles. During resistance exercise training, ventilatory effort rises and greater inspiratory pleural pressure is required to maintain ventilation in pace with metabolic demands. Therefore, an increase in negative pleural pressure would increase both the left ventricular (LV) transmural pressure gradient and LV afterload [4]. Previous studies have demonstrated that positive airway pressure decreases the large variations in pleural pressure during the effort and, consequently, reduces LV afterload, thereby improving contractile performance of the heart during exercise [7, 8].

Another mechanism that may be involved with changes in hemodynamic behavior during NIV is the decrease in LV preload. During a regular ventilation cycle, within two pressure levels, the increase in intrathoracic pressure elevates right atrial pressure, which results in decreased venous return, followed by a reduction in LV filling. This results in enhanced LV performance in patients with HF [9]. Therefore, it is suggested that improvements in cardiac function with the application of positive airway pressure is the result of augmented LV filling and decreased LV afterload [10].

During a submaximal evaluation (6-min walk test), Chermont et al. [11] and Lima Eda et al. [12] did not report significant modifications in systolic blood pressure and heart rate in patients with HF when continuous positive airway pressure (CPAP) was applied before the exercise. However, in agreement with our study [13], which demonstrated a cardiorespiratory improvement during a resistance protocol when bi-level positive airway pressure (BPAP) was applied during the exercise, O'Donnell et al. [14] has also demonstrated that BPAP improves cardiorespiratory responses during a maximum cardiopulmonary test in the same population. These differences in responses between CPAP and BPAP may reflect additional beneficial effects of BPAP and the application during exercise, which can produce a lower pulmonary capillary wedge pressure and expiratory flow limitation during exercise.

26.2.2 Effects of NIV on Functional Performance

Silva et al. [13] demonstrated that NIV reduces quadriceps fatigability (lower Δ peak torque (PT), Δ total work (TW), and Δ peak work (Pw), $p<0.05$) during an isokinetic resistance exercise protocol. Bhorgi-Silva et al. [15] previously demonstrated similar results in fatigability reduction in patients with chronic obstructive pulmonary disease (COPD) utilizing the same ventilatory strategy.

This improvement could be explained by the increase in perfusion to working skeletal muscle during ventilatory unloading. Previous studies have shown augmentation of total respiratory work increases noradrenaline levels and reduces leg blood flow during exercise [16]. Moreover, other studies have demonstrated an increase in blood flow to active skeletal muscle during diaphragm muscle unloading [17]. As an example, Harms et al. [18] previously demonstrated ventilatory muscle unloading with a different NIV approach (proportional assisted ventilation that increased leg blood flow).

In addition, increased metabolic stimulation of small afferent fibers (types III and IV) from the respiratory musculature, especially from the diaphragm [19], may contribute to physical activity limitations in this patient population. Activation of this mechanism during exercise seems to induce inspiratory muscle fatigue and may also contribute to the reduction in blood flow to the active skeletal muscle [20]. Therefore, the application of NIV during exercise could possibly attenuate the inspiratory metaboreflex impact on physical performance, but this hypothesis requires further investigation.

26.2.3 NIV for Dynamic Hyperinflation

The dynamic hyperinflation (DH) observed in patients with COPD leads to dyspnea and limits the capacity to perform exercise training. The use of NIV to decrease DH during exercise has been documented [21]. The mechanism thought to promote this attenuation in exercise DH is the reduction of expiratory dynamic airway compression. Application of expiratory positive airway pressure (EPAP) may increase bronchial pressure and consequently transmural pressure, leading to a diminution of airway collapse [22]. Additionally, EPAP should reduce the inspiratory threshold load on the inspiratory muscles of patients with COPD with hyperinflation and enhance neuromuscular coupling [22]

26.2.4 Level of Evidence

Two recent meta-analyses demonstrated that NIV increases functional capacity (evaluated by a 6-min walk test, Figs. 26.1 and 26.2) and quality of life in patients with HF and also those with COPD [23, 24]. However, the methodological quality and sample size is low and new studies should be encouraged to investigate

	NIV			Control				Mean Difference
Study or Subgroup	Mean	SD	Total	Mean	SD	Total	Weight	IV, Fixed, 95% CI
1.3.1 Percentage change peak work rate								
Hawkins 2002	32.9	17.4	10	14.5	10.1	9	64.8%	18.40 [5.76, 31.04]
Johnson 2002	50	35.4	11	38	35	11	12.0%	12.00 [-17.42, 41.42]
Reuxeny 2005	24.5	20.7	9	8.8	26.2	10	23.2%	15.70 [-5.43, 36.83]
Subtotal (95% CI)			**30**			**30**	**100.0%**	**17.01 [6.83, 27.19]**
Heterogeneity: Chi² = 0.17, df = 2 (P = 0.92); I² = 0%								
Test for overall effect: Z = 3.27 (P = 0.001)								
1.3.2 Percentage change constant work rate endurance time								
Hawkins 2002	123	97.2	10	74	50.1	9	64.2%	49.00 [-19.56, 117.56]
xan't Hul 2006	164	124	15	88	128	14	35.8%	76.00 [-15.83, 167.83]
Subtotal (95% CI)			**25**			**23**	**100.0%**	**58.66 [3.72, 113.60]**
Heterogeneity: Chi² = 0.21, df = 1 (P = 0.64); I² = 0%								
Test for overall effect: Z = 2.09 (P = 0.04)								

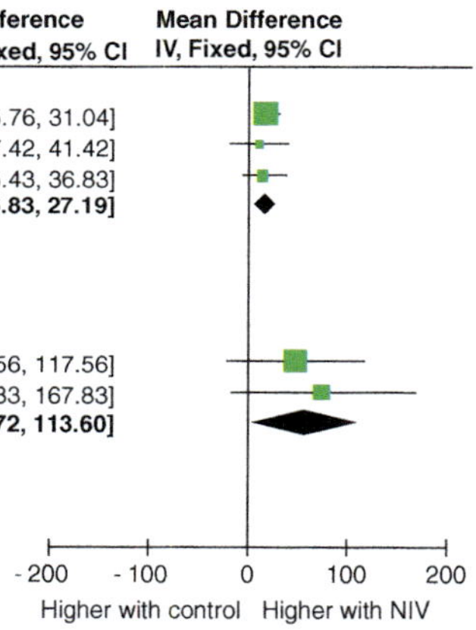

Fig. 26.1 Forest plot comparing exercise capacity in protocols with NIV during exercise training versus exercise training in patients with COPD (Withdraw from Ricci et al. [23])

	CPAP			Control/Sham				
Study or subgroup	Mean	SD	Total	Mean	SD	Total	Weig	Mean difference IV, Fixed, 95% CI
Chermont et al.[4] 2009	507	33	12	446	36	12	91.9%	61.00 [33.37, 88.63]
Lima et al.[5] 2011	534	89.9	6	420	73.8	6	8.1%	114.00 [20.93, 207.07]
Total (95% CI)			**18**			**18**	**100%**	**65.29 [38.80, 91.78]**
Heterogeneity: Chi2 = 1.14, df = 1 (P = 0.28): I² = 13%;								
Test for overall effect: Z = 4.83 (P < 0.00001)								

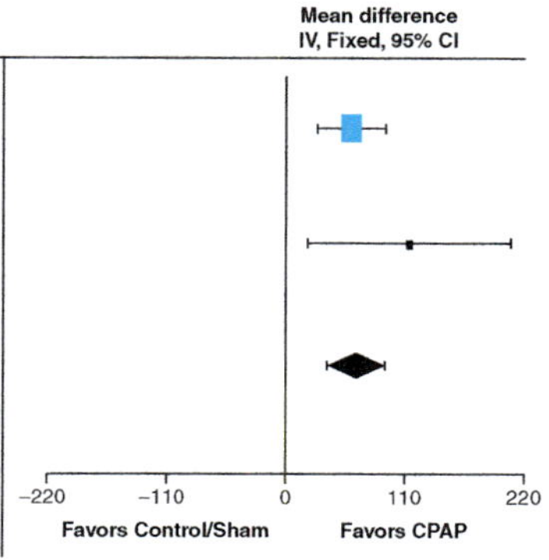

Fig. 26.2 Forest plot comparing 6-min walk test in two different protocols: CPAP×control/sham group in patients with HF (Withdraw from: Bundchen et al. [24])

physiological effects, best parameters, and NIV modalities to allow successful use of NIV during exercise.

Conclusion

NIV has emerged as a complementary therapy during cardiovascular rehabilitation programs to improve exercise tolerance and possibly optimize skeletal muscle and cardiopulmonary benefits during cardiovascular rehabilitation.

Key Major Recommendations

- Despite the growing body of the literature about NIV during cardiac rehabilitation protocols, the actual available evidence supports this application to improve exercise tolerance and walking distance.
- Clinicians must have expertise in the implementation NIV during exercise to choose the best NIV modality, pressure level, and application to achieve better responses in patients with HF and also those with COPD.

The authors have no conflicts of interest to disclose.

References

1. Clark AL, Harrington D, Chua TP, Coats AJ. Exercise capacity in chronic heart failure is related to the aetiology of heart disease. Heart. 1997;78:569–71.
2. Harrington D, Coats AJ. Skeletal muscle abnormalities and evidence for their role in symptom generation in chronic heart failure. Eur Heart J. 1997;18:1865–72.
3. Harrington D, Clark AL, Chua TP, Anker SD, Poole-Wilson PA, Coats AJ. Effect of reduced muscle bulk on the ventilatory response to exercise in chronic congestive heart failure secondary to idiopathic dilated and ischemic cardiomyopathy. Am J Cardiol. 1997;80:90–3.
4. Yan AT, Bradley TD, Liu PP. The role of continuous positive airway pressure in the treatment of congestive heart failure. Chest. 2001;120:1675–85.
5. Guazzi M, Adams V, Conraads V, Halle M, Mezzani A, Vanhees L, Arena R, Fletcher GF, Forman DE, Kitzman DW, Lavie CJ, Myers J, EACPR, AHA. EACPR/AHA Joint Scientific Statement. Clinical recommendations for cardiopulmonary exercise testing data assessment in specific patient populations. Eur Heart J. 2012;33:2917–27.
6. Naughton MT, Rahman MA, Hara K, Floras JS, Bradley TD. Effect of continuous positive airway pressure on intrathoracic and left ventricular transmural pressures in patients with congestive heart failure. Circulation. 1995;91:1725–31.
7. Lalande S, Luoma CE, Miller AD, Johnson BD. Effect of changes in intrathoracic pressure on cardiac function at rest and during moderate exercise in health and heart failure. Exp Physiol. 2012;97:248–56.
8. Lalande S, Johnson BD. Breathing strategy to preserve exercising cardiac function in patients with heart failure. Med Hypotheses. 2010;74:416–21.
9. Grace MP, Greenbaum DM. Cardiac performance in response to PEEP in patients with cardiac dysfunction. Crit Care Med. 1982;10:358–60.
10. Pinsky MR, Matuschak GM, Klain M. Determinants of cardiac augmentation by elevations in intrathoracic pressure. J Appl Physiol. 1985;58:1189–98.
11. Chermont S, Quintao MM, Mesquita ET, Rocha NN, Nobrega AC. Noninvasive ventilation with continuous positive airway pressure acutely improves 6-minute walk distance in chronic heart failure. J Cardiopulm Rehabil Prev. 2009;29:44–8.

12. Lima Eda S, Cruz CG, Santos FC, Gomes-Neto M, Bittencourt HS, Reis FJ, Aras R, Guimaraes AC, Rodrigues-Junior ES. Effect of ventilatory support on functional capacity in patients with heart failure: a pilot study. Arq Bras Cardiol. 2011;96:227–32.
13. da Silva VZ, Lima A, Cipriano GB, da Silva ML, Campos FV, Arena R, Martins WR, Chiappa G, Bottaro M, Cipriano G. Noninvasive ventilation improves the cardiovascular response and fatigability during resistance exercise in patients with heart failure. J Cardiopulm Rehabil Prev. 2013;33:378–84.
14. O'Donnell DE, D'Arsigny C, Raj S, Abdollah H, Webb KA. Ventilatory assistance improves exercise endurance in stable congestive heart failure. Am J Respir Crit Care Med. 1999;160:1804–11.
15. Borghi-Silva A, Di Thommazo L, Pantoni CB, Mendes RG, Salvini Tde F, Costa D. Noninvasive ventilation improves peripheral oxygen saturation and reduces fatigability of quadriceps in patients with COPD. Respirology. 2009;14:537–44.
16. Ribeiro JP, Chiappa GR, Callegaro CC. The contribution of inspiratory muscles function to exercise limitation in heart failure: pathophysiological mechanisms. Rev Bras Fisioter. 2012;16:261–7.
17. Harms CA, Wetter TJ, McClaran SR, Pegelow DF, Nickele GA, Nelson WB, Hanson P, Dempsey JA. Effects of respiratory muscle work on cardiac output and its distribution during maximal exercise. J Appl Physiol. 1998;85:609–18.
18. Harms CA, Babcock MA, McClaran SR, Pegelow DF, Nickele GA, Nelson WB, Dempsey JA. Respiratory muscle work compromises leg blood flow during maximal exercise. J Appl Physiol. 1997;82:1573–83.
19. Hill JM. Discharge of group IV phrenic afferent fibers increases during diaphragmatic fatigue. Brain Res. 2000;856:240–4.
20. Callegaro CC, Ribeiro JP, Tan CO, Taylor JA. Attenuated inspiratory muscle metaboreflex in endurance-trained individuals. Respir Physiol Neurobiol. 2011;177:24–9.
21. Stather DR, Stewart TE. Clinical review: mechanical ventilation in severe asthma. Crit Care. 2005;9:581–7.
22. Pessoa IM, Costa D, Velloso M, Mancuzo E, Reis MA, Parreira VF. Effects of noninvasive ventilation on dynamic hyperinflation of patients with COPD during activities of daily living with upper limbs. Rev Bras Fisioter. 2012;16:61–7.
23. Ricci C, et al. Physical training and noninvasive ventilation in COPD patients: a meta-analysis. Respir Care. 2014;59(5):709–17.
24. Bundchen D, et al. Noninvasive ventilation and exercise tolerance in heart failure: a systematic review and meta-analysis. Braz J Phys Ther. 2014;18(5):385–94.

Noninvasive Ventilation: Factors Influencing Carbon Dioxide Rebreathing – Key Practical Implications

27

Jacek Nasiłowski

Contents

Abbreviations

CO_2	Carbon dioxide
EPAP	Expiratory positive airway pressure
$FiCO_2$	Fraction of inspiratory CO_2
ICU	Intensive care unit
NIV	Noninvasive ventilation
Vte	Exhaled tidal volume
Vti	Inspiratory tidal volume

J. Nasiłowski, MD, PhD
Department of Internal Medicine, Pneumology and Allergology, Medical University of Warsaw, ul. Banacha 1a, Warsaw 02-097, Poland
e-mail: jnasilowski@wum.edu.pl

A.M. Esquinas (ed.), *Noninvasive Mechanical Ventilation: Theory, Equipment, and Clinical Applications*, DOI 10.1007/978-3-319-21653-9_27

27.1 Introduction

Noninvasive ventilation (NIV) may increase the risk of carbon dioxide (CO_2) rebreathing for two reasons: firstly, the single-limb circuit that is preferentially used for NIV causes patients to exhale into the same space from which they inhale, and, secondly, the interfaces used for NIV increase dead space.

As the main indication for NIV is hypoventilation resulting in hypercapnia [1], whether the side effects of ventilation will overcome the aim of the therapy seems to be a crucial issue. This question is particularly important in the treatment of the acute episodes of chronic disease, when hypercapnia is usually much greater and can cause life-threatening respiratory acidosis. Moreover, in the acute setting, interfaces covering the nose and mouth with a larger volume of dead space (oronasal masks, total face masks, and helmets) are the interfaces of choice [2].

There are a few issues concerning CO_2 rebreathing. Firstly, it is not clear whether CO_2 rebreathing is only a theoretical problem or if it has an important clinical significance, translating into failure of NIV. There is no conclusive proof, for example, reported cases, that CO_2 rebreathing during NIV caused a need of intubation. However, as a potential drawback of NIV, it must be always a concern of the physician. Secondly, the assessment of fraction of inspiratory CO_2 ($FiCO_2$) is not technically an easy procedure and physicians are not able to measure it during everyday practice. Thirdly, there are only a few studies that have evaluated this issue, and most of them were carried out in lung models [3–6] or healthy volunteers [4, 7], which cannot perfectly imitate *in vivo* conditions. The most informative study on patients was that of Szkulmowski et al. [8]. They evaluated $FiCO_2$ in patients with respiratory failure hospitalized in an intensive care unit (ICU). Seven subjects were ventilated noninvasively with oronasal mask and 11 invasively. All of them used a single-limb circuit with a leak port and pressure support mode of ventilation (mean inspiratory positive airway pressure (IPAP) 23.9 ± 6.0 mmHg; mean expiratory positive airway pressure (EPAP) 7.3 ± 1.8 mmHg). The authors found that only 19 % of all inhaled breaths had $FiCO_2 > 0.1$ %. The mean $FiCO_2$ of those breaths was 0.27 ± 0.33 %, whereas the average $FiCO_2$ of all breaths was 0.072 ± 0.17 %, which is close to the concentration of CO_2 in the air (0.03 %). Four factors were significantly correlated with higher $FiCO_2$:

1. High level of end tidal CO_2
2. Low EPAP
3. High respiratory rate
4. And, surprisingly, invasive versus noninvasive ventilation

NIV should provoke higher CO_2 rebreathing due to larger dead space, caused by an interface comparable to an endotracheal tube, which reduces dead space. However, lower $FiCO_2$ may be easily explained by the presence of unintentional leaks during NIV. And it seems to be a self-correcting mechanism, which can protect against CO_2 rebreathing [9].

27.2 Mask Ventilation

Treatment with NIV can be performed by three different circuit systems: dual-limb circuit, single-limb circuit with exhalation valve, and single-limb circuit with exhalation port (leak port).

27.2.1 Dual-Limb Circuit

A dual-limb circuit is a traditional ventilator system used broadly in ICUs with invasive ventilation. It consists of one inhalation limb that introduces air into the patient's airways and one exhalation limb that leads exhaled gas outside of the airways. This system prevents the mixing of exhaled gas with inhalation gas. The risk of rebreathing of exhaled CO_2 comes from the enlarged dead space created by an interface and the part of the circuit situated distally from Y-piece valve. To prevent CO_2 rebreathing, one must take care to increase the exhaled tidal volume (Vte) by the amount of the volume of additional dead space. Increasing only an inspiratory tidal volume (Vti) may not effectively reduce the risk of reinhalation due to an unknown volume of inhaled gases escaping with unintentional leaks, which to a larger or smaller extent are always present between the mask and the skin of the patient's face.

27.2.2 Single-Limb Circuit with Exhalation Valve

A single-limb circuit with an exhalation valve is rarely used in acute settings but is quite popular in chronic ventilation. A unidirectional valve is located in the patient's end of a limb. The valve is closed on inspiration and opens on expiration, allowing the exhaled gas to leave the respiratory circuit. A unidirectional valve system prevents mixing of inhaled and exhaled gases and prevents CO_2 rebreathing [10]. As in a double-limb circuit, this circuit enlarges dead space by the volume of interface and the distal part of the circuit situated between the valve and interface. The clinician must be aware of the additional volume and increase Vte accordingly.

27.2.3 Single-Limb Circuit with Exhalation Port (Leak Port)

A single-limb circuit with an exhalation port is most frequently used at home and in the hospital. The exhalation port located within an interface or in a distal part of a tube is open throughout the entire respiratory cycle. In this scenario, inhaled and exhaled gases mix easily during every breath in the inner space of the interface and the risk of CO_2 rebreathing has to be taken into consideration. The empting of the exhaled gas from the interface space depends on

1. The expiratory flow
2. The distance between the exhalation port and nose and/or mouth (dynamic dead space)

Table 27.1 Factors increasing the risk of CO_2 rebreathing during mask ventilation with a single-limb circuit with exhalation port

Domain	Factor
Ventilatory settings	Low CPAP
	Low inspiratory:exspiratory ratio
	Short inspiratory time
	High respiratory rate
Interface	High inner volume
Exhalation port	Large distance from nose and mouth
	High resistance of the holes
Patient	High $PaCO_2$
	Rapid pattern of breathing

3. The volume of the interface (static dead space)
4. The patient's breathing pattern (the time of expiration)

In practice, unintentional leaks also play a role, but they cannot be taken into consideration, although the aim is to reduce them as much as possible. To clear the mask space of exhaled CO_2, it is necessary to set the EPAP to provide an intentional leak that exceeds patient expiratory flow. In the mid-1990s, Lofaso et al. [11] studied the flow-though Whisper Swivel connector, which is located between a mask and the distal end of a circuit. They found that, at the level of EPAP 5 cmH_2O, the intentional leak was 200 ml/s, which means that during respiration with higher tidal volume (e.g., 500 ml) or shorter expiratory time (e.g., 1 s), expiratory gas cannot be fully washed out at this setting. EPAP had to be increased in such a respiratory pattern scenario. The higher the EPAP level, the faster the venting of the interface space and the lower the risk of CO_2 rebreathing. Ferguson et al. [10] proved that EPAP below 4–6 cmH_2O markedly increased CO_2 rebreathing. The EPAP level is the factor that can most easily be corrected by a physician, and it should be adjusted according to the static and dynamic dead space, breathing pattern, and actual level of $PaCO_2$.

The second relatively easily modifiable element of mask ventilation is the location of the leak port. Saatci et al. [12] proved that an exhalation port over the nasal bridge reduces dynamic (effective) dead space to a higher extent than ports positioned elsewhere within the mask. The dynamic dead space was the largest when the port was situated between the mask and circuit. Moreover, the relationship between static dead space (inner volume of the interface) and dynamic dead space is quite poor. This means that even an interface with a larger volume, for example, a total face mask, can have small dynamic dead space if the flow of gas through the mask is effective. Table 27.1 lists the factors that increase the risk of CO_2 rebreathing. Up-to-date ventilators and interfaces strive to protect against rebreathing. The pressure support ventilation setting and circuits with an exhalation port do not allow reduction of EPAP below a certain level (2–4 cmH_2O), and an alarm sounds if too little leakage occurs. Masks have a leak port located close to the nose to reduce effective dead space.

27.3 Helmet Ventilation

A helmet is an interface that has an extremely large internal volume, up to 10 l, which constitutes a huge dead space, promoting CO_2 rebreathing [4, 13]. In fact, a helmet cannot be considered as an interface *sensu stricto*. It is rather a kind of hermetic tent over the patient's head, with the aim of creating a high-pressure environment for the respiratory system. The pressure is maintained by the constant flow of gas that enters by the inspiratory limb and exits by the exhalation limb. The internal volume of a helmet is much larger than the patient's tidal volume. The patient takes a breath from the gas located under the helmet and then exhales into this specific semi-closed atmosphere. However, the volume of a helmet does not correspond to effective dead space. Fodil et al. [14], using a mathematical model, estimated the effective dead space of a helmet by analyzing the pressure field/flow pattern. They found that effective dead space consists of only 4 % of helmet gas volume due to the streaming effect. Exhaled CO_2 is diluted in internal gas volume and inhaled gas may be only slightly enriched with CO_2. To correctly perform NIV with a helmet, sufficient gas flow has to be provided. The flow is aimed not only to maintain adequate expiratory and inspiratory pressures but also to constantly extract CO_2 from the inner space. The concentration of CO_2 in the helmet gas is dependent on $PaCO_2$ [6]. Thereupon, the flow must be adjusted according to the level of patient's hypercapnia and generally should exceed 30 l/min.

Antonelli et al. [15] published one of the first studies comparing efficacy of helmet NIV and NIV with mask in hypercapnic respiratory failure. In this matched case control study, the efficacy of helmet NIV was worse in terms of reducing $PaCO_2$, which may confirm the important role of CO_2 rebreathing in the treatment effects. However, lesser efficacy of ventilation could partly be attributed to worse patient-ventilator synchronization in comparison with mask ventilation. In a randomized study published in 2015 by Pisani et al. [16], a new model of helmet, specifically designed to improve performance in hypercapnic patients, was tested in comparison with oronasal mask. The novel helmet (CaStar R Next, StarMed, Mirandola, Italy) has less internal volume than standard ones. Moreover, the authors used ventilator settings specifically focused on optimization of patient-ventilator synchronization: fast rate of pressurization and a cycling-off threshold between 25 and 50 % of maximal inspiratory flow. The pressures were titrated to provide a flow inside the helmet >30 l/min. The mean inspiratory and expiratory pressures were 19.6 ± 5.7 cmH_2O and 7.7 ± 1.9 cmH_2O, respectively, which was ~30 % higher than in mask ventilation. The results showed the same efficacy in improving hypercapnia and respiratory acidosis in both groups.

Current evidence authorizes the use of helmet ventilation in hypercapnic respiratory failure. However, a physician must take into account the higher risk of CO_2 rebreathing than with ventilation with a mask. Higher pressures, proportionally to $PaCO_2$ of the patient, are needed and close monitoring should be applied.

Key Recommendations

- CO_2 rebreathing occurs during mask ventilation with a single-limb circuit with exhalation port and during helmet ventilation.
- In spite of a lack of convincing evidence, CO_2 rebreathing must be treated as a potential risk factor of NIV failure.
- To avoid CO_2 rebreathing, adequate EPAP (mask ventilation) and flow-by (helmet ventilation) must be provided, adjusted to $PaCO_2$, respiratory rate, and effective dead space of the interface.

References

1. Muir J-F, Molano C, Cuvelier A. NIV and obstructive lung diseases. Eur Respir Mon. 2008;41: 203–23.
2. Crimi C, Noto A, Princi P, et al. A European survey of noninvasive ventilation practices. Eur Respir J. 2010;36:362–9.
3. Loeppky JA, Icenogle MV, Caprihan A, et al. CO2 rebreathing model in COPD: blood-to-gas equilibration. Eur J Appl Physiol. 2006;98:450–60.
4. Taccone P, Hess D, Caironi P, et al. Continuous positive airway pressure delivered with a "helmet": effects on carbon dioxide rebreathing. Crit Care Med. 2004;32:2090–6.
5. Schettino GP, Chatmongkolchart S, Hess DR, et al. Position of exhalation port and mask design affect CO2 rebreathing during noninvasive positive pressure ventilation. Crit Care Med. 2003;31:2178–82.
6. Mojoli F, Iotti GA, Gerletti M, et al. Carbon dioxide rebreathing during non-invasive ventilation delivered by helmet: a bench study. Intensive Care Med. 2008;34:1454–60.
7. Samolski D, Calaf N, Güell R, et al. Carbon dioxide rebreathing in non-invasive ventilation. Analysis of masks, expiratory ports and ventilatory modes. Monaldi Arch Chest Dis. 2008;69: 114–8.
8. Szkulmowski Z, Belkhouja K, Le QH, et al. Bilevel positive airway pressure ventilation: factors influencing carbon dioxide rebreathing. Intensive Care Med. 2010;36:688–91.
9. Hill NS, Carlisle C, Kramer NR. Effect of a nonrebreathing exhalation valve on long-term nasal ventilation using a bilevel device. Chest. 2002;122:84–91.
10. Ferguson GT, Gilmartin M. CO_2 rebreathing during BiPAP ventilatory assistance. Am J Respir Crit Care Med. 1995;151:1126–35.
11. Lofaso F, Brochard L, Hang T, et al. Home versus intensive care pressure support devices. Experimental and clinical comparison. Am J Respir Crit Care Med. 1996;153:1591–9.
12. Saatci E, Miller DM, Stell IM, et al. Dynamic dead space in face masks used with noninvasive ventilators: a lung model study. Eur Respir J. 2004;23:129–35.
13. Esquinas AM, Papadakos PJ, Carron M, et al. Clinical review: helmet and non-invasive mechanical ventilation in critically ill patients. Crit Care. 2013;17:223.
14. Fodil R, Lellouche F, Mancebo J, et al. Comparison of patient–ventilator interfaces based on their computerized effective dead space. Intensive Care Med. 2011;37:257–62.
15. Antonelli M, Pennisi MA, Pelosi P, et al. Noninvasive positive pressure ventilation using a helmet in patients with acute exacerbation of chronic obstructive pulmonary disease: a feasibility study. Anesthesiology. 2004;100:16–24.
16. Pisani L, Mega C, Vaschetto R, et al. Oronasal mask versus helmet in acute hypercapnic respiratory failure. Eur Respir J. 2015;45:691–9.

Part III

Clinical Applications: Pre and Intra Hospital

Noninvasive Mechanical Ventilation in Hypoxemic Respiratory Failure: Determinants of Response and Patients' Flow Chart Recommendations – Key Topics and Clinical Implications

28

Roberto Cosentini and Tommaso Maraffi

Contents

Abbreviations

ACPE Acute cardiogenic pulmonary edema
DNI Do not intubate
ETI Endotracheal intubation
IBW Ideal body weight

R. Cosentini, MD (✉)
Fondazione IRCCS Ca' Granda Ospedale Maggiore Policlinico, Pronto Soccorso e Medicina d'Urgenza, Milan, Italy

Gruppo NIV_UOC Pronto Soccorso e Pronto Soccorso e Medicina d'Urgenza, Milan, Italy
e-mail: r.cosentini@gmail.com

T. Maraffi, MD
Dipartimento di Fisiopatologia Medico-Chirurgica e dei Trapianti, Universita' degli Studi di Milano, Milan, Italy
e-mail: tommaso.maraffi@gmail.com

A.M. Esquinas (ed.), *Noninvasive Mechanical Ventilation: Theory, Equipment, and Clinical Applications*, DOI 10.1007/978-3-319-21653-9_28

NPPV	Non-invasive positive pressure ventilation
NPPV	Noninvasive positive pressure ventilation
PEEP	Positive end-expiratory pressure
PS	Pressure support
Vt	Tidal volume

28.1 Introduction

Acute hypoxemic respiratory failure (AHRF) is one of the most common conditions of severe dyspnea seen in the emergency department. This chapter summarizes the main indications for noninvasive positive pressure ventilation (NPPV) in AHRF, with a focus on evidence, clinical recommendations, and practical points.

28.2 Acute Cardiogenic Pulmonary Edema

The literature and rationale for noninvasive ventilation (NIV) use in acute cardiogenic pulmonary edema (ACPE) are discussed in detail in Chap. 27 of this book; we summarize it briefly here:

- NIV treatment in ACPE significantly reduces endotracheal intubation (ETI) and mortality, as evidenced by several systematic reviews and a meta-analysis.
- The number needed to treat (NNT) for ETI is 8 and is 13 for mortality. Therefore, there is a strong recommendation for NIV in ACPE, based on a high level of evidence.
- ACPE is also effectively treated with NIV in the prehospital setting.

When treating a patient with ACPE in the emergency department, two main clinical questions must be answered:

1. Should the patient with hypercapnia be treated with bi-level NPPV rather than CPAP?
2. Does the patient with hypertensive ACPE have a different prognosis compared with a patient who is nonhypertensive?

28.2.1 Bi-level NPPV Versus CPAP: Are Two Better than One?

As many as 50 % of patients treated with NIV for ACPE present with acute respiratory failure. This is due to muscle fatigue induced by a remarkable decrease of compliance resulting from sudden alveolar flooding. The theoretical advantage for muscle workload of the addition of pressure support (PS) to positive end-expiratory pressure (PEEP) versus continuous positive airway pressure (CPAP) is not demonstrated in the literature. Several randomized studies and a meta-analysis showed faster relief of respiratory acidosis; however, neither ETI nor mortality differed significantly between the two modalities. The Cochrane Review on NPPV efficacy in ACPE concludes, "CPAP may be considered the first option in selection of NPPV due to more robust evidence for its effectiveness and safety and lower cost compared with bilevel NPPV" [1]. This may be explained by the rapid favorable effects of PEEP application on both respiration (alveolar recruitment + compliance increase) and circulation (venous return decrease + left ventricle transmural pressure decrease). In summary, in patients with ACPE who have acute respiratory acidosis, NIV and CPAP are equivalent; hence, our advice is to use the treatment that you prefer and are most familiar with.

28.2.2 Hypertensive Versus Nonhypertensive ACPE: Blood Pressure Matters

As many as 50 % of patients treated with NIV for ACPE present with hypertensive crisis, that is, arterial blood pressure ≥140/90 mmHg. Cardiogenic shock associated with ACPE has a much greater mortality. The question is whether nonhypertensive ACPE patients have a worse prognosis than those with hypertensive ACPE. Several studies observed that mortality significantly increases in patients presenting to the emergency department with blood pressure <140/90 mmHg when treated either with NIV or standard therapy. This means that, especially in these patients, the search for a possibly reversible cause of ACPE is mandatory [2]. The comprehensive approach to patients with ACPE should include the assessment of lung involvement, volemia, and heart dysfunction to identify reversible causes such arrhythmias, myocardial ischemia, or valvular dysfunction with bedside ultrasound.

Summary

1. NIV is effective in the treatment of ACPE (Evidence A; NNT = 8 for ETI, NNT = 13 for mortality).
2. NIV can be started effectively in the prehospital setting.
3. Patients with acute respiratory acidosis can be treated with either CPAP or NPPV, provided that the patient does not have any preexisting respiratory muscle overload.
4. Reversible causes (e.g., ischemia, arrhythmias, valvular disease) should be identified.
5. Patients without hypertensive response have a worse prognosis.

28.2.3 NIV for ACPE in Practice

- An initial PEEP level of 10 cmH_2O is probably the best choice.
- If CPAP is used, high-flow stand-alone devices are preferred.
- If bi-level NPPV is used, apply a PS of 10–15 cmH_2O on top of PEEP 8–10 cmH_2O, closely monitoring patient-ventilator interaction, respiratory rate (RR), and tidal volume (Vt).

- Titrate FiO_2 to a SpO_2 >94 %.
- Titrate PS level to obtain a Vt ≤6 ml/kg ideal body weight (IBW) and a RR <25 bpm.
- Increase PEEP up to 12–15 cmH_2O if necessary.
- Set the minimal inspiratory trigger to avoid auto-triggering.
- Set a short rise time according to RR.
- Set a late expiratory trigger (e.g., 20–40 %).
- After 30 min of NIV, reassess arterial blood gases to evaluate both oxygenation and ventilation.

During NIV, serial monitoring of clinical and laboratory values is mandatory:

- Search for any reversible cause (e.g., ischemia, arrhythmias, valvular disease).
- Chose a mask or helmet according to patient preference.
  - Assess patient comfort and leaks.
  - Assess patient-ventilator interaction and synchrony (ineffective efforts, double triggering, auto-triggering).
  - Measure RR and adjust ventilator settings, aiming for a RR ≤25 bpm.
  - Monitor Vt, aiming for ≤6 ml/kg IBW.
  - Repeat arterial blood gas tests for oxygenation and CO_2 monitoring.

28.3 Acute Respiratory Distress Syndrome

Evidence for the use of NPPV in acute respiratory distress syndrome (ARDS) is scant and heterogeneous, however sound knowledge of the pathophysiology of ARDS and ventilator-induced lung injury (VILI) may guide clinicians in deciding whether to apply NIV. The literature and the rationale for NIV use in ARDS are discussed in detail in Chap. 50 of this book, but we summarize it briefly below:

1. In the case of NIV in AHRF, patients with ARDS have worse outcomes [7, 8].
2. NIV in ARDS is accompanied by a high failure rate (up to 70 % [6]), and NIV failure is associated with increased mortality [10].
3. Patients with successful NIV have a low mortality rate (around 20 %) [10], but this may be due to selection of less severe patients.

The main clinical goals for the use of NIV in ARDS should be the following:

- Reversal of hypoxemia
- Prevention of muscle fatigue and severe hypercapnia
- Attenuation of dyspnea and respiratory distress
- Prevention of VILI

Table 28.1 Berlin definition of ARDS from Ferguson et al. [10]

	Acute respiratory distress syndrome		
Timing	Within 1 week of a known clinical insult or new/worsening respiratory symptoms		
Chest imaging[a]	Bilateral opacities—not fully explained by effusions, lobar/lung collapse, or nodules		
Origin of edema	Respiratory failure not fully explained by cardiac failure or fluid overload; need objective assessment (e.g., echocardiography) to exclude hydrostatic edema if no risk factor present		
	Mild	Moderate	Severe
Oxygenation[b]	200< PaO_2/FiO_2 ≤300 with PEEP or CPAP ≥5 cmH_2O[c]	100< PaO_2/FiO_2 ≤200 with PEEP ≥5 cmH_2O	PaO_2/FiO_2 ≤100 with PEEP ≥5 cmH_2O

ARDS acute respiratory distress syndrome, *PaO_2* partial pressure of arterial oxygen, *FiO_2* fraction of inspired oxygen, *PEEP* positive end-expiratory pressure, *CPAP* continuous positive airway pressure, *N/A* not applicable

[a]Chest X-ray or CT scan

[b]If altitude is higher than 1000 m, a correction factor should be applied as follows: $PaO_2/FiO_2 \times$(barometric pressure/760)

[c]This may be delivered noninvasively in the mild ARDS group

According to the Berlin definition of ARDS [9], patients can be stratified into three different categories based on their initial PaO_2/FiO_2 ratio while on at least 5 cmH_2O of PEEP (see Table 28.1). Given the above considerations, we recommend considering NIV only in patients not requiring immediate intubation (approximately 15 % of ARDS patients) [10] and those without significant hemodynamic impairment or severe metabolic acidosis [6].

In patients considered for a NPPV trial:

- Ensure the appropriate environment for NPPV delivery (intensive care unit or high dependency unit) and appropriate ventilator availability (no home ventilators).
- Use an oronasal mask as interface to minimize leaks.
- NIV is preferred over CPAP use, especially in patients with marked distress and hypercapnia. ARDS is generally accompanied by an increased respiratory drive and places great stress on the respiratory muscles. Attenuation of inspiratory effort with PS is advisable. Another important advantage of NIV over CPAP is the ability to closely monitor Vt, which must be maintained below 6 ml/kg IBW.
- Start with a low PEEP level: 5 cmH_2O is probably the best choice, as it allows for subsequent reassessment of the degree of hypoxemia and appears to improve patient stratification [11].
- Apply a PS of 10–15 cmH_2O, closely monitoring patient-ventilator interaction, RR, and Vt.
- Titrate FiO_2 to a SpO_2 >94 %.

- After 30 min of NIV, reassess arterial blood gases.
  - If PaO_2/FiO_2 ratio is <200, the patient has moderate to severe ARDS. Invasive mechanical ventilation is indicated [11].
  - If PaO_2/FiO_2 ratio is >200, the patient has mild ARDS and may be treated with NIV in this phase.
  - If hypercapnia with respiratory acidosis has developed or worsened (i.e., pH <7.3 with $PaCO_2$ >50 mmHg), consider invasive mechanical ventilation.

Once it has been established that a patient has mild ARDS on NIV with 5 cmH_2O of PEEP and does not have significant or worsening respiratory acidosis:

1. Titrate PS level to obtain a Vt ≤6 ml/kg IBW and a RR <25.
2. Titrate FiO_2 to maintain a SpO_2 ≥94 %.
3. Increase PEEP up to 10 cmH_2O if necessary.

During NIV, serial monitoring of clinical and laboratory values is mandatory:

- Assess patient comfort and leaks.
- Assess patient-ventilator interaction and synchrony (ineffective efforts, double triggering, auto-triggering).
- Measure respiratory rate and adjust ventilator settings, aiming for a RR ≤25 bpm.
- Monitor Vt, aiming for ≤6 ml/kg IBW.
- Repeat arterial blood gases for oxygenation and CO_2 monitoring.

Maintain a low threshold for ETI and invasive mechanical ventilation in ARDS patients. Delaying a necessary intubation may harm patients and increase mortality [10].

28.4 Pneumonia

The scant literature on randomized and observational studies in the immunocompetent population does not allow for a strong recommendation for NIV for the treatment of acute respiratory failure in the course of pneumonia. The explanation for the difference of success in comparison with ACPE is twofold: (1) the effects of medical treatment on pneumonia takes much longer; and (2) the favorable effect of PEEP on oxygenation depends on the pattern of lung involvement (greater recruitment in interstitial than in consolidation), and its cardiovascular effects may be remarkably deleterious.

The results of randomized and observational trials in the immunocompromised population are more encouraging, because ETI – the alternative to NIV for severe acute respiratory failure – is frequently complicated by severe infections and a high mortality. Hence, NIV use in the immunocompromised population may decrease intubation rate and improve outcome.

According to the literature, the following suggestions can be made on the probability of NIV success in pneumonia in the immunocompetent population. The outcome is significantly better in patients with preexisting chronic cardiocirculatory or obstructive lung disease than in those with de novo acute respiratory failure [3]. Finally, early treatment of severe hypoxemic pneumonia with helmet CPAP may effectively reduce the risk of meeting ETI criteria compared with oxygen therapy [4].

Summary
1. NIV is effective in the immunocompromised population.
2. NIV is more effective in acute-on-chronic versus de novo respiratory failure.
3. In immunocompetent patients without a do not intubate (DNI) order, a cautious early NIV trial may be attempted (the interface is a key factor).
4. In immunocompetent patients with a DNI order, NIV is a possible ceiling treatment (the interface is a key factor).

28.4.1 NPPV for Pneumonia in Practice

- An initial PEEP level of 5–8 cmH_2O is probably the best choice.
- If your choice is CPAP, high-flow stand-alone devices are preferred.
- The interface is crucial; helmet CPAP may be better tolerated because treatment is generally longer than two days.
- If your choice is bi-level NPPV, apply a PS of 10–15 cmH_2O on top of PEEP 5–8 cmH_2O, closely monitoring patient-ventilator interaction, RR, and Vt.
- Titrate FiO_2 and PEEP to a SpO_2 >94 %.
- Test the best PEEP, according to PaO_2/FiO_2 ratio, pCO_2, and vital signs responses.
- Titrate PS level to obtain a Vt ≤6 ml/kg IBW and a RR <25 bpm.
- Increase PEEP up to 10–12 cmH_2O if necessary, according to PEEP test.
- Set the minimal inspiratory trigger to avoid auto-triggering.
- Set a short rise time according to respiratory rate.
- Set a late expiratory trigger (e.g., 20–40 %).
- After 30 min of NIV, reassess arterial blood gases to evaluate both oxygenation and ventilation.

During NIV, serial monitoring of clinical and laboratory values is mandatory:

- Treat and monitor clinical response to sepsis (antibiotics, fluids, lactate clearance, etc.).
- Chose the interface according to patient preference; a long NIV course is expected, therefore, a helmet might be preferable.
  - Assess patient comfort and leaks.
  - Assess patient-ventilator interaction and synchrony (ineffective efforts, double triggering, auto-triggering).
  - Measure RR and adjust ventilator settings, aiming for a RR ≤25 bpm.
  - Monitor Vt, aiming for ≤6 ml/kg IBW.
  - Repeat arterial blood gases for oxygenation and CO_2 monitoring

Maintain a low threshold for ETI and invasive mechanical ventilation.

28.5 Blunt Chest Trauma and Atelectasis

NIV in atelectasis is reviewed in detail elsewhere in this book. Trauma patients frequently develop acute respiratory failure resulting from ventilation perfusion mismatching and shunt because of lung contusion, atelectasis, inability to clear secretions, or pneumothorax and/or hemothorax. The rationale for NIV is alveolar recruitment and chest stabilization to prevent ETI and its complications that may lead to adverse outcomes. Randomized trial excluded patients with either severe hypoxemia (PaO_2/FiO_2 <200), respiratory acidosis, or multiorgan dysfunction because they are usually unable to cooperate or protect the airway or clear secretions [5]. Time is a key factor, inasmuch as early treatment is associated with better outcome; further, a lack of response at 1–4 h should promptly lead to intubation and invasive mechanical ventilation. Patient selection seems to be the most important prognostic factor for improved outcome of NPPV treatment of acute respiratory failure due to blunt chest trauma.

Summary

- NIV may decrease both ETI and mortality provided that:
  Patients are treated during early acute respiratory failure
- NIV is used only in hypoxemic non-hypercapnic patients
- NIV is used only in patients without other organ failures
- Other medical and surgical treatments are added to NIV

28.6 Acute Respiratory Failure After Drowning

Acute respiratory failure after drowning is a common event, but its severity spans from rapidly reversible mild hypoxemia to full-blown ARDS. For an in-depth review of the pathophysiology of drowning and the applications of NIV, see Chap. 50 in this book.

Drowning involves aspiration of water into the airways, which directly damages alveolar surface, washes surfactant, and increases lung weight determining atelectasis. Additionally, reflex bronchospasm contributes to hypoxia and respiratory distress while increased permeability in the lung induces pulmonary edema (Szpilman D Drowning *NEJM* 2012). Interestingly, drowning appears to be associated with rapidly reversible respiratory failure [14], thus often requiring short-term ventilatory support. After rescue from water, patients may present with cardiac arrest, generally associated with pulseless electrical activity. Cardiac arrest in this situation is generally hypoxic in nature (especially in the young population) and thus mandates rapid administration of oxygen and ventilatory assistance as well as reversal of hypothermia.

In hemodynamically stable patients, respiratory symptoms may vary from cough and rales (presentation associated with low mortality rates) to severe hypoxemia, cough, and foamy secretions (mortality around 20 % [13]).

Administration of oxygen and SpO_2 monitoring for at least 8 h are advisable in all patients, but those presenting SpO_2 <94 % and signs of respiratory distress may deserve treatment with NIV before considering ETI [15]. NIV may be applied in the prehospital period if indications for emergency ETI are not met.

The main concerns with NIV use in drowned patients are the inability to fully protect the airway and sudden vomiting and aspiration. Given the pathophysiology of drowning, it seems logical to start with noninvasive CPAP, which is usually more widely available and easier to manage. Helmet or full face mask may be used according to availability and staff experience. We recommend starting CPAP with a continuous high-flow delivery system (Venturi system) to avoid CO_2 rebreathing and maximize oxygen delivery to the patient, starting with a PEEP of 10 cmH_2O and titrating FiO_2 to achieve a SpO_2 >94 %. Alternatively, NIV can be started with a PEEP of 10 cmH_2O and a PS level titrated to the patient's need, aiming for a Vt of 6–8 ml/kg IBW (usually around 10 cmH_2O). NIV may be better than CPAP in patients presenting with hypoxic-hypercapnic respiratory failure, provided no alterations in neurologic status exist. Foamy secretions certainly represent a challenge, but clinicians must remember that they are the result of increased permeability in the lung and may thus be controlled or reduced with positive airway pressure.

After NIV or CPAP initiation, neurologic status, RR, blood pressure, and SpO_2 should be closely monitored during the first 1–2 h. Arterial blood gas tests should then be performed. If oxygenation is improving after 60–120 min of CPAP or NIV and no hypercapnia has developed, patients may continue treatment. However, if oxygenation fails to improve or signs of respiratory muscle fatigue are present (including respiratory acidosis), ETI must be performed and invasive mechanical ventilation started. Prognostic factors associated with favorable outcome after drowning are short submersion time and symptom severity after rescue, with worse prognosis in case of cardiac arrest (up to 90 % mortality).

Key Major Recommendations (Fig. 28.1)

- Patients with ACPE should be treated with either CPAP or NIV (strong recommendation).
- In patients with ARDS, NIV is preferred over CPAP. If a cautious trial fails within 1 h, prompt intubation is required.
- In immunocompromised patients with pneumonia, early treatment with NIV may avoid the need for intubation.
- In immunocompetent patients with pneumonia, early treatment is recommended with NIV. The interface is crucial (a helmet is better tolerated). Test a short trial. Pay attention to sepsis.
- In patients with blunt chest trauma: start early, only in hypoxaemic patients and those without other organ failures.

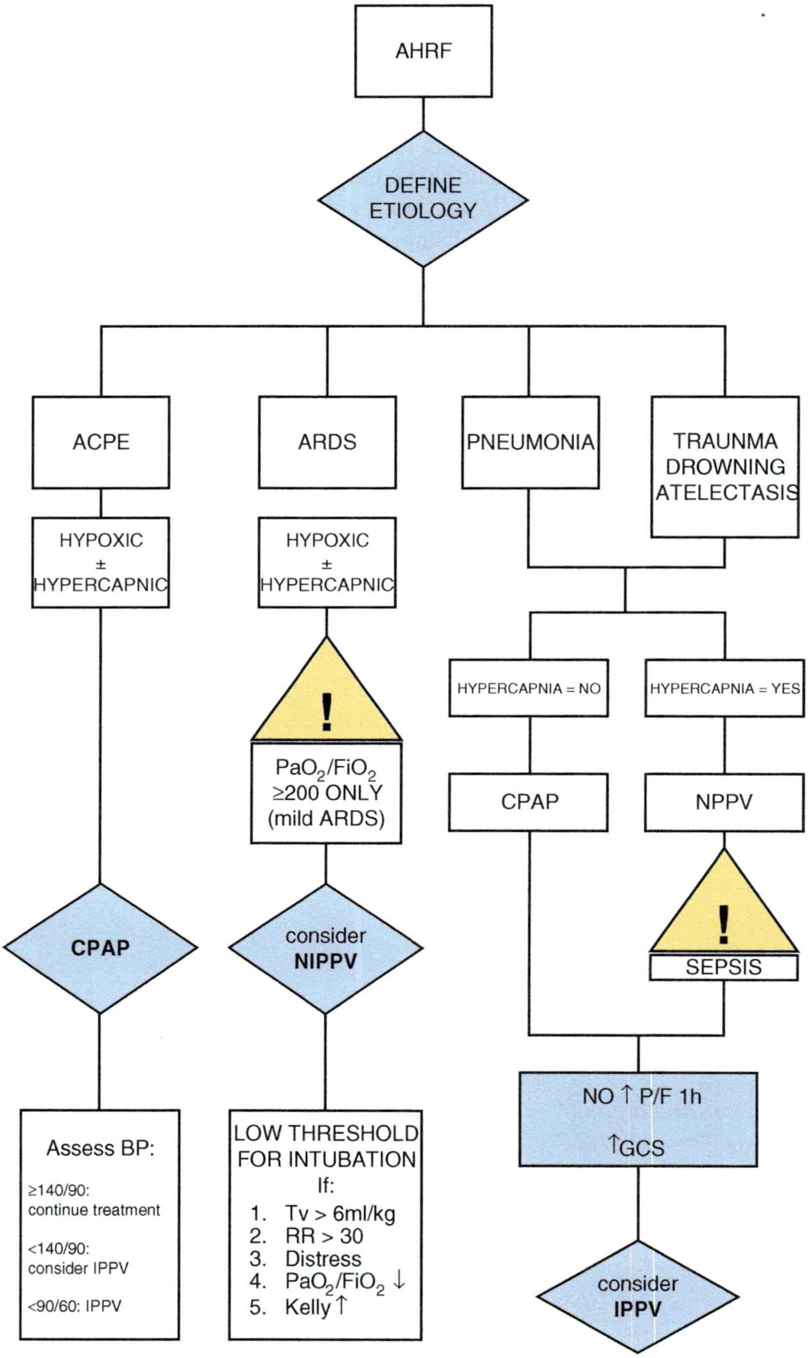

Fig. 28.1 Algorithm for initial management of acute hypoxaemic respiratory failure with NIPPV

References

ACPE

1. Vital FMR, Ladeira MT, Atallah AN. Non-invasive positive pressure ventilation (CPAP or bilevel NPPV) for cardiogenic pulmonary oedema. Cochrane Database Syst Rev. 2013;5:CD005351. doi:10.1002/14651858.CD005351.pub3.
2. McMurray JJV, Adamopoulos S, Anker SD, et al. ESC Guidelines for the diagnosis and treatment of acute and chronic heart failure 2012. Eur Heart J. 2013;33:1787–847.

Pneumonia

3. Carrillo A, Gonzalez-Diaz G, Ferrer M, Martinez-Quintana ME, Lopez-Martinez A, Llamas N, et al. Non-invasive ventilation in community-acquired pneumonia and severe acute respiratory failure. Intensive Care Med. 2012. doi:10.1007/s00134-012-2475-6.
4. Brambilla AM, Aliberti S, Prina E, et al. Helmet CPAP vs. oxygen therapy in severe hypoxemic respiratory failure due to pneumonia. Intensive Care Med. 2014;40:942–9. doi:10.1007/s00134-014-3325-5.

Trauma

5. Karcz MK, Papadakos PJ. Noninvasive ventilation in trauma. World J Crit Care Med. 2015;4(1):47–54.

ARDS

6. Rana S, Jenad H, Gay PC, et al. Failure of noninvasive ventilation in patients with acute lung injury: observational cohort study. Crit Care. 2006;10:R79.
7. Ferrer M, Esquinas A, Leon M, et al. Noninvasive ventilation in severe hypoxemic respiratory failure: a randomized clinical trial. Am J Respir Crit Care Med. 2003;168:1438–44.
8. Agarwal R, Agarwal AN, Gupta D. Role of noninvasive ventilation in acute lung injury/acute respiratory distress syndrome: a proportion meta-analysis. Respir Care. 2010;55:1653–60.
9. ARDS Definition Task Force. Acute respiratory distress syndrome: the Berlin Definition. JAMA. 2012;307:2526–33.
10. Antonelli M, Conti G, Esquinas A, et al. A multiple-center survey on the use in clinical practice of noninvasive ventilation as a first-line intervention for acute respiratory distress syndrome. Crit Care Med. 2007;35:18–25.
11. Ferguson N, Fan E, Camporota L, et al. The Berlin definition of ARDS: an expanded rationale, justification, and supplementary material. Intensive Care Med. 2012;38:1573–82.
12. Caironi P, Carlesso E, Cressoni M, et al. Lung recruitability is better estimated according to the Berlin definition of acute respiratory distress syndrome at standard 5 cm H_2O rather than higher positive end-expiratory pressure: a retrospective cohort study. Crit Care Med. 2015;43:781–90.

Drowning

13. Szpilman D. Near-drowning and drowning classification: a proposal to stratify mortality based on the analysis of 1831 cases. Chest. 1997;112(3):660–5.
14. Gregorakos L, Markou N, Psalida V, et al. Near-drowning: clinical course of lung injury in adults. Lung. 2009;187(2):93–7.
15. Dottorini M, Eslami A, Baglioni S, et al. Nasal-continuous positive airway pressure in the treatment of near-drowning in freshwater. Chest. 1996;110(4):1122–4.

Noninvasive Mechanical Ventilation in Acute Exacerbations of Chronic Obstructive Pulmonary Disease: Key Determinants of Early and Late Failure

29

Oya Baydar and Ezgi Ozyilmaz

Contents

Abbreviations

ABG	Arterial blood gas
ARF	Acute respiratory failure
COPD	Chronic obstructive pulmonary disease
CPAP	Continuous positive airway pressure
ETI	Endotracheal intubation
FiO_2	Fraction of inspired oxygen
HES	Hypercapnic encephalopathy
ICU	Intensive care unit
IMV	Invasive mechanical ventilation
IPV	Intrapulmonary percussive ventilation
NIV	Noninvasive ventilation
NNT	Number needed to treat
OR	Odds ratio
RCTs	Randomized controlled trials
UMC	Usual medical care

O. Baydar, MD (✉) • E. Ozyilmaz, MD
Department of Chest Diseases, Cukurova University Faculty of Medicine, Adana, Turkey
e-mail: oyabaydarr@yahoo.com.tr; ezgiozyilmaz@hotmail.com

A.M. Esquinas (ed.), *Noninvasive Mechanical Ventilation: Theory, Equipment, and Clinical Applications*, DOI 10.1007/978-3-319-21653-9_29

29.1 Introduction

Acute exacerbations of chronic obstructive pulmonary disease (COPD) are a frequent cause of admission to the hospital and the intensive care unit (ICU). During these episodes, a major deterioration in gas exchange is accompanied by a worsening in the clinical condition of the patient, characterized by a rapid and shallow breathing pattern, severe dyspnea, right ventricular failure, and encephalopathy. The pathophysiological pathway of all these features is the inability of the respiratory system to maintain adequate alveolar ventilation in the presence of major abnormalities in respiratory mechanics. Hypercapnia, acidosis, and hypoxemia all ensue, leading to clinical deterioration in cardiovascular and neurological functions [1]. Estimates of inpatient mortality range from 4 to 30 %, but patients admitted due to acute respiratory failure (ARF) experience a higher rate, in particular elderly patients with comorbidities (up to 50 %) and those requiring ICU admission (11–26 %) [2].

What triggers the abnormal breathing pattern of the patient remains unclear [1]. The key element during decompensation seems to be the shortening of the inspiratory time, inducing both a decrease in tidal volume and an increase in respiratory frequency. Because this is associated with, or is secondary to, excessive respiratory loads, treatment should be directed at reducing the loads imposed on the respiratory muscles. Unfortunately, the ability of medical treatment to reverse severe respiratory failure in these patients is limited. When hypoventilation becomes so severe that several organ dysfunctions occur, there is no choice other than to provide "artificial" ventilation to avoid a fatal outcome [1]. The traditional manner of artificial ventilation was invasive mechanical ventilation (IMV), but today the role of noninvasive ventilation (NIV) in the management of acute hypercapnic respiratory failure secondary to COPD is well established [3]. Several randomized controlled trials (RCTs) have demonstrated that adding NIV to standard medical therapy improves dyspnea as well as reduces mortality, intubation rate, and hospital length of stay [3, 4]. A previous study using NIV in respiratory failure secondary to exacerbations of COPD demonstrated reductions in respiratory rate and transdiaphragmatic activity with increases in tidal volume and minute ventilation. Thus, NIV not only rapidly improves gas exchange but also allows respiratory muscle rest, reducing respiratory muscle work in respiratory failure [5].

29.2 Discussion and Analysis

How does NIV work? There are three important characteristics of NIV in this setting that must be understood to answer this question. The first concerns ventilation itself. The success of the technique is based on the ability of assisted ventilation (or synchronized ventilation) to improve alveolar ventilation by increasing tidal volume. The widely accepted pressure-targeted modes deliver support in synchrony with the patient's inspiratory effort, which usually results in an increase in tidal volume, subsequently associated with a reduction in the amount of effort performed by the patient [6]. The ability of these modes to improve the volume delivered to the lung explains the ability of NIV to reverse other clinical and gas exchange abnormalities. The second characteristic of NIV is that it is an intermittent mode of support. NIV is usually delivered for only a few hours during a 24-h period (usually 6–12 h) and is rarely delivered as a continuous support. These patients have a highly stimulated and active respiratory drive and can therefore sustain prolonged periods of spontaneous breathing. However, the treatment should provide a reduction in the amount of effort needed and intermittent support seems to be adequate. When the need for ventilatory support becomes permanent, tolerance of the mask becomes a limitation and is frequently a cause of failure. The third characteristic of NIV is the use of a face mask in place of an endotracheal tube. Although the use of these masks is associated with specific problems such as leaks and limited clinical tolerance, they have been shown to replace endotracheal intubation (ETI) advantageously as a first-line treatment [1].

Chandra et al. [7] reported outcome data over a 10-year period, from 1998 to 2008, including more than 7.5 million COPD admissions from a database of 1,000 hospitals in the United States. These data demonstrated a four-fold increase in the use of NIV, which represented an increase from 1.0 to 4.5 % of all admissions. There was a corresponding 42 % decrease in invasively ventilated patients, from 6.5 to 3.5 % of all admissions.

Lindanauer reported a retrospective cohort study of 25,628 patients hospitalized for exacerbation of COPD who received mechanical ventilation on the first or second hospital day. Those initially treated with NIV had a lower risk of death or of developing pneumonia during the hospitalization, a shorter length of stay, and lower costs compared with those who initially underwent invasive ventilation. The relative advantage of NIV was attenuated among patients with higher comorbidity burden and in the subgroup of patients who had pneumonia present at the time of hospital admission [8]. NIV has been shown to improve acute respiratory acidosis (increases pH and decreases $PaCO_2$) and decrease respiratory rate, work of breathing, severity of breathlessness, complications such as ventilator-associated pneumonia, and length of hospital stay (evidence level A). More importantly, mortality and intubation rates are reduced by this intervention (evidence level A) [9].

However, NIV is not successful in all cases of acute or chronic respiratory failure due to COPD when compared with usual medical care, with reported failure rates of between 9 and 50 %. There has also been concern that NIV may delay ETI and mechanical ventilation, resulting in a worse outcome [10].

Prediction of outcomes, specifically negative predictors, following acute NIV is essential to assisting the physician with decisions regarding the use of NIV in the acute setting. Patient selection is the cornerstone of NIV. Among the patient-related predictors of NIV failure, based on data from RCTs, three temporal moments were identified: (1) immediate failure (within minutes to <1 h), (2) early failure (1–48 h), and (3) late failure (after 48 h); these three types of failures were associated with 15, 68, and 17 % of failures, respectively.

29.2.1 Patient-Related Risk Factors

Immediate Risk Factors

1. Weak cough reflex and/or excessive secretions
2. Hypercapnic encephalopathy and coma
3. Intolerance and psychomotor agitation
4. "Fighting with the machine": patient-ventilator asynchrony

Early Risk Factors: Hypoxemic ARF

1. Baseline arterial blood gas (ABG) and inability to correct gas exchange (pH < 7.25)
2. Increased severity of disease
3. Increased respiratory rate (>35 breaths/min)
4. Miscellaneous: poor nutritional status, increased heart rate, higher baseline C-reactive protein/white blood cell count, lower serum potassium, airway colonization by nonfermenting gram-negative bacilli

Late Risk Factors

1. Sleep disturbance
2. Functional limitation
3. Possible initial improvement in pH
4. Hyperglycemia

29.2.2 Immediate NIV Failure

Immediate NIV failure refers to failure within minutes and not beyond the first hour of treatment. About 15 % of all NIV failures were defined as "immediate" in RCTs, irrespective of the underlying causes of respiratory failure.

29.2.2.1 Weak Cough Reflex and/or Excessive Secretions

NIV does not allow direct access to the airways. A weak cough reflex leading to inefficient clearance of excessive secretions from airways is a common cause of immediate NIV failure. The inability to spontaneously remove secretions is considered a relative contraindication for NIV, especially in patients with impaired consciousness and depressed cough. Some data indicate that specific "manual" or "mechanical" physiotherapeutic techniques may improve mucociliary clearance during NIV, and NIV can still be used in these circumstances. Intrapulmonary percussive ventilation (IPV) is a technique that delivers small bursts of high-flow respiratory gas at high rates for mobilization of secretions. Two clinical studies demonstrated that IMV used before or in combination with NIV may reduce the risk of ETI in COPD patients with difficulties removing secretions. Early fiber-optic bronchoscopy is another potential intervention that can be used to minimize the burden of respiratory secretions [11].

29.2.2.2 Hypercapnic Encephalopathy and Coma

Hypercapnic encephalopathy (HES) is often considered a cause of immediate NIV failure because of poor compliance due to confusion and/or agitation. Additionally, it is viewed as a relative contraindication because of the increased risk of aspiration. The risk of aspiration has been shown to be minimized by the rapid improvement of neurological status under NIV, and NIV failure rates were reported to be comparable among patients with and without HES. The use of a relatively high back-up rate and/or pressure control ventilation may also help to "capture" the patient better. Another key factor in patients with HES is the rebound effect of fraction of inspired oxygen (FiO_2) on the $PaCO_2$ and pH, known as the "Haldane effect." This effect can be prevented by a simple intervention: decreasing the FiO_2 level [11].

29.2.2.3 Intolerance and Psychomotor Agitation

Patient tolerance has been shown to be critical for NIV success, especially in the first few minutes while the patient adapts to this "new mode" of breathing. The use of judicious sedation may be valuable to achieve a sedation level that keeps the patient awake, easily arousable, and comfortable. Ideal sedatives should be short acting and have no significant effects on respiratory drive and hemodynamics. It has to be kept in mind that oversedation during NIV can be potentially dangerous. Thus, close monitoring with evaluation of ABG, cardiopulmonary and ventilator parameters, adverse events, and the level of sedation is mandatory [11].

29.2.2.4 Patient-Ventilator Asynchrony

Asynchrony has rarely been cited as a direct cause of NIV immediate failure. Asynchrony can easily be detected by a physical examination (e.g., number of spontaneous breaths vs ventilator-delivered breaths, accessory muscle use) of the patient and symptoms (e.g., dyspnea). Two main causes of asynchrony are a high level of ventilator support and an increased number of leaks. A number of strategies can be implemented to avoid "gross asynchronies," such as optimization of ventilator settings using the screen ventilator waveforms, adjusting trigger sensitivity, increasing positive end-expiratory pressure, minimizing leaks, and using different modes or more sophisticated ventilators. New modes of ventilation, such as neutrally adjusted ventilator assist, have been documented to reduce asynchrony [11].

29.2.3 Early NIV Failure

Nearly 65 % of NIV failures occur within 1–48 h of NIV use. This time interval has received more attention in assessments of predictors of failure. It has two main subtypes, hypoxemic and hypercapnic respiratory failure, and we will discuss hypercapnic failure in detail, as it is our main concern.

Although hypercapnic ARF includes ARF due to neurological disorders (such as neuromuscular disorders) and other acute or chronic lung disorders (such as restrictive lung disease), most of the studies done in this field have involved patients with COPD exacerbations [11].

29.2.3.1 Baseline ABG and Inability to Correct Gas Exchange

The pH level, which is an indicator of the severity of hypercapnia, has been reported to be a critical factor in determining the success of NIV. Although some reports failed to show any relationship between baseline ABGs and the success of NIV, a large body of evidence clearly indicated that a lower baseline pH is a risk factor for NIV failure in COPD patients. In nearly 50–60 % of patients with a baseline pH of <7.25, NIV was unsuccessful. A subgroup analysis of COPD patients with mild to moderate acidosis revealed that NIV improved patient outcomes only if the baseline pH was ≥7.30. Three studies with 320 patients were included in the 7.35–7.30 subgroup and five studies with 221 patients in the <7.30 subgroup. Studies in both pH subgroups showed treatment failure to be significantly less with NIV (RR 0.63; 95 % CI 0.43, 0.95 and RR 0.37; 95 % CI 0.25, 0.54, respectively). There were no significant differences between the two pH subgroups [5].

In addition to baseline levels, pH values 1 h after the application of NIV were shown to be strong predictors of the success of NIV, with high sensitivity and good specificity (93 and 82 %, respectively) [9]. In a study of more than 1,000 COPD patients, Confalonieri et al. pointed out that a pH <7.25 after 1 h of NIV use was associated with an increased risk of failure and that the risk of failure was even greater than when the pH levels were <7.25 at admission [12]. For the above-mentioned reasons, we do not recommend routine use of NIV in patients with a pH <7.25 outside a "protected" environment [11].

29.2.3.2 Increased Severity of Disease

The relationship between NIV failure and the severity scores, including Acute Physiology and Chronic Health Evaluation II (APACHE II) and Simplified Acute Physiology Score II (SAP II), has been documented in a number of reports. Several researchers found an association, whereas others failed to find any association.

29.2.3.3 Increased Respiratory Rate

An initial high respiratory rate and its reduction after 1 h of NIV have been shown to be associated with successful NIV outcomes in COPD patients. A respiratory rate of 30–34 and ≥35 breaths/min at admission were demonstrated to lead to NIV failure, with an OR of 1.83 and 2.66, respectively, whereas the ratios increased to 2.67 and 4.95, respectively, for the same breathing frequency after 2 h of NIV [11].

29.2.3.4 Miscellaneous Risk Factors of NIV Failure

Miscellaneous risk factors for NIV failure in hypercapnic ARF are poor nutritional status, a high white blood cell count, low serum potassium, and an increased heart rate. Two additional issues may merit specific consideration. Old age has never been shown to be a "negative" variable in determining NIV outcomes, and older patients with hypercapnic ARF may respond even better than younger ones to NIV [11].

29.2.3.5 Late NIV Failure

Although the definition of late NIV failure has not been standardized, it is usually defined as failure that occurs 48 h after initiation of NIV, following an initial successful response. It occurs in a considerable subset of patients (about 15 % of NIV failures).

The occurrence of late failure in COPD patients admitted with hypercapnic ARF to ICUs when NIV was used >24 h was found to be associated with functional limitation before admission, the presence of hyperglycemia, and a lower pH at admission. $PaCO_2$ and pH values improved gradually and similarly within the first 24 h in both success and late failure groups. This is of particular importance because initial good responses to NIV may decrease attention and monitoring by clinicians in the following hours. During a hospital stay, pneumonia was more frequently observed as a complication in a late failure group compared with a success group (12.9 % vs 0 %). The mortality of a late failure group was extremely high compared with a successful group in another study (68 % vs 0 %). In a recent study, sleep disturbance (classified as an abnormal electroencephalographic pattern, greater circadian sleep-cycle disruption, and less nocturnal rapid eye movement sleep) and increased delirium during an ICU stay were also associated with late NIV failure in hypercapnic patients. NIV patients should be continuously monitored (including their sleep patterns and state of delirium), even if their initial clinical and ABG responses are good, because late NIV failure can lead to high mortality [11].

The global rise in obesity has impacted on the COPD population. Of further interest, obese COPD patients were protected from adverse outcomes and were less likely to develop late NIV failure or require hospital readmission at 1 year. Patients with COPD and obesity are also more likely to receive long-term ventilatory support in the form of either NIV or continuous positive airway pressure (CPAP) to treat COPD–obstructive sleep apnea overlap syndrome. It is unclear from the data whether the improved outcomes in obese patients with COPD are a reflection of enhanced interaction between opposing pulmonary mechanics or whether it simply reflects the higher incidence of home NIV and CPAP as a treatment, which increases overall health-care support.

Concerning the efficiency of NIV in COPD patients with severe community acquired pneumonia, one randomized study including COPD patients with hypercapnic ARF and pneumonia reported by Confalonieri et al. showed that NIV may reduce the rate of intubation and complications in comparison with medical therapy. The same advantages were not achieved when NIV was compared with conventional mechanical ventilation [13].

We have discussed the patient-related risk factors of NIV failure; there are also some non-patient-related risk factors, too. The timing of the application of NIV is a critical factor. A longer delay between admission and NIV use was shown to be an independent risk factor for NIV failure, probably due to the progression of the underlying disease. Therefore, early use of NIV is recommended. It is also critical not to unduly delay the decision to intubate a patient with failed NIV, because the risk of unanticipated respiratory or cardiac arrest could lead to increased morbidity and mortality [5, 11].

The location of the NIV therapy is another important determinant in the success of NIV. The decision about where to perform NIV should be based on matching the capabilities of the units and teams with the patient's clinical severity and the need for monitoring. Five studies with 414 patients were conducted outside the ICU and three studies with 127 patients in the ICU. Both subgroups showed significant improvements in treatment failure with NIV, with the results being slightly better in the ICU subgroup. However, the difference did not reach statistical significance, as can be seen with the overlapping 95 % CIs for the two point estimates [5].

The experience and the skills of the staff are other key components of NIV success. Training in NIV implementation is an important factor in reducing nosocomial infections and improving survival in critically ill patients with COPD [11].

Although much attention has been paid to the development of new interfaces to increase tolerance and patient comfort, mask intolerance remains a major cause of NIV failure. An oronasal mask is generally the most commonly preferred one in ARF, followed by nasal masks, helmets, and mouthpieces [11].

How to withdraw the patient from NIV is also critical. A pilot prospective, single-center, open-labeled randomized study comparing stepwise versus immediate withdrawal of NIV in patients with COPD exacerbation recovering from acute hypercapnic respiratory failure revealed no statistically significant difference in the success rate, with NIV successfully stopped in 74.3 % and 56 % in the stepwise and immediate withdrawal groups, respectively ($p=0.139$).

Conclusion

In summary, a review of 14 RCTs with 758 patients shows clear benefit of NIV as an adjunct therapy to usual medical care (UMC) (compared with UMC alone) in the management of patients admitted to hospital with respiratory failure secondary to an acute exacerbation of COPD. NIV compared with UMC showed significant improvements in pH, $PaCO_2$, respiratory rate, treatment failure, mortality, intubation rate, complications, and length of hospital stay. Studies conducted in the ICU or outside the ICU were also not significantly different. With NIV, the risk of treatment failure was reduced by more than 50 % and the number needed to treat was 5. Therefore, for every five patients treated with NIV, we would avoid one patient failing treatment. Treatment failure was significantly reduced, whether the study was conducted in the ICU or the wards. However, as with the pH subgroups, greater reduction in the risk of treatment failure was seen with studies in ICUs (risk reduction of 71 %) than in studies conducted in the ward (risk reduction of 39 %). There was a significant reduction in risk of mortality with NIV of 48 % compared with UMC. For every 10 patients treated with NIV, we would avoid one death. There has been debate as to whether NIV would delay ETI, leading to an increase in mortality. It is shown that mortality is significantly decreased with NIV use. With admission pH less than 7.30, risk reduction was 49 %; with admission pH between 7.35 and 7.30, risk reduction was 55 %. With NIV, the risk of ETI was more than halved (59 %), and by treating four patients with NIV we would avoid one patient being intubated. Length of hospital stay was significantly reduced by more than 3 days with NIV. Acidosis has been shown to be an important prognostic factor in survival from respiratory failure in COPD, and thus early correction of acidosis is an essential goal of therapy [5].

Recommendations

Studies show that NIV offers better outcomes to patients admitted with acute exacerbations of COPD than either medical treatment alone or ICU management with ETI as second-line treatment (approximately 75 % of patients). Three complementary interventions can therefore now be proposed in a stepwise approach to these patients, and their combination should become a new standard of care. The first step is based on drug treatment and appropriate management of oxygen. The second step is the early use of NIV to prevent further worsening and clinical deterioration. How soon this treatment should be applied is still a matter of debate and may be difficult to base solely on objectively quantified criteria. The final treatment step is ETI and mechanical ventilation. This should be reserved for patients in whom NIV is contraindicated, for those meeting intubation criteria despite NIV, or those requiring immediate ETI on admission.

References

1. Brochard L. Non-invasive ventilation for acute exacerbations of COPD: a new standard of care. Thorax. 2000;55:817–8.
2. American Thoracic Society. Standards for the diagnosis and care of patients with chronic obstructive pulmonary disease. Am J Respir Crit Care Med. 1995;152:77–120.
3. Plant PK, Owen JL, Elliott MW. Early use of noninvasive ventilation for acute exacerbations of chronic obstructive pulmonary disease on general respiratory wards: a multicentre randomised controlled trial. Lancet. 2000;355:1931–5.
4. Conti G, Antonelli M, Navalesi P, et al. Noninvasive vs. conventional mechanical ventilation in patients with chronic obstructive pulmonary disease after failure of medical treatment in the ward: a randomized trial. Intensive Care Med. 2002;28:1701–7.
5. Ram FSF, Picot J, Lightowler J, Wedzicha JA. Non-invasive positive pressure ventilation for treatment of respiratory failure due to exacerbations of chronic obstructive pulmonary disease (Review). Cochrane Database Syst Rev. 2003;326:185–190.
6. Brochard L, Isabey D, Piquet J, et al. Reversal of acute exacerbations of chronic obstructive lung disease by inspiratory assistance with a face mask. N Engl J Med. 1990;323:1523–30.
7. Chandra D, Stamm JA, Taylor B, et al. Outcomes of noninvasive ventilation for acute exacerbations of chronic obstructive pulmonary disease in the United States, 1998–2008. Am J Respir Crit Care Med. 2012;185:152–9.
8. Lindenauer PK, Stefan MS, Shieh MS, et al. Outcomes associated with invasive and noninvasive vertilation among patients hospitalized with exacerbations of chronic obstructive pulmonary disease. JAMA Intern Med. 2014;174(12):1982–93.
9. Global Intiative for Chronic Obstructive Lung Disease (GOLD). Global strategy for diagnosis, management, and prevention of Chronic Obstructive lung disease. Updated 2014. Global initiative for chronic obstructive lung disease, Inc. Available from: http://www.goldcopd.org/uploads/users/files/GOLD_Report2014_Feb07.pdf. Accessed July 12, 2015.
10. Ambrosino N, Foglio K, Rubini F, Clini E, Nava S, Vitacca M. Non-invasive mechanical ventilation in acute respiratory failure due to chronic obstructive pulmonary disease: correlates for success. Thorax. 1995;50:755–7.
11. Ozyilmaz E, et al. Timing of noninvasive ventilation failure: causes, risk factors, and potential remedies. BMC Pulm Med. 2014;14:19.
12. Confalonieri M, Garuti G, Cattaruzza MS, et al. A chart of failure risk for non-invasive ventilation in patients with COPD exacerbation. Eur Respir J. 2005;25(2):348–55.
13. Confalonieri M, Potena A, Cosbone G, et al. Acute respiratory failure in patients with severe community-acquired pneumonia. Am J Respir Crit Care Med. 1999;160:1585–91.

Noninvasive Ventilation in the Prehospital Setting: Key Applications

30

Patrick Chaftari, Maria Teresa Cruz Carreras, and Jayne Viets-Upchurch

Contents

Abbreviations

ACPE	Acute cardiogenic pulmonary edema
COPD	Chronic obstructive pulmonary disease
NIV	Noninvasive ventilation

30.1 Respiratory Emergencies

In normal respiration, the contraction of external intercostal muscles and the diaphragm increases the lung volume, creating negative pressure that results in the movement of air to the alveoli. The relaxation of the external intercostal muscles

P. Chaftari, MD (✉) • M.T.C. Carreras, MD • J. Viets-Upchurch, MD
Emergency Medicine, The University of Texas MD Anderson Cancer Center, Houston, TX, USA
e-mail: pchaftari@mdanderson.org; mcruz3@mdanderson.org; jviets@mdanderson.org

A.M. Esquinas (ed.), *Noninvasive Mechanical Ventilation: Theory, Equipment, and Clinical Applications*, DOI 10.1007/978-3-319-21653-9_30

and diaphragm restores the thoracic cavity to preinspiratory volume, increasing pressure in the lungs and generating exhalation. This movement of air in and out of the lungs, known as pulmonary ventilation, provides the necessary oxygen to the alveoli and eliminates carbon dioxide. Pulmonary ventilation maintains optimal partial pressure of each gas, allowing gas exchange at the level of the alveoli and pulmonary capillaries.

Some of the most common calls to emergency medical services are associated with respiratory complaints [1–4]. Differential diagnosis includes neurological issues (e.g., head trauma, drugs, and cerebrovascular accidents), upper airways (e.g., swelling, blockage by a foreign body, and trauma), lower airways (e.g., asthma and chronic obstructive pulmonary disease (COPD)), alveoli, and possible impairment in pulmonary circulation resulting from pulmonary embolism. Congestive heart failure and COPD make up the largest percentage of respiratory emergencies. In the United States, approximately one million patients per year are treated by paramedics for acute congestive heart failure [5].

Dyspnea, or shortness of breath, accounts for 10–13 % of emergency medical service calls [6]. Standard care for dyspnea in the prehospital setting typically involves supplemental oxygen and beta agonist nebulizer therapy. Vasopressors and diuretics may also be employed, depending on the emergency medical service protocol and responder skill level.

Respiratory failure occurs when the lungs can no longer provide adequate oxygenation, generally resulting in tachypnea, hypoxemia, hypercapnia, and perceived dyspnea. Severe respiratory failure has been managed in the prehospital setting by endotracheal intubation, an invasive procedure that requires sedation and advanced skills. Endotracheal intubation may be difficult and dangerous because of the presence of contact-protective airway reflexes [7] and is associated with multiple complications, such as oral lacerations, aspiration, tube malposition, barotrauma, and ventilator-associated pneumonia. The poorly controlled environment of the prehospital setting increases the likelihood of these complications.

Trauma and pneumothorax may present with the symptom of dyspnea. The presence of trauma is generally easily discerned, and presentation of significant pneumothorax typically involves tracheal deviation and unilateral loss of breath sounds. More perplexing are the life-threatening medical causes of dyspnea, such as exacerbations of COPD, asthma, pneumonia, pulmonary embolism, cardiac ischemia, and acute cardiogenic pulmonary edema (ACPE) (COPD and ACPE are the most common). The uncertain etiology of medically induced dyspnea complicates its management in the prehospital setting.

30.2 Noninvasive Ventilation Techniques and Mechanisms

Improving alveolar ventilation is a critical step for delivering oxygenated blood to the tissue. Different techniques for accomplishing this have been introduced over the years, ranging from provision of supplemental oxygen to endotracheal intubation. With recent advances, noninvasive positive-pressure ventilation (NIV), a technique introduced in 1981 by Sullivan and colleagues to provide alveolar ventilation without creation of an invasive airway, has emerged as an efficient alternative to endotracheal intubation with mechanical ventilation; NIV also has a lower rate of complications such as pneumonia, vocal injury, and tracheal stenosis than invasive techniques [8].

Unlike bag valve mask ventilation, the most basic form of NIV, which is typically used for pre-oxygenation of a patient prior to endotracheal intubation, two types of NIV are used in lieu of endotracheal intubation. The first type, continuous positive airway pressure, applies supportive pressure in a uniform fashion during both the inspiratory phase and the expiratory phase. The second type, bi-level positive airway pressure, alternates different levels of inspiratory and expiratory pressure. Both types typically provide pressure support of 4–20 cmH_2O, usually via a face mask, although helmets and nasal cannulas can also be used [9]. Because BiPaP matches the patient's spontaneous respiratory drive, in certain patients NIV may be more efficient than endotracheal intubation and controlled mechanical ventilation [10]. In addition, the training required to deliver NIV is less extensive than the training required for endotracheal intubation.

Over the past several years, NIV modalities have proven to be effective in management of acute respiratory failure. NIV decreases the effort required for breathing through several mechanisms. It improves pulmonary compliance and reduces the ventilation/perfusion mismatch. Smaller, pliable airways are stented open. This allows for recruitment and ventilation of atelectatic alveoli. The increased intrathoracic pressure decreases venous return, transmural pressure, and afterload, which improves cardiac function. Edema is shifted back into the vascular system [10].

30.3 Indications

30.3.1 Hospital Setting

Common indications for NIV in hospital patients include COPD exacerbation, ACPE, acute respiratory failure in immunosuppressed patients, post-intubation weaning, and post-extubation support in patients at high risk for reintubation [9]. Patients with nontraumatic chest wall deformity, neuromuscular disease, obstructive sleep apnea, cystic fibrosis, or pneumonia may benefit as well [11]. The evidence supporting routine use of NIV for asthma is limited, although small studies indicate that NIV may be of value [2, 9, 11]. The British Thoracic Society recommends NIV for chest trauma if analgesia and high-flow oxygen fail to maintain adequate oxygenation; in such cases, patients should be monitored closely for pneumothorax [11].

NIV may obviate the need for endotracheal intubation [12]. Recent reviews and guidelines have suggested that NIV be considered the first option for ventilatory support in patients with COPD or ACPE, citing decreased mortality and shorter hospital stays [9, 12–14]. Evidence supporting the use of continuous positive airway pressure is more robust than that supporting the use of bi-level positive airway pressure [15]. Because NIV does not require sedation, it provides the advantage of keeping the patient alert and capable of making health-care decisions.

30.3.2 Prehospital Setting

Although there is now compelling evidence of the benefits of the early initiation of NIV as an adjunct to medication for COPD and ACPE, the use of NIV for respiratory failure in the prehospital setting remains limited [16]. Paramedics in the field can improve the effectiveness of their treatment of respiratory failure by becoming more familiar with the indications for and methods of NIV so that NIV can be used appropriately and in all cases that warrant it.

NIV should be carefully considered in patients with respiratory failure. The best candidate for NIV is an awake patient in respiratory distress who is alert and cooperative and has an intact gag reflex [17]. It is appropriate to consider NIV in patients with respiratory failure with oxygen saturation less than 90 % despite oxygen delivery at 15 l/m. It is also appropriate to use NIV in patients with do-not-intubate orders or when the patient's wishes regarding advanced life support are unknown and cannot be discussed on the scene.

30.4 Outcomes

Acute respiratory failure must be treated promptly for optimal outcome. Given the positive results for NIV in inpatients, it follows that administering NIV to patients in the field would also improve outcomes. Inpatient studies suggest that COPD and ACPE patients are the most likely to benefit from prehospital NIV.

Several studies and meta-analyses have attempted to clarify the value of NIV in the prehospital setting [2, 3, 15, 18–21]. Most of these studies have focused on ACPE. Primary endpoints included mortality, need for subsequent intubation, length of hospital stay, length of intensive care unit stay, vital sign stability, and patients' subjective assessment of symptom control. Studies like this are fraught with challenges. Because double-blind studies are impractical, the potential for treatment bias is high. Ethically, the care of a patient experiencing respiratory failure should not be delayed for the purpose of obtaining consent for treatment.

Compared with standard medical care, prehospital NIV is generally associated with lower mortality and lower rates of intubation [2, 3, 15, 19–21]. Patients treated with NIV reported symptomatic relief [18, 19]. Whereas some studies reported clear improvement in vital signs [19, 20], others did not find this to be the case [18]. Improvements were most pronounced with regard to the heart rate and respiratory rate, not oxygen saturation [22]. Despite such improvements, most studies did not show a decrease in the length of stay in the intensive care unit or in the length of hospitalization [2, 19].

30.5 Contraindications and Complications

NIV is contraindicated in comatose patients. Patients with hemodynamic instability, decreased respiratory drive, or severe respiratory distress mandate immediate endotracheal intubation to secure the airway. As with endotracheal intubation, pneumothorax should be treated prior to initiation of NIV therapy. Structural facial abnormalities, trauma, and burns can hinder mask-to-face sealing and preclude the use of NIV. Patients with fixed upper airway obstructions do not respond to NIV. Altered mentation, agitation, or somnolence can decrease a patient's ability to cooperate with NIV therapy. Decreased gag reflexes put patients at a higher risk of aspiration of digestive tract contents through NIV. Gastrointestinal contraindications include active vomiting, distention, and bowel obstruction, which also increase the risk of aspiration. Patients with recent facial or upper gastrointestinal tract surgery should not receive NIV [10, 11].

Patients should be monitored for response to NIV. As a patient's subjective comfort level improves, objective findings such as oxygenation, vital signs, and work of breathing should stabilize. Successfully treated patients should continue to receive therapy. Treatment should be coordinated with the receiving emergency department so that the treatment is not interrupted. Progressive deterioration, intolerance to therapy, or development of treatment-related complications mandate an alternative strategy (e.g., intubation or construction of a surgical airway).

NIV is generally well tolerated, but in the prehospital setting, emesis and claustrophobia are frequent complications of NIV [2, 23]. Other NIV-associated complications include nasal abrasion, rhinitis, nose pain, gastric distention, and poor sleep [24]. There are also challenges when it comes to mask leakage and poor mask fit. One study suggested an increase in mortality from acute myocardial infarction in hospital patients treated with NIV [25]. Subsequent meta-analyses have not supported this finding [13, 26]. In cases of trauma, there is a risk for pneumocephalus, subcutaneous emphysema, pneumothorax, hypotension, and infection [10].

Oxygen toxicity has been cited as detrimental in critically ill patients, particularly in patients with myocardial infarction and cerebrovascular disease. NIV has traditionally been used with high oxygen concentrations, but a recent study has shown low oxygen concentrations to be effective in patients with these conditions [23].

Conclusions

Acute respiratory distress is a common diagnostic dilemma for paramedics and can be due to various conditions. The goals of care include identifying the cause, promptly initiating targeted management, stabilizing the airway, and observing for ventilatory improvement or deterioration. When advanced directives are not clear and the patient has an advanced illness or a poor prognosis, administering noninvasive ventilation to a patient in respiratory distress provides the time needed to explore the patient's wishes by communicating directly with the patient, family members, or medical personnel who might be familiar with the patient, while en route to the hospital.

In the prehospital setting, diagnostic testing is challenging and transport times can be long. Prior to arrival at a hospital, options are limited for patients whose condition is rapidly deteriorating. In patients with severe respiratory distress, prehospital NIV has been shown to reduce the need for intubation or mechanical ventilation upon admission to a hospital as well as in-hospital mortality in several randomized controlled trials reviewed by Mal and colleagues [2]. NIV is generally safe, especially when the provider is knowledgeable of the contraindications for prolonged NIV such as excessive somnolence, respiratory fatigue, agitation, or facial anomalies.

Key Recommendations

- The best candidates for NIV are patients in respiratory distress who are awake and cooperative. It is appropriate to consider NIV in patients with respiratory failure with oxygen saturation less than 90 % despite oxygen delivery at 15 l/m.
- NIV can be administered by means of continuous positive airway pressure or bi-level positive airway pressure via a ventilator, at the discretion of the emergency medical service personnel at the scene or of a physician [27].
- Consider NIV and early initiation of ventilation for COPD and ACPE as an adjunct to medication.
- Progressive deterioration, intolerance to therapy, or development of treatment-related complications mandates intubation or construction of a surgical airway.
- Patients with facial abnormalities, decreased respiratory drive, or evidence of cognitive impairment should not be treated with NIV.

References

1. Clawson J, Olola C, Heward A, Patterson B, Scott G. Profile of emergency medical dispatch calls for breathing problems within the medical priority dispatch system protocol. Prehosp Disaster Med. 2008;23(5):412–9.
2. Mal S, McLeod S, Iansavichene A, Dukelow A, Lewell M. Effect of out-of-hospital noninvasive positive-pressure support ventilation in adult patients with severe respiratory distress: a systematic review and meta-analysis. Ann Emerg Med. 2014;63(5):600–7.e601.
3. Thompson J, Petrie DA, Ackroyd-Stolarz S, Bardua DJ. Out-of-hospital continuous positive airway pressure ventilation versus usual care in acute respiratory failure: a randomized controlled trial. Ann Emerg Med. 2008;52(3):232–41, 241.e231.
4. Bakke SA, Botker MT, Riddervold IS, Kirkegaard H, Christensen EF. Continuous positive airway pressure and noninvasive ventilation in prehospital treatment of patients with acute respiratory failure: a systematic review of controlled studies. Scand J Trauma Resusc Emerg Med. 2014;22(1):69.
5. Dib JE, Matin SA, Luckert A. Prehospital use of continuous positive airway pressure for acute severe congestive heart failure. J Emerg Med. 2012;42(5):553–8.
6. Maio RF, Garrison HG, Spaite DW, Desmond JS, Gregor MA, Cayten CG, Chew Jr JL, Hill EM, Joyce SM, MacKenzie EJ, et al. Emergency medical services outcomes project I (EMSOP I): prioritizing conditions for outcomes research. Ann Emerg Med. 1999;33(4):423–32.
7. Wang HE, Davis DP, O'Connor RE, Domeier RM. Drug-assisted intubation in the prehospital setting (resource document to NAEMSP position statement). Prehosp Emerg Care. 2006;10(2):261–71.
8. Sullivan CE, Issa FG, Berthon-Jones M, Eves L. Reversal of obstructive sleep apnoea by continuous positive airway pressure applied through the nares. Lancet. 1981;1(8225):862–5.

9. Keenan SP, Sinuff T, Burns KE, Muscedere J, Kutsogiannis J, Mehta S, Cook DJ, Ayas N, Adhikari NK, Hand L, et al. Clinical practice guidelines for the use of noninvasive positive-pressure ventilation and noninvasive continuous positive airway pressure in the acute care setting. Can Med Assoc J. 2011;183(3):E195–214.
10. Daily JC, Wang HE. Noninvasive positive pressure ventilation: resource document for the National Association of EMS Physicians position statement. Prehosp Emerg Care. 2011;15(3):432–8.
11. British Thoracic Society Standards of Care C. Non-invasive ventilation in acute respiratory failure. Thorax. 2002;57(3):192–211.
12. McCurdy BR. Noninvasive positive pressure ventilation for acute respiratory failure patients with chronic obstructive pulmonary disease (COPD): an evidence-based analysis. Ont Health Technol Assess Ser. 2012;12(8):1–102.
13. Winck JC, Azevedo LF, Costa-Pereira A, Antonelli M, Wyatt JC. Efficacy and safety of non-invasive ventilation in the treatment of acute cardiogenic pulmonary edema–a systematic review and meta-analysis. Crit Care. 2006;10(2):R69.
14. Budweiser S, Jorres RA, Pfeifer M. Treatment of respiratory failure in COPD. Int J Chron Obstruct Pulmon Dis. 2008;3(4):605–18.
15. Goodacre S, Stevens JW, Pandor A, Poku E, Ren S, Cantrell A, Bounes V, Mas A, Payen D, Petrie D, et al. Prehospital noninvasive ventilation for acute respiratory failure: systematic review, network meta-analysis, and individual patient data meta-analysis. Acad Emerg Med. 2014;21(9):960–70.
16. Sellmann T, Conty C, Treschan T, Kindgen-Milles D. [Prehospital non-invasive ventilation in Germany: results of a nationwide survey of ground-based emergency medical services]. Anaesthesist. 2014;63(3):217–24.
17. Brunner ME, Lyazidi A, Richard JC, Brochard L. [Non-invasive ventilation: indication for acute respiratory failure]. Revue Med Suisse. 2012;8(366):2382–7.
18. Schmidbauer W, Ahlers O, Spies C, Dreyer A, Mager G, Kerner T. Early prehospital use of non-invasive ventilation improves acute respiratory failure in acute exacerbation of chronic obstructive pulmonary disease. Emerg Med J. 2011;28(7):626–7.
19. Simpson PM, Bendall JC. Prehospital non-invasive ventilation for acute cardiogenic pulmonary oedema: an evidence-based review. Emerg Med J. 2011;28(7):609–12.
20. Taylor DM, Bernard SA, Masci K, MacBean CE, Kennedy MP, Zalstein S. Prehospital noninvasive ventilation: a viable treatment option in the urban setting. Prehosp Emerg Care. 2008;12(1):42–5.
21. Williams TA, Finn J, Perkins GD, Jacobs IG. Prehospital continuous positive airway pressure for acute respiratory failure: a systematic review and meta-analysis. Prehosp Emerg Care. 2013;17(2):261–73.
22. Aguilar SA, Lee J, Dunford JV, Castillo E, Lam B, Choy J, Patel E, Pringle J, Serra J. Assessment of the addition of prehospital continuous positive airway pressure (CPAP) to an urban emergency medical services (EMS) system in persons with severe respiratory distress. J Emerg Med. 2013;45(2):210–9.
23. Bledsoe BE, Anderson E, Hodnick R, Johnson L, Johnson S, Dievendorf E. Low-fractional oxygen concentration continuous positive airway pressure is effective in the prehospital setting. Prehosp Emerg Care. 2012;16(2):217–21.
24. Vitacca M, Nava S, Confalonieri M, Bianchi L, Porta R, Clini E, Ambrosino N. The appropriate setting of noninvasive pressure support ventilation in stable COPD patients. Chest. 2000;118(5):1286–93.
25. Mehta S, Jay GD, Woolard RH, Hipona RA, Connolly EM, Cimini DM, Drinkwine JH, Hill NS. Randomized, prospective trial of bilevel versus continuous positive airway pressure in acute pulmonary edema. Crit Care Med. 1997;25(4):620–8.
26. Peter JV, Moran JL, Phillips-Hughes J, Warn D. Noninvasive ventilation in acute respiratory failure–a meta-analysis update. Crit Care Med. 2002;30(3):555–62.
27. Duchateau FX, Beaune S, Ricard-Hibon A, Mantz J, Juvin P. Prehospital noninvasive ventilation can help in management of patients with limitations of life-sustaining treatments. Eur J Emerg Med. 2010;17(1):7–9.

Equipment Technology for Noninvasive Ventilation in the Pre-hospital Setting

31

Steven C. LeCroy

Contents

Noninvasive ventilation (NIV) is the delivery of ventilatory support without the need for an artificial airway. NIV is provided using either positive or negative pressure. However, since the early 1980s, noninvasive positive pressure ventilation (NIPPV) has emerged as an important advance in respiratory care. In 2000, the National Association of EMS Physicians (NAEMSP) issued a position statement on pre-hospital NIPPV: "Non-invasive positive pressure ventilation is a viable pre-hospital therapeutic option for acute dyspnea" [1]. The NAEMSP position statement was based on the work of Kosowsky [2], titled "Pre-hospital use of continuous positive airway pressure (CPAP) for presumed pulmonary edema: a preliminary case series," also published in 2000.

NIPPV has proved effective in the pre-hospital setting for a variety of cardiopulmonary conditions, from congestive heart failure (CHF) to chronic obstructive pulmonary disease (COPD). In fact, it is not uncommon to see pre-hospital medical protocols directing emergency medical services (EMS) clinicians to

S.C. LeCroy, MA, CRTT, EMTP
Emergency Medical Services, St. Petersburg College, St. Petersburg, FL, USA

Hillsborough Community College, Plant City, FL, USA
e-mail: slecroy@mercurymed.com

A.M. Esquinas (ed.), *Noninvasive Mechanical Ventilation: Theory, Equipment, and Clinical Applications*, DOI 10.1007/978-3-319-21653-9_31

consider NIPPV for any patient in respiratory distress regardless of underlying pathology. A common technique for NIPPV pre-hospital is continuous positive airway pressure (CPAP). Another option can be the use of bi-level positive airway pressure (BiPAP). Of the two, CPAP has a proven track record when used pre-hospital; support for BiPAP is still lacking. In addition, current technology for providing BiPAP requires a more complex device or ventilator; neither is well suited for prehospital use. In contrast, simple disposable and non-disposable CPAP devices designed specifically for pre-hospital are available, as well as a variety of transport ventilators with NIV capabilities. This chapter will cover the current technology and equipment to provide NIPPV in the out-of-hospital emergency environment.

Historically, NIPPV use in the field was limited by the available technology. Limitations of using hospital NIV devices included size, cost, durability, and oxygen consumption. Over time and with feedback from the field, each of these limitations has been addressed with new and innovative technology. Before looking at current devices available for use in the pre-hospital setting and to help determine the appropriate device for a particular agency, there are a few fundamental questions that providers should ask before selecting a device: First, what constitutes a good pre-hospital NIPPV device? Second, what capabilities are required to meet the needs of a particular agency? EMS agencies share some basic fundamental protocols and equipment types, but, if you have seen one EMS agency then you have seen one EMS agency; no two are alike.

There are a variety of devices available for clinicians to choose from when providing NIPPV, from fully disposable to capital equipment. All medical devices have variations in performance and design. Providers of NIPPV should be aware of these differences and the effect the differences may have on the care provided.

31.1 Important Components of a Pre-hospital NIV Device

Patient Interface NIPPV is only effective if the patient is compliant with the treatment; patient comfort is key, as a patient is rarely compliant when not comfortable. The choice of interface is a crucial issue in NIV. Available interfaces include nasal, oronasal, and facial masks, mouthpieces, and helmets, with full face mask being common. Interfaces come in different sizes, and having the correct size makes the device more comfortable and improves the seal, requiring less pressure from the head strap or harness. Another option to improve comfort is to have some mechanism to take pressure off the bridge of the nose, reducing the incidence of pressure sores, a common complaint of patients receiving NIV.

Manometer Applying positive pressure to the airway is not without risk and may lead to a wide range of problems, including pneumothorax, reduced cardiac output, and even death. As with every therapy, keeping a balance between risk and reward is important. To help manage the risk, it is recommended that all patients receiving NIPPV should have the pressure continuously monitored. A manometer also allows the clinician to document pressures used, information that will be valuable in the event of a bad outcome.

Few Parts/Compact EMS units have limited, space not only in their vehicles but in the equipment bags/cases taken to the patient. It is imperative that any equipment designed for EMS be compact and simple, with minimal parts. Historically, EMS providers have an aversion to any equipment with lots of parts that require assembly before use. Because the number of parts increases confusion, application error and reduction in use increases.

Oxygen Consumption Unlike a hospital, EMS crews or ambulances have a limited supply of oxygen. Many agencies have converted to D cylinders because of their size and weight as a trade-off for less oxygen. Those agencies with longer transport times have to be concerned with oxygen consumption rates.

Nebulizer Capable With the expanded use of NIV for patients in respiratory distress, including COPD and asthma, the ability to provide nebulized medications is no longer an option but a necessity.

Capnography/Capnometry Capable The measuring of end tidal CO_2 ($EtCO_2$) should be a standard for any patient in respiratory distress or failure. With current $EtCO_2$ technology, all critical patients should be continuously monitored.

Anti-asphyxia Capabilities With EMS's limited oxygen carrying capabilities and potential long transport times or delays, a NIV device should have anti-asphyxia capabilities. Anti-asphyxia or anti-suffocation protection is commonly provided by an anti-asphyxia valve if the device is of a closed design. Open systems do not require an anti-asphyxia valve because the device is open to room air.

Adequate Inspiratory Flow Rates Patients in respiratory distress often require the air/oxygen to be provided at a fast enough speed to meet their demand. It is often not the volume of air/oxygen that is the problem, but the velocity at which it arrives. Inadequate inspiratory flow rates will cause shortness of breath, difficulty breathing, and an increase in work of breathing. Patients in respiratory distress may need flow rates as high as 65 l/min or greater.

Fraction of Inspired Oxygen (FiO_2) The administration of high oxygen concentrations has been the subject of great debate for several years. The outdated theory that oxygen administration is risk free has been shown to be false. However, at this time the only way to treat hypoxia is with oxygen. A NIV device with low oxygen concentration capabilities is limited when treating hypoxic patients. Clinicians are left with few options when a device has a maximum FiO_2 of 30 % and the patient is still hypoxic but needs the positive pressure to reduce the work of breathing.

Pressure Pop-Off or Relief Because high airway pressures are dangerous, a NIV device should incorporate a mechanism to relieve excessive pressure. Common causes of excessive pressure are blocked exhalation valves or blocked exhalation openings, commonly found with open systems.

31.2 Types of Pre-hospital NIPPV Systems

Commercially available systems provide portable NIPPV through either a conventional external pressure regulator, disposable CPAP system, demand-flow, or a transport ventilator. All four designs contain key features that influence selection and implementation.

Regulator-based portable NIPPV systems generate continuous pressure from oxygen flow, directly controlling inspiratory and expiratory pressure. Regulator-based NIPPV systems allow different inhaled oxygen fractions with reduced oxygen consumption.

Some disposable devices are open systems and use a different NIPPV approach, accelerating oxygen flow through a series of channels to create turbulence. The turbulence acts as a virtual valve, generating positive airway pressure.

Demand-flow devices have a variety of pressure levels and built-in manometers. Transport ventilators may be designed to provide NIPPV. Depending on the individual brand and model, the process can be somewhat complicated and beyond standard EMS training.

31.2.1 Conventional External Pressure Regulator NIPPV Systems

Regulator-based portable NIPPV systems generate continuous pressure from oxygen flow, directly controlling inspiratory and expiratory pressure. Regulator-based NIPPV systems allow different inhaled oxygen fractions with reduced oxygen consumption. In 1981, J.B. Downs invented a new Venturi device called the Downs Flow Generator. The flow generators were the first pre-hospital devices used on a large scale and come in two types, adjustable flow and fixed flow. Devices using the Downs Flow Generator design incorporate controls to adjust flow rates as well as the inspired oxygen percentage (FiO_2). Positive end-expiratory pressure (PEEP) is determined by a PEEP valve found in the mask.

31.2.1.1 WhisperFlow® and Vital Signs CPAP Systems

The first Downs Flow Generator devices were the WhisperFlow (Philips Respironics; http://whisperflow.respironics.com/) and the Vital Signs (http://www.obex.co.nz/Product/Index/137) CPAP systems. Both devices are reuseable flow generators with disposable circuits that attach to the high-pressure side of a flow meter or regulator. These devices are solely powered by gas flow and entrain room air through a Venturi device. Each produces high gas flow rates ranging from 100 to 140 l/min. The gas flow leaves the device and enters a breathing circuit, exiting through a spring-loaded valve; all pressure adjustments are made by changing valves. Neither unit incorporates a pressure manometer, and they both have high oxygen consumption rates [3].

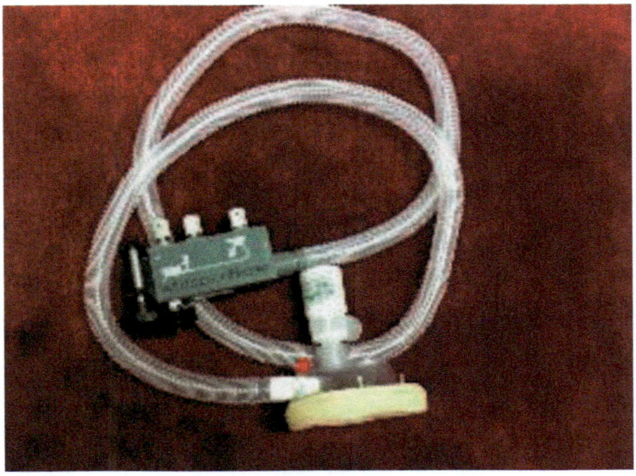

Variable flow Whisperflow, Photograph by Steve LeCroy

31.2.2 Disposable CPAP Devices

Disposable devices attach to the low-pressure side of the regulator or flow meter (Boussignac®, Flow-Safe®, O-Two Controlled Ventilation™, and Rescuer® Emergency CPAP System) or to the high-pressure side (O2-RESQ™).

31.2.2.1 Boussignac

The disposable Boussignac CPAP device (Vygon; https://www.vygon.com/catalog/vygon-boussignac-cpap_572_00557013), first described by Dr. George Boussignac in 1989, was the first completely disposable CPAP devices. The principle behind the Boussignac valve is to increase the forward velocity of a gas by narrowing the flow through a cylinder. By increasing the velocity, turbulence is created within the device. It is the turbulence and friction within the cylinder that creates the resistance the patient must breathe against. All pressure adjustments are made by adjusting the flow rate to either increase or decrease the turbulence. This process eliminates the need for valves or moving parts. The valve is open, meaning that it is open to the atmosphere, allowing the patient to breath in room air as needed. The device incorporates a measuring port to add a manometer if needed. The manufacturer reports that CPAP of 10 cmH_2O can be achieved with approximately 25 l/min of oxygen flow.

31.2.2.2 Flow-Safe

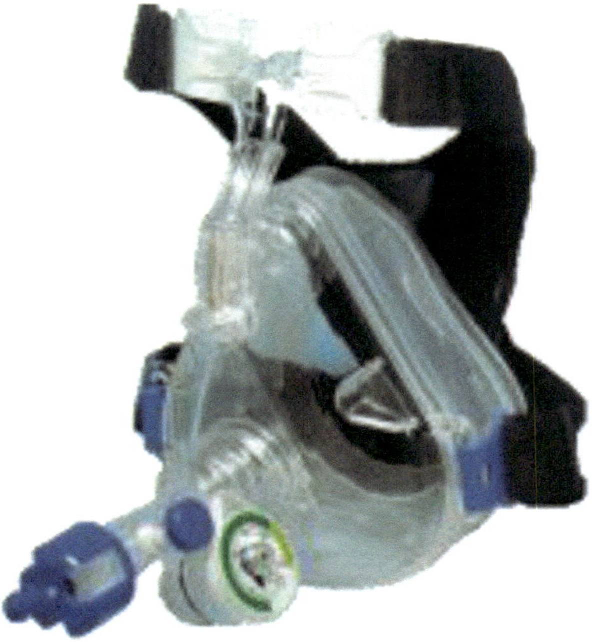

Photograph courtesy of Mercury Medical

Flow-Safe (Mercury Medical; http://mercurymed.com/home/) is a completely disposable CPAP device featuring a built-in manometer to monitor airway pressure and a pressure relief valve for patient safety. There are three versions of Flow-Safe: the original Flow-Safe, Flow-Safe II, and Flow-Safe II EZ. Each device uses the same principle to create pressure. Similar to the Boussignac, the Flow-Safe device changes the velocity of the gas by narrowing the flow. The increased gas flow creates the inspiratory pressure to assist the patient to inhale and also provides the PEEP during exhalation. Pressure adjustments are made by increasing or decreasing the gas flow rate from the flow meter or regulator and monitoring the built-in manometer. According to the manufacturer, the original Flow-Safe achieves pressures from 1.5 to 10 cmH_2O with oxygen flow rates of 10–25 l/min. Flow-Safe II achieves the same pressures as the original Flow-Safe using lower flow rates, however, the trade-off is a slightly lower FiO_2. Flow-Safe II EZ incorporates a built-in nebulizer, allowing both the valve and the nebulizer to be powered from a single gas source.

31.2.2.3 O-Two Controlled Ventilation

The O-Two Single-Use CPAP device (O-Two Medical Technologies; http://otwo.com/emergency-cpap/o_two-single-use-cpap/) is completely disposable. Adjustment of pressure levels occurs by adjusting the flow rate from the flow meter or regulator. Pressure and flow rate settings are found on the body of device.

According to the manufacturer, the CPAP range is between 5 and 20 cmH_2O at flow rates of 8–25 l/min.

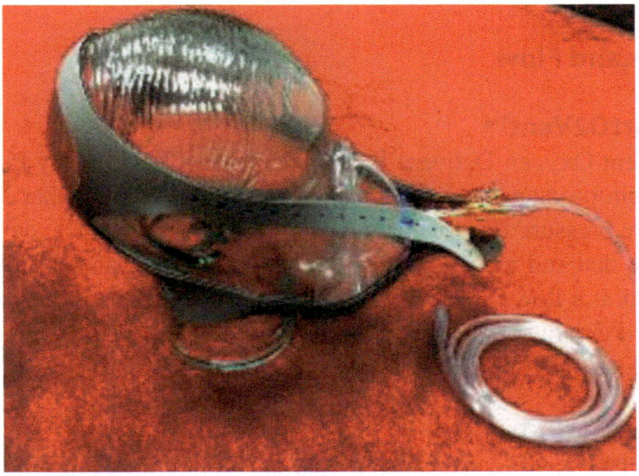

Photograph by Steve LeCroy

31.2.2.4 O2-RESQ

The O2-RESQ (Pulmodyne; http://www.pulmodyne.com/products/pre-hospital-and-emergency-medicine/o2-resq-product-information/) is an expansion chamber with a Venturi air entrainment port. The basic unit provides approximately 30 % FiO_2 at a continuous flow up to 140 l/min to meet patient demand. CPAP valves are available from 2.5 to 20 cmH_2O and provide constant pressures at any flow rate. With the addition of the O_2-MAX™ Trio adaptor, FiO_2 can be adjusted from 30% to 60% or 90%. CPAP valves, snapped onto the anti-asphyxia housing end of the circuit, are used to maintain PEEP pressures.

31.2.2.5 Rescuer Emergency CPAP System

Rescuer Emergency CPAP (BLS Systems; http://blssystemsltd.com/cpap_em.html) incorporates an oxygen reservoir that, according to the manufacturer, allows higher FiO_2 levels with low flow rates, saving oxygen. The device also has filters on both the inhalation and exhalation side to reduce exposure to airborne pathogens. With the addition of the Rescuer II compact, a smaller version than the original BLS Rescuer, BLS Systems now offers a version with a built-in manometer. The device can also be configured to power a small volume nebulizer directly off the CPAP device.

31.2.2.6 Smith Oxy-PEEP™

Oxy-PEEP (Smiths Medical; http://www.smiths-medical.com/catalog/oxygen-medication-delivery/oxygen-delivery/oxygen-masks/oxy-peep.html) is a high-concentration, high-flow oxygen diluter with adjustable PEEP. However, the device should not be considered a CPAP or BiPAP device inasmuch as there is no inspiratory pressure. Only when the patient attempts to breathe out is there any pressure within the circuit. This device allows for variable flows, variable O_2 concentrations, and variable PEEP.

31.2.3 Demand Flow

31.2.3.1 PortO2Vent™

The PortO2Vent Oxygen Delivery System (Emergent Respiratory Products; http://www.eresp.com/products/porto2vent/) is a gas-powered device that delivers noninvasive positive pressure to spontaneously breathing patients. The device features a nondisposable demand valve that delivers oxygen during inhalation through a disposable circuit at a flow rate determined by the patient's inspiratory effort. A specially designed expiratory valve is pressure balanced to precisely maintain pressure levels and reduce patient effort to open and exhale through the valve.

31.2.3.2 MACS CPAP System

The MACS CPAP System (Airon; http://aironusa.com/macs-cpap-system/)provides infinitely variable PEEP, a built-in pressure gauge, and only flows oxygen during inspiration, for reduced oxygen consumption and easier patient monitoring. The device is non-disposable and uses a disposable circuit. It also incorporates a calibrated knob that sets the CPAP level and a switch selects either 65 % or 100 % oxygen.

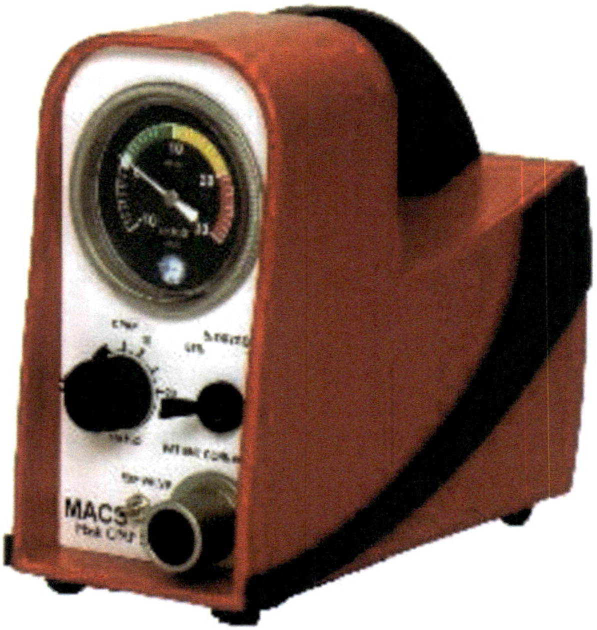

Photograph Courtesy of Airon Corporation

31.2.4 Transport Ventilators with NIV Functionality

Most transport ventilators are complex mechanical ventilation devices and provide most forms of ventilation, including both CPAP and BiPAP. However, many were not designed to provide facemask NIV; the CPAP/BiPAP modes are for patients with protected airways. Transport ventilators that do provide NIV have capabilities well beyond those found on other types of pre-hospital NIV devices and are considered capital equipment, with an average starting price of approximately $5,000 per unit with a disposable circuit and mask. The following is a noninclusive list of transport ventilators that offer NIV capabilities:

CAREvent® ALS+ CPAP (O-Two ™ Medical Technologies; http://otwo.com/wp-content/uploads/O-Two_CAREvent-ALS-CPAP_2012.pdf)

Flight 60 (Flight Medical®; http://www.flight-medical.com/flight-60-3)

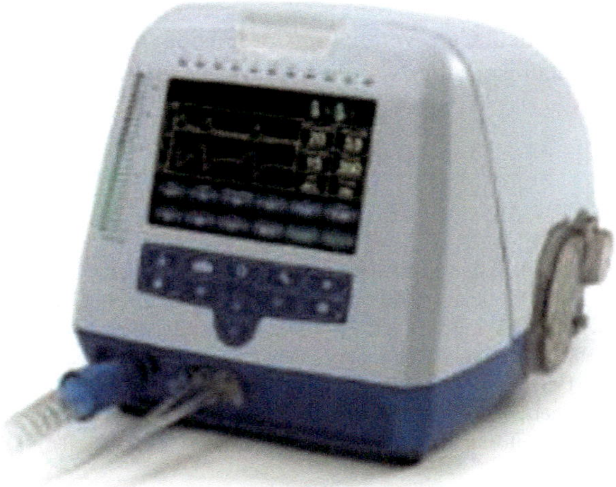

Photograph Courtesy of Mercury Medical

LSP AutoVent™ 4000 CPAP (Allied Healthcare Products Inc.; http://www.alliedhpi.com/images/z90-00-0008.pdf)

Newport HT70® Ventilator (Covidien™; http://www.covidien.com/rms/products/portable-ventilation/newport-ht70-plus)

Pneupac® paraPAC plus™ (Smiths Medical; http://www.smiths-medical.com/catalog/mechanical-ventilation/pneupac/para-pac/pneupac-parapac-mri-p200d.html)

pNeuton® Model S Ventilator (Airon; http://aironusa.com/ems-products/ems-pneuton-model-s/)

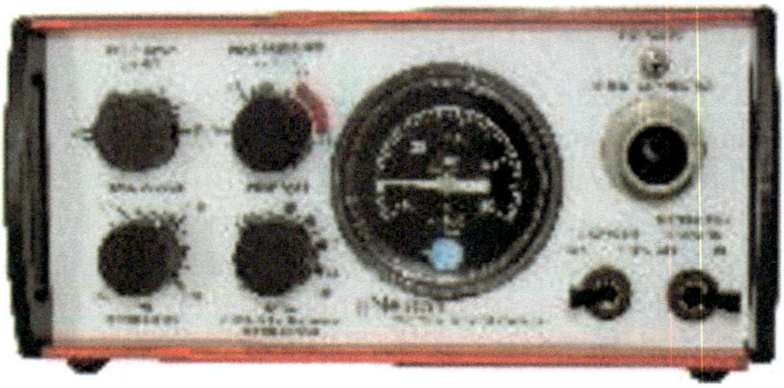

Photograph Courtesy of Airon Corporation

Oxylog® 3000 Plus (Drager Medical; http://www.draeger.com/sites/en_aunz/Pages/Hospital/Oxylog-3000-plus.aspx)

Uni-Vent® 731 Series Model EMV+® and AEV® (Zoll®; http://www.impactii.com/Vents.html)

ReVel® Portable Critical Care Ventilator (CareFusion; http://www.carefusion.com/medical-products/respiratory/ventilation/revel-ventilator-system/)

Work Cited

1. Daily J, Wang H. Noninvasive positive pressure ventilation: resource document for the National Association of EMS Physicians position statement. Prehosp Emerg Care. 2011;15(3):432–8.
2. Kosowsky J, Stephanides S, Branson R, Sayre M. Prehospital use of continuous positive airway pressure (CPAP) for presumed pulmonary edema: a preliminary case series. Prehosp Emerg Care. 2001;5(2):190–6.
3. Glover GW, Fletcher SJ. Assessing the performance of the Whisperflow continuous positive airway pressure generator: a bench study. Br J Anaesth. 2009;102(6):875–81.

Resources

Branson R, Johannigman J. Pre-hospital oxygen therapy. Respir Care. 2013;58(1):86–97.

Eisenman A, Rusetski V, Sharivker D, Avital RN. Role of the Boussignac continuous positive pressure mask in the emergency department. Israeli J Emerg Med. 2008;8(2):6–11.

Fisher GC. The Downs' adjustable flow generator. Anaesthesia. 1988;43:766–9. The Association of Anaesthetists of Gt Britain and Ireland.

Hubble M, Richards M, Jarvis R, Millikan T, Young D. Effectiveness of prehospital continuous positive airway pressure in the management of acute pulmonary edema. Prehosp Emerg Care. 2006;10(4):430–9.

Mosesso V, Dunford J, Blackwell T, Griswell J. Prehospital therapy for acute congestive heart failure: state of the art. Prehosp Emerg Care. 2003;7(1):13–23.

Simpson PM, Bendall JC. Prehospital non-invasive ventilation for acute cardiogenic pulmonary oedema: an evidence-based review. Emerg Med J. 2011;28(7):609–12.

Templier F, Dolveck F, Baer M, Chauvin M, Fletcher D. 'Boussignac' continuous positive airway pressure system: practical use in a prehospital medical care unit. Eur J Emerg Med. 2003;10:87–93.

Intra-hospital Transport of Patients during Noninvasive Ventilatory Support: Key Topics

32

Antonio Javier Domínguez Petit and Antonio M. Esquinas

Contents

Abbreviations

ECG Electrocardiography
ED Emergency department
ICU Intensive care unit
IMV Invasive mechanical ventilation
NIV Noninvasive mechanical ventilation

A.J. Domínguez Petit, MD, Ph (✉)
Emergency Department of the General Hospital, Hospital Universitario Virgen del Rocío, Seville, Spain
e-mail: antoniodominguezpetit@gmail.com

A.M. Esquinas, MD, PhD, FCCP
Intensive Care and Non Invasive Ventilatory Unit, Hospital Morales Meseguer, Murcia, Spain

International School of Non-invasive mechanical Ventilation, Murcia, Spain
e-mail: antmesquinas@gmail.com

A.M. Esquinas (ed.), *Noninvasive Mechanical Ventilation: Theory, Equipment, and Clinical Applications*, DOI 10.1007/978-3-319-21653-9_32

32.1 Introduction

Noninvasive mechanical ventilation (NIV) has proven to be effective in patients with acute respiratory failure of various etiologies. Its application in both the pre-hospital and hospital settings decreases the need for invasive mechanical ventilation (IMV) and admission to the intensive care unit (ICU), especially in selected cases of acute cardiogenic pulmonary edema or chronic obstructive pulmonary disease exacerbations [1, 2], but evidence is growing regarding its efficacy in different conditions, such as pulmonary contusion, pneumonia, and near-fatal drowning [3]. In recent years, NIV has gained a growing role in emergency departments (EDs) and their acute care areas, as there is a greater understanding of the practice and evidence of its benefits in selected groups of patients.

Intra-hospital transports of noninvasively ventilated patients usually are made (1) from the ED to the ICU or other hospital wards with experience in handling NIV (e.g., the respiratory intermediate care unit), (2) between the ED and the radiology facilities, and (3) between different areas of these unit [4, 5]

32.2 Discussion and Analysis

The architecture of hospitals and the location of the different destinations significantly affect the time spent in performing such movements and exposure to potential adverse effects during treatment [5–7]. Ideally, the transfer of a patient on NIV to another hospital area should not exceed 10–15 min once the circuit transfer is activated. Some recommendations on some specific points may be useful.

Staff All patients on NIV should be accompanied by at least one physician and one nurse, well trained in airways management and cardiopulmonary resuscitation, and one technician or medical transport guard. It is, of course, of pivotal importance that the personnel involved in the transfer are competent with noninvasive ventilatory support modalities, accessories, and interfaces and will recognize any problems and act accordingly. The team receiving the patient should be warned in advance, to allow sufficient staff available to implement the transfer to bed, prepare the NIV system change (if necessary), and minimize the occurrence of complications. On arrival at the receiving unit, there must be a direct communication between the accompanying team and the one expected to assume responsibility for the patient's care after the transport is complete. A specifically dedicated record reporting the patient's medical history, treatment initiated, ventilator settings, vital signs, and major events suffered during transport should be part of the entire medical file. The authors strongly suggest the implementation of a clear clinical flowchart, readily accessible to all staff members involved, reflecting their role in the transfer process.

Equipment Equipment should be light, strong, and able to be easily transported through corridors and lifts. A wide range of devices capable of administering NIV is available. We recommend devices specifically designed for NIV because there is less trouble in administering noninvasive support. To minimize the problems related to the transfer of devices, it is important to use dedicated equipment, eventually placed on stands with wheels or directly attached to the bed for easy movement.

Should the duration of the transport be extended, as in the case of multiple imaging evaluation, a key consideration is the provision of adequate battery and oxygen supply. It is therefore crucial to check the status of the battery and the oxygen cylinders before moving the patient. It is also necessary to carry the electrical connections of the devices and appropriate extensions to connect the ventilator to the wall oxygen jacks. NIV and transport ventilators generally have an internal battery life of 5 h or longer. The authors strongly recommend that the operators involved in the transfer know in-depth the functions and settings of the ventilator in use.

Masks and interfaces deserve separate consideration. Different types of interfaces have been validated for NIV. While ventilator modalities are set to a specific clinical goal, the choice of a particular interface affects prevention of leaks and patient comfort and is closely related to the success of the technique [8]. Therefore, in the absence of specific evidence on this subject, it seems logical that a patient who is well adapted on a particular interface before being transferred should continue on NIV with the same interface during the transfer, which could also reduce hospital costs. This peculiar requirement must be matched to the features of the ventilator system adopted for the transport. In any case, it is important to ensure a proper fit of the mask before the transfer and to check it continuously during the transfer because accidental displacements and air leaks frequently occur in this setting.

Although a discussion of ventilator modalities is beyond the scope of this chapter, during the transport it is important to maintain the patient on the same parameters that he or she is well adapted to. This may require a correction of the settings when switching a patient from a different ventilatory algorithm so that the same level of ventilatory support is maintained. For this and the aforementioned reasons, as a general rule, one should avoid replacing a NIV system, as this may result in the loss of the benefit obtained.

Finally, although thorough stabilization of the patient must precede the decision to transfer (see below), one must be prepared for the eventuality of an abrupt worsening of the patient's clinical condition during the transfer. Therefore, adequate instrumentation and medications for advanced airways control and cardiopulmonary resuscitation must be part of the equipment for intra-hospital transports.

Monitoring Patient monitoring during transfers should address the main potential complications described for this condition (Table 32.1) [9, 10]. During the transport,

Table 32.1 Major complications and contraindications during intra-hospital transport

Major complications:
1. The loss of PEEP/CPAP can lead to hypoxemia
2. The changes in the patient's position may involve hypotension and hypoxemia
3. Arrhythmias associated with transporting critically ill
4. Malfunction of the equipment used, which can result in loss of patient monitoring or collecting of incorrect variables
5. The movement can cause the disconnection of ventilatory support and compromise the patient's respiratory function
6. The movement may cause the accidental withdrawal of catheters and intravenous administration interruption medications which the patient is receiving
Major contraindications for transferring patients on NIV:
1. Inability to provide adequate oxygenation and ventilation during transport through the chosen NIV system
2. Inability to maintain adequate hemodynamics during transport (hemodynamic instability, shock, unstable ischemic heart disease, arrhythmias, poorly controlled)
3. Inability to monitor the patient's cardiopulmonary status during transfer
4. Inability to maintain control of the airway during transport (respiratory arrest, upper gastrointestinal bleeding, excessive secretions, airway obstruction, increased risk of pulmonary aspiration, severe encephalopathy with GCS <10 points, burn, trauma, or facial surgery)
5. Shortage of staff to perform the transfer under optimal conditions
6. Insufficient knowledge in the transfer of critically ill members appointed to do
7. Lack of communication and coordination between the various departments involved

NIV should be monitored objectively and subjectively (improvement of dyspnea and comfort). Consequently, the authors recommend the provision of the following points:

1. Continuous electrocardiography (ECG) tracing
2. Intermittent noninvasive blood pressure
3. Continuous oxygen saturation
4. Respiratory rate and exhaled tidal volumes
5. Patient-ventilator synchrony (physical signs or pressure and flow curves)
6. Clincal surveillance for the entire duration of the transfer, with particular attention to the level of consciousness, auscultation, inspection, and detection of displacement of the mask and air leaks

Selection of Patients to be Transported on NIV Hemodynamic stability, spontaneous breathing, and the ability to protect the airways are definite requirements for the application of NIV. Patients who have only a partial response to the technique or those in whom the indication for a NIV approach is debatable, are poor candidates to be transferred on NIV. Patients who display poor synchronization with the system or continue to be severely dyspneic despite efforts to optimize ventilator settings, along with those who are agitated and uncooperative or have severe and difficult-to-handle bronchorrhea, require further evaluation and to be stabilized before transfer. Table 32.2 summarized the key major elements of intra-hospital transport of patients on NIV.

Table 32.2 Key major elements and equipment to intra-hospital transport

1. Ensure proper indication of NIV
2. Assess the risks and benefits to the patient of alternatives (high-flow oxygen therapy, IMV)
3. Decide whether or not to maintain NIV
4. Equipment and practical checking:
(a) Before starting the transfer, verify the availability and correct functioning of intubation, ventilation bag, and proper equipment to perform intubation if the patient's respiratory status deteriorates
(b) Presence of a source of oxygen with sufficient volume for the secured transfer
(c) Presence of a portable monitor that provides ECG monitoring and heart rate and allows measurement of arterial pressure
(d) Capacity to perform pulse oximetry (always) and capnography (desirable)
(e) If a non-mechanical NIV device is used (continuous positive airway pressure (CPAP) high-flow devices):
(i) Check the correct operation of the manometer to maintain desired level of CPAP:
1. Checking that the flowmeter is suitable, that is, can provide 30 l/min instead of 15 l/min to get the virtual CPAP valve effect
2. Evaluating and adjusting the position of the interface and the correct connection of the hose, filter, and oxygen source
(ii) If a mechanical NIV device is used:
1. Check the battery charge status
2. Monitor tidal volume, respiratory rate, level of positive end-expiratory pressure, leaks, and the FiO_2 system provided
3. Set system alarms
4. Evaluate the tightness of interfaces and the correct connection between the different parts
(f) Appropriate medication (sedatives, opioids, nitrites, etc.)

Key Major Recommendations

- Conduct a comprehensive assessment of the patient and proceed to stabilize the patient prior to transfer, assuring perfect coordination between the various teams participating in the transfer, avoiding delays and limiting the exposure of the patient to the possibility of adverse events.
- Provide a clear flowchart (printed or digital), readily accessible to all staff, reflecting the role of every member of the transport team.
- Define the monitoring equipment necessary to carry out the transport.
- Know in-depth the characteristics and functioning of the devices in use during transport, providing an adequate training of staff on NIV, airways management, and cardiopulmonary resuscitation.
- Review the problems encountered during transport to avoid their repetition in the future (production of records and audits), and establish periodical retraining programs on NIV for staff.

Appendix 1: Inter-hospital Transport of Patients Receiving NIV Algorithm

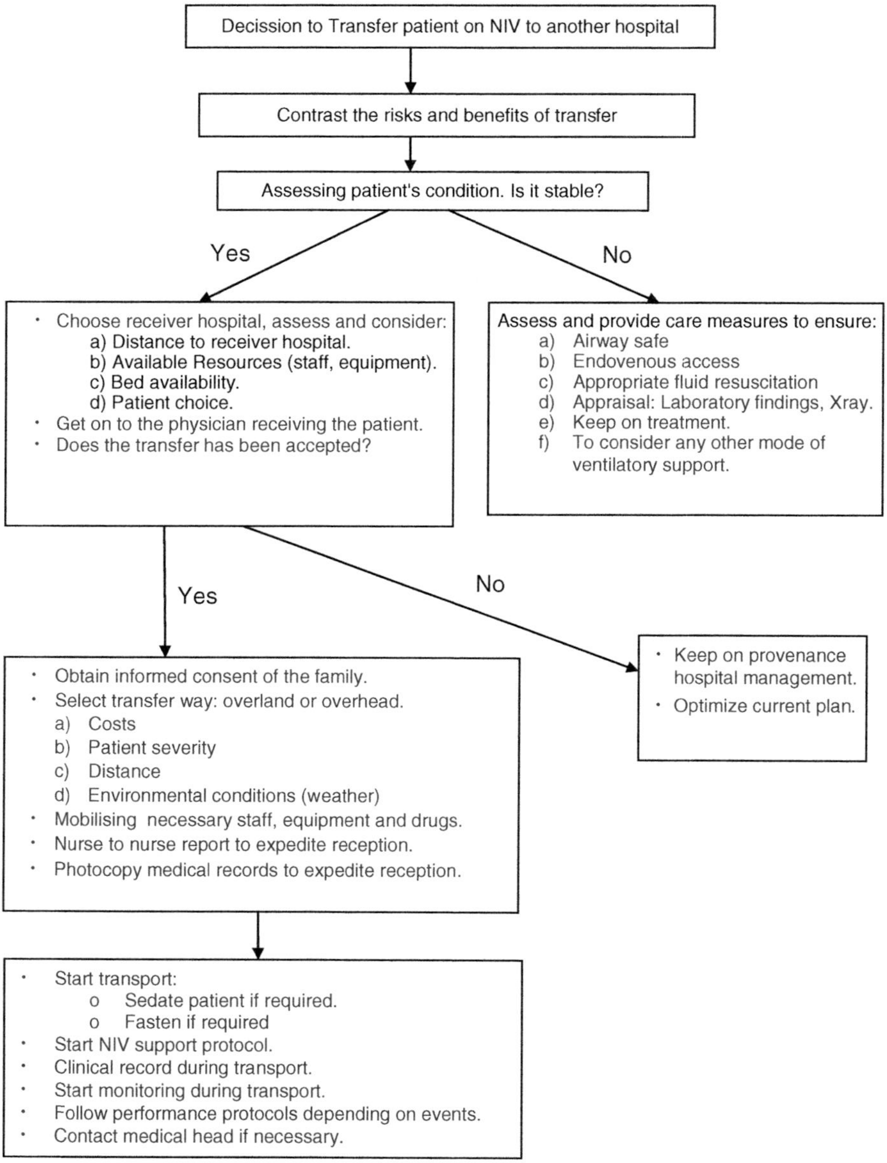

References

1. Esquinas RAM. Desarrollo de la VMNI: del reto clínico a la evidencia científica. In: Esquinas RA, editor. Tratado de ventilación mecánica no invasiva. Madrid: Grupo Aula Médica SL; 2006. p. 3–5.
2. Esquinas R, et al. Guía Esencial de Metodología en Ventilación no Invasiva. Editorial Médica Panamericana; 2010.
3. Carrillo A, Gonzalez-Diaz G, Ferrer M, Martinez-Quintana ME, Lopez-Martinez A, Llamas N, Alcazar M, Torres A. Non-invasive ventilation in community-acquired pneumonia and severe acute respiratory failure. Intensive Care Med. 2012;38(3):458–66.
4. Fanara B, Manzon C, Barbot O, Desmettre T, Capellier G. Recommendations for the intra-hospital transport of critically ill patients. Crit Care. 2010;14:R87.
5. European Society of Intensive Care Medicine. Update patient transport skills and techniques. 2011. Available at: http://pact.esicm.org/media/Patient%20transportation%201Feb2011%20final.pdf. Consultado el 10.06.2011.
6. Warren J, Fromm R, Orr R, Rotello L, Horst M. Guidelines for the inter- and intrahospital transport of critically ill patients. Crit Care Med. 2004;32:256–62.
7. Schwebel C, Clec'h C, Magne S, et al. Safety of intrahospital transport in ventilated critically ill patients: a multicenter cohort study*. Crit Care Med. 2013;41:1919–28.
8. Storre JH, Bohm P, Dreher M, Windisch W. Clinical impact of leak compensation during non-invasive ventilation. Respir Med. 2009;103:1477–83.
9. Gillman L, Leslie G, Williams T, et al. Adverse events experienced while transferring the critically ill patient from the emergency department to the intensive care unit. Emerg Med J. 2006;23:858–61.
10. Papson JPN, Russell KL, Taylor D. Unexpected events during the intrahospital transport of critically ill patients. Acad Emerg Med. 2007;14:544–7.

Part IV

Hospital Critical Care Applications: Acute Chronic Exacerbations

Respiratory Mechanics in COPD Patients Who Failed Noninvasive Ventilation

33

Vittorio Antonaglia, Massimo Ferluga, and Umberto Lucangelo

Contents

33.1 Introduction

First-line intervention with noninvasive positive pressure ventilation (NPPV) can adequately treat acute respiratory failure in a significant number of patients, in particular those with an acute exacerbation of chronic obstructive pulmonary disease (COPD), but in some instances NPPV treatment fails [1, 2]. These patients failed NPPV essentially for respiratory reasons or, after an initial rapid improvement of blood pH and gas exchange, they may require tracheal intubation and sedation for intolerance of the face mask or claustrophobia, due to the almost continuous application of NPPV. The latter can be considered as responders to NPPV in terms of improvement in gas exchange and reduction of respiratory rate and dyspnea. In these patients, the main cause of subsequent intubation is increased ventilation/perfusion mismatching, which is amplified by the decrease in mixed venous partial pressure of oxygen resulting from greater oxygen consumption due to the increased work of the respiratory muscles subsequent to lung dynamic hyperinflation. The partial dissipation of inspiratory pressure in the NPPV device, which thwarts the patient-machine synchrony, a delay in pressurization

V. Antonaglia, MD (✉) • M. Ferluga, MD • U. Lucangelo, MD, PhD
Laboratory of Respiratory Biomechanics, Department of Anesthesia and Intensive Care, Cattinara Hospital, University of Trieste, Strada di Fiume 447, Trieste I-34139, Italy
e-mail: v.antonaglia@libero.it; m.ferluga@me.com; umbyluca@libero.it

A.M. Esquinas (ed.), *Noninvasive Mechanical Ventilation: Theory, Equipment, and Clinical Applications*, DOI 10.1007/978-3-319-21653-9_33

of the interface that is incompatible with the high inspiratory drive, and difficulties in managing copious tracheal secretions can prevent NPPV from effectively increasing alveolar ventilation and improving gas exchange.

The elevated mechanical load and, particularly, the high intrinsic positive end-expiratory pressure (PEEPi) were found to be the major determinants of COPD patients' ventilator dependence [3]. In this line, a correlation between the severity of COPD and the ratio between dynamic and static intrinsic positive end-expiratory pressure (PEEPi,dyn/PEEPi,stat) has been reported in mechanically ventilated patients [4]. PEEPi,stat represents the average PEEPi of the pulmonary regions with different time constants reached after a sufficient equilibration time between regional alveolar and airway opening pressure has elapsed. PEEPi,dyn corresponds to the lowest PEEPi resulting from the lung region with the shortest time constant, and will underestimate PEEPi,stat in the presence of significant time constant inequalities [4]. As a result, the discrepancy between PEEPi,dyn and PEEPi,stat has been introduced as an index of pulmonary mechanical inequality, reflecting an inhomogeneous time constant distribution and/or viscoelastic behavior [5].

33.2 Discussion

PEEPi,dyn is believed to represent the "best" mechanical condition in a sick inhomogeneous lung in relation to an imposed ventilatory pattern; the static intrinsic PEEP reflects the mean time constant of the system [4]. During artificial ventilation, the values of PEEPi must be taken into account; naturally, they should tend to decrease with the improvement in respiratory mechanics. In patients who failed NPVV for respiratory causes, the trend to find higher values of PEEPi,stat at zero end-expiratory pressure (ZEEP) reflects a more important lung hyperinflation, and the lower value of PEEPi,dyn/PEEPi,stat represents a potential increase in the inhomogeneous time constant distribution and/or viscoelastic behavior [5]. Indeed, a small value of PEEPi,dyn/PEEPi,stat indicates an inhomogeneous system [4], whereas the closer the ratio is to unity, a more homogeneous gas distribution is obtained.

In a group of COPD patients with acute exacerbation, a mean value of PEEPi,dyn of 5.3 cmH_2O during noninvasive pressure support ventilation was reported [3]. In a recent investigation, lower values of PEEPi,dyn under zero end-expiratory pressure (ZEEP) were found, but this difference can be attributed to the technique of measurement used during mechanical ventilation [6]. Moreover, Appendini et al. [3] found that the diaphragmatic effort was reduced by the use of low-level external PEEP (80–90 % of PEEPi,dyn). During noninvasive ventilation, Rossi et al. [7] used similar values of external PEEP, obtaining an improvement in gas exchange without either changes in mechanical load or hemodynamic effects. In the study of Antonaglia et al. [6], PEEPi,dyn/PEEPi,stat increased after external PEEP application in line with the improvement in PaO_2/FiO_2 in both groups of patients, but the difference between them remained significant. Thus, external PEEP improved gas exchange, reducing the inequalities between the time constants present in each group of patients [7], but it was not able to reduce the differences between the groups. In fact, in the presence of external PEEP, PEEPi,stat remained substantially unchanged, reflecting potential flow limitation, whereas the PEEPi,dyn increased in both groups, indicating a reduction in inhomogeneous time constant distribution and/or viscoelastic behavior.

Many methods have approached gas distribution during invasive mechanical ventilation in heterogeneous lung using static and dynamic computed tomography scanning and different experimental lung injury models, but the respiratory mechanical modifications induced by NPPV have been scantly studied. Diaz et al. [8], using the multiple inert gas elimination technique, found that the improvement in respiratory blood gases during NPPV was essentially caused by a higher alveolar ventilation and not an improvement in the ventilation/perfusion relationship. In the study of Antonaglia et al. [6], the patients who failed NPPV for respiratory causes or intolerance presented similar elastic and resistive loads, and intolerant patients can be considered as responders to NPPV in terms of improvement in gas exchange and reduction in respiratory rate and dyspnea. It follows that the less important lung mechanical inhomogeneities in the latter, as reflected by a higher PEEPi,dyn/PEEPi,stat, can be considered responsible for the improvement in arterial blood gases. In this group of patients, pH and $PaCO_2$ presented a remarkable trend of improvement with respect to the start values, whereas, in the group of patients who failed NPPV for respiratory reasons, the pH remained unchanged and the reduction in $PaCO_2$ was slight. Before intubation, only pH was different between the two groups. $PaCO_2$ levels were also different, but the sample size was probably not large enough to make this difference statistically significant.

Moreover, in the group of patients who responded to NPPV but failed because of intolerance, PEEPi,dyn/PEEPi,stat was lower when the use of NPPV was shorter and increased nonlinearly when the duration of NPPV was augmented (Fig. 33.1). After a limited period of continuous use of NPPV, a sequential use of NPPV was applied with different modalities. In a clinical trial where NPPV was proposed as an alternative to invasive mechanical ventilation (in patients with similar clinical characteristics to those of Antonaglia et al. [6]), the patients successfully treated with NPPV received it continuously for at least 18 h/day during the first 48 h [2]. In another study, the control group treated with mask NPPV received a mean value of 30 h of NPPV before allowing sequential use [9]. According to Fig. 33.1, PEEPi,dyn/PEEPi,stat increased and become stable after about 30 h of continuous NPPV. Thus, a potential relationship between the improvement in PEEPi,dyn/PEEPi,stat and the duration of NPPV, applied as first-line intervention in patients with acute severe COPD exacerbation, is conceivable. In similar clinical conditions, the application of NPPV beyond 30 h should not promote further decrease in pulmonary mechanical inequality, essentially inducing intolerance and potential NPPV failure. In the study of Antonaglia et al. [6], 35 % of intolerant patients failed NPPV after 30 h. Therefore, after this period it can be useful for the clinician to implement short periods of NPPV with other strategies like oxygen therapy and chest physiotherapy.

Another important finding in the latter study was that the time dependency disappeared after the measurements were made at PEEP, which was able to reduce the differences in time constants of lung districts. External PEEP changed the value of

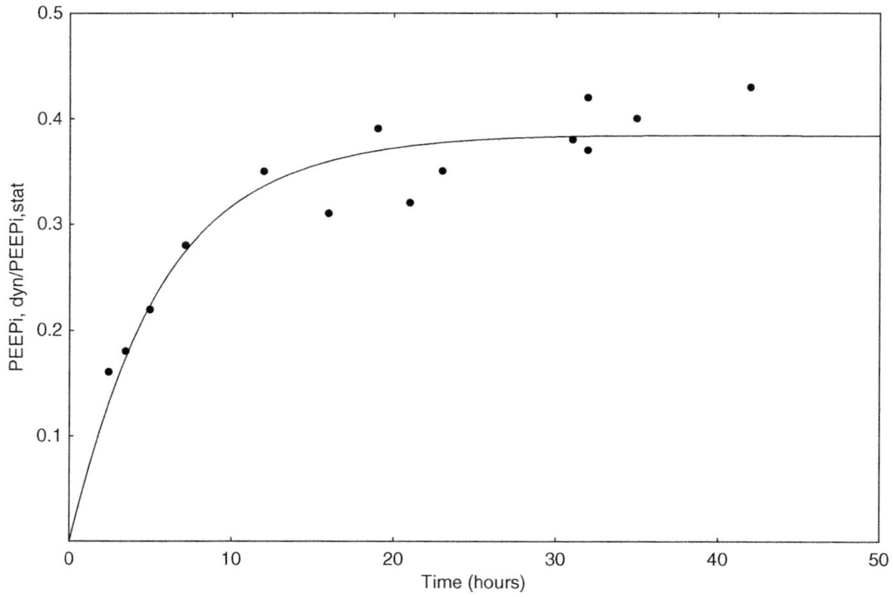

Fig. 33.1 Relationship between duration of NPPV and the ratio between dynamic and static measurements of intrinsic PEEP (PEEPi,dyn/PEEPi,stat) at ZEEP (●) and PEEP (Δ) in patients who failed NPPV because of intolerance

PEEPi,dyn in both groups in comparison to ZEEP, while the PEEPi,stat remained substantially unchanged. The small difference between dynamic and static PEEP did not permit assessment of the relationship between duration of NPPV and PEEPi,dyn/PEEPi,stat.

In the first day of treatment of patients with severe exacerbation of COPD it may be necessary to apply NPPV continuously, and intolerance to the interface may be a complication. A subgroup of patients, after an initial rapid improvement in blood pH and gas exchange, may require tracheal intubation and sedation owing to intolerance to the face mask. Conti et al. [1] reported a percentage of success of NPPV by facial mask of 38 %, similar to those found by Squadrone et al. [2]. Among the patients who failed NPPV, 46 % failed due to intolerance [9].

In the study of Antonaglia et al. [6], respiratory mechanical parameters were assessed within 6 h of invasive mechanical ventilation under the same conditions, that is, they were sedated, paralyzed, and ventilated with a similar ventilatory setting and PEEP was used during NPPV. The mechanical parameters were measured again after a short period of stabilization at ZEEP and were within the range reported in the literature pertaining to COPD patients [7].

Peak tracheal pressure (Ptr,max) was followed by a rapid initial drop in Ptr (Pi) and by a slow decay of Ptr to an apparent plateau value. This plateau pressure, recorded 5 s after the occlusion, was taken to represent the static end-inspiratory elastic recoil pressure of the respiratory system (Pst). By dividing (Ptr,max−Pi) by the flow (V') immediately preceding the occlusion, the Newtonian resistance of the respiratory system (Rint) was obtained. The static elastance of the respiratory system (Est) was computed by dividing the corresponding values of (Pst − PEEPi,stat − PEEP) by tidal volume (VT). ΔP was calculated as (Pi − Pst) and represents the pressure dissipated against viscoelastic properties and mechanical inhomogeneities in the respiratory system. We considered the change in end-expiratory lung volume (ΔEELV) relative to the relaxation volume of the respiratory system [6].

ΔP is an indicator of the degree of inhomogeneous time constant distribution and/or viscoelastic behavior within the respiratory system, and it also encompasses the pressure used to overcome the viscoelastic properties of the system. In this line, ΔP tended to be lower in patients intubated owing to intolerance to NPPV than in those who failed due to respiratory causes. In the study of Antonaglia et al. [6], PEEPi,dyn/PEEPi,stat was found to be inversely correlated with ΔP, thus supporting the aforementioned notion of the existence of more important mechanical inequalities in the lungs of these patients.

The methods for approaching gas distribution during noninvasive mechanical ventilation present some limitations. Firstly, the measurements were usually made in sedated, paralyzed patients and the results, therefore, must be cautiously extended to spontaneously breathing patients. Secondly, the increase in PEEPi,dyn with external PEEP reflects the mode of measurement of dynamic PEEPi (value of tracheal pressure at zero flow). If the measurement of dynamic PEEPi were made using esophageal pressure, this increase could possibly be smaller. Moreover, the data obtained by partitioning the respiratory mechanics by esophageal pressure would be useful for accurate interpretation of our data. If the measures were performed in paralyzed patients and no significant pleural effusions or parietal abnormalities were found in chest X-rays and no obese patients were studied, we believe that the analysis could be sufficiently appropriate.

Conclusions

The patients who failed NPPV owing to intolerance had a smaller amount of inhomogeneous time constant distribution and/or viscoelastic behavior, but similar impairment of the mechanical properties as the subjects requiring invasive ventilation due to respiratory reasons. In the former patients, the degree of pulmonary mechanical inequality was correlated with the duration of NPPV, providing a hypothetical explanation for the effects of NPPV on the lungs of patients with COPD.

Key Major Recommendations

- NPPV can fail for different reasons related to gas exchange impairment or intolerance.
- The patients who failed NPPV because of intolerance present a smaller mechanical inequality, expressed as PEEPi,dyn/PEEPi,stat.
- PEEPi,dyn/PEEPi,stat is correlated with the duration of NPPV.

References

1. Conti G, Antonelli M, Navalesi P, et al. Noninvasive vs. conventional mechanical ventilation in patients with chronic obstructive pulmonary disease after failure of medical treatment in the ward: a randomized trial. Intensive Care Med. 2002;28:1701–7.
2. Squadrone E, Frigerio P, Fogliati C, Gregoretti C, Conti G, Antonelli M, Costa R, Baiardi P, Navalesi P. Noninvasive vs invasive ventilation in COPD patients with severe acute respiratory failure deemed to require ventilatory assistance. Intensive Care Med. 2004;30:1303–10.
3. Appendini L, Purro A, Patessio A, Zanaboni S, Carone M, Spada E, Donner CF, Rossi A. Partitioning of inspiratory muscle workload and pressure in ventilator-dependent COPD patients. Am J Respir Crit Care Med. 1996;154:1301–9.
4. Maltais F, Reissmann H, Navalesi P, Hernandez P, Gursahaney A, Ranieri VM, Sovilj M, Gottfried SB. Comparison of static and dynamic measurements of intrinsic PEEP in mechanically ventilated patients. Am J Respir Crit Care Med. 1994;150:1318–24.
5. Koutsoukou A, Bekos B, Sotiropoulou C, Koulouris NG, Roussos C, Milic-Emili J. Effects of positive end-expiratory pressure on gas exchange and expiratory flow limitation in adult respiratory distress syndrome. Crit Care Med. 2002;30:1941–9.
6. Antonaglia V, Ferluga M, Capitanio G, et al. Respiratory mechanics in COPD patients who failed non-invasive ventilation: role of intrinsic PEEP. Respir Physiol Neurobiol. 2012;184:35–40.
7. Rossi A, Santos C, Roca J, Torres A, Felez MA, Rodriguez-Roisin R. Effects of PEEP on VA/Q mismatching in ventilated patients with chronic airflow obstruction. Am J Respir Crit Care Med. 1994;149:1077–84.
8. Diaz O, Iglesia R, Ferrer M, Zavala E, Santos C, Wagner PD, Roca J, Rodriguez-Roisin R. Effects of noninvasive ventilation on pulmonary gas exchange and hemodynamics during acute hypercapnic exacerbations of chronic obstructive pulmonary disease. Am J Respir Crit Care Med. 1997;156:1840–5.
9. Antonelli M, Pennisi MA, Pelosi P, Gregoretti C, Squadrone V, Rocco M, Cecchini L, Chiumello D, Severgnini P, Proietti R, Navalesi P, Conti G. Noninvasive positive pressure ventilation using a helmet in patients with acute exacerbation of chronic obstructive pulmonary disease. Anesthesiology. 2004;100:16–24.

Impact of Comorbidities on Noninvasive Mechanical Ventilation Response: Key Practical Implications

34

Szymon Skoczyński

Contents

Abbreviations

ALS	Amyotrophic lateral sclerosis
ARF	Acute respiratory failure
CAP	Community-acquired pneumonia
CHS	Central hypoventilation syndromes
COPD	Chronic obstructive pulmonary disease
CPAP	Continuous positive airway pressure
CRF	Chronic respiratory failure
DNI	Do not intubate

S. Skoczyński, MD, PhD
Department of Pneumology, School of Medicine in Katowice, Medical University of Silesia, Medyków 14 Street, Katowice 40-752, Poland

Institute of Occupational Medicine and Environmental Health, Kościelna 13 Street, Sosnowiec 41-200, Poland
e-mail: simon.mds@pocyta.fm, s.skoczynski@imp.sosnowiec.pl

A.M. Esquinas (ed.), *Noninvasive Mechanical Ventilation: Theory, Equipment, and Clinical Applications*, DOI 10.1007/978-3-319-21653-9_34

EPAP	Expiratory positive airway pressure
FEV_1	Forced expiratory volume in 1 second
FiO_2	Fraction of inspired oxygen
ICU	Intensive care unit
IPAP	Inspiratory positive airway pressure
NIV	Noninvasive mechanical ventilation
OHS	Obesity hypoventilation syndrome
OSA	Obstructive sleep apnea
PaO_2/FiO_2	Ratio of arterial oxygen partial pressure to fractional inspired oxygen
PCF	Peak cough flow
PCO_2	Partial pressure of carbon dioxide
PEEP	Positive end-expiratory pressure
PS	Pressure support
PVT	Peak velocity time
RF	Respiratory failure
RR	Respiratory rate
S/T	Spontaneous over timed mode
SCI	Spinal cord injuries
T	Timed mode
TV	Tidal volume

34.1 Introduction

Noninvasive mechanical ventilation (NIV) is a universally recognized, effective method for type-2 respiratory failure (RF) treatment. Ventilator settings and treatment success rates vary, depending on machine configuration, provider experience, patient compliance, and, last but not least, the underlying condition and/or overlapping diseases. NIV is accepted by evidence-based medicine as a good treatment option for the following chronic diseases: amyotrophic lateral sclerosis (ALS), central hypoventilation syndromes (CHS), chronic obstructive pulmonary disease (COPD), kyphoscoliosis, obesity hypoventilation syndrome (OHS), Duchenne muscular dystrophy, and other muscular dystrophies and myopathies, as well as for patients with post-polio syndrome [1] and after spinal cord injuries (SCI) (usually level A of evidence). In acute respiratory failure (ARF), NIV is indicated in COPD exacerbations with $pH < 7.35$ (acute or acute-on-chronic respiratory failure), pneumonia in immunocompromised patients, cardiogenic pulmonary edema disqualified from interventional treatment, high-risk recurrent ARF after planned extubation or weaning from mechanical ventilation, ARF in declared "do not intubate" patients, and in acute respiratory deteriorations of patients on NIV due to chronic conditions (usually level A of evidence) [2].

Along with increasing knowledge and NIV development, the number of clinical indications proved by guidelines is constantly rising. On the other hand, international guidelines are usually disease specific; therefore, in clinical practice, it may be difficult to apply disease-specific ventilator settings and choose patients adequately. Recently, especially in aging Western populations, overlapping of frequent diseases, such as COPD, obstructive sleep apnea (OSA), OHS, and/or CHS secondary to cardiovascular complications, is often observed, but there is still insufficient high-level evidence on precise NIV applications and settings. Therefore, in overlapping diseases, the most important advice is watchful observation of the patient's respiratory pattern, including rate and depth of use of additional respiratory muscles, as well as careful monitoring of measured variables such as minute ventilation, respiratory rate (RR), tidal volume (TV), and arterial blood gases in case of hospitalized patients. If possible, it is recommended to preset TV at 6-8 ml/kg (ideal body weight) in all adult patients, if different values are not indicated on the basis of pulmonary functional tests (spirometry and/or body plethysmography). As stated above, it is important to remember that overlapping is poorly addressed in the literature but may be frequently observed in real life, such as in the case of COPD and OSA/OHS overlapping, in which, if it is well tolerated by the patient and not previously determined by other anatomical and/or pathophysiological factors, pressure support (PS) should be primarily set on the basis of COPD guidelines, and expiratory positive airway pressure (EPAP) set on the basis of previous continuous positive airway pressure (CPAP) titration.

34.2 Discussion and Analysis

34.2.1 Chronic Respiratory Failure

Pure COPD has been accepted as one of the leading indications for home NIV [3]. With aging, a substantial number of patients with COPD may suffer from stroke or other cardiovascular complications. In these patients, there is a great likelihood of clinically significant bulbar syndrome. Therefore, it must be emphasized that, besides COPD-typical NIV settings, cough-assist devices may have to be implemented, which is not routinely done in patients with COPD. In these patients, maximal inspiratory positive airway pressure (IPAP) may be limited by the risk secondary to air-trapping gastric extension, which, if not considered in ventilator settings, can lead to increased risk for regurgitation and aspiration.

Another important comorbidity that may increase risk of death in patients with COPD is lower respiratory tract infections such as severe COPD exacerbation and/or pneumonia. Although these clinical situations are accepted as NIV susceptible, the increased risk might be caused by delay in medical consultation and antibiotic administration, resulting from the patient's self-assurance. Another possible scenario, which should also be taken into account, is chest injury complicated by pneumothorax or spontaneous pneumothorax. In such situations, NIV application without chest tube insertion, even in a minor lung injury, may result in tension pneumothorax and death.

Chest deformation, such as scoliosis in the course of neuromuscular diseases, is not a real overlapping disease but rather a disease manifestation or complication, which should be taken into account in home treatment. In these patients, TV should be accordingly adjusted, from volumes calculated initially on the basis of ideal body weight, to smaller values adjusted according to slowly decreasing total lung capacity.

34.2.2 Acute Respiratory Failure

In most clinical guidelines, NIV patients undergoing acute and chronic respiratory failure are subject to single organ failure (lung/skeletal frame/respiratory muscle/ventilatory central drive). Those disease-related groups are well defined and should be treated according to disease-specific guidelines. In the course of these chronic conditions, overlapping diseases are primarily lower respiratory tract infections. The additional NIV settings are not yet sufficiently described in the literature, but it is usually underlined that NIV is effective and provides survival benefit. To deal with this problem, it is recommended that NIV settings be adjusted according to the severity of clinical disease condition (basic indication or overlapping disease). In case of lobar pneumonia or pulmonary cardiogenic edema, to improve alveolar recruitment and, therefore, oxygenation, it is suggested to increase positive end-expiratory pressure/ expiratory positive airway pressure (PEEP/EPAP) above standard COPD/OHS overlapping baseline (5–10 cmH_2O), with or without inspiratory time prolongation. In patients with bronchial pneumonia or bronchial obstruction, such as in cases of acute bronchitis or COPD acute exacerbation, it is recommended to increase the driving pressure, which means increasing PS or IPAP above baseline value. In acute-on-chronic and, more importantly, in ARF, close patient monitoring is vital. In case of observed NIV therapy ineffectiveness 4 h after treatment onset, urgent intubation and transfer to the intensive care department/intermediate care department should be undertaken, especially because intubation after initial NIV failure is a greater risk factor for death than direct intubation without a preceding NIV trial [4]. This might be even of greater importance in patients with overlapping diseases, and, therefore, it should be taken under consideration for appropriate patient selection when considering NIV treatment.

A large group of "good candidates" in acute setting are patients with "do not intubate" (DNI) orders, however, in this group the most common clinical indication is severe COPD complicated by disease exacerbation or overlapping diseases such cancer (particularly lung cancer) and advanced heart failure. Therefore, in most cases, the NIV device can be set according to standard NIV disease-specific guidelines, with the main difference being that the major treatment goal should be achieving patient comfort and dyspnea relief rather than pushing treatment efficacy in terms of partial pressure of carbon dioxide (PCO_2) reduction by high-intensity NIV. In this group, it is more likely that there will be consciousness problems requiring more nursing stuff assistance, airway clearance, and physiotherapy maneuvers. NIV in patients with DNI orders is accepted as cost effective, especially when there are intensive care bed shortages.

Contrary to the above-mentioned standard ARF NIV indications, sepsis, acute respiratory distress syndrome, and other non-pulmonary systemic inflammatory response syndromes generally represent multiorgan failure caused by systemic capillary leak syndrome, which results in hypoperfusion, increased oxygen consumption, and CO_2 and lactate accumulation, indicating probable (≈50 %) NIV failure

[5]. Another important but frequently forgotten concomitant disease that should be taken into account while applying NIV is anemia. In both acute and chronic RF, in cases of patient's paleness and/or difficult-to-explain tachycardia, tissue hypoxemia mirrored by hemoglobin lactate level should be assessed. If confirmed and indicated, red cell transfusion should be considered rather than increasing positive end-expiratory pressure (PEEP) and/or fraction of inspired oxygen (FiO_2) to the limit. If NIV is applied in immunocompromised patients suffering from ARF, it is most effective if the underlying cause is a hematological condition, even though high Acute Physiology and Chronic Health Evaluation (APACHE) II score, need for catecholamine administration, and low ratio of arterial oxygen partial pressure to fractional inspired oxygen (PaO_2/FiO_2) ratio at admission are known as independent risk factors for NIV failure [5].

In community-acquired pneumonia (CAP), NIV is known to be beneficial; however, in patients with large secretion volume, the application may be difficult. Nevertheless, patients with CAP and hypercapnia benefit more than those with pure hypoxemia. Interestingly, NIV administered in patients with overlapping COPD is more effective in terms of the intubation rate and mortality decrease [6].

Another frequently observed "comorbidity situation" is encountered in a wide group of patients with a few mild, underlining medical conditions such as COPD, OSA, and heart failure. These patients often undergo various surgical procedures that are not necessarily related to the above-mentioned impairing respiratory conditions. In this group, risk of postoperative hypoxemia resulting from atelectasis or pulmonary edema is especially high. The risk is especially high after pulmonary, cardiac, or abdominal procedures or surgeries.

It was found that not only NIV but also CPAP treatment at a level from 7.5 to 10 cmH_2O may decrease pneumonia morbidity, intubation rates, and days in intensive care unit (ICU) [7].

34.2.3 Comorbidities and Age Groups

Coexistence of the most common NIV indication, hypercapnic respiratory failure in COPD with mild airflow obstruction (FEV_1>40%N), is frequently caused by overlapping OSA and/or OHS. These patients should be assessed with polysomnography, and their treatment should start with CPAP titration along with oxygen therapy. The number of elderly patients with multiple comorbidities and consciousness disturbances is increasing, especially in the inpatient setting. Consequently, agitation or confusion may lead to difficulties with mask administration and secretion management, resulting in significant risk for aspiration pneumonia.

On the other hand, in elderly patients with muscle wasting, there is a considerable risk for weaning problems and MV complications. Bearing in mind the significantly higher risk for endotracheal intubation, cautious NIV initiation may be considered by experienced caregivers in a closely monitored setting with an ICU backup [8].

34.2.4 Facial Oronasal Comorbidities and Airway Clearance

Facial oronasal comorbidities are especially important in home NIV treatment. Patients with a dental prosthesis qualified for home NIV program in hospital settings should be informed that, during home treatment, the denture should be used the same as at the time of qualification and hospital treatment. Denture removal may cause excessive leakage due to secondary facial softening and mask-induced facial deformation. To prevent such situations, the patient should be informed that, during NIV therapy, dentures should not be removed, or, if effective and well tolerated, it may be reasonable to supply the patient with different types of masks, such as nasal prongs which are tolerated and effective when IPAPmax settings are <20 cmH_2O. In contrary to nasal and oro-nasal masks nasal prongs do not require facial bone support.

Another significant and often observed comorbidity is chronic and/or acute sinusitis. In chronic conditions, positive airway pressure application may lead to secondary nasal congestion and upper airway disease exacerbation. In these cases, nasal congestion should be proactively treated, for example, with nasal glucocorticosteroids, as in atopic rhinitis. Poor compliance due to nasal congestion is likely to stop patients NIV treatment. To facilitate NIV continuation, an oronasal mask should be preferred over nasal masks in patients with nasal congestion and sinusitis. In those patients with Chronic respiratory failure (CRF), humidification in NIV may greatly improve patient compliance as a result of a decrease in nasal congestion.

With bacterial sinusitis, the patient should be informed that positive airway treatment may aggravate the disease and cause potential purulent complications. Therefore, in cases of acute sinusitis, the patient should be advised to seek help from the home-care provider and/or their general practitioner, depending on the local NIV system.

ALS and lower respiratory tract infection overlapping in a patient already treated with NIV may cause problems with effective airway clearance leading to NIV ineffectiveness, respiratory failure exacerbation, and potential complications such as pneumonia. To prevent such situations, patients with stable disease should be assessed with the Norris bulbar scale (<29; 39 = normal value), peak cough flow (PCF) (<4.25 l/s), or peak cough flow/peak velocity time (PCF/PVT < 28.88 l/s). If at least one borderline point is met, assisted airway clearance techniques should be introduced [9]. In ALS, congestive heart failure (periodic breathing), or COPD/OHS overlapping, there is a significant probability of the co-presence of central apneas and hypopneas; therefore, the spontaneous over timed (S/T) ventilation mode is recommended. Similarly, patients on chronic NIV after SCI have significant risk of respiratory complications such as atelectasis, difficulties in secretion clearance, and higher pneumonia morbidity. Lifelong maneuvers dedicated to maintaining airway clearance are recommended to prevent complications that are accepted as leading causes of death in patients with high-level tetraplegia. Patients presenting with SCI are usually young and therefore initially do not have significant overlapping diseases. Chest deformities predisposing to progressive respiratory impairment are frequently observed after longer treatment.

Mask-related complications such as facial bruises are accepted as some of the most important NIV contraindications and side effects, and proactive screening should be implemented. To avoid this complication, patients and their families should be well trained and informed of the need to change the interface or even obtain a mask customized to the patient. This applies to selected cases of home-treated patients, especiallychildren with neuromuscular diseases.

34.2.5 Metabolic Comorbidities and Obesity

Type-2 diabetes is often observed in patients with OHS/OSA and obese patients with COPD. It should be taken into consideration that NIV may promote weight loss and decrease insulin resistance. This may result in glycemia level reduction, which is, from a long-term perspective, beneficial for the patient. On the other hand, an uninformed patient, especially on insulin treatment, may suffer potentially life-threatening hypoglycemia episodes. Therefore, patients with diabetes should be advised that more attentive glucose control and potential anti-diabetic drug dosage modification may be necessary.

Accordingly, in patients with poorly controlled hypertension, effective NIV treatment may lead to secondary blood pressure decrease and hypotonia related complications such as fainting. In both clinical conditions, hypoglycemia and hypotension are clinically positive features, but caution is needed to adjust the patient's drug dosages accordingly. Moreover, significant weight loss in patients with overlapping OSA/OHS may allow for a decrease in treatment intensity from NIV to CPAP. Therefore, a ventilation program in obese patients should always be enhanced by weight loss consulting and/or a treatment program.

Conclusion

There is a deficit of prospective randomized studies that assess the impact of comorbidities on noninvasive mechanical ventilation response. Moreover, currently, even in single-disease guidelines, there are huge gaps in knowledge, even in basic recommendations such as ventilation mode, triggering, interface, and humidification [10]. Therefore, more random controlled trials are needed in basic diseases in most fields of NIV. Patients with overlapping diseases may undergo NIV treatment, but they require carefully monitoring and alternative treatment options, such intubation and mechanical ventilation, should be readily available. In these situations, the staff should have significant experience, as treatment outcomes rely significantly on personal experience and watchful patient observation.

Generally it is easier and more feasible to treat obese patients with a slow respiratory rate than lean patients with fast shallow breathing. In cases where a few diseases overlap, the presence of COPD should be considered a positive prognostic factor. Standard NIV contraindications seem to have a stronger impact on treatment results than in single-disease scenarios, with exception of patients with DNI orders, where the treatment is dedicated to comfort than effectiveness.

The role of comorbidities may be crucial but different in acute and in chronic settings. The role of diseases not directly correlated with ventilation should be taken into account when applying NIV. Most importantly, the patient and the patient's family should be involved in the process of therapeutic decision making. The most important factors influencing RF treatment efficacy are precise understanding of overlapping disease pathophysiology, medical team dedication, and an ethics-based approach. Currently, it seems impossible to create a universal flowchart or table to guide the treatment protocol in all patients with RF caused by overlapping diseases. Therefore, clinicians are encouraged to publish their own observations in this important area of clinical research.

Key Major Recommendations

- NIV should be attempted in all patients (without absolute NIV contraindications) with type-2 chronic respiratory failure, even in cases with significant overlapping diseases.
- NIV should be attempted in most patients with type-2 acute or acute-on-chronic respiratory failure, even in cases of significant overlapping diseases.
- NIV settings should be always adjusted on the basis of combined pathophysiology of overlapping diseases and the patient's treatment tolerance.
- In overlapping diseases, the final result of the treatment is more dependent on the combination of contraindications than the treatment indications.
- In overlapping diseases, the presence of COPD, especially in patients with decreased respiratory drive, should be considered as a positive prognostic factor.

References

1. McKim DA, Road J, Avendano M, et al. Canadian Thoracic Society Home Mechanical Ventilation Committee, Canadian Thoracic Society Home Mechanical Ventilation Committee. Home mechanical ventilation: a Canadian Thoracic Society clinical practice guideline. Can Respir J. 2011;18:197–215.
2. Non-invasive ventilation guidelines for adult patients with acute respiratory failure. Available at: http://www.aci.health.nsw.gov.au/. Downloaded on 20 Mar 2015.
3. Köhnlein T, Windisch W, Köhler D, et al. Non-invasive positive pressure ventilation for the treatment of severe stable chronic obstructive pulmonary disease: a prospective, multicentre, randomised, controlled clinical trial. Lancet Respir Med. 2014;2:698–705.
4. Walkey AJ, Wiener RS. Use of noninvasive ventilation in patients with acute respiratory failure, 2000–2009: a population-based study. Ann Am Thorac Soc. 2013;10:10–7.
5. Razlaf P, Pabst D, Mohr M, et al. Non-invasive ventilation in immunosuppressed patients with pneumonia and extrapulmonary sepsis. Respir Med. 2012;106:1509–16.

6. Mandell LA, Wunderink RG, Anzueto A, et al. Infectious Diseases Society of America/American Thoracic Society consensus guidelines on the management of community-acquired pneumonia in adults. Clin Infect Dis. 2007;44 Suppl 2:S27–72.
7. Squadrone V, Coha M, Cerutti E, et al. Continuous positive airway pressure for treatment of postoperative hypoxemia: a randomized controlled trial. JAMA. 2005;293:589–95.
8. Scala R. Non-invasive ventilation in acute respiratory failure with altered consciousness syndrome: a bargain or an hazard? Minerva Anestesiol. 2013;79:1291–9.
9. Sancho J, Servera E, Díaz J, Marín J. Predictors of ineffective cough during a chest infection in patients with stable amyotrophic lateral sclerosis. Am J Respir Crit Care Med. 2007;175:1266–71.
10. Keenan SP, Sinuff T, Burns KE, et al.; Canadian Critical Care Trials Group/Canadian Critical Care Society Noninvasive Ventilation Guidelines Group. Clinical practice guidelines for the use of noninvasive positive-pressure ventilation and noninvasive continuous positive airway pressure in the acute care setting. CMAJ. 2011;183:E195-214.

Noninvasive Continuous Positive Airway Pressure Response in Bronchiectasis Exacerbations: Key Practical Aspects and Topics

35

Annia Schreiber, Andrea Antonelli, and Cesare Gregoretti

Contents

Abbreviations

CF	Cystic fibrosis
CPAP	Continuous positive airway pressure
COPD	Chronic obstructive pulmonary disease
FEV_1	Forced expiratory volume in one second
FRC	Functional residual capacity
FVC	Forced vital capacity

A. Schreiber, MD (✉)
Terapia Subintensiva Respiratoria e Pneumologia Riabilitativa, IRCCS Fondazione Salvatore Maugeri, Pavia, Italy
e-mail: annia.schreiber@icloud.com

A. Antonelli, MD
Allergologia e Fisiopatologia Respiratoria, ASO Santa Croce e Carle, Cuneo, Italy
e-mail: andrea-antonelli@tiscali.it

C. Gregoretti, MD
Dipartimento di Anestesia, Città della Salute e della Scienza, Torino, Italy
e-mail: c.gregoretti@gmail.com

A.M. Esquinas (ed.), *Noninvasive Mechanical Ventilation: Theory, Equipment, and Clinical Applications*, DOI 10.1007/978-3-319-21653-9_35

FiO_2	Fraction of inspired oxygen
HFNC	High-flow nasal cannula oxygen
NIV	Noninvasive ventilation
NPPV	Noninvasive positive pressure ventilation
$PaCO_2$	Partial pressure of carbon dioxide
PaO_2	Partial pressure of oxygen
PEEPi	Intrinsic positive end-expiratory pressure
PEP	Positive expiratory pressure
Pdi	Transdiaphragmatic pressure
Pes	Esophageal pressure
PTPes/b	Pressure time product of the esophageal pressure per breath
PTPes/min	Pressure time product of the esophageal pressure per minute
RV	Residual volume
TPEP	Temporary positive expiratory pressure
VO_2	Oxygen consumption
WOB	Work of breathing

35.1 Introduction

Non-cystic fibrosis bronchiectasis is a chronic, debilitating condition characterized by persistent cough and chronic excessive sputum production. This term refers to the permanent abnormal dilatation of the airways associated with parenchymal destruction [1]. The precise prevalence of bronchiectasis is unknown due to a lack of cross-sectional community surveys. In addition, different diseases causing bronchiectasis vary across different countries and different historical periods, and the techniques used to diagnose and define this condition have changed over the years. It has been estimated that in 2005 in the United States it affected at least 110,000 adults [2], but it is likely to be underdiagnosed. As a matter of fact, many of the affected patients are misdiagnosed, suffering from other conditions, particularly chronic obstructive pulmonary disease (COPD) or asthma. However, there is an overlap with COPD, with a reported incidence of bronchiectasis in COPD of between 29 and 50 % [3]. Bronchiectasis is typically complicated by poor mucus clearance, resulting in bacterial colonization with recurrent infections and excessive airway inflammation in response to the infection. An ongoing cycle of infection and inflammation may then be established and contribute to lung damage [4]. The natural history is a progressive lung disease with parenchymal destruction, resulting in poor gas exchange and progressive respiratory failure. Infective exacerbations are a significant cause of morbidity in non-cystic fibrosis bronchiectasis and often necessitate utilization of health-care resources including in-patient admissions for intravenous antibiotic therapy and for the management of the consequent respiratory failure [5]. Respiratory failure is the cause of death in more than 90 % of patients with cystic fibrosis (CF) and it also represents the leading cause of death in diffuse bronchiectasis [6, 7].

In the initial stages of the disease or in case of localized disease, patients with bronchiectasis may be characterized by a preserved pulmonary function. As the disease evolves, spirometry usually shows some degree of airway obstruction with a high prevalence of bronchial hyperreactivity [8]. Obstruction is mainly related to thickening of the bronchial wall due to infiltration of the airway walls by inflammatory cells [9]. The inflammation within the bronchial walls causes structural damage and airways dilatation with lack of structural support, which determines distal airway collapse during expiratory maneuvers. The peculiar accumulation of mucus plugging also contributes to the obstructive pattern; large airways plugging was found to be most closely associated with alterations in the forced expiratory volume in one second (FEV_1) and partial pressure of oxygen (PaO_2), whereas changes in small airways plugging were shown to be most strongly associated with a decrease in forced vital capacity (FVC) [9, 10]. The association with a restrictive disease, related to the presence of small atelectasis, may configure a mainly restrictive lung disease or a mixed obstructive and restrictive clinical condition [11].

Acute respiratory failure commonly arises because of alveolar flooding caused by new infections or exacerbations of previous colonizations. Also, an acute event such as abdominal surgery or chest trauma, causing pain, could impair cough and expectoration and worsen atelectasis and consequently hypoxemia [12]. The final result is an increase in the ventilation-perfusion mismatch, a fall in FEV_1, a decrease in functional residual capacity (FRC) and lung compliance, with a consequent increase in the work of breathing (WOB) [12]. Progressive hypoxemia with the establishment of chronic respiratory failure can be a consequence of a chronic progression of the lung disease. At a later stage of the disease, beyond a worsening of ventilation-perfusion mismatch, alveolar hypoventilation and hypercapnia may occur.

Similarly to what happens in CF, hypoxemia and hypercapnia first become clinically significant during sleep and during situations that require an increase in alveolar ventilation such as during the exercise, chest physiotherapy, and exacerbations. Hypercapnia could eventually become diurnal as disease progresses over time [13, 14].

Bronchiectasis treatment and management guidelines are still not clearly defined. Initial ventilatory strategies should aim to decrease ventilation-perfusion mismatch, correct hypoxemia, improve lung function, increase compliance, and limit atelectasis formation. In the more advanced stages, when the respiratory load is increased due to progressive airflow, obstruction and hypoventilation occur, and an additional goal is to correct hypercapnia.

Studies of bronchiectasis have generally included fewer than 20 patients and few of them have been randomized or blinded. Furthermore, the vast majority of recommendations existing were based on the management of the microbiological aspect, on infection control, and on the treatment of pulmonary exacerbations with medical therapies, prevalently antibiotics [15].

35.2 Discussion and Analysis

Continuous positive airway pressure (CPAP) consists of the application of positive airway pressure throughout the entire respiratory cycle in a spontaneously breathing subject. This distinguishes CPAP from noninvasive positive pressure ventilation (NPPV), which supplies real ventilatory support and allows an increase in effective alveolar ventilation with a consequent decrease in partial pressure of carbon dioxide ($PaCO_2$). NPPV is generally considered part of the treatment of advanced disease, sometimes at the end-stage and as a bridge to transplant. When alveolar hypoventilation occurs and a progressive hypercapnic respiratory failure is established, NPPV is able to unload the respiratory muscles, thereby improving alveolar ventilation and gas exchange. Little is known about the role of CPAP in bronchiectasis, and the limited knowledge available is based on evidence from studies in CF. CPAP has been used in exacerbations of bronchiectasis with the aim of improving ventilation-perfusion mismatch [16], promoting airway clearance as a part of chest physiotherapy [17] or assisting chest physiotherapy [18]. Both during and after exacerbations, there may be value for CPAP use during exercise, as has been shown in other conditions [19].

35.2.1 CPAP in Acute Respiratory Failure

The primary indication for CPAP should be severe hypoxemia (type I respiratory failure), when the patient is refractory to high-concentration oxygen therapy. In fact, CPAP may deliver a constant fraction of inspired oxygen (FiO_2) in comparison with conventional supplementary oxygen, when used with dedicated devices.

In bronchiectasis, it may promote recruitment of the flooded alveoli, increasing the number of functioning units and re-expanding dependent areas of the lung in which airway opening occurs late in inspiration or does not occur at all. In the prevalent restrictive pattern, CPAP may lead to an increase in FRC and residual volume (RV), thereby improving respiratory mechanics [16]. The increase in RV also contributes to more effective clearance of bronchial secretions.

By reversing hypoxemia and reducing respiratory rate together with improved respiratory mechanics, CPAP will contribute to decrease the ventilation-perfusion mismatch and relief of dyspnea. Last but not least, by countering intrinsic positive end-expiratory pressure (PEEPi), particularly in case of airways obstruction, as during acute exacerbations of chronic obstructive pulmonary disease (COPD) patients, CPAP may also reduce the WOB [20–23].

A novel way to supply a continuous positive pressure is the humidified high-flow nasal cannula oxygen (HFNC). HFNC is a technique that can deliver heated and humidified gas, up to 100 % oxygen, at a maximum flow of 60 l/min of gas via nasal cannula [24, 25]. Previous studies have demonstrated that this method of supplying high-flow humidified oxygen is associated with the generation of a low level of CPAP. It has also been shown that the degree of CPAP is flow dependent and also reliant on the way of breathing (the higher the leak from an open mouth, the lower the pressure) [26, 27]. A study by Vargas and coworkers [28] evaluated the effects of HFNC compared with CPAP and oxygen therapy delivered via facemask in patients with acute hypoxemic respiratory failure. Compared with the conventional oxygen therapy device and similarly to CPAP, HFNC resulted in less inspiratory effort, as indicated by a significant reduction in esophageal pressure (Pes), pressure time product of the esophageal pressure per breath and per minute (PTPes/b and

PTPes/min), and in a slight but significant increase in the PaO_2/FIO_2 ratio. In addition, HFNC led to a significant reduction in median respiratory rate compared with standard oxygen therapy, without a significant difference compared with CPAP. Both HFNC and CPAP decreased dyspnea, although not significantly. Tolerance was similar for both methods.

Besides the effect of generating a CPAP, HFNC delivers heated and humidified gas, which *per se* appears to play a role in bronchiectasis. Inspired air humidification has, in fact, been reported to show some benefit in bronchiectasic patients. Hasani and coworkers [29] used a radioaerosol technique to measure lung mucociliary clearance before and after 7 days of domiciliary humidification. They found that following warm air humidification, lung mucociliary clearance significantly improved compared with baseline assessment. This appears to be of a crucial relevance in bronchiectasis, especially during an exacerbation.

A preliminary study by Storgaard and coworkers [30] showed that, in patients affected by COPD and chronic respiratory failure who were receiving long-term oxygen therapy, HFNC reduced the number of acute exacerbations in comparison with controls. Furthermore, patients treated with HFNC had fewer hospital admissions than the control patients. This could be partly due to the effect of promoting mucus clearance and it seems reasonable to surmise that this result could be replicated in bronchiectasis. Further studies are needed to demonstrate this theory. The use of HFNC may also play a role in preserving lung function, as we know that secretions and the vicious cycle of inflammation and infection contribute to the functional decline. Hasani and coworkers found that all lung function indices slightly improved following a short period of HFNC therapy, even if not significantly. We could hypothesize that these data could become significant in the long term.

35.2.2 CPAP in Promoting Airway Clearance and During Chest Physiotherapy

Despite the lack of physiotherapy guidelines advocating specific techniques and outcome measures [31], bronchiectasic patients, except those with virtually no sputum, appear to benefit from airway clearance strategies and should therefore undertake regular chest physiotherapy, particularly during exacerbations. In fact, effective clearance of excessive mucus from the airways appears to be important as it can potentially break the vicious cycle of the disease by minimizing the stagnation of mucus, mucus plug formation, bacterial load, inflammation, and recurrent infections. Treatment methods that improve mucus clearance are therefore considered essential in optimizing respiratory function and reducing the progression of the disease. Moreover, recent studies have provided evidence that regular physiotherapy improves quality of life [32]. This is particularly true during pulmonary exacerbations when the amount of sputum is typically increased and sputum clearance may be further impaired by more severe airway inflammation and obstruction and by the greater viscosity of secretions [33]. Chest physiotherapy has been used for many years with the aim of promoting lung re-expansion, improving clearance of mucus, and facilitating its expectoration. Several techniques that involve positive pressure are available, such as positive expiratory pressure (PEP) and oscillatory PEP devices (e.g., the so-called flutter device), but few controlled studies have documented a clinical benefit in bronchiectasis [34]. PEP consists of cycles of active expiration against a variable expiratory orifice flow-resistor. It is usually applied via a face mask or mouthpiece. The mucus clearing effect is thought to be due to the widening of the airways because of the increased expiratory pressure [17].

A new modality to deliver a low positive pressure level during spontaneous breathing for a fraction of the expiratory phase is now available. Called temporary positive expiratory pressure (TPEP), this technique was developed to assist patients with chronic mucus hypersecretion, such as patients with bronchiectasis. Preliminary studies have shown that, in the long term, a low positive pressure (less than or equal to 1 cmH_2O) applied for a fraction of the expiratory phase may improve the distribution of alveolar ventilation, symptoms, and lung volumes [35]. A more recent study [36] demonstrated that, in the short-term (after 10 days of treatment), there were significant increases in FEV_1, FVC, tidal volume, and inspiratory capacity in comparison with a control group treated by manually assisted breathing techniques. The effect on inspiratory capacity appears to be correlated with the concomitant reduction in airways obstruction and the recruitment of collapsed lung parenchyma. TPEP was also associated with an improvement in both the perceived bronchial encumbrance and the effective reduction of expectoration, as well as with an improvement in secretion density and purulence, compared with the control group. The effect on lung function appears to be common to other types of positive expiratory pressure-based techniques. The benefit of all these techniques is in their ability to enhance mucus clearance by stenting the airways and preventing airway collapse, or increasing intrathoracic pressure and collateral ventilation distal to retained secretions, or decreasing functional residual capacity [37].

The continuous administration of positive airway pressure (i.e., CPAP) has been evaluated in promoting mucus clearance, and its effect has been compared with PEP delivered via a face mask (PEP mask) and to NPPV [17]. Placidi and coworkers [17] compared the short-term effects of these three techniques in 17 patients with CF and severe airway obstruction admitted for pulmonary exacerbation. There were no statistically significant differences in sputum clearance and the dry weight of sputum collected between CPAP, mask PEP, and NPPV. At the same time, they did not find any differences in terms of pulmonary-function measures, pulse-oximetry values, and patients' subjective efficacy scores. Less fatigue was reported after CPAP and NPPV than after mask PEP. The authors concluded that CPAP and NPPV could be considered as an alternative airway-clearance regimen that might be clinically relevant in patients who feel tired and uncomfortable using conventional airway-clearance techniques during a lung-disease exacerbation.

Although chest physiotherapy is a critical component of the care of patients with bronchiectasis, especially during exacerbations, it should be remembered that it may increase energy expenditure and cause oxygen desaturation, respiratory muscle fatigue, and dyspnea [38]. This could occur particularly when there is a greater need to promote airway clearance, such as during exacerbations.

In this context, NPPV has been shown to decrease respiratory muscle work and improve oxygenation, thereby decreasing the occurrence of respiratory failure and dyspnea [18]. We can postulate that CPAP may play a role similar to that of NIV, at least in preventing or limiting desaturations, improving oxygenation, and in alleviating dyspnea during chest physiotherapy [16]. It has, in fact, been demonstrated that both CPAP and NPPV could decrease inspiratory muscle WOB [39]. An alternating application of CPAP and chest physiotherapy could therefore be hypothesized with the purpose of optimizing the duration and effectiveness of physiotherapy sessions.

35.2.3 CPAP During Exercise

A relevant proportion of patients with CF have a marked decrease in exercise tolerance, which can be mainly related to lung disease, as well as to impaired muscle function and decreased physical activity levels in daily life [40]. Preliminary findings suggest that patients with non-CF bronchiectasis face the same problems and share the same mechanisms [41].

Previous studies have evaluated the role of CPAP during exercise in chronic obstructive lung diseases. In these patients, the sensation of dyspnea is mostly related to the increased WOB, a consequence of an increased resistive load, hyperinflation, and of the deleterious effect of intrinsic positive end-expiratory pressure (PEEPi) [40]. As previously mentioned, the administration of low-level CPAP provides a means of counteracting the effect of PEEPi in patients with severe hyperinflation [20–22, 42].

CPAP has been associated with an improvement in exercise tolerance in CF patients, particularly in those with more severe lung disease [43]. Indeed, in these patients, CPAP seemed to significantly reduce oxygen consumption (VO_2), the respiratory effort assessed by the transdiaphragmatic pressure (Pdi) and dyspnea; these values tended to increase only slightly in patients with mild lung disease [43]. The decreases in VO_2, Pdi, and dyspnea score suggest that CPAP can reduce the work of breathing and increase exercise tolerance [19]. The beneficial effects during exercise were more important in the patients with severe lung disease because, in these patients, the presence of PEEPi may be favorably counteracted by CPAP. However, because upper airway loading with complete or partial obstruction and PEEPi are not the sole mechanisms of hypoventilation, CPAP alone may be insufficient in patients with significant respiratory function abnormalities. In this case, NPPV should be used.

Conclusion

In conclusion, there is a physiologic rationale for the use of CPAP in bronchiectasis exacerbations and as an airway clearance technique. However, CPAP is not a true ventilator mode and therefore is not suitable for the treatment of hypercapnic respiratory failure. Close monitoring of patients treated with CPAP for a hypoxemic episode is to be recommended to switch to true ventilatory support in the occurrence of hypercapnia. Further studies are needed to define the most pertinent criteria to propose CPAP in patients with bronchiectasis as well as the best ventilatory regimens for each situation.

Key Recommendations

In patients affected by bronchiectasis:

CPAP should be recommended in patients with acute exacerbation of hypoxemic respiratory failure, unless there are contraindications.

CPAP may promote lung recruitment, reverse hypoxemia, improve respiratory mechanics, reduce the WOB, and alleviate dyspnea.

CPAP could play a role in promoting airway clearance, limiting desaturations during chest physiotherapy, and increasing tolerance during exercise.

References

1. Hill AT, Pasteur M, Cornford C, et al. Primary care summary of the British Thoracic Society guideline on the management of non-cystic fibrosis bronchiectasis. Prim Care Respir J. 2011;20(2):135–40.
2. Weycker D, Edelsberg J, Oster G, et al. Prevalence and economic burden of bronchiectasis. Clin Pulm Med. 2005;4:205–9.
3. Patel IS, Vlahos I, Wilkinson TM, et al. Bronchiectasis, exacerbation indices, and inflammation in chronic obstructive pulmonary disease. Am J Respir Crit Care Med. 2004;170:400–7.
4. King P. Pathogenesis of bronchiectasis. Paediatr Respir Rev. 2011;12(2):104–10.
5. Kelly MG, Murphy S, Elborn JS. Bronchiectasis in secondary care: a comprehensive profile of a neglected disease. Eur J Intern Med. 2003;14:488–92.
6. Gibson RL, Burns JL, Ramsey BW. Pathophysiology and management of pulmonary infections in cystic fibrosis. Am J Respir Crit Care Med. 2003;168:918–31.
7. Sood N, Paradowski LJ, Yankaskas JR. Outcomes of intensive care unit care in adults with cystic fibrosis. [see Comment]. Am J Respir Crit Care Med. 2001;163:335–8.
8. Pang J, Chan HS, Sung JY. Prevalence of asthma, atopy and bronchial hyperactivity in bronchiectasis: a controlled study. Thorax. 1989;44:948–51.
9. Sheehan RE, Wells AU, Copley SJ, et al. A comparison of serial computed tomography and functional change in bronchiectasis. Eur Respir J. 2002;20:581–7.
10. King P, Holdsworth S, Freezer N. Bronchiectasis. Intern Med J. 2006;36(11):729–37.
11. Barker AF. Bronchiectasis. N Engl J Med. 2002;346:1383–93.
12. Sprague K, Graff G, Tobias JD. Noninvasive ventilation in respiratory failure due to cystic fibrosis. South Med J. 2000;93:953–61.
13. Tepper RS, Skatrud JB, Dempsey JA. Ventilation and oxygenation changes during sleep in cystic fibrosis. Chest. 1983;84:388–93.
14. Muller NL, Francis PW, Gurwitz D, et al. Mechanism of hemoglobin desaturation during rapid-eye-movement sleep in normal subjects and in patients with cystic fibrosis. Am Rev Respir Dis. 1980;121:463–9.
15. Murray MP, Turnbull K, MacQuarrie S, et al. Assessing response to treatment of exacerbations of bronchiectasis in adults. Eur Respir J. 2009;33:312–7.

16. Linder KH, Lotz P, Ahnefeld FW. Continuous positive airway pressure effect on functional residual capacity, vital capacity and its subdivisions. Chest. 1987;92:66–70.
17. Placidi G, Cornacchia M, Polese G, et al. Chest physiotherapy with positive airway pressure: a pilot study of short-term effects on sputum clearance in patients with cystic fibrosis and severe airway obstruction. Respir Care. 2006;51(10):1145–53.
18. Holland AE, Denehy L, Ntoumenopoulos G, et al. Non-invasive ventilation assist chest physiotherapy in adults with acute exacerbations of cystic fibrosis. Thorax. 2003;58:880–4.
19. Regnis JA, Donnelly PM, Robinson M, et al. Ventilatory mechanics at rest and during exercise in patients with cystic fibrosis. Am J Respir Crit Care Med. 1996;154(5):1418–25.
20. Coussa ML, Guerin C, Eissa NT, et al. Partitioning of work of breathing in mechanically ventilated COPD patients. J Appl Physiol (1985). 1993;75:711–1719.
21. Goldberg P, Reissmann H, Maltais F, et al. Efficacy of noninvasive CPAP in COPD with acute respiratory failure. Eur Respir J. 1995;8:1894–900.
22. Appendini L, Patessio A, Zanaboni S, et al. Physiologic effects of positive end-expiratory pressure and mask pressure support during exacerbations of chronic obstructive pulmonary disease. Am J Respir Crit Care Med. 1994;149:1069–76.
23. Katz JA, Marks JD. Inspiratory work with and without continuous airway pressure in patients with acute respiratory failure. Anesthesiology. 1985;63:598–607.
24. Roca O, Riera J, Torres F, et al. High-flow oxygen therapy in acute respiratory failure. Respir Care. 2010;55:408–13.
25. Parke RL, McGuinness SP, Eccleston ML. A preliminary randomized controlled trial to assess effectiveness of nasal high-flow oxygen in intensive care patients. Respir Care. 2011;56: 265–70.
26. Groves N, Tobin A. High flow nasal oxygen generates positive airway pressure in adult volunteers. Aust Crit Care. 2007;20:126–31.
27. Parke RL, McGuinness SP, Eccleston ML. Nasal high-flow therapy delivers low level positive airway pressure. Br J Anaesth. 2011;107(9):98–1004.
28. Vargas F, Saint-Leger M, Boyer A, et al. Physiologic effects of high-flow nasal cannula oxygen in critical care subjects. Respir Care. 2015. pii: respcare.03814. [Epub ahead of print].
29. Hasani A, Chapman TH, McCool D, et al. Domiciliary humidification improves mucociliary clearance in patients with bronchiectasis. Chron Respir Dis. 2008;5:81–6.
30. Storgaard LH, Frystyck RN, Hockey H, et al. Exacerbations in COPD patients on LTOT treated with a nasal high flow system. Poster Session ERS Congress. 2014.
31. O'Neill B, Bradley JM, McArdle N, et al. The current physiotherapy management of patients with bronchiectasis: a UK survey. Int J Clin Pract. 2002;56:34–5.
32. Mutalithas K, Watkin G, Willig B, et al. Improvement in health status following bronchopulmonary hygiene physical therapy in patients with bronchiectasis. Respir Med. 2008;102:1140–4.
33. Murray MP, Pentland JL, Hill AT. A randomised crossover trial of chest physiotherapy in non-cystic fibrosis bronchiectasis. Eur Respir J. 2009;34:1086–92.
34. King PT, Daviskas E. Management of bronchiectasis. Breathe. 2010;6(4):353–60.
35. Bott J, Blumenthal S, Buxton M, et al. On behalf of the British Thoracic Society Physioterapy Guideline Development Group. Guidelines for the physiotherapy management of the adult, medical, spontaneously breathing patient. Thorax. 2009;64:i1–52.
36. Venturelli E, Crisafulli E, DeBiase A, et al. Efficacy of temporary positive expiratory pressure (TPEP) in patients with lung diseases and chronic mucus hypersecretion. The UNIKO® project: a multicentre randomized controlled trial. Clin Rehabil. 2013;27(4):336–46.
37. Nunn JF. Nunn's applied respiratory physiology. 5th ed. Oxford: Butterworth-Heinemann; 2000.
38. Cecins N, Jenkins S, Pengelly J, et al. The active cycle of breathing techniques: to tip or not to tip? Respir Med. 1999;93:660–5.
39. Fauroux B, Boule M, Lofaso F, et al. Chest physiotherapy in cystic fibrosis: improved tolerance with nasal pressure support ventilation. Pediatrics. 1999;103(3), E32.

40. Williams CA, Saynor ZL, Tomlinson OW, et al. Cystic fibrosis and physiological responses to exercise. Expert Rev Respir Med. 2014;8(6):751–62.
41. Burtin C, Hebestreit H. Rehabilitation in patients with chronic respiratory disease other than chronic obstructive pulmonary disease: exercise and physical activity interventions in cystic fibrosis and non-cystic fibrosis bronchiectasis. Respiration. 2015;89(3):181–9.
42. Janssens JP, de Muralt B, Titelion V. Management of dyspnea in severe chronic obstructive pulmonary disease. J Pain Symptom Manage. 2000;19(5):378–92.
43. Henke KG, Regnis JA, Bye PTP. Benefits of continuous positive airway pressure during exercise in cystic fibrosis and relationship to disease severity. Am Rev Respir Dis. 1993;148: 1272–6.

Noninvasive Mechanical Ventilation in Asthma Exacerbation: Key Practical Aspects and Clinical Evidence

36

Guniz M. Koksal and Emre Erbabacan

Contents

Abbreviations

BiPAP	Bi-level positive airway pressure
COPD	Chronic obstructive pulmonary disease
CPAP	Continuous Positive Airway Pressure
FEV1	Forced expiratory volume in 1 s
GINA	Global initiative for asthma
NIV	Noninvasive mechanical ventilation
PEEP	Positive end-expiratory pressure

G.M. Koksal, MD (✉) • E. Erbabacan, MD
Department of Anesthesiology and Reanimation, Cerrahpasa Medical School, Istanbul University, Istanbul, Turkey
e-mail: gunizkoksal@hotmail.com; emreerbabacan@hotmail.com

A.M. Esquinas (ed.), *Noninvasive Mechanical Ventilation: Theory, Equipment, and Clinical Applications*, DOI 10.1007/978-3-319-21653-9_36

36.1 Introduction

Asthma is highly prevalent worldwide (estimated to account for 1 in every 250 deaths) and its exacerbations can lead to acute respiratory failure. A mortality rate of 27 % has been reported in invasively ventilated patients. Approximately 5–10 % of asthmatic patients experience at least one severe acute asthma episode in a given year, and there are approximately 2 million emergency department visits and 500,000 hospital admissions annually worldwide [1].

The major physiological changes in severe acute asthma are associated with the onset or worsening of limitation of the air flow as a result of bronchospasm, mucosal edema, and mucus hyperproduction, which are triggered by bronchial flogosis and hyperresponsiveness. Like in COPD exacerbations, the increase in airway resistance prolongs the exhalation time required to empty the lung, producing air trapping (dynamic hyperinflation with increased auto-positive end-expiratory pressure (PEEP)), reduced FEV_1 (<60 %), and reduced lung elastic recoil [2].

The severity assessment of an asthma attack has been suggested by the Global Initiative for Asthma (GINA) [3]

36.2 Criteria for Defining Severe Acute Asthma

36.2.1 Clinical Signs

Clinical signs include the following: breathlessness at rest; wheezing (life-threatening respiratory arrest is imminent if the chest is silent); use of accessory respiratory muscles (life-threatening respiratory arrest is imminent if paradoxical thoracoabdominal movement is present); limited ability to talk; and agitation (life-threatening respiratory arrest is imminent if confusion or coma are present).

36.2.2 Physiologic Signs

Physiologic signs include the following: respiratory rate > 30 breaths/min; heart rate > 120 beats/min (life-threatening respiratory arrest is imminent if bradycardia is present); pulsus paradoxus >25 mmHg (life-threatening respiratory arrest is imminent if pulsus paradoxus is present); post-bronchodilator peak expiratory flow <60 % of patient's best or predicted, or <100 l/m; $FEV_1 < 30$ % of patient's best or predicted Level; and $SpO_2 < 90$ %, $PaO_2 < 60$ mmHg, and $PaCO_2 > 45$ mmHg on room air.

The NIV therapy is used routinely in the acute exacerbations of COPD, and its efficiency has been proved. It is known that the efficacy of bronchodilator therapy also increases as the airways and alveoli open during NIV application [4]. It is curious that even the physiopathologies of COPD and asthma exacerbations are so alike; NIV therapy is not used routinely during the asthma attacks. A reason for this is the lack of strong prospective, randomized clinical studies with large number of patients that suggest the use of NIV in asthma exacerbations. Although all clinical studies show that administration of NIV during asthma exacerbations increases FEV_1, PaO_2, and peripheral oxygen saturation values and decreases the work of breathing, none of those studies recommend use of NIV during exacerbations strictly [5–9].

Gupta et al. [5] randomized 53 patients hospitalized in an intensive care unit with severe acute asthma attacks into two groups. Twenty-five of the patients received only medical therapy whereas 28 patients received NIV with oronasal mask in addition to medical therapy. NIV therapy was started with inspiration/expiration pressures values of 8/4 cmH_2O and they were increased 2 cmH_2O according to peripheral oxygen saturation and arterial blood gas sample follow-ups. Maximum pressure values administered were 20/10 cmH_2O. Bronchodilator therapy was given via T-piece with ultrasonic nebulizer. They found that NIV was of similar efficacy to standard medical treatment in improving respiratory rate, FEV_1, pH, PaO_2/FiO_2, and $PaCO_2$ in every acute asthma. A limitation of their study was the small number of patients included in the study.

Soma et al. [6] prospectively randomized 44 patients with acute mild and moderate asthma suffering an attack into two main groups: (a) a group receiving NIV (bi-level positive airway pressure (BiPAP)) therapy via a nasal or face mask (n = 30), which was divided into two subgroups, receiving high (8/6) and low pressure (6/4), or (b) a control group (n = 14). They suggested that NIV, even if delivered at lower pressures than are usually recommended to support acute respiratory failure patients, might help acute asthma attacks, even without inhaled bronchodilators.

Brandao et al. [7] evaluated the effects of bronchodilators administered via jet nebulization during either spontaneous breathing or NIV with inspiratory/expiratory pressures of 15/5 or 15/10 cmH_2O and showed an improvement in peak expiratory flow, FEV_1, and forced vital capacity in comparison with the control group. They speculated that this synergic effect of NIV in adjunct to the nebulized bronchodilator might be due to a better drug penetration into the peripheral airways.

Soroksky et al. [8] reported a pilot study where they applied BiPAP to severely asthmatic patients who were refractory to standard medical treatment. BiPAP was applied for 3 h in the emergency ward. They found that use of BiPAP significantly improved lung function tests in 80 % of the patients in the BiPAP group who reached the predetermined primary endpoints (an increase of at least 50 % in FEV_1 compared with baseline) versus 20 % in control group. However, a major limitation of the study was its small sample size.

Tokioka et al. [9] showed that application of pressure support may decrease auto-PEEP and work of breathing in asthmatic patients. This may unload inspiratory muscles and decrease muscle fatigue.

36.3 Discussion and Analysis

When studies of asthma attacks were considered, different understandings and approaches were found. Exact information on the timing and duration for NIV application is absent. For example, should NIV be delivered in the beginning of the attack when the steroid dose is increased as the patients are unresponsive to steroid therapy (prophylactic), delivered when hypoxia emerges, or even only when silent lung is observed and just before intubation? NIV administration should possibly be started when respiratory rate increases and when drug doses need to be increased. By this means, the airways and alveoli will stay open and the bronchodilator therapy will be able to reach to the terminal points where its efficiency will be secured. Most of the patients with asthma diagnosis are not hypoxic or hypercarbic except during the attacks. In this sense, it is important to differentiate COPD with asthma. Patients with COPD are resistant to hypoxia and hypercarbia and hence they have longer time for NIV application [10]. In an asthma attack, as the arterial blood gas samples start to deteriorate in the later periods, using them as a predictor for NIV might be erroneous. As the occurrence of hypoxia and hypercarbia will worsen the clinical state of the patient, administration of NIV could be slow and patients' synchronization could be more difficult. Accordingly, by delivering NIV at the beginning of the attack, we may increase our chance of success [1].

It is important to clarify the parameters that will be used during asthma attacks, as these are directly related to the success of NIV administration. In an asthma attack, inspiratory flow and airway resistance increases, expiration time decreases, air trapping occurs, and these increase auto-PEEP, which results with an increase in the work of breathing. The patient needs to make more effort to start the inspiration. To reduce all these pathologies and thereby work of breathing, external PEEP should be applied via NIV and auto-PEEP can be offset. The type of ventilation mode that can be used is not clarified in these studies. Although recovery was faster and FEV_1 values increased in patients receiving CPAP, it might be inappropriate to use the same airway pressures during inspiration and expiration to overcome inspiratory flow increase and airway resistance during an asthma attack. The main issue that increases the work of breathing during an asthma attack is increase in the inspiratory flow and airway resistance, and, hence, higher pressure support levels are needed during inspiration compared with expiration [7, 8]. Using the same levels during expiration and inspiration can cause overdistention, as the emptying of the alveoli can be even less sufficient with the already shortened expiration time. For that matter, it might be more appropriate to use BiPAP that has two different pressure support parameters or pressure support modes that use decelerating flow in patients with asthma attacks. Patients synchronized with NIV will not be in need of sedation [8].

NIV administration during asthma attacks can be done via nasal mask, oronasal mask, or full face mask. These options can be chosen according to the facial features of the patients or to availability. In patients with excessive secretions who cannot excrete them successfully, or in agitated patients with coughing attacks, synchronization with ventilation fails, causing failure in NIV therapy. Humidification of the air given during NIV administration can be problematic and needs extra consideration [10].

Patients with acute asthma attacks should be monitored and must be followed closely. Although this follow-up is most efficient in intensive care units, NIV therapy can be applied in emergency departments by experienced health-care workers.

NIV therapy should never delay intubation. NIV is never an alternative to intubation. NIV prevents the occurrence of the factors that lead to intubation and avoid intubation [10].

Conclusion

During asthma attacks, administration of NIV with the appropriate parameters and modes at the right time can increase efficacy of the medical therapy, resulting in a shorter hospital stay and positive effects on mortality. Prospective, randomized clinical trials with larger numbers of patients are needed to determine these effects.

Key Major Recommendations

- An acute asthma attack is pathophysiologically similar to COPD. NIV can be used during asthma attacks.
- Choosing the appropriate patient and time to start to NIV therapy affects the success of the therapy. NIV can be started with the first signs of an asthma attack.
- Two different levels of pressure support can increase patient synchronization and NIV success.

References

1. Scala R. Noninvasive ventilation in severe acute asthma? Still far from the truth. Respir Care. 2010;55(5):630–7.
2. Brenner B, Corbridge T, Kazzi A. Intubation and mechanical ventilation of the asthmatic patient in respiratory failure. J Allergy Clin Immunol. 2009;124(2 Suppl):S19–28.
3. Global Initiative for Asthma. Global strategy for asthma management and prevention. NIH publication 02–3659. Revised 2007. http://www.ginasthma.com/guidelineItem.asp?intid=1389. Accessed 5 Mar 2010.
4. Nowak R, Corbrigde T, Brenner B. Noninvasive ventilation. J Allergy Clin Immunol. 2009;124(2 Suppl):S15–8.
5. Gupta D, Nath A, Ritesh A, Behera D. A prospective randomized controlled trial on the efficacy of noninvasive ventilation in severe acute asthma. Respir Care. 2010;55(5):536–43.
6. Soma T, Hino M, Kida K, Kudoh S. A prospective and randomized study for improvement of acute asthma by non-invasive positive pressure ventilation. Intern Med. 2008;47(6):493–501.
7. Brandao DC, Lima VM, Filho VG. Reversal of bronchial obstruction with bi-level positive airway pressure and nebulization in patients with acute asthma. J Asthma. 2009;46(4):356–61.
8. Soroksky A, Stav D, Shpirer I. A pilot prospective, randomized, placebo-controlled trial of bilevel positive airway pressure in acute asthmatic attack. Chest. 2003;123:1018–25.
9. Tokioka H, Saito S, Saeki S, et al. The effect of pressure support ventilation on auto-PEEP in a patients with asthma. Chest. 1992;101:285–6.
10. Brochard L, Mancebo J, Wysocki M, et al. Noninvasive ventilation for acute exacerbations of chronic obstructive pulmonary disease. N Engl J Med. 1995;333:817–22.

Acute Applications of Noninvasive Ventilation in Obesity Hypoventilation Syndrome: Evidence and Key Practical Recommendations

37

Malcolm Lemyze

Contents

Abbreviations

ARF	Acute respiratory failure
BMI	Body mass index
EPAP	Expiratory positive airway pressure
IPAP	Inspiratory positive airway pressure
NIV	Noninvasive ventilation
OHS	Obesity hypoventilation syndrome
OSAS	Obstructive sleep apnea syndrome

37.1 Introduction

Obesity hypoventilation syndrome (OHS) refers to the form of chronic respiratory failure specifically resulting from obesity. The diagnostic criteria include obesity (body mass index (BMI) > 30 kg/m^2), alveolar hypoventilation ($PaCO_2$ > 45 mmHg),

M. Lemyze, MD
Department of Respiratory and Critical Care Medicine, Schaffner Hospital, Lens, France
e-mail: malcolmlemyze@yahoo.fr

A.M. Esquinas (ed.), *Noninvasive Mechanical Ventilation: Theory, Equipment, and Clinical Applications*, DOI 10.1007/978-3-319-21653-9_37

and sleep-disordered breathing, without any common cause of respiratory failure (e.g., chronic obstructive pulmonary disease (COPD), chest wall deformity, or neuromuscular disease) [1]. Given the current epidemic of obesity, OHS is expected to become the second leading cause of chronic respiratory failure worldwide [2, 3]. The higher the BMI, the higher the incidence of OHS [2]. The diagnosis is usually made during an episode of acute respiratory failure (ARF), which is the most common life-threatening complication of OHS. Over the last two decades, noninvasive ventilation (NIV) has emerged as the most effective treatment for ARF in obese patients [1].

37.2 Discussion

37.2.1 Main Indications for NIV

37.2.1.1 Type 2 (Hypercapnic) Respiratory Failure

Hypercapnic ARF is the most meaningful indication for NIV especially in morbidly obese patients. During a 13-year study period, Carillo et al. [4] have prospectively evaluated the benefit of NIV in 173 patients with OHS versus 543 patients with COPD in hypercapnic ARF. NIV was more effective in preventing intubation in decompensated OHS than in COPD (NIV failure 7 % vs 13 %, $p=0.037$), resulting in a lower in-hospital mortality in the OHS group compared with COPD patients (6 % vs 18 %, $p<0.001$). In our prospective study including 76 morbidly obese patients weakened by malignant OHS and admitted to the intensive care unit (ICU) for ARF, NIV was constantly successful in patients with idiopathic hypercapnic ARF [5]. The severity of respiratory acidosis, the level of hypercapnia, and the depth of encephalopathy were not reliable criteria for predicting NIV failure. Along the same lines, Dias et al. [6] clearly demonstrated that NIV is safe and successful in reversing hypercapnic coma in patients in acute-on-chronic respiratory failure. In this series, the success rate reached 80 % in comatose patients (Glasgow Coma Score <7, $n=95$) as compared with 70 % in non-comatose patients (Glasgow Coma Score >8, $n=863$, $p=0.04$). Response to NIV may be delayed, especially in hypercapnic obese patients on respiratory depressant drugs or diuretics promoting alveolar hypoventilation [5].

37.2.1.2 Type 1 (Hypoxemic) Respiratory Failure

If the use of NIV for patients in hypoxemic ARF is still questionable, at best it avoids intubation and at worst it can be used for patient preoxygenation because it has been demonstrated effective in the preoperative management of morbidly obese patients before abdominal surgery [7]. In all cases, NIV must be initiated in a suitable environment (an emergency room, ICU, or at least a respiratory step-down unit) with a large, well-trained team capable of providing close monitoring and quick intubation if the patient's condition worsens. In cases of persistent refractory hypoxemia ($PaO_2/FiO_2<200$) after a 1–2 h NIV trial, escalation to intubation should be immediately discussed, especially when the cause of ARF is not easily and rapidly reversible (e.g., pneumonia, ARDS, or gravitational atelectasis).

37.2.1.3 Preoxygenation Before Intubation

A combination of preoxygenation with NIV before intubation and a lung recruitment maneuver, consisting of applying CPAP at 40 cmH_2O for 40 s immediately after intubation, reduces the risk of desaturation and improves lung volume during and after intubation [7].

37.2.1.4 Post-extubation Respiratory Distress

Morbidly obese patients are usually difficult to wean from mechanical ventilation and are prone to post-extubation ARF. In a randomized controlled study, El-Solh et al. [8] demonstrated that the systematic use of prophylactic NIV immediately after extubation can significantly reduce the risk of ARF in the first 48 h following extubation.

37.2.2 Positioning Morbidly Obese Patients for NIV

Positioning is too often overlooked in massively obese patients, although it is a priority issue and an essential prerequisite for the management of these patients. Sitting position prevents gravitational atelectasis, unloads the diaphragm from the pressure exerted by the abdomen, thus facilitating its piston-like downward capacity, and reduces work of breathing by reversing both expiratory flow limitation and auto-PEEP [9]. Poor positioning of obese patients in ARF may result in NIV failure and death [10].

37.2.3 Ventilator Settings

Pressure-limited ventilatory modes are preferred over flow-limited modes. PEEP (or expiratory positive airway pressure (EPAP)) prevents upper airway collapse and nocturnal arterial desaturation [1]. By maintaining a positive transpulmonary pressure at expiration, PEEP increases functional residual capacity, averts gravitational atelectasis, reverses expiratory flow limitation, and, finally, decreases work of breathing by counterbalancing auto-PEEP [9]. The pressure support level increases alveolar ventilation and thus corrects respiratory acidosis by improving CO_2 removal. In clinical practice, obese patients in ARF usually need high levels of inspiratory positive airway pressure (IPAP) (mean, 18 cmH_2O; from 12 to 25 cmH_2O) and PEEP (mean, 9 cmH_2O; from 5 to 13 cmH_2O) [1, 4, 5]. Polysomnography can help identify sleep-disordered breathing (obstructive sleep apnea syndrome (OSAS), hypoventilation alone, or a combination of OSAS and OHS) to better adapt the ventilator settings for long-term NIV [1].

Conclusion

NIV and sitting position are the two cornerstones of the initial therapeutic management of morbidly obese patients in ARF. NIV is consistently successful in hypercapnic decompensation of OHS. Refractory hypoxemia is the main determinant of NIV failure in these patients.

Key Major Recommendations

- Good positioning (in the sitting position) is an essential prerequisite for NIV success in the obese patient.
- In type 2 (hypercapnic) respiratory failure of obese patients, bi-level positive airway pressure should be advanced, as it is consistently successful,
- NIV can be cautiously used in type 1 (hypoxemic) respiratory failure, especially if the underlying cause is rapidly reversible, but only in an environment allowing close monitoring and rapid performance of intubation.
- NIV is helpful in preoxygenating the obese patient before intubation.
- NIV should be systematically performed immediately after extubation to prevent post-extubation ARF in morbidly obese patients

References

1. Mokhlesi B. Obesity hypoventilation syndrome: a state-of-the-art review. Respir Care. 2010;55:1347–62.
2. Nowbar S, Burkart KM, Gonzales R, et al. Obesity-associated hypoventilation in hospitalized patients: prevalence, effects, and outcome. Am J Med. 2004;116:1–7.
3. Finucane MM, Stevens GA, Cowan MJ, et al. National, regional, and global trends in body-mass index since 1980: systematic analysis of health examination surveys and epidemiological studies with 960 country-years and 9.1 million participants. Lancet. 2011;377:557–67.
4. Carrillo A, Ferrer M, Gonzalez-Diaz G, et al. Noninvasive ventilation in acute hypercapnic respiratory failure caused by obesity hypoventilation syndrome and chronic obstructive pulmonary disease. Am J Respir Crit Care Med. 2012;186:1279–85.
5. Lemyze M, Taufour P, Duhamel A, et al. Determinants of noninvasive ventilation success or failure in morbidly obese patients in acute respiratory failure. PLoS One. 2014;9(5), e97563.
6. Futier E, Constantin JM, Pelosi P, et al. Noninvasive ventilation and alveolar recruitment maneuver improve respiratory function during and after intubation of morbidly obese patients: a randomized controlled study. Anesthesiology. 2011;114:1354–63.
7. Díaz GG, Alcaraz AC, Talavera JC, Pérez PJ, Rodriguez AE, Cordoba FG, Hill NS. Noninvasive positive-pressure ventilation to treat hypercapnic coma secondary to respiratory failure. Chest. 2005;127:952–60.
8. El-Solh AA, Aquilina A, Pineda L, et al. Noninvasive ventilation for prevention of post-extubation respiratory failure in obese patients. Eur Respir J. 2006;28:588–95.
9. Lemyze M, Mallat J, Duhamel A, et al. Effects of sitting position and applied positive end-expiratory pressure on respiratory mechanics of critically ill obese patients receiving mechanical ventilation. Crit Care Med. 2013;41:2592–9.
10. Lemyze M, Guerry MJ, Mallat J, Thevenin D. Obesity supine death syndrome revisited. Eur Respir J. 2012;40:1568–9.

Noninvasive Ventilation in Chest Wall Deformities: When and Why

38

Dhruva Chaudhry and Rahul Roshan

Contents

Abbreviations

EPAP	Expiratory positive airway pressure
ICU	Intensive care unit
IPAP	Inspiratory positive airway pressure
LTOT	Long-term oxygen therapy

D. Chaudhry, MD, DNB(Med), DM(PCCM), FICCM, FICP (✉)
R. Roshan, MD, DNB, FCCP
Pulmonary & Critical Care Medicine, Pt. B.D. Sharma PGIMS,
Pt. B.D. Sharma University of Health Sciences, Rohtak, Haryana 124001, India
e-mail: dhruvachaudhry@yahoo.co.in; rahul.roshan81@gmail.com

A.M. Esquinas (ed.), *Noninvasive Mechanical Ventilation: Theory, Equipment, and Clinical Applications*, DOI 10.1007/978-3-319-21653-9_38

NIV	Noninvasive ventilation
NREM	Non-rapid eye movement
$PaCO_2$	Arterial carbon dioxide tension
PaO_2	Arterial oxygen tension
PI_{max}	Maximal inspiratory pressure
Pdi	Transdiaphgramatic pressure
Pdi_{max}	Maximal transdiaphgramatic pressure
P_{pl}	Pleural pressure
REM	Rapid eye movement

38.1 Introduction

Diseases affecting the chest wall reduce the functional capacity of the diaphragm and lung, invariably leading to ventilatory failure. Chest wall or thoracic cage deformities can be primary, like idiopathic kyphoscoliosis, ankylosing spondylitis, pectus excavatum, and pectus carinatum, or secondary to pleural fibrosis, thoracoplasty (after lobectomy or pneumonectomy), or poliomyelitis. These restrictive diseases can affect the components of the inspiratory pump, including the bony rib cage, respiratory musculature, and the spine and its articulations, as well as the soft tissue comprising the abdomen. Respiratory muscle weakness is the most common factor leading to chest infections, hospital admissions, and early mortality in these patients. Most of these patients gradually develop nocturnal hypoventilation, initially during rapid-eye-movement (REM) sleep before progressing to non-REM (NREM) sleep, eventually leading to daytime chronic ventilatory failure. Management of chronic ventilatory failure with noninvasive ventilation (NIV) is standard recommended care. Nocturnal nasal intermittent positive pressure ventilation (NIPPV) has been shown to increase survival and improve blood gases, respiratory function, sleep architecture, and quality of life in patients with chest wall diseases.

38.2 Pathophysiology of Respiratory Failure in Chest Wall Diseases

Restrictive chest wall disease leads to altered pulmonary pathophysiology, with reduction in total lung capacity, vital capacity, and functional residual capacity but without changes in residual volume [1, 2]. Diseases like pectus excavatum and pectus carinatum do not appear to have important effects on respiratory pump, whereas ankylosing spondylitis occasionally leads to severe ventilatory failure as total lung capacity and functional residual capacity are not reduced. Patients with kyphoscoliosis, post-tuberculosis sequelae, and post-thoracoplasty have higher risk of ventilatory failure, being dependent on the degree of deformity and age of onset. The severity of deformity can be quantified by measuring the angle of primary curves (Cobb's angle). An angle greater than 100° suggests severe deformity with increased risk of respiratory failure, alveolar hypoventilation, and cor pulmonale. Anomalous muscle insertion due to thoracic deformity in diseases like kyphoscoliosis may lead to muscle weakness. Inspiratory muscle strength is significantly impaired. Chest wall deformity leads to increased respiratory load due to a fall in chest wall and lung compliance. A fall in inspiratory capacity is seen due to mechanical disadvantage as a result of the altered geometry of the rib cage. Increase workload and a decrease in the ability to generate the force with increased oxygen consumption can lead to greater risk of respiratory failure due to muscle fatigue. The increase in the respiratory load leads to a breathing pattern characterized by low tidal volumes and very high respiratory rates with increased dead space, alveolar hypoventilation, and disordered sleep.

Patients with chest wall deformities have a reduced ability to generate maximal inspiratory pressures (PI_{max}). Severe reductions in the maximal transdiaphgramatic pressures (Pdi_{max}) along with an increase in pleural pressure (P_{pl}) and transdiaphgramatic pressure (Pdi) deflections during normal breathing is observed. These pressure changes lead to higher P_{pl}/ Pdi_{max} and Pdi/ Pdi_{max} ratios, suggesting respiratory fatigue. In addition to altered pulmonary pathophysiology, hypoventilation and central or obstructive sleep apneas also contribute to respiratory failure. A negative correlation has been noted between $PaCO_2$ and PI_{max}, possibly demonstrating that inspiratory muscle restriction plays a vital role in the occurrence of respiratory failure in kyphoscoliosis patients. The increased work of respiration and decreased respiratory muscle activity during REM sleep contributes to hypercapnia being seen at this time, before it manifests during the deeper stages of NREM sleep and, later, in wakefulness.

38.3 Mechanism of Action of NIV

The mechanism behind the benefit of NIV in chest wall diseases is not yet fully understood [2, 3] (Fig. 38.1). Various factors have been postulated to elaborate these effects. First, NIV allows chronically fatigued inspiratory muscles to rest and time to recover, leading to improvement in inspiratory muscle function, ventilation, and arterial blood gases during the daytime. Second, nocturnal application of NIV attenuates hypoventilation during sleep, resets central response to hypercapnia, and improves ventilation and gas exchange during the day. Third, NIV improves lung function by recruiting micro-atelectatic lung zones, improving pulmonary distensibility, and providing better ventilation perfusion exchange. Finally, NIV improves sleep architecture. It alleviates the symptoms mostly related to sleep fragmentation subsequent to apneas, such as daytime sleepiness, fatigue, morning headache, cognitive dysfunctions, and dyspnea.

NIV has been shown to improve sleep quality, to lead to a rise in PaO_2 and a fall in $PaCO_2$, and to decrease the number of hospitalizations and cost of treatment. Further, NIV has been found to alleviate daytime sleepiness, improve nocturnal hypoventilation, increase maximal respiratory pressures, provide greater ability to perform activities of daily living and better quality of life, and prolong survival.

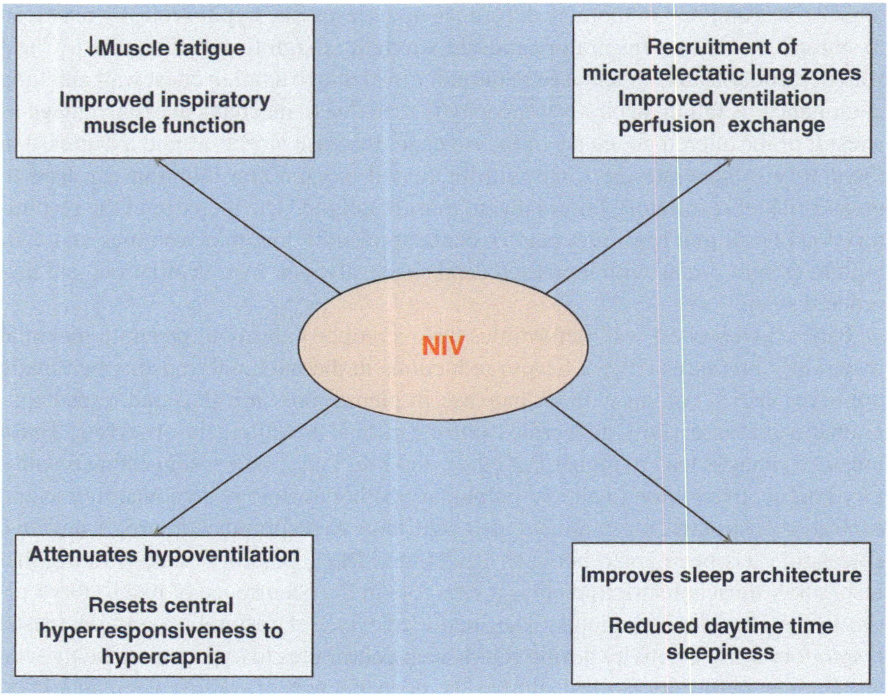

Fig. 38.1 Mechanism of action of NIV in chest wall diseases

38.4 NIV in Chest Wall Diseases

A Cochrane review suggests that the therapeutic benefit of mechanical ventilation in patients with neuromuscular and chest wall disease is weak but consistent, indicating short duration relief in the symptoms of chronic hypoventilation [4]. Buyse et al. [5] found that in kyphoscoliosis, NIPPV demonstrated an increase in PaO_2 by 54 %, a fall in $PaCO_2$ by 21 %, and a rise in vital capacity and maximal static inspiratory mouth pressure by 47 % and 33 %, respectively, but these improvements were not present in patients who received long-term oxygen therapy (LTOT). In the NIV group, the 1-year survival was higher compared with the LTOT group (100 % versus 66 %).

Budweiser and coworkers [6] found that pressure support > 15 cmH_2O accentuated the fall in $PaCO_2$ during long-term follow-up in patients with restrictive chest wall diseases. They showed that the inspiratory positive airway pressure (IPAP)–expiratory positive airway pressure (EPAP)/weight ratio correlated with the fall in $PaCO_2$ at the first visit after hospital discharge with long-term NIV. Domiciliary NIV significantly improves quality of life, including dyspnea, fatigue, and emotional status in patients with chest wall disease. Application of NIV improves clinical and physiological response to exercise by alleviating acidosis, hypoxia, and hypercapnia along with a reduction in perception of breathlessness and effort. NIV leads to marked improvement in diurnal arterial oxygen and carbon dioxide tensions (PaO_2 and $PaCO_2$) along with a decrease in the days for hospital admission for respiratory failure in patients with kyphoscoliosis or sequelae of previous tuberculosis. Better quality of sleep was reported by 62 % of the patients and 70 % reported improvements in activities of daily living [7].

Significant improvement in respiratory and peripheral muscle endurance along with improvement in arterial blood gases has been seen after administration of NIV for 3 months among patients with post-tuberculosis sequelae and scoliosis [8]. An increase in maximal inspiratory pressure of 33–80 % along with a rise in maximal expiratory pressures by 16 % has been observed in patients with chest wall diseases.

In a randomized cohort study in an intensive care unit (ICU), the success rate of NIV in kyphoscoliosis patients with acute respiratory failure was found to be 76.4 % [9]. The frequency of sepsis and septic shock in patients with NIV failure was greater than in patients with NIV success. The mortality rate was higher in patients in the ICU with NIV failure compared with those patients who were initially put on invasive ventilation. The predictors of NIV failure were significantly higher Acute Physiology and Chronic Health Evaluation (APACHE) II score and increased respiratory rate, with lower Glasgow Coma Scale and pH values. Lung functions and 6-min walk distance were found to improve with pressure support of around 15 cm H_2O with pressure-cycled NIV devices during long-term treatment. $PaCO_2 \geq 50$ mmHg at 1 month of home ventilation and comorbidity (Charlson comorbidity index ≥3) were independent predictors of mortality in chest wall disease treated with noninvasive home mechanical ventilation [10].

Newer modes of ventilation such as average volume-assured pressure support are an effective treatment option in kyphoscoliotic patients with chronic respiratory failure, leading to an immediate and long-term improvement of daytime and nocturnal blood gas exchange. This mode has shown a significant improvement of diurnal PaO_2 and $PaCO_2$, mean blood oxygen saturation during sleep on the 5th day of NIV and after 1 year of NIV, along with increase in forced vital capacity after 1 year [11]. Petitjean et al. [12] found that discontinuation of NIV in patients, initially stabilized on NIV, with chronic ventilatory failure ($PaCO_2 > 50$ mmHg) due to restrictive chest wall diseases (total lung capacity ≤ 65 % of predicted), subjects them rapidly to nocturnal respiratory failure and, within days, to diurnal respiratory failure. Withholding of NIV for more than 24 – 48 h is not recommended.

Patients are usually compliant with NIV, with average daily use significantly higher in post-tuberculosis sequelae and post-poliomyelitis patients in comparison with patients with kyphoscoliosis (9 vs 6 h per day). At present, the compliance rate of NIV in patients with kyphoscoliosis and polio is reported to be around 80–90 %. Mortality rate in patients with kyphoscoliosis on long-term home NIV has been reported as 21 % over 4 years.

38.5 Who Should Receive NIV?

38.5.1 Prophylaxis Therapy in High-Risk Patients

Though there is a little evidence in the literature, NIV may be given as a prophylactic therapy in asymptomatic high-risk patients having greater chances of ventilatory failure (vital capacity of 1–1.5 l, early development of scoliosis before the age of 8 years, and a high thoracic curve). In patients with normal daytime blood gas tensions, the amount of nocturnal hypoxia and hypercapnia, along with presence of complications such as polycythemia or a high pulmonary artery pressure, may benefit from nocturnal NIV, but the decision to apply depends upon the physician [3, 13].

38.5.2 Definite Therapy for Respiratory Failure

Patients who are symptomatic and have abnormal blood gas tensions have been more strongly suggested to benefit from NIV (Table 38.1).

38.6 How to Deliver NIV

Since the 1980s, volume-targeted NIV has been the predominant mode of NIV used in chest-wall deformity presenting with chronic ventilatory failure. In the last decade, however, pressure-targeted NIV emerged as a popular alternative because it is less expensive and is associated with fewer gastrointestinal side effects. Recent studies have shown equal efficacy of volume-targeted and pressure-targeted modes

Table 38.1 Indications for NIV in chest wall diseases

Clinical
Fatigue, morning headache, hypersomnolence, nightmares, enuresis
Tiredness, dyspnea, cognitive changes
Cor pulmonale
Physiological
$PaCO_2 > 45$ mmHg
Vital capacity <50 % of the predicted value
Maximal inspiratory pressure < 60 cmH_2O
Nighttime arterial desaturation: $SaO_2 < 90$ %; for > 5 min, or > 10 % of the total recording time
Other indications
Recovering from acute respiratory failure with persistent hypercapnia
Frequent hospital admissions for acute respiratory failure
Failure to respond to CPAP alone if obstructive sleep apnea

$PaCO_2$ arterial carbon dioxide tension, *SaO_2* arterial oxygen saturation, *CPAP* continuous positive airway pressure

of long-term NIV with relation to improvements in gas exchange, sleep architecture, physical activity, and quality of life in patients with chest-wall deformity, although the pressure-targeted mode has greater leak than volume ventilation. Benefits of NIPPV by volumetric ventilator or a bi-level positive airway pressure (BIPAP) device have been found to be equal for patients with kyphoscoliosis, however, subjective response and tolerance may be slightly better with BIPAP. No significant difference has been observed in time needed to successfully adapt to volume-targeted NIV compared with pressure-targeted NIV in patients with chest-wall deformity. There is a subgroup of patients who respond well to volume ventilators after failure of initial pressure support modes. NIPPV via a mask has mostly replaced negative pressure ventilation, but among the patients who cannot tolerate nasal mask negative pressure ventilation, tracheostomy ventilation can be the only substitute.

38.6.1 Negative Pressure Ventilation

A cuirass or jacket type of negative pressure ventilator is mostly preferred over a tank ventilator. These negative pressure ventilators have a major drawback as patients need to lie on their back throughout the night and have a restricted area of movement. This becomes especially difficult in patients with a kyphosis, where the sharp angulation of the spine can become uncomfortable. It can also be cumbersome to mould a cuirass in patients with a severe thoracic scoliosis. One of the greatest disadvantages of negative pressure ventilation is greater patient ventilator asynchrony and its tendency to induce obstructive apneas due to upper airway collapse. The minimum inspiratory and expiratory times are similar to those required for positive pressure ventilation.

38.6.2 NIPPV

A nasal mask is generally preferred over a full face mask or a mouthpiece (Fig. 38.2). Patients with kyphoscoliosis are no more prone to NIV complications – mask displacement, nasal ulcers, air leaks, or upper airway obstruction – than other diseases of ventilatory failure. Both pressure- and volume-preset modes of ventilation can be used. In the pressure preset mode, a peak inspiratory pressure of 20–25 cmH_2O is often desired with an inspiratory time of 0.8–1 s and an expiratory time of 2 s. The fast respiratory rate in patients with restrictive chest wall disease mandates a sensitive triggering system with a short response time. Positive end-expiratory pressure can be beneficial at a pressure of 2–4 cmH_2O, but is not absolutely necessary except in some bi-level pressure-support modes in which it is essential to flush the dead space. Adequate IPAP-EPAP difference should be ensured for movement of the chest wall. Because of the rapid, shallow breathing pattern seen in kyphoscoliosis, the ventilator triggering system should have a short response time to minimize patient ventilator asynchrony. Failure of trigger on the spontaneous mode during

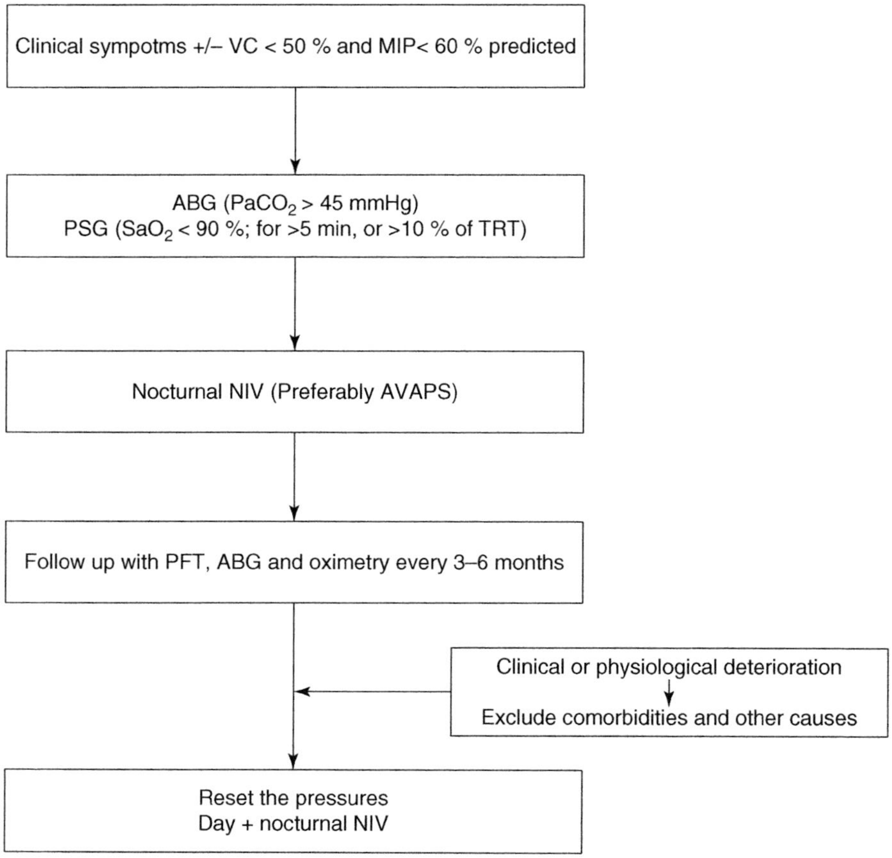

Fig. 38.2 NIV protocol in chest wall diseases. *VC* vital capacity, *MIP* maximal inspiratory pressure, *ABG* arterial blood gas analysis, *PaCO2* arterial carbon dioxide tension, *PSG* polysomnography, *SaO2* arterial oxygen saturation, *TRT* total recording time, *NIV* noninvasive ventilation, *AVAPS* average volume-assured pressure support, *PFT* pulmonary function test

sleep warrants a trial with spontaneous timed mode if air leak has been ruled out. Supplemental oxygen may be required if the partial pressure of oxygen in arterial blood is low.

38.6.3 Contraindications of NIV

The contraindications of noninvasive ventilation in chest wall deformities are no different than in the other diseases. Difficulty in application of the headgear, cuirass, or jacket can be an important issue. Lack of motivation along with psychological factors, such as claustrophobia, are also significant (Table. 38.2).

Table 38.2 Contraindications for NIV in chest wall diseases

Failure to protect the airway
Poor cough
Impaired swallowing with chronic aspiration
Excess tracheobronchial secretions
Continuous or nearly continuous ventilation requirement
Anatomical facial deformities preventing appropriate mask fitting
Poor patient or family motivation
Uncooperative patient

38.7 Special Conditions

38.7.1 Pregnancy in Chest Wall Diseases

Pregnancy may aggravate type II respiratory failure in the presence of a restrictive thoracic wall disorder. Risk factors appear to be a vital capacity of < 1 l, thoracic scoliosis > 100°, hypercapnia, the presence of bilateral diaphragm weakness, or extensive intercostals muscle weakness in addition to the chest wall disorder. In normal women, the gravid uterus affects lung function by upward displacement of the diaphragm, leading to a fall in functional residual capacity and residual volume. These lung function changes and the raised metabolic needs are offset by rise in cardiac output and rapid breathing. However, pregnancy in patients with severe kyphoscoliosis may lead to failure of these adaptive mechanisms, with an increase in the dependant airway closure causing ventilation perfusion abnormalities and increased respiratory workload that may contribute to nocturnal and subsequent daytime respiratory failure. Such patients generally respond well to noninvasive ventilatory support.

Conclusion

NIV is beneficial in patients with kyphoscoliosis with ventilatory failure. It improves arterial blood gas abnormalities and provides better lung functions and quality-of-life sleep architecture. However, predictors of failure and the relative contraindications should be kept in mind during application of NIV. Positive pressure ventilators are now preferred over negative pressure ventilators. The volume-assured pressure support mode may be preferred over conventional pressure support modes. Guidelines need to be developed regarding the use of this noninvasive mode in restrictive chest wall diseases.

References

1. Casas A, Pavía J, Maldonado D. Respiratory muscle disorders in chest wall diseases. Arch Bronconeumol. 2003;39(8):361–6.
2. Lisboa C, Díaz O, Fadic R. Noninvasive mechanical ventilation in patients with neuromuscular diseases and in patients with chest restriction. Arch Bronconeumol. 2003;39(7):314–20.

3. Shneerson JM, Simonds AK. Noninvasive ventilation for chest wall and neuromuscular disorders. Eur Respir J. 2002;20(2):480–7.
4. Annane D, Orlikowski D, Chevret S. Nocturnal mechanical ventilation for chronic hypoventilation in patients with neuromuscular and chest wall disorders. Cochrane Database Syst Rev. 2014;(12): CD001941.
5. Buyse B, Meersseman W, Demedts M. Treatment of chronic respiratory failure in kyphoscoliosis: oxygen or ventilation? Eur Respir J. 2003;22(3):525–8.
6. Budweiser S, Heinemann F, Fischer W, et al. Impact of ventilation parameters and duration of ventilator use on noninvasive home ventilation in restrictive thoracic disorders. Respiration. 2006;73(4):488–94.
7. Leger P, Bedicam JM, Cornette A, et al. Nasal intermittent positive pressure ventilation: long-term follow-up in patients with severe chronic respiratory insufficiency. Chest. 1994;105(1):100–5.
8. Schonhofer B, Wallstein S, Wiese C, et al. Noninvasive mechanical ventilation improves endurance performance in patients with chronic respiratory failure due to thoracic restriction. Chest. 2001;119(5):1371–8.
9. Adıgüzel N, Karakurt Z, Gungor G, et al. Management of kyphoscoliosis with respiratory failure in the intensive care unit and during long term follow up. Multidiscip Respir Med. 2012;7(1):30.
10. Martí S, Pallero M, Ferrer J, et al. Predictors of mortality in chest wall disease treated with noninvasive home mechanical ventilation. Respir Med. 2010;104(12):1843–9.
11. Piesiak P, Brzecka A, Kosacka M, et al. Efficacy of non invasive volume targeted ventilation in patients with chronic respiratory failure due to kyphoscoliosis. Adv Exp Med Biol. 2015;838:53–8.
12. Petitjean T, Philit F, Germain-Pastenne M, et al. Sleep and respiratory function after withdrawal of noninvasive ventilation in patients with chronic respiratory failure. Respir Care. 2008;53(10):1316–23.
13. Consensus Conference Report. Clinical indications for noninvasive positive pressure ventilation in chronic respiratory failure due to restrictive lung disease, COPD and nocturnal hypoventilation. Chest. 1999;116(2):521–34.

Noninvasive Mechanical Ventilation in Duchenne Muscular Dystrophy: What Have We Learned?

39

Giuseppe Fiorentino, Antonio Pisano, and Anna Annunziata

Contents

Abbreviations

DMD	Duchenne muscular dystrophy
FVC	Forced vital capacity
IPAP	Inspiratory positive airway pressures
$PaCO_2$	Arterial partial pressure of CO_2
REM	Rapid eye movement
RR	Respiratory rate

G. Fiorentino, MD (✉) • A. Annunziata, MD
Division of Respiratory Physiopathology and Rehabilitation,
A.O.R.N. "Dei Colli" – Monaldi Hospital, Naples, Italy
e-mail: giuseppefiorentino1@gmail.com; anna.annunziata@gmail.com

A. Pisano, MD
Cardiac Anesthesia and Intensive Care Unit,
A.O.R.N. "Dei Colli" – Monaldi Hospital, Naples, Italy
e-mail: antoniopisanoMD@libero.it

A.M. Esquinas (ed.), *Noninvasive Mechanical Ventilation: Theory, Equipment, and Clinical Applications*, DOI 10.1007/978-3-319-21653-9_39

SDB	Sleep disordered breathing
VC	Vital capacity
V_T	Tidal volume

39.1 Introduction

Pulmonary complications in Duchenne muscular dystrophy (DMD) are usually more predictable than in other neuromuscular diseases because they correlate with overall muscle strength. Respiratory failure in DMD is primarily associated with restrictive pulmonary disease caused by inspiratory muscle weakness, severe scoliosis, reduced lung and chest wall compliance, and ineffective cough because of respiratory muscle weakness. The majority of patients also develop cardiomyopathy. Respiratory disease is a nearly inevitable complication in adult DMD patients, and it represents the underlying cause of death in 70 % of DMD patients younger than 25 years [1].

39.2 Discussion and Analysis

39.2.1 Diurnal and Nocturnal Respiratory Function in DMD

Because, in healthy subjects, vital capacity (VC) increases with growth during the first decade of life, early respiratory muscle dysfunction may be masked until VC does not reach its plateau. Accordingly, in DMD patients, VC progressively decreases by about 5–6 % per year, usually starting around 12 years of age. However, the rate of this decline may be variable: in particular, a sudden reduction in VC can be occasionally precipitated by intercurrent events such as a worsening of scoliosis or infective complications leading to the development of hypoventilation. A forced vital capacity (FVC) $\leq$1 l is a predictor of poor outcome, with a survival rate at 5 years of only 8 % if assisted ventilation is not provided [2].

Reductions in maximum inspiratory pressure occur early in the clinical course of DMD and may precede the reduction in VC. However, despite significant weakness of the respiratory muscles, pulmonary symptoms are often minimal in the early stages of the disease. Particularly, hypercapnia is uncommon in patients with DMD in the absence of pulmonary infections. This is believed to be due to a relative preservation of diaphragm function until the later stages of the disease. Anyhow, once hypercapnia develops, the course is rapidly progressive [1].

Sleep-related respiratory disturbances are frequent in DMD. Symptoms of sleep-disordered breathing (SDB) (headache, somnolence, etc.) should be actively investigated when VC is less than 30 % of predicted. Sleep-related hypoxemia may contribute to respiratory failure and to the development of pulmonary hypertension. To minimize the work and perception of breathing, patients progressively accelerate their respiratory rate (RR), leading to higher RR/tidal volume (V_T) ratio.

Nevertheless, once this compensatory mechanism no longer allows the patient to maintain adequate alveolar ventilation, arterial partial pressure of CO_2 ($PaCO_2$) rises [2, 3].

In summary, hypercapnic chronic respiratory failure in DMD patients typically evolves through four stages: stage 1, SDB without hypercapnia; stage 2, SDB with severe nocturnal hypoventilation and hypercapnia during rapid eye movement (REM) sleep; stage 3, SDB with hypercapnia during REM and non-REM sleep; stage 4, diurnal hypercapnia. At stage 4, mean survival is less than 1 year if ventilatory support is not started. When applied at stages 2 and 3, NIV corrects hypercapnia and improves both quality of life and survival [3].

39.2.2 When to Start Noninvasive Mechanical Ventilation

The primary goals of noninvasive mechanical ventilation in DMD are to improve alveolar ventilation, reduce the shunt effect due to hypoxic pulmonary vasoconstriction, and decrease the risk of pulmonary complications. This may lead to reduction in the rate of hospitalization, prolonged survival, and improvement in quality of life, and could attenuate the decline in both FVC and maximum voluntary ventilation, thus delaying the need for tracheostomy and invasive mechanical ventilation [4].

However, the criteria to initiate ventilatory support in DMD patients are not well defined. Raphael et al. [5] found that prophylactic NIV in normocapnic, asymptomatic DMD patients was poorly tolerated and provided no survival benefit. However, this study has been criticized, primarily due to the lack of information about secretion clearance and nocturnal hypercapnia.

Early initiation of NIV is an increasingly used approach. The initial objective of prophylactic NIV is to counteract the unavoidable worsening of VC associated with disease progression. Initiation of night-time NIV before the development of daytime hypercapnia is beneficial to the patient; in fact, it may relieve symptoms and improve quality of life, reduce daytime hypercapnia, slow the decline in pulmonary function, and reduce the risk of intensive care unit admission. In particular, when NIV is started in the presence of nocturnal hypercapnia alone, the onset of daytime hypercapnia is delayed, and it usually does not develop until 4–5 years after NIV initiation [6]. Once patients require NIV, the pressures to be set should be established in the sleep laboratory to eliminate nocturnal apneas and hypopneas [7].

As time passes, patients with DMD develop a constant hypoventilation and need respiratory support 24 h a day. The use of NIV in the daytime is also, mostly, empirically guided. Mechanical ventilation for 18–20 h a day has been described in patients with VC < 300 ml, whereas a daily ventilator-free time of less than 15 min has been reported in patients with VC < 10 % of predicted [4]. Worsening of symptoms (primarily dyspnea) during the day suggests high energy expenditure in the attempt to maintain normocapnia, and reversal of symptoms may be expected after a few hours on daytime NIV. However, evidence in this regard is lacking.

Finally, an obvious indication for late initiation of NIV is daytime hypercapnia. In fact, NIV is well tolerated in DMD patients with established respiratory failure, resulting in improved daytime arterial blood gases, and can be maintained for a relatively long time (up to 5–7 years) without the need for invasive mechanical ventilation [8].

39.2.3 Choice of Ventilator, Interfaces, and Settings

39.2.3.1 Ventilator

The most commonly used noninvasive technique is mouthpiece intermittent positive pressure ventilation. It has been used successfully, over a period of more than 8 years, in DMD patients with mean FVC of 0.6 l (5 % of predicted) [1, 6]. Two types of positive pressure ventilators were used: volume ventilators and pressure support ventilators. Both systems have similar effects on alveolar hypoventilation and on (partial) respiratory muscle unloading. Newer ventilators combine the advantages of pressure and volume modalities, providing air leak compensation, targeted volume, and sensitive triggering for optimal synchronization and comfort. During the daytime, volume modalities are preferable due to the benefits of air-stacking and the absence of leak compensations, thus enabling mouthpiece ventilation on demand. Moreover, many patients with DMD have central sleep apnea and need NIV machines that allow a respiratory rate to be set [8, 9].

39.2.3.2 Interfaces

The nasal mask remains the first choice as interface for nocturnal ventilation. Mouthpiece ventilation is well tolerated and does not interfere with eating or speaking. Both nasal and mouthpiece ventilation are a safe and effective form of respiratory support for DMD patients who require NIV for 24 h a day [1].

39.2.3.3 Settings

Ventilator parameters may vary widely among individuals. Effective ventilation is usually achieved with relatively low inspiratory positive airway pressures (IPAP), between 10 and 15 cm H_2O, although the use of inspiratory pressures higher than 20 cm H_2O may be needed and have been reported [1, 4]. For volume modalities, high RR (between 14 and 22 breaths per minute) and V_T (up to 10–14 ml/kg of actual body weight) have been described as initial settings in DMD patients [1, 4].

39.2.4 Complications and Contraindications of NIV

Complications of nasal intermittent positive pressure ventilation include eye irritation, conjunctivitis, skin ulceration, gastric distention, and emesis into a full face mask. Facial complications can be avoided by regular follow-up to assess mask fit. In fragile patients, mask displacement can rapidly lead to severe hypoxemia and hypercapnia. Contraindications are rare. Education of caregivers and families on airway clearance techniques during home mechanical ventilation is an important factor in the success of NIV [8].

39.2.5 Causes of NIV Failure

Failure of NIV may occur due to technical issues, patient reluctance, or disease progression. Air leaks are a main problem leading to inefficacy of NIV. Air can leak between the mask and the skin, or through the mouth. Leaks may be associated with a high mask pressure, for instance, when the patient and the ventilator are uncoordinated, or with a low mask pressure, when the muscles controlling the velolingual and lip sphincters fail to provide an airtight seal. Mouth leaks may also be secondary to high pharyngeal pressures, for instance, during complete glottic closure (external leaks). Another possibility to be considered is the presence of internal leaks: air entering the esophagus and stomach rather than the trachea, or air being accommodated in the compliant upper (pharyngeal) airway acting as a shunt compliance. The amount of leaks will depend to a great extent on upper airway pressure, which in turn will partly depend on glottic resistance or, in other words, on glottic narrowing in response to NIV [1, 4]. The strategies to reduce air leaks include raising RR, decreasing IPAP or V_T, or increasing inspiratory to expiratory ratio [4, 8].

However, pulmonary function continues to deteriorate, with patients requiring increasingly more hours a day of mechanical ventilation and, finally (usually after 3–4 years after NIV initiation), the transition to tracheostomy and invasive positive pressure ventilation [9].

Conclusions

Chronic respiratory failure is inevitable throughout the disease progression in patients with DMD. Without NIV, morbidity and mortality are highly likely toward the end of the second decade of life. Respiratory interventions, particularly the institution of nocturnal noninvasive ventilation, have a major beneficial effect on survival in DMD.

Key Major Recommendations

- A FVC < 1 l in DMD patients is a predictor of poor outcome within a short time and should prompt the initiation of NIV. In fact, 5-year survival rate is only 8 % in these patients if assisted ventilation is not provided.
- Nasal nocturnal ventilation is a safe and effective treatment in hypercapnic DMD patients.
- No effective care is possible without skilled caregivers and adequate training and dedication of the patient's family.

References

1. Finder JD, Birnkrant D, Carl J, et al. Respiratory care of the patient with Duchenne muscular dystrophy: ATS consensus statement. Am J Respir Crit Care Med. 2004;170(4):456–65.

2. Phillips MF, Quinlivan CM, Edwards RH, et al. Changes in spirometry over time as a prognostic marker in patients with Duchenne muscular dystrophy. Am J Respir Crit Care Med. 2001;164:2191–4.
3. Fauroux B, Aubertin G, Clement A, et al. Which tests may predict the need for noninvasive ventilation in children with neuromuscular disease? Respir Med. 2009;103:574–81.
4. Toussaint M, Chatwin M, Soudon P. Mechanical ventilation in Duchenne patients with chronic respiratory insufficiency: clinical implications of 20 years published experience. Chron Respir Dis. 2007;4(3):167–77.
5. Raphael J-CC, Chevret S, Chastang C. Randomised trial of preventive nasal ventilation in Duchenne muscular dystrophy. Lancet. 1994;343(8913):1600–4.
6. Villanova M, Brancalion B, Mehta AD. Duchenne muscular dystrophy: life prolongation by noninvasive ventilatory support. Am J Phys Med Rehabil. 2014;93(7):595–9.
7. Annane D, Orlikowski D, Chevret S. Nocturnal mechanical ventilation for chronic hypoventilation in patients with neuromuscular and chest wall disorders. Cochrane Database Syst Rev. 2014;12:CD001941.
8. Hamada S, Ishikawa Y, Aoyagi T, et al. Indicators for ventilator use in Duchenne muscular dystrophy. Respir Med. 2011;105:625–9.
9. Bach JR, Martinez D. Duchenne muscular dystrophy: continuous noninvasive ventilatory support prolongs survival. Respir Care. 2011;56(6):744–50.

Noninvasive Ventilation in Amyotrophic Lateral Sclerosis: Key Technical and Practical Applications

40

Bart Vrijsen, Dries Testelmans, and Bertien Buyse

Contents

Abbreviations

AAN	American Academy of Neurology
ALS	Amyotrophic lateral sclerosis
FVC	Forced vital capacity
MI-E	Mechanical in-exsufflation
MIP	Maximal inspiratory mouth pressure
NIV	Noninvasive ventilation
PCF	Peak cough flow
PEG	Percutaneous endoscopic gastrostomy
PSG	Polysomnography

B. Vrijsen, PT, MSc (✉)
Department of Pulmonology, Leuven University Centre for Sleep/Wake Disorders (E352), University Hospitals, Herestraat 49, Leuven 3000, Belgium

Faculty of Kinesiology and Rehabilitation Sciences, KULeuven, Leuven, Belgium
e-mail: bart.vrijsen@uzleuven.be

D. Testelmans, MD, PhD • B. Buyse, MD, PhD
Department of Pulmonology, Leuven University Centre for Sleep/Wake Disorders (E352), University Hospitals, Herestraat 49, Leuven 3000, Belgium

Department of Clinical and Experimental Medicine, KULeuven, Leuven, Belgium
e-mail: dries.testelmans@uzleuven.be; bertien.buyse@uzleuven.be

A.M. Esquinas (ed.), *Noninvasive Mechanical Ventilation: Theory, Equipment, and Clinical Applications*, DOI 10.1007/978-3-319-21653-9_40

40.1 Introduction

Amyotrophic lateral sclerosis (ALS) is the most frequently occurring progressive neurodegenerative disease in adults, affecting approximately 1.5 out of every 100,000 people per year [1]. ALS is characterized by progressive muscle weakness of the voluntary muscles. At a certain point in the disease progression, alveolar hypoventilation occurs because of further progressive weakness of the respiratory muscles. At that time, noninvasive ventilation (NIV) can be suggested to relieve symptoms of alveolar hypoventilation.

NIV has been shown to improve survival and quality of life in patients with ALS [2]. However, with the use of NIV in ALS patients, several difficulties can occur, such as bulbar weakness, immobility, and sialorrhea, and the question of when and how to start NIV to assure an appropriate treatment has not been definitively answered. The rapidly evolving devices coming to the market also confront us with new treatment modalities, and whether they can improve the treatment in the ALS population is uncertain. Finally, although they show an enormous willingness, we often see patients in whom NIV is not tolerated at all.

40.2 Discussion

Whether bulbar weakness is present or not in patients with ALS is often a major difference at the initiation of NIV. Bulbar-affected patients often have problems with sialorrhea and swallowing. When initiating NIV in patients with sialorrhea, it is important to reduce the amount of salivary secretions. Medication, such as oxybutynin and amitriptyline, and botulinum toxin injections can help patients in the management of their saliva. Speech therapists can provide useful information on effective swallowing. During nocturnal NIV, however, the possibility of aspiration of saliva remains, certainly during use of oronasal interfaces.

The choice of mask is an important issue at initiation of NIV. Oronasal interfaces can be a solution when mouth leakages are persistent (even after the use of nasal mask plus chin strap), however, oronasal interfaces can increase the chance of aspiration. Furthermore, oronasal masks can induce obstructive events by causing backward movement of the tongue during inspiration [3].

One of the new modalities in the recently developed devices is target-volume ventilation. Research on this topic has been performed in patients with chronic obstructive pulmonary disease, obesity hypoventilation syndrome, and kyphoscoliosis. To our knowledge, this research has not been performed in ALS patients. Theoretically, target-volume ventilation could be an addition to pressure support ventilation as it could change its pressure during different sleep stages or even in the further rapid progression of the disease. By increasing pressure, though, the chance of causing leaks increases, especially in the occurrence of bulbar progression.

The criteria of the American Academy of Neurology (AAN) to initiate NIV in ALS patients were updated in 2009 [4]. Patients with ALS could be started on NIV in the presence of symptoms of nocturnal hypoventilation and one of the following criteria: predicted forced vital capacity (FVC) <50 % predicted, maximal inspiratory mouth pressure (MIP) <60 cm H_2O, sniff nasal inspiratory pressure (SNIP) <40 cm

H_2O, or abnormal nocturnal oximetry. The most recent European guidelines suggest starting NIV when one or more symptoms of respiratory failure are occurring and at least one parameter similar to the AAN guidelines, except for FVC <80 % predicted or a morning arterial carbon dioxide >45 mmHg [5]. It is most important to consider the rapid, and sometimes even unexpected, onset of respiratory failure. Therefore, routine follow-up of the above-mentioned parameters is necessary so that NIV treatment can be discussed with the patient and family and NIV can be initiated at the right time. The chance of having an unanticipated emergency tracheostomy can thereby be strongly reduced. However, the correct timing of starting NIV in severe bulbar patients should still be studied because these patients often have difficulties in performing FVC, MIP, and SNIP measurements, and the complaint of orthopnea because of respiratory muscle impairment in these patients is often confused with shortness of breath caused by difficulties in managing salivary secretions in the supine position.

The discussion about how to monitor NIV titration and follow-up afterwards, not only in ALS patients, is ongoing. NIV parameters set according the patient's comfort during daytime may not ensure adequate nocturnal ventilatory support, because being asleep influences the ventilatory pattern by inducing modifications of ventilatory control, upper airway patency, and respiratory muscle recruitment. Until now, no uniform strategy has been stated regarding how to monitor ALS patients with NIV. Monitoring can range from a single arterial blood gas measurement to full video-polysomnography (PSG). Nocturnal oxygen saturation measurement is now generally accepted as a minimal measurement during NIV titration, although nocturnal transcutaneous carbon dioxide measurement can have great additional value because some patients can have normal oxygen saturation with an increased carbon dioxide level. Nevertheless, these measurements do not provide any information about some important interactions between patient and ventilator. Therefore, polygraphy (thoracic-abdominal belts combined with nocturnal oximetry and flow and pressure recordings) provides additional information on the synchrony between patient and ventilator and perhaps explain why NIV is not effective at a certain moment. As alveolar hypoventilation typically occurs first during rapid-eye-movement sleep, PSG combined with nocturnal transcutaneous carbon dioxide measurement can ensure NIV initiation in time, at the earliest moment of carbon dioxide retention. Furthermore, because sleep is often disturbed in patients with ALS, the use of PSG during NIV titration could give evidence of improvement in sleep structure and sleep quality.

NIV improves survival and quality of life in ALS patients, but as NIV is initially used during the night, it is important to improve sleep quality and sleep structure in these patients. Until recently, only two studies reported on objective sleep parameters in ALS patients with NIV treatment [6, 7]. NIV seemed to have no effect on sleep because sleep structure did not improve during PSG measurement shortly after initiation [6]. In a group of ALS patients, already on NIV for 8.3 ± 4.8 months, a high patient-ventilator asynchrony index and time spent in asynchrony were observed [7]. No data were reported on sleep architecture in this study, but asynchrony between patient and ventilator could cause an increase in arousals and awakenings with deterioration of sleep structure and sleep quality. It is important to notice that, in both studies, NIV is initiated at home according to patient comfort, awake efficacy, and awake oxygen saturation. However, a prospective study using in-hospital PSG to titrate NIV in ALS patients showed an improvement in sleep structure immediately after NIV initiation in patients with none to mild bulbar involvement. This improvement remained after 1 month of NIV use [8].

At the beginning, NIV is used during the night. But as the disease progresses and daytime alveolar hypoventilation develops, patients become dependent on NIV during the daytime. Mouthpiece ventilation could be tried, but as most of patients have at least a minimal deterioration of bulbar muscle strength, it becomes difficult to keep the mouthpiece in place. An alternative is to use a different interface during daytime. Nasal prongs have minimal contact with the patient's face and have the advantage that patients still have good vision and can keep their glasses on. Alternating interfaces between night and day also ensures different pressure points on the face, resulting in less chance of skin lesions.

Patients with ALS eventually reach the level of total inability to move or speak, meaning that they will become unable, if not already at NIV initiation, to solve problems with the ventilator independently. Therefore, assuring adequate alarms and a battery, to which the device cycles during power supply failure, seem necessary. The battery cycle life time also becomes important once patients become dependent of their ventilator during daytime. NIV devices can be placed on the back of the wheelchair, ventilating the patient via mouthpiece or mask and assuring the highest possible independence and quality of life.

Patients with ALS, and certainly those with bulbar involvement and those with daytime NIV, are confronted with nutritional problems and excessive weight loss. Placement of a percutaneous endoscopic gastrostomy (PEG) is a possible solution, but being in supine position with a gastrostomy scope in the esophagus for several minutes can cause major problems in the oxygen saturation and carbon dioxide levels. Therefore, in these patients, PEG placement can be performed during NIV use with an adapted mask with an entrance for the gastrostomy scope. In our center, we always use a volume-controlled mode during the procedure and put the patient back on the normal settings immediately at the end of the procedure until the effects of the sedatives are fully dissipated.

Adequate NIV and respiratory physiotherapy are inseparably connected. Clearing bronchopulmonary secretions is essential for a cooperative performance between the ventilator and the patient and preventing sputum retention and lower respiratory tract infections. A cough is sufficient if a peak cough flow (PCF) of 160 l/min is reached. However, once ALS patients perform a PCF <270 l/min, cough augmentation techniques should be taught to prevent secretion accumulation and respiratory infections. Several techniques are described to improve cough efficiency: thoracic (abdominal) thrust, air stacking, and mechanical insufflation-exsufflation (MI-E). Thrust can be performed during the expiratory phase of the cough, improving PCF. Air stacking, performed by a resuscitation balloon or volume-controlled ventilator, increases the inspiratory capacity before coughing but also, because of the elastic recoil of the lungs, increase PCF. Air-stacking can also be performed preventively on daily base to avoid atelectasis and respiratory infection. The combination of both techniques often results in a higher PCF than each separately. Once thrust and air-stacking become insufficient, MI-E may be required. In severe bulbar patients though, these cough augmentation techniques may have no clinical effect and other methods of clearing airway secretions are necessary. Suctioning or placement of tracheostomy can then be discussed.

NIV is initially started during the nighttime and is mostly followed by daytime ventilation. However, ALS progresses in a way that NIV will not be able to compensate for the respiratory muscle weakness and respiratory impairment or (certainly severe bulbar) patients become intolerant of their ventilation. At that time, one can choose between two options: palliative sedation using benzodiazepines or opioids if patients decide to end their life, or tracheal ventilation if patients decide to continue their life. The decision concerning end-of-life care should be taken in advance as unwanted tracheostomies should be avoided when patients are admitted to the emergency unit with respiratory failure.

Conclusion

Initiation of NIV in patients with ALS often is accompanied by difficulties. Bulbar involvement is one of the major issues, having consequences on mask choice, increasing the risk of aspiration, and defining the appropriate time of NIV initiation. As patients are not able to move and become completely dependent on their ventilator, ventilators should be carefully selected and a battery is necessary. The choice of mask should also be made with caution, especially as patients become increasingly more dependent on their ventilator.

A large diversity is found in monitoring NIV during the start-up procedure, but nocturnal oximetry measurement is found to be minimal. Polygraphy and PSG seem to have important additional effects, especially when trying to improve patient-ventilator synchrony and sleep quality.

Key Recommendations

- When starting patients with ALS on NIV, one should control hypersaliva to minimize the risk of aspiration and respiratory tract infections.
- It is generally agreed that NIV titration during the daytime is insufficient as the ventilatory pattern is different between day and night. Nocturnal oxygen saturation measurement should be a minimum, but transcutaneous carbon dioxide measurement and polygraphy are excellent additions in titrating and following-up NIV, as these measurements assure the efficiency and the synchrony between patient and ventilator.
- Advanced care planning is of major importance in ALS, as ALS is a rapid progressive disease with an uncertain course. Unwanted tracheostomies should especially be avoided, and the wishes of the patient (and family) concerning the end of life should be discussed in advance.
- Ventilators and interfaces should be chosen with great care. To assure the best possible independence and safety, a battery is necessary. As patients develop daytime hypoventilation and the ventilator is used during daytime, different interfaces will be necessary to decrease the risk of skin lesions.
- To assure a successful treatment with NIV, a respiratory physiotherapist should be included in the NIV team.

References

1. Radunovic A, Mitsumoto H, Leigh PN. Clinical care of patients with amyotrophic lateral sclerosis. Lancet Neurol. 2007;6:913–25.
2. Bourke S, Tomlinson M, Williams T, et al. Effects of non-invasive ventilation on survival and quality of life in patients with amyotrophic lateral sclerosis. Lancet Neurol. 2006;5:140–7.
3. Vrijsen B, Buyse B, Belge C, et al. Upper airway obstruction during noninvasive ventilation induced by the use of an oronasal mask. J Clin Sleep Med. 2014;10:1033–5.
4. Miller RG, Jackson CE, Kasarskis EJ, et al. Practice parameter update: the care of the patient with amyotrophic lateral sclerosis: multidisciplinary care, symptom management, and cognitive/behavioral impairment (an evidence-based review): report of the Quality Standards Subcommittee of the American Academy of Neurology. Neurology. 2009;73:1227–33.
5. Andersen PM, Abrahams S, Borasio GD, EFNS Task Force on Diagnosis and Management of Amyotrophic Lateral Sclerosis, et al. EFNS guidelines on the clinical management of amyotrophic lateral sclerosis (MALS) – revised report of an EFNS task force. Eur J Neurol. 2012;19:360–75.
6. Katzberg HD, Selegiman A, Guion L, et al. Effects of noninvasive ventilation on sleep outcomes in amyotrophic lateral sclerosis. J Clin Sleep Med. 2013;9:345–51.
7. Atkeson A, RoyChoudhury A, Harrington-Moroney G, et al. Patient-ventilator asynchrony with nocturnal non-invasive ventilation in ALS. Neurology. 2011;77:549–55.
8. Vrijsen B, Buyse B, Belge C, et al. Noninvasive ventilation improves sleep in amyotrophic lateral sclerosis: a prospective polysomnographic study. J Clin Sleep Med. 2015;11(5):559–66.

Noninvasive Ventilation in Myasthenic Crises

41

Susana Pinto and Mamede de Carvalho

Content

Abbreviations

EPAP	Expiratory positive airway pressure
ICU	Intensive care unit
IMV	Invasive mechanical ventilation
IPAP	Inspiratory positive airway pressure
MC	Myasthenic crisis
MG	Myasthenia gravis
NIV	Noninvasive ventilation
$PaCO_2$	Partial pressure of carbon dioxide in arterial blood
RI	Respiratory insufficiency
SpO_2	Saturation level of oxygen in hemoglobin by arterial puncture

S. Pinto (✉)
Neuromuscular Unit, Institute of Molecular Medicine, University of Lisbon, Lisbon, Portugal
e-mail: susana.c.pinto@sapo.pt

M. de Carvalho
Faculdade de Medicina, Translational and Clinical Physiology Unit, Institute of Molecular Medicine, Universidade de Lisboa, Lisbon, Portugal

Neuroscience Department, Centro Hospitalar Lisboa Norte – Hospital de Santa Maria, Lisbon, Portugal

A.M. Esquinas (ed.), *Noninvasive Mechanical Ventilation: Theory, Equipment, and Clinical Applications*, DOI 10.1007/978-3-319-21653-9_41

Myasthenic crisis (MC) has long been described as acute neuromuscular respiratory insufficiency (RI) requiring mechanical ventilation in patients with myasthenia gravis (MG) [1–3]. MC occurs in about 15–20 % of patients with MG, although 30 % of MG patients experience some degree of respiratory distress [2, 4, 5]. After the first MC episode, a second crisis occurs in one-third of patients [6]. Respiratory infection is the main precipitating factor, occurring in 40 % of cases (bacterial pneumonia, viral upper respiratory infection, and bronchitis) [4]. Other factors include acute aspiration pneumonitis (10 %) and changes in medication (8 %), namely withdrawal of steroids or anticholinesterase medication, initiation of steroids, or aminoglycoside administration [4]. In 30 % of patients, no precipitating factor is identifiable [4]. MC tends to occur early in the course of MG, when the disease is more severe [6]. The advent of newer and more efficacious therapies, including thymectomy and immunotherapies [7, 8], has diminished MC events, with fewer cases occurring in patients with longstanding, poorly controlled MG [6].

MC episodes in MG patients have been traditionally managed using intubation and invasive mechanical ventilation (IMV), which was responsible for an important reduction in mortality in the 1970s [9]. However, pulmonary complications, namely atelectasis and pneumonia, are frequent, increasing morbidity and health-care costs with longer length stays in the intensive care unit (ICU) [4, 10].

The advent of noninvasive ventilation (NIV) brought a new care approach for these patients. NIV has been successfully used in treating RI from acute to chronic settings, in patients with primary pulmonary diseases [11] or with different neuromuscular diseases [12, 13]. Bi-level NIV allows the delivery of different inspiratory and expiratory positive pressures in conscious patients, each cycle being triggered by the patient's breathing effort. The inspiratory positive airway pressure (IPAP) is higher than the expiratory positive airway pressure (EPAP). By overcoming the upper airway resistance and expanding the lungs with lower work effort, IPAP ensures an adequate air volume and maintains gas exchange. EPAP prevents the collapse of the alveoli and lower airways at the end of each breathing cycle, preventing microatelectasis. Different facial or nasal masks allow a personalized choice for each patient, increasing comfort and tolerance to NIV. In patients with bulbar weakness, facial masks are chosen so that patients can successfully receive the necessary inspiratory pressure support.

In MG patients with respiratory fatigue, MC can be effectively handled by NIV, as an alternative to and preventing IMV [14]. In 2002, in the first work to approach the benefits of NIV in MG, Rabinstein and Wijdicks [14] report that NIV prevented IMV in 70 % of the trials (7 out of 11 episodes of MC) but failed to alleviate dyspnea in patients with established hypercapnia. Presence of hypercapnia ($PaCO_2 > 50$ mmHg) at the time of NIV institution predicted its failure ($p < 0.01$), which occurred mostly within the first 24 h of NIV usage. Seneviratne and coworkers [15] also found that $PaCO_2 > 45$ mmHg on NIV initiation was the only predictor of its failure ($p = 0.04$). In their work, 60 episodes of MC were identified in 52 patients; 40 % (24 episodes) were adapted to NIV and the remaining 46 episodes to IMV (77 %, initially in 36 plus 10 episodes that required IMV after NIV).

Although the working definition of MC used by these authors was acute neuromuscular RI in MG patients requiring either IMV or NIV, no criteria for the option of IMV versus NIV was established [15].

IPAP and EPAP parameters reported in the literature for NIV pressure support in MC care are usually low, averaging 14/6 mmHg [15], 13/5 mmHg (range 10–16/4–6 mmHg) [14], and 15/6 mmHg in a case study [16]. Oxygen supplementation is provided as necessary to keep $SaO_2 > 90$ mmHg (range 2–10 l/min) [14]. In the works by Seneviratne et al. [15] and Rabinstein and Wijdicks [14], mean duration of NIV usage in the hospital was about 5 days (4.3 ± 2.9 days in the study by Seneviratne et al. [15] and 5 days in the study by Rabinstein and Wijdicks [14], ranging from 4 h to 16 days). In both studies, length of stay was significantly lower for episodes successfully treated with NIV when compared with those treated with IMV (5.6 days, range 1.5–21 days vs 13.6 days, range 3–60 days [15] and 7 ± 5 days vs 23 ± 16 days, $p = 0.03$ [10], respectively). NIV usage also significantly shortened ICU stay with decreased rates of pulmonary complications. Despite these results, patients continue today to be offered NIV less frequently (6.5 %, 141 patients vs 21.5 %, 433 patients, in a total of 37 % of MC patients studied by Alshekhlee et al. [17]).

Patients included in the published articles were discontinued from NIV after the MC. It is not clear in the article published by Rabinstein and Wijdicks [14] whether the four patients who were discharged under NIV continued with it thereafter. In our center, three patients with MG were unable to sleep without NIV support after MC. The three female patients (ages at diagnosis 26, 56, and 51 years) have a long evolution of generalized myasthenia gravis (14, 8, and 19 years, respectively) with poor pharmacological control. They had positive acetylcholine receptor antibodies (AChR) and were thymectomized. One had a previous history of pulmonary sequestration culminating in pulmonary surgery with secondary iatrogenic unilateral diaphragm paresis. After MC, patients continued nocturnal NIV (GoodKnight® 420G, Puritan Bennet® Tyco Healthcare) with facial masks, switching to nasal masks in periods of bulbar weakness improvement. The patient with unilateral diaphragm paresis progressively extended the use of NIV through the day due to dyspnea for progressive lower efforts and presently uses NIV 24 h a day. These three cases clarify some of the factors that can contribute to the impossibility of achieving a nocturnal NIV-free period after MC, namely generalized myasthenia with difficult pharmacological control and preexisting respiratory function limitations, as in the case with diaphragm paresis. Additionally, previously existing pulmonary obstructive disorders can be aggravated by atelectasis. These result from inadequate secretion clearance due to expiratory muscle weakness and inadequate cough. Deficient gas exchange is improved by the pulmonary expansion provided by NIV. Other reasons can be speculated. Sleep is highly demanding for the respiratory function, even in healthy subjects. In particular, there is a decrease in the respiratory center output, the upper airways become more flaccid, and the external intercostals and other inspiratory accessory muscles do not support the functioning of the diaphragm during REM sleep. Therefore, the physiologic respiratory stress of sleep on ventilation can become more demanding following a MC.

In conclusion, there are few studies in the literature addressing the use of NIV in MC. However, it is the consensus that NIV should be initiated soon after MC diagnosis because it improves gas exchange, reduces patient fatigue, and decreases respiratory complications as well as the duration of the ventilatory support when compared with IMV. In MC, multicentric randomized trials comparing NIV with IMV should be initiated to establish firm guidelines for treating MC.

Key Major Recommendations

- NIV should be initiated soon after the diagnosis of MC, as it improves gas exchange (lowering respiratory work effort and fatigue), decreases respiratory complications, and decreases duration of respiratory support when compared with IMV.
- Facial masks are preferred over nasal masks in MC with bulbar weakness.
- IPAP and EPAP should be adjusted individually, although the usual average values are 14/6 mmHg (IPAP/EPAP).
- In MC, randomized trials comparing NIV with IMV should be performed.

References

1. Lacomis D. Myasthenic crisis. Neurocrit Care. 2005;3(3):189–94.
2. Bedlack RS, Sanders DB. On the concept of myasthenic crisis. J Clin Neuromusc Dis. 2002;4(1):40–2.
3. Keesey JC. “Crisis” in myasthenia gravis: an historical perspective. Muscle Nerve. 2002;26(1):1–3.
4. Thomas CE, Mayer SA, Gungor Y, et al. Myasthenic crisis: clinical features, mortality, complications, and risk factors for prolonged intubation. Neurology. 1997;48(5):1253–60.
5. Fink ME. Treatment of the critically ill patient with myasthenia gravis. In: Ropper AH, editor. Neurological and neurosurgical intensive care. 3rd ed. New York: Raven; 1993. p. 351–62.
6. Mayer SA. Intensive care of the myasthenic patient. Neurology. 1997;48 Suppl 5:S70–5.
7. Qureshi AI, Choudhry MA, Akbar MS, et al. Plasma exchange versus intravenous immunoglobulin treatment in myasthenic crisis. Neurology. 1999;52(3):629–32.
8. Stricker RB, Kwiatkowska BJ, Habis JA, Kiprov DD. Myasthenic crisis: response to plasmapheresis following failure of intravenous gamma-globulin. Arch Neurol. 1993;50(8):837–40.
9. Cohen MS, Younger D. Aspects of the natural history of myasthenia gravis: crisis and death. Ann N Y Acad Sci. 1981;377:670–7.
10. Varelas PN, Chua HC, Natterman J, et al. Ventilatory care in myasthenia gravis crisis: assessing the baseline adverse event rate. Crit Care Med. 2002;30(12):2663–8.
11. Keenan SP, Brake D. An evidence-based approach to noninvasive ventilation in acute respiratory failure. Crit Care Clin. 1998;14(3):359–72.
12. Simonds AK, Muntoni F, Heather S, et al. Impact of nasal ventilation on survival in hypercapnic Duchenne muscular dystrophy. Thorax. 1998;53(11):949–52.
13. Pinto AC, Evangelista T, Carvalho M, et al. Respiratory assistance with a non-invasive ventilator (Bipap) in MND/ALS patients: survival rates in a controlled trial. J Neurol Sci. 1995;129:S19–26.
14. Rabinstein A, Wijdicks EF. BiPAP in acute respiratory failure due to myasthenic crisis may prevent intubation. Neurology. 2002;59(10):1647–9.

15. Seneviratne J, Mandrekar J, Wijdicks EFM, Rabinstein AA. Noninvasive ventilation in myasthenic crisis. Arch Neurol. 2008;65(1):54–8.
16. Agarwal R, Reddy C, Gupta D. Noninvasive ventilation in acute neuromuscular respiratory failure due to myasthenic crisis: case report and review of literature. Emerg Med J. 2006;23(1):e6.
17. Alshekhlee A, Miles JD, Katirji B, et al. Incidence and mortality rates of myasthenia gravis and myasthenic crisis in US hospitals. Neurology. 2009;72:1548–54.

Part V

Hospital Critical Care Applications: Critical Care Acute Hypoxemic Respiratory Failure

Noninvasive Ventilation in Acute Cardiogenic Pulmonary Edema

42

Chiara Lazzeri, Serafina Valente, Adriano Peris, and Gian Franco Gensini

Contents

Abbreviations

ACPE	Acute cardiogenic pulmonary edema
ACS	Acute coronary syndrome
COPD	Chronic obstructive pulmonary disease
CPAP	Continuous positive airway pressure
NIV	Noninvasive ventilation
NPPV	Noninvasive positive pressure ventilation
PEEP	Positive end-expiratory pressure
RCT	Randomized controlled trial

C. Lazzeri, MD (✉) • S. Valente, MD
Intensive Care Unit of Heart and Vessels Department, Azienda Ospedaliero-Universitaria Careggi, Florence, Italy
e-mail: lazzeric@libero.it

A. Peris
Anesthesia and Intensive Unit of Emergency Department, Azienda Ospedaliero-Universitaria Careggi, Florence, Italy

G.F. Gensini, MD
Intensive Care Unit of Heart and Vessels Department, Azienda Ospedaliero-Universitaria Careggi, Florence, Italy

Department of Experimental and Clinical Medicine, University of Florence, AOU Careggi, Fondazione Don Carlo Gnocchi IRCCS, Florence, Italy

A.M. Esquinas (ed.), *Noninvasive Mechanical Ventilation: Theory, Equipment, and Clinical Applications*, DOI 10.1007/978-3-319-21653-9_42

Acute cardiogenic pulmonary edema (ACPE) is a life-threatening medical emergency. International guidelines recommend the use of noninvasive ventilation (NIV) (continuous positive airway pressure (CPAP) or noninvasive positive pressure ventilation (NPPV)) in dyspneic patients with ACPE and a respiratory rate >20 breaths/min to improve breathlessness and reduce hypercapnia and acidosis (Class IIa recommendation) [1–3]. In fact, ACPE is one of four NIV applications based on randomized controlled trials (RCTs) and a meta-analysis that have provided NIV grade A evidence regarding this condition [4], together with chronic obstructive pulmonary disease (COPD) exacerbation, immunocompromised conditions, and ventilator weaning in patients with COPD.

The Canadian clinical practice guidelines recommend NPPV or CPAP as the first option for ventilator support for patients with ACPE and respiratory failure in the absence of shock or acute coronary syndrome requiring acute coronary revascularization (grade 1A recommendation) and state that CPAP delivered by mask is just as effective as NPPV [5]. Similar conclusions were reached by reviews and a meta-analysis [6–11].

42.1 Respiratory and Hemodynamic Effects of Noninvasive Ventilation: Key Elements

The terms CPAP and NPPV are sometimes used interchangeably, but they are different. With noninvasive CPAP, an interface (usually a face mask) is used to apply a pressure greater than atmospheric to the proximal airway throughout spontaneous breathing, thus splinting open the upper airway, increasing lung volume and intrathoracic pressure. The work of breathing is entirely assumed by the patient and the tidal ventilation is completely dependent on the respiratory muscles. NPPV differs from CPAP because it has two pressure levels, an inspiratory positive airway pressure (which provides mechanical breaths) and an expiratory positive airway pressure, acting as positive end-expiratory pressure (PEEP).

Acute cardiogenic pulmonary edema is characterized by an increase in left ventricle filling pressures, causing a rise in pulmonary capillary pressure, and thereafter fluid overload toward the pulmonary interstitial compartment and alveolar spaces [12]. All these factors lead to an increase in airway resistance, a decrease in lung diffusion capacity, a drop in functional residual capacity, and an increased intrapulmonary shunt effect. Hypoxemia develops, associated with an increase in respiratory effort.

The application of intrathoracic positive pressure in patients with ACPE, particularly with PEEP, has the following *cardiovascular effects:* (a) a decrease in venous return and in right ventricle preload; (b) a decrease in transmural pressure (transmural pressure = intraventricular pressure − intrathoracic pressure); and (c) a reduction in left ventricle afterload [13–15]. Cardiac output and myocardial contractility may increase. Moreover, the application of positive pressure produces also *respiratory effects*. In particular, it favors alveolar recruitment and increases functional residual capacity, lung compliance, and alveolar ventilation, with a reduction of the intrapulmonary shunt and respiratory effort, thus improving oxygenation [16].

Compared with conventional oxygen therapy, the application of NIV (both CPAP and NPPV) [17–20] was associated with faster clinical (reduction of respiratory frequency and of dyspneic sensation) and blood gas improvements (increased PaO_2, reduction of $PaCO_2$ and acidosis) [21]. NPPV has the potential advantage over CPAP of assisting the respiratory muscles during inspiration, resulting in faster alleviation of dyspnea [22–24].

In a retrospective observational study in consecutive patients admitted for ACPE, neither acidemia nor the type of acidosis on admission was a risk factor for adverse outcome in ACPE patients treated with CPAP [25]. Similar results were reported by our group [26] in 65 consecutive patients with ACPE treated with NIV, characterized by a more severe hemodynamic impairment as inferred by the high percentage of devices used and administration of inotropes.

42.2 NIV Versus Conventional Treatment

CPAP was reported to improve survival and avoid intubation in ACPE patients compared with conventional treatment plus oxygen therapy [8, 27–35], and five systematic reviews [6–8, 31, 36] consistently demonstrated a significant reduction in endotracheal intubation with both types of NIV.

The 3CPO trial (Three Interventions in Cardiogenic Pulmonary Oedema), a large randomized controlled trial including 1069 patients, showed no difference in short- or long-term mortality rates between standard oxygen therapy and NIV treatments in patients presenting to emergency departments with severe ACPE [21]. This finding was not confirmed in a subsequent meta-analysis [9] (including the 3CPO and five meta-analyses) [6, 8, 33, 37], which reported a significant mortality benefit of NPPV in ACPE (fixed effect model, risk ratio 0.75, CI 0.61–0.92).

In a Cochrane review [38], including 21 studies and 1,071 subjects, NIV, compared with standard care, significantly reduced the need for endotracheal intubation, with a RR of 0.53 (95 % CI 0.34–0.83) and a NNT (number needed to treat) of 8. There was also a significant reduction in hospital mortality (RR 0.6, 95 % CI 0.45–0.84) and a NNT of 13. Similar results were reported by Winck et al. [31], in their meta-analysis, which showed that, in ACPE patients, CPAP and NPPV both significantly decrease the need for endotracheal intubation, and CPAP significantly reduces mortality when compared with standard medical therapy. A reduction in mortality was also reported by Mariani et al. [27], with NIV delivered through either NPPV or CPAP in ACPE patients.

A recent meta-analysis [39] (including 78 randomized controlled trials) was specifically focused on the effect of NIV on mortality in acute care settings. In the subanalysis of patients with ACPE, NIV showed a beneficial effect on survival when applied to treat acute respiratory failure (RR 0.64, 95 % CI 0.45–0.90, $p = 0.01$, NNT = 16). However, in trials allowing crossover, with NIV used a rescue therapy, this benefit was not confirmed. This finding strongly suggests the need to focus future research on the best timing for NIV treatment in ACPE.

42.3 NIV in ACPE Following Acute Coronary Syndrome

Inclusion and exclusion criteria varied among the trials. All 15 trials from 2000 to 2009 excluded patients with cardiogenic shock. In addition, 9 of these 15 trials, and 8 of the 10 trials in the period 2005–2009, also excluded patients who required acute coronary revascularization [19–22, 40–42], or who had acute coronary syndrome [43, 44].

An early RCT suggested that NPPV was associated with a greater risk of myocardial infarction than was CPAP [45], but many subsequent RCTs did not confirm this finding [8, 15, 22, 38, 41, 43, 44]. In the Cochrane review by Vital et al. [38], NIV was not associated with an increased risk in the incidence of myocardial infarction (RR 1.24, 95 % CI 0.79–1.95) when compared with standard medical care. In the meta-analysis by Weng et al. [28], NIV was not associated with an incidence of new myocardial infarction and, likewise, in the meta-analysis of Li H et al. [46], which included 12 RCTs with a total of 1,433 ACPE patients, the occurrence of new cases of myocardial infarction and length of stay were also not significantly different between CPAP and NPPV.

According to the available evidence, NIV can be safely used in patients with acute coronary syndrome (ACS) complicated by acute respiratory failure due to ACPE. In clinical practice, the use of NIV in these patients seems to still be related to local practices. In the FINN AKVA study group, including 620 acute heart failure (AHF) patients [47], NIV was used more frequently in the ACS-AHF than in the non-ACS-AHF patients (38 % vs 18 %, respectively, $p<0.001$) [48], but only half of patients with cardiogenic shock and pulmonary edema were treated with NIV [47].

Key Major Recommendations

- NIV is indicated in patients with ACPE and acute respiratory failure because it reduces the need for endotracheal intubation and lowers mortality rates.
- The choice between NPPV and CPAP is often related to the expertise and skills of the medical team. NPPV offers the advantage of reducing the work of respiratory muscles, thereby quickly reducing the sensation of dyspnea.
- NIV can be safely used in patients with ACS complicated by acute respiratory failure resulting from ACPE.

References

1. Nieminen MS, Böhm M, Cowie MR, et al. Executive summary of the guidelines on the diagnosis and treatment of acute heart failure: the Task Force on Acute Heart Failure of the European Society of Cardiology. Eur Heart J. 2005;26:384–416.
2. Dickstein K, Cohen-Solal A, Filippatos G, et al. ESC Committee for Practice Guidelines (CPG). ESC guidelines for the diagnosis and treatment of acute and chronic heart failure 2008: the Task Force for the diagnosis and treatment of acute and chronic heart failure 2008

of the European Society of Cardiology. Developed in collaboration with the Heart Failure Association of the ESC (HFA) and endorsed by the European Society of Intensive Care Medicine (ESICM). Eur J Heart Fail. 2008;10:933–89.

3. McMurray JJ, Adamopoulos S, Anker SD, et al. ESC Committee for Practice Guidelines. ESC guidelines for the diagnosis and treatment of acute and chronic heart failure 2012: The Task Force for the Diagnosis and Treatment of Acute and Chronic Heart Failure 2012 of the European Society of Cardiology. Developed in collaboration with the Heart Failure Association (HFA) of the ESC. Eur J Heart Fail. 2012;14:803–69.
4. Nava S, Hill N. Non-invasive ventilation in acute respiratory failure. Lancet. 2009; 374(9685):250–9.
5. Keenan SP, Sinuff T, Burns KEA, et al. Clinical practice guidelines for the use of noninvasive positive-pressure ventilation and noninvasive continuous positive airway pressure in the acute care setting. CMAJ. 2011;183:E195–214.
6. Masip J, Roque M, Sanchez B, et al. Noninvasive ventilation in acute cardiogenic pulmonary edema: systemic review and meta-analysis. JAMA. 2005;294:3124–30.
7. Ho KM, Wong K. A comparison of continuous and bi-level positive airway pressure noninvasive ventilation in patients with acute cardiogenic pulmonary oedema: a meta-analysis. Crit Care. 2006;10:R49.
8. Peter JV, Moran JL, Phillips-Hughes JK, et al. Effect of non-invasive positive pressure ventilation (NIPPV) on mortality in patients with acute cardiogenic pulmonary edema: a meta-analysis. Lancet. 2006;367:1155–63.
9. Potts JM. Noninvasive positive pressure ventilation. Effect on mortality in acute cardiogenic pulmonary edema: a pragmatic meta-analysis. Pol Arch Med Wewn. 2009;119(6):349–53.
10. Hess DR. Noninvasive ventilation for acute respiratory failure. Respir Care. 2013;58(6):950–69.
11. Ferrer M, Torres A. Non invasive ventilation for acute respiratory failure. Curr Opin Crit Care. 2015. doi:10.1097/MCC.0000000000000173.
12. Rialp Cervera G, del Castillo Blanco A, on behalf of the GT-IRA of the SEMICYUC, et al. Noninvasive mechanical ventilation in chronic obstructive pulmonary disease and in acute cardiogenic pulmonary edema. Med Intensiva. 2014;38(2):111–21.
13. Baratz DM, Westbrook PR, Shah PK. Effect of nasal continuous positive airway pressure on cardiac output and oxygen delivery in patients with congestive heart failure. Chest. 1992;102:1397–401.
14. Lenique F, Habis M, Lofaso F. Ventilatory and hemodynamic effects of continuous positive airway pressure in left heart failure. Am J Respir Crit Care Med. 1997;155:500–5.
15. Park M, Lorenzi-Filho G, Feltrim MI, et al. Oxygen therapy, continuous positive airway pressure, or noninvasive bilevel positive pressure ventilation in the treatment of acute cardiogenic pulmonary edema. Arq Bras Cardiol. 2001;76:221–30.
16. International Consensus Conference in Intensive Care Medicine. Noninvasive positive pressure ventilation in acute respiratory failure. Am J Respir Crit Care Med. 2001;163:283–91.
17. Bersten AD, Holt AW, Vedig AE, et al. Treatment of severe cardiogenic pulmonary edema with continuous positive airway pressure delivered by face mask. N Engl J Med. 1991;325:1825–30.
18. Räsänen J, Heikkilä J, Downs J, et al. Continuous positive airway pressure by face mask in acute cardiogenic pulmonary edema. Am J Cardiol. 1985;55:296–300.
19. Nava S, Carbone G, DiBattista N, et al. Noninvasive ventilation in cardiogenic pulmonary edema: a multicenter randomized trial. Am J Respir Crit Care Med. 2003;168:1432–7.
20. Masip J, Betbesé AJ, Páez J, et al. Non-invasive pressure support ventilation versus conventional oxygen therapy in acute cardiogenic pulmonary oedema: a randomised trial. Lancet. 2000;356:2126–32.
21. Gray A, Goodacre S, Newby DE, et al. Noninvasive ventilation in acute cardiogenic pulmonary edema. N Engl J Med. 2008;359:142–51.
22. Rusterholtz T, Kempf J, Berton C, et al. Noninvasive pressure support ventilation (NIPSV) with face mask in patients with acute pulmonary edema (ACPE). Intensive Care Med. 1999;25:21–8.
23. Takeda S, Nejima J, Takano T, et al. Effect of nasal continuous positive airway pressure on pulmonary edema complicating acute myocardial infarction. Japan Circ J. 1998;62:553–8.

24. Liesching T, Nelson DL, Cormier KL, et al. Randomized trial of bilevel versus continuous positive airway pressure for acute pulmonary edema. J Emerg Med. 2014;46(1):130–40.
25. Aliberti S, Piffer F, Brambilla AM, et al. Acidemia does not affect outcomes of patients with acute cardiogenic pulmonary edema treated with continuous positive airway pressure. Crit Care. 2010;14:R196. doi:10.1186/cc9315.
26. Lazzeri C, Gensini GF, Picariello C, et al. Acidemia in severe acute cardiogenic pulmonary edema treated with noninvasive pressure support ventilation: a single-center experience. J Cardiovasc Med (Hagerstown). 2015;16(9):610–5. doi:10.2459/JCM.0000000000000079.
27. Mariani J, Macchia A, Beziti C, et al. Noninvasive ventilation in in acute cardiogenic pulmonary edema: a meta-analysis of randomized controlled trials. J Card Fail. 2011;17:850–9.
28. Weng CL, Zhao YT, Liu QH, et al. Meta-analysis: noninvasive ventilation in acute cardiogenic pulmonary edema. Ann Intern Med. 2010;152(9):590–600.
29. Mehta S, Al-Hashim AH, Keenan SP. Noninvasive ventilation in patients with acute pulmonary edema. Respir Care. 2009;54(2):186–95.
30. Masip J. Noninvasive ventilation in acute cardiogenic pulmonary edema. Curr Opin Crit Care. 2008;14(5):531–5.
31. Winck JC, Azevedo LF, Costa-Pereira A, et al. Efficacy and safety of non-invasive ventilation in the treatment of acute cardiogenic pulmonary edema–a systematic review and meta-analysis. Crit Care. 2006;10:R69.
32. Chadda K, Annane D, Hart N, et al. Cardiac and respiratory effects of continuous positive airway pressure and noninvasive ventilation in acute cardiac pulmonary edema. Crit Care Med. 2002;30(11):2457–61.
33. Ferrer M, Esquinas A, Leon M, et al. Noninvasive ventilation in severe hypoxemic respiratory failure: a randomized clinical trial. Am J Respir Crit Care Med. 2003;68:1438–44. Kelly CA, Newby DE, McDonagh TA, et al. Randomised controlled trial of continuous positive airway pressure and standard oxygen therapy in acute pulmonary oedema. Eur Heart J. 2002;23:1379–86.
34. L'Her E, Duquesne F, Girou E, et al. Noninvasive continuous positive airway pressure in elderly cardiogenic pulmonary edema patients. Intensive Care Med. 2004;30:882–8.
35. Salman A, Milbrandt EB, Pinsky MR. The role of noninvasive ventilation in acute cardiogenic pulmonary edema. Crit Care. 2010;14:303–6.
36. Collins SP, Mielnicznik LM, Whittingham HA, et al. The use of noninvasive ventilation in emergency department patients with acute cardiogenic pulmonary edema: a systematic review. Ann Emerg Med. 2006;48:260–9.
37. João CW, Luís FA, Altamiro CP, et al. Efficacy and safety of non-invasive ventilation in the treatment of acute cardiogenic pulmonary edema – a systematic review and meta-analysis. Crit Care. 2006;10:R69.
38. Vital FMR, Saconato H, Ladeira MT, et al. Non-invasive positive pressure ventilation (CPAP or bilevel NPPV) for cardiogenic pulmonary edema (review). Cochrane Collaboration. 2008;3:1–99.
39. Cabrini L, Landoni G, Oriani A, et al. Noninvasive ventilation and survival in acute care settings: a comprehensive systematic review and meta-analysis of randomized controlled trials. Crit Care Med. 2015;43(4):880–8.
40. Park M, Sangean MC, Volpe M, et al. Randomized, prospective trial of oxygen, continuous positive airway pressure, and bilevel positive airway pressure by face mask in acute cardiogenic pulmonary edema. Crit Care Med. 2004;32:2407–15.
41. Moritz F, Brousse B, Gellee B, et al. Continuous positive airway pressure versus bilevel noninvasive ventilation in acute cardiogenic pulmonary edema: a randomized multicenter trial. Ann Emerg Med. 2007;50:666–75.
42. Crane SD, Elliott MW, Gilligan P, et al. Randomised controlled comparison of continuous positive airways pressure, bilevel non-invasive ventilation, and standard treatment in emergency department patients with acute cardiogenic pulmonary oedema. Emerg Med J. 2004;21:155–61.

43. Bellone A, Monari A, Cortellaro F, et al. Myocardial infarction rate in acute pulmonary edema: noninvasive pressure support ventilation versus continuous positive airway pressure. Crit Care Med. 2004;32:1860–5.
44. Ferrari G, Olliveri F, De Filippi G, et al. Noninvasive positive airway pressure and risk of myocardial infarction in acute cardiogenic pulmonary edema: continuous positive airway pressure vs noninvasive positive pressure ventilation. Chest. 2007;132:1804–9.
45. Mehta S, Jay GD, Woolard RH, et al. Randomized, prospective trial of bilevel versus continuous positive pressure in acute pulmonary edema. Crit Care Med. 1997;25:620–8.
46. Li H, Hu C, Xia J, et al. A comparison of bilevel and continuous positive airway pressure noninvasive ventilation in acute cardiogenic pulmonary edema. Am J Emerg Med. 2013;31:1322–7.
47. Tarvasmäki T, Harjola VP, Tolonen J, FINN-AKVA Study Group, et al. Management of acute heart failure and the effect of systolic blood pressure on the use of intravenous therapies. Eur Heart J Acute Cardiovasc Care. 2013;2(3):219–25. doi:10.1177/2048872613492440.
48. Tarvasmäki T, Harjola VP, Nieminen MS, FINN-AKVA Study Group, et al. Acute heart failure with and without concomitant acute coronary syndromes: patient characteristics, management, and survival. J Card Fail. 2014;20(10):723–30.

Is NIV Safe and Effective in Patients with ACPE Due to Diastolic Dysfunction?

43

Andrea Bellone, Massimiliano Etteri, Guido Caironi, Giorgio Gadda, and Roberto Rossi

Contents

43.1 Introduction

A large number of patients presenting with acute cardiogenic pulmonary edema (ACPE) have preserved left ventricular (LV) systolic function and as a result are affected by diastolic dysfunction. In these patients, survival is similar to that of patients with reduced ejection fraction [1, 2]. However, no previous studies have classified patients with ACPE according to a different pathophysiological class before continuous positive airway pressure (CPAP) treatment. Therefore, the role of noninvasive ventilation (NIV) in ACPE with preserved systolic function is not well known. Agarwal and colleagues [3] suggested that CPAP should be used with

A. Bellone, MD (✉) • M. Etteri, MD • G. Caironi, RN • R. Rossi, LN
Emergency Department, Azienda Ospedaliera Sant'Anna (Presidio di Como), Via Ravona 1, San Fermo della Battaglia, 22100 Como, Italy
e-mail: andreabellone@libero.it; max.etteri@alice.it; caironiguido@gmail.com; roberto.rossi73@hsacomo.org

G. Gadda, LN
Emergency Unit, Azienda Ospedaliera Salvini (Presidio di Rho), 20100 Milan, Italy
e-mail: gadda.giorgio@gmail.com

A.M. Esquinas (ed.), *Noninvasive Mechanical Ventilation: Theory, Equipment, and Clinical Applications*, DOI 10.1007/978-3-319-21653-9_43

caution in patients with diastolic heart failure because a positive airway pressure may compromise venous return and decrease LV end-diastolic volume, further limiting stroke volume. On the other hand, one open prospective study demonstrated that the benefit of CPAP in patients with diastolic heart failure could be due to a decrease in LV end-diastolic volume (preload) [4]. Moreover, another study showed that resolution time is not significantly different in patients with ACPE with preserved or impaired systolic function submitted to CPAP [5].

To define the safety of NIV in ACPE with preserved ejection fraction, we evaluated, in the emergency setting, the response to NIV according to two different dosages of nitrate.

43.2 Materials and Methods

Data were collected from September 2013 to June 2014. Twenty patients affected by ACPE and diastolic dysfunction admitted to two emergency departments (Como and Milan, Italy) were enrolled. The protocol was approved by the institutional review boards at each institution and written informed consent was obtained for each patient. Inclusion criteria were the presence of clinical signs of ACPE with preserved left ventricular ejection fraction (LVEF) and respiratory distress (peripheral oxygen saturation (SpO_2) <90 % while breathing room air or <92 % while breathing oxygen (>35 % of inspiratory oxygen concentration (FiO_2), respiratory frequency >25 breaths/min, and active accessory respiratory muscles). Exclusion criteria were: (1) unstable clinical conditions (need for vasopressor more than 24 h, acute coronary syndrome, life-threatening arrhythmias); (2) refusal of treatment; (3) weak cough reflex; (4) agitation or non-cooperation; (5) failure of more than two organs; (6) cardiac arrest; (7) respiratory arrest requiring tracheal intubation; (8) recent trauma or burns of neck and face; (9) pregnancy; and (10) LV systolic dysfunction.

ACPE patients underwent a morphological bedside cardiac ultrasound investigation to exclude those with depressed LV function or valvular abnormalities. The remaining patients were submitted to NIV for 1 h plus pharmacological therapy and they were randomly divided according to two different dosages of nitrate:

- Group A = 20 mg of nitrate/50 ml of saline at 4 ml/1 h (total 1.6 mg)
- Group B = 20 mg of nitrate/50 ml of saline at 14 ml/1 h (total 4.8 mg).

Diuretics were similar between the two groups of patients = 60 mg of furosemide. Patients' baseline characteristics are shown in Tables 43.1 and 43.2.

43.2.1 Ventilator and Interfaces

All patients received NIV via a standard intensive care unit ventilator with double-tube circuit in pressure support mode for 1 h after the initial evaluation. They were randomly assigned to perform NIV with the nitrate lower than 2 mg = Group A or nitrate greater than 4.5 mg = Group B.

Table 43.1 Baseline values versus 1 h

Baseline vs 1 h (mean ± SD)

	Group A	Group A 1 h	*p*	Group B	Group B 1 h	*p*
Respiratory rate (breaths/min)	42 ± 6.5	29.6 ± 9	<0.01	39 ± 4.3	27.2 ± 4	<0.01
Arterial pH	7.29 ± 0.13	7.33 ± 0.5	<0.01	7.30 ± 0.11	7.33 ± 0.6	<0.01
$PaCO_2$ (mmHg)	54.7 ± 12.6	43.7 ± 8	<0.01	52.1 ± 14.9	44.0 ± 9	<0.01
PaO_2/FiO_2 ratio	163 ± 74	269 ± 72	<0.01	169 ± 63	249 ± 66	<0.01
Bicarbonate (Meq)	19 ± 5	21 ± 7	ns	20 ± 7	22 ± 6	ns
Heart rate (beats/min)	97 ± 26	88 ± 42	ns	106 ± 29	89 ± 38	<0.05

Table 43.2 Patients' outcomes

	Group A (*n* = 10)	Group B (*n* = 10)	*p* value
Endotracheal intubation	1 (2.5 %)	0 (0 %)	ns
In-hospital death	0 (0 %)	0 (0 %)	ns
Transient arterial hypotension (<3 min)	1 (10 %)	5 (50 %)	0.05
Prolonged arterial hypotension to need saline infusion/NIV withold	0 (0 %)	1 (10 %)	ns

The oronasal mask assigned to each patient was chosen according to anthropometric characteristics, minimization of air leaks, and tolerance of the patients. Among the interfaces available in the two units were the Ultra Mirage™ FFM-NV (ResMed, San Diego, CA, USA) and the PerforMax Face Mask (Philips Respironics, Murrysville, PA, USA).

The ventilator settings were decided according to the usual practice: maximal tolerated inspiratory pressure support to obtain a tidal volume of 6–8 ml/kg of body weight (never greater than 20 cmH_2O) and 5 cmH_2O positive end-expiratory pressure (PEEP).

43.2.2 Bedside Ultrasound

All patients underwent a morphological cardiac ultrasound investigation shortly before NIV. Two-dimensional echocardiogram (SONOS 2000, Hewlett-Packard, Andover, MA, USA) was performed to qualitatively estimate the LV systolic function. Patients were considered as having LV systolic dysfunction if the ejection fraction was estimated <45 %. In the absence of this condition and significant valvular abnormalities, patients were considered to have preserved systolic function. Competency of emergency physician ultrasonographers was demonstrated through multiple steps. Initially, they underwent a training course of fast echography in an emergency setting and then they performed at least 100 noncardiac and 75 cardiac ultrasounds with credentialed supervision. In addition, before the start of this study, all emergency physicians were given a course in goal-directed echocardiography.

43.2.3 Randomization

Patients were randomly assigned to one of the two treatment groups using opaque, sealed, numbered envelopes. We used a computer-generated randomization sequence, which was generated by an independent biostatistician who was not otherwise involved in the trial. The envelopes were kept in the head nurses' offices in each institution's critical care unit. The nurses who opened the envelopes were those on shift that day or night and totally independent of the enrolment process. They communicated the random treatment allocation to the attending physician that assigned the patients to the study group.

43.3 Discussion

The results of the preliminary study show that, in patients with ACPE and preserved LV systolic function, NIV was safe and effective. In group B, with a higher dosage of nitrate, there was significant transient hypotension, although in-hospital mortality, adverse events, and the need for invasive mechanical ventilation were similar in all treated patients regardless of the nitrate dosage.

In our study, patients with ACPE (clinical signs, chest X-ray, and interstitial syndrome by ultrasound evaluation) and preserved systolic function and no valvular abnormalities were supposed to be affected by LV diastolic dysfunction. The strength of our study is the use of cardiac echoes to assess LV function by emergency department physicians just before bi-level positive airway pressure begins in patients with acute respiratory distress.

Gudmunsson and colleagues [6] have suggested that eyeballing ejection fraction may be the most accurate echocardiographic method for the assessment of LV systolic function and could be used for routine echocardiography instead of formal methods.

Aurigemma et al. [7] suggested that the effects of positive pressure therapy compromise venous return and decrease LV end diastolic volume, further limiting stroke volume and, hence, cardiac output because of the steep curve for LV diastolic pressure in relation to volume with resultant deterioration in hemodynamics. In contrast, Gutierrez-Chico and colleagues [8] suggested that chronic diastolic heart failure is different from ACPE due to diastolic dysfunction, where transthoracic echocardiography underestimates LV end diastolic volume.

For this reason, we decided to evaluate patients with ACPE and diastolic dysfunction with a different nitrate dosage. In this way, we could stress the potential negative effects of positive airway pressure in these patients, but the results of this preliminary study shows that the application of NIV in patients with ACPE due to diastolic dysfunction seems to be safe and effective regardless of nitrate dosage.

In conclusion, we suggest:

1. NIV is safe and effectiveness in diastolic cardiogenic pulmonary edema
2. The transient arterial hypotension caused by the combination of NIV and nitrate therapy in patients with diastolic dysfunction does not compromise the beneficial effects.

Conflict of Interest The authors declare that they have no conflicts of interest.

References

1. Owan TE, Hodge DO, Herges RM, et al. Trends in prevalence and outcome of heart failure with preserved ejection fraction. N Engl J Med. 2006;355:251–9.
2. Bhatia RS, Tu JV, Lee DS, et al. Outcome of heart failure with preserved ejection fraction in a population-based study. N Engl J Med. 2006;355:260–9.
3. Agarwal R, Agarwal AN, Gupta D, Jindal SK. Evidence based review: non-invasive ventilation in acute cardiogenic pulmonary edema. Postgrad Med J. 2005;81:637–43.
4. Bendjelid K, Shutz N, Suter PM, et al. Does continuous positive airway pressure by face mask improve patients with acute cardiogenic pulmonary edema due to left ventricular diastolic dysfunction. Chest. 2005;127:1053–5.
5. Bellone A, Monari A, Cortellaro F, et al. Myocardial infarction rate in acute pulmonary edema: non-invasive pressure support ventilation versus continuous positive airway pressure. Crit Care Med. 2004;32:1860–5.
6. Gudmundsson P, Ryberg E, Winter R, Willenheimer R. Visually estimated left ventricular ejection fraction by echocardiography is closely correlated with formal quantitative methods. Intern J Cardiol. 2005;101:209–12.
7. Aurigemma GP, Gaasch WH. Diastolic heart failure. N Engl J Med. 2004;351:1097–105.
8. Gutierrez-Chico JL, Zamorano JL, Perez de Isla L, et al. Comparison of left ventricular volumes and ejection fractions measured by three-dimensional echocardiography versus two-dimensional echocardiography and cardiac magnetic resonance in patients with various cardiomyopathies. Am J Cardiol. 2005;95:809–13.

Noninvasive Mechanical Ventilation in Acute Cardiogenic Pulmonary Edema and Cardiac Procedures: How to Choose the Most Appropriate Mode and Improve Its Programming

44

Javier Mendoza Vázquez

Contents

44.1 Introduction

Acute cardiogenic pulmonary edema (ACPE) is a life-threatening situation with 10–20 % risk of in-hospital mortality, especially when it is associated with acute myocardial infarction [1]. Thus, it is important to treat it appropriately. While treating the trigger for the ACPE (i.e., fast ventricular rate atrial fibrillation or myocardial ischemia), treatment must simultaneously be started with intravenous diuretics (which have an immediate venodilator action that reduces preload and subsequent removal of fluid), opiates (which reduce anxiety, relieve distress associated with dyspnea, reduce preload by venodilator effect, and reduce sympathetic drive), and possibly a vasodilator if systolic blood pressure is >110 mmHg or inotropics for patients with hypotension or severe reduction in cardiac output [2].

While these measures take effect, blood oxygenation must be improved (and CO_2 elimination in case of global respiratory failure) and respiratory muscular fatigue

J. Mendoza Vázquez
Acute Cardiac Care Unit, Arnau De Vilanova University Hospital, Lleida, Spain
e-mail: jamevaz@hotmail.com

A.M. Esquinas (ed.), *Noninvasive Mechanical Ventilation: Theory, Equipment, and Clinical Applications*, DOI 10.1007/978-3-319-21653-9_44

reduced to avoid endotracheal intubation (ETI) and invasive mechanical ventilation (IMV) that is related to significant morbidity and mortality. Finally, the suffering of patients with ACPE must be reduced. To achieve all these objectives, noninvasive mechanical ventilation (NIMV) can be used to apply positive pressure and oxygen into the airway through an external interface (usually a mask).

44.2 Modes of NIMV and Therapeutic Effects

There are two modes of NIMV:

Continuous positive airway pressure (CPAP): fixed positive pressure is applied throughout the entire respiratory cycle, increasing oxygenation by alveolar recruitment. Strictly speaking, CPAP is not a true mode of ventilation because it does not provide any inspiratory support [3]. It is used in hypoxemic respiratory failure.

Bi-level positive airway pressure (BIPAP): there is an expiratory positive airway pressure (EPAP) that recruits alveoli and prevents their collapse, increasing oxygenation and inspiratory positive airway pressure (IPAP), which reduces the inspiratory effort and diaphragm fatigue, increasing the tidal volume. This is the mode that should be used in patients with hypercapnia and global respiratory failure and even in patients without hypercapnia but with signs of significant respiratory fatigue. Compared with CPAP, BIPAP produces greater improvements in oxygenation and CO_2 clearance and a greater reduction in the work of breathing in patients with ACPE [1]. However, the superiority of BIPAP over CPAP has not been demonstrated in reducing mortality in the treatment of ACPE [4].

In summary, application of positive airway pressure with NIMV in ACPE has positive respiratory effects, improving alveolar ventilation and gas exchange and reducing respiratory muscular fatigue. It also has hemodynamic effects, by reducing preload and afterload, which, in patients with ACPE (who are usually "afterload dependent"), improve cardiac performance and myocardial oxygen imbalance [5] (Fig. 44.1).

44.3 NIMV Versus Standard Medical Treatment in ACPE

In 2013, a meta-analysis was published that included 32 studies (2,916 participants) to determine the effectiveness and safety of NIMV in the treatment of ACPE. NIMV added to standard medical treatment (SMT) has several benefits compared with SMT alone [4]:

- Reduction in the need for ETI, with risk difference (RD) of −12 % (95 % CI −0.19 to −0.04) and a number needed to treat (NNT) of 8 [4]. Lower ETI favored BIPAP-treated patients (RR 0.45, 95 % CI 0.26–0.80) [4]. This effect is

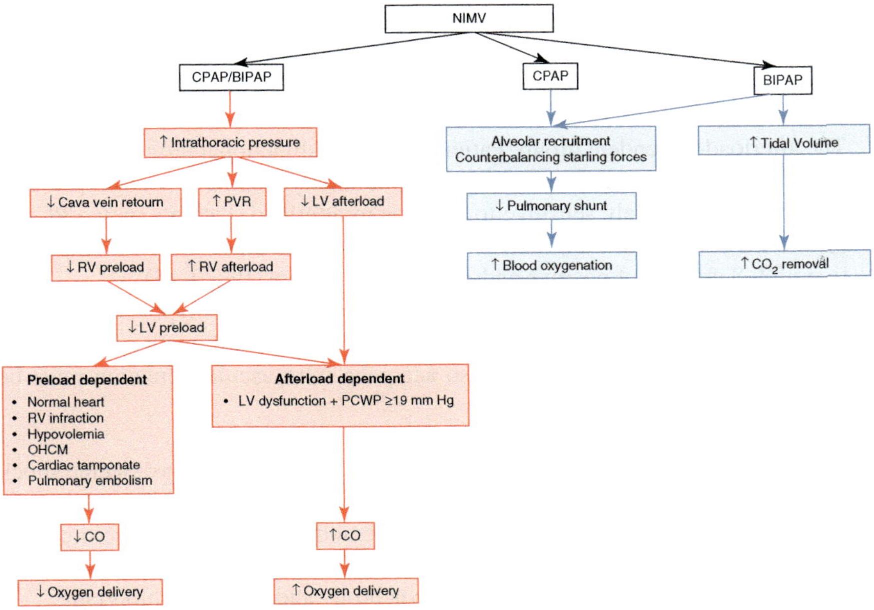

Fig. 44.1 *BIAP* bilevel positive airway pressure, *CO* cardiac output, *CPAP* continuous positive airway pressure, *LV* left ventricle, *NIMV* non invasive mechanical ventilation, *OHCM* obstructive hypertrophic cardiomyopathy, *PRV* pulmonary vascular resistance, *RV* right ventricle. Colors: haemodynamic effects (in *red*); respiratory effects (in *blue*) (Modified from Wiesen et al. [5] with permission)

important because of the related complications of IMV. Patients with hypoxic respiratory failure due to ACPE treated with NIMV have the lowest intubation rate (10 %) compared with other etiologies [6].

- The impact on mortality remains controversial [3]. The largest randomized trial [1], with a total of 1,069 patients, did not show an effect on short-term mortality. This trial was included in the Cochrane meta-analysis [4], which showed significantly reduced hospital mortality (RR 0.66, 95 % CI 0.48–0.89). However, the evidence for this potential benefit is derived from small trials. No difference was found in hospital mortality comparing CPAP and BIPAP directly [4].
- Reduction in intensive care unit length of stay by 1 day [4].
- There were no significant increases in the incidence of acute myocardial infarction with NIMV during its application [4], an adverse outcome that was found in some previous studies.
- Less progressive respiratory distress and neurological failure (coma) [4].

In summary, the use of NIMV is an important part of the treatment of ACPE, and the sooner it is started, the better. We need to "ventilate the patient" instead of "oxygenate the patient."

44.4 NIMV in APCE and Cardiogenic Shock

There are two groups depending on the haemodynamic effect of the NIMV [5]:

- The afterload-dependent group: Patients with a dysfunctional left ventricle (even with myocardial infarction) with high pulmonary capillary wedge pressure (PCWP) are extremely sensitive to changes in afterload. Patients with a PCWP ≥ 19 mmHg experience improvement in their cardiac output (CO) with the addition of 3–8 cmH_2O of positive end-expiratory pressure (PEEP) [5].
- The preload-dependent group: Patients with normal heart, hypovolemia, right ventricular infarction, or obstructive hypertrophic myocardiopathy. In all these patients, NIMV can decrease CO, so adequate intravascular repletion must be ensured.

Thus, patients with ACPE with left ventricule dysfunction and cardiogenic shock can have positive hemodynamic effects by using NIMV with moderate levels of PEEP and CPAP. These patients have tenuous hemodynamic status, therefore inappropriate ventilation settings could have severe deleterious effects [5]. Careful programming and close monitoring to avoid asynchrony and leaks are important.

44.5 CPAP or BIPAP?

According to blood gas analyses, one should choose CPAP in hypoxemic patients and BIPAP in patients who are hypercapnic or in global respiratory failure. But one should also be mindful of clinical factors, and it is not always possible to wait for blood gas analyses to decide, initially, the modality of NIMV. The initial choice and programming should be guided by physical signs (e.g., breathing pattern, respiratory fatigue signs), comorbidity, patient´s physical features and pressure, flow curve analysis, and blood gas analysis. Cardiac wasting syndrome, pleural effusion, and ascites (three common conditions in advanced heart failure patients) and chronic obstructive pulmonary disease (COPD), a common comorbidity in heart failure patients, should be kept in mind.

Patients who should preferably be ventilated with BIPAP include those with

- COPD: These patients have greater work of breathing than others and have a tendency to hypercapnia. CPAP can increase the work of breathing working like an expiratory obstacle that increase hyperinsuflation. Thus, CPAP could aggravate autoPEEP and consequently increases inspiratory effort. In BIPAP model, an adecuate level of EPAP counterbalances auto-PEEP and decrease inspiratory effort. EPAP must be carefully titrated from 4 cmH_2O (lower than in other patients) because an excessive level of EPAP can increase the inspiratory effort (for the same reason as CPAP); excessive IPAP that could aggravate hyperinsufflation should be avoided.
- Significant obesity and ascites: Both increase the diaphragm's effort to inspire, so they benefit from BIPAP.

- Cardiac cachexia: The muscular weakness in these patients makes more tendency to appear respiratory fatigue, that could be treated and prevent with IPAP.
- Significant pleural effusion, which increases inspiratory effort.
- Important signs of inspiratory fatigue: These include thoracoabdominal dissociation and sternocleidomastoid activation.
- Inspiratory failure during CPAP: Low volume/min with correct respiratory rate or correct but with persisting inspiratory fatigue signs and/or hypercapnia.

44.6 Programming of NIMV

General rules for initial programming of NIMV are available, including how to change it depending of blood gas analyses, physical signs, and analysis of flow-pressure waveforms and leaks [7]. For patients with ACPE who are treated with CPAP (hypoxemic patients, those without important fatigue signs or COPD):

- Begin with 5 cmH_2O CPAP and with FiO_2 required to achive a pulse oximetry saturation (Sat O_2) < 90 %, increase CPAP in 2 cmH_2O increments in order to reduce the FiO_2 below 60 % (preferably <50 %) to avoid oxygen toxicity.
- Remember that the maximum CPAP level is 12 cmH_2O. If hypoxemia is not corrected, consider increasing FiO_2.
- Progressively decrease in 2 cmH_2O increments when the patient is ameliorating.
- If hypercapnia, respiratory fatigue signs, or tidal volume (TV) <7 ml/kg is present, change to BIPAP.

Patients treating with BIPAP:

- Begin with 10 cmH_2O IPAP and 5 cmH_2O EPAP. The goal is to achieve Sat O_2 >90 % in chronic hypercapnic patients or >92–95 % in others.
- Program a slope pressure as steep as possible to prolong the expiration cycle to remove CO_2.
- Increase IPAP in 2 cmH_2O increments until a TV of 7–8 ml/kg is achieved. Consider increasing further if the sternocleidomastoid contraction persists, with a maximum of 25 cmH_2O. Rule out excessive EPAP that could lead to increasing inspiratory effort.
- If saturation <90 % and there is no bradypnea (which can be corrected with assisted mode) with low VT, consider increasing IPAP. If it is correct, increase EPAP or FiO_2, as with the previous option.
- If abdominal contraction appears (expiratory effort by excessive IPAP), decrease IPAP. Rule out excessive EPAP also.
- If there is an auto-PEEP pattern in the flow curve: First, consider whether the dyspnea could be undertreated (opiates). This generates tachypnea, which in

COPD leads to auto-PEEP. Consider bronchodilators if bronchospasm is present. Second, rule out hyperinsufflation, in which case one should decrease IPAP. Finally, if the previous possibilities are ruled out, change EPAP until the auto-PEEP pattern disappears. Keep in mind that the repetitive failed inspirations is usually secondary to auto-PEEP.

In both modalities one should avoid excessive leaks, adjusting the mask and procuring a 30–45° position. Nasal masks are not adequate in ACPE because the mouth is usually open. An oronasal mask is the most commonly used interface.

44.7 NIMV in Cardiac Procedures

Decubitus is required to perform the following cardiologic procedures: catheterization, percutaneous valve implantation, definitive and transitory pacemaker implantation, intra-aortic balloon counterpulsation (IABCP), transesophageal echocardiography (TEE), and electrophysiologic studies. Decubitus reduces the functional residual capacity and cannot be tolerated by patients with chronic respiratory failure, either COPD or restrictive respiratory failure (i.e., obesity or neuromuscular disease) and orthopneic heart failure patients [8]. Furthermore, decubitus increases the venous return that increases preload and leads to a rise of PCWP. Therefore, decubitus is not tolerated in acute respiratory failure and can lead on to acute respiratory failure in some stable patients.

One should not pospone some cardiac procedures because it worsen prognosis,as in the case of urgent catheterization in acute myocardial infarction, urgent transitory pacemaker implantation, or IABCP implantation. To achieve decubitus toleration and avoid general anesthesia, one can use NIMV [9]. Furthermore, in case of femoral artery percutaneous interventions, several hours of decubitus–semi-decubitus after the procedure may be necessary to ensure correct hemostasis and it could be required more time during venous femoral transitory pacemaker stimulation or arterial femoral intra-aortic balloon counterpulsation.

Finally, in orthopneic cardiac patients needing TEE, NIMV can be performed with the TEE probe passed through a modified face mask [9].

Bibliography

1. Gray A, Goodacre S, Newby DE, Masson M, Sampson F, Nicholl J, 3CPO Trialists. Noninvasive ventilation in acute cardiogenic pulmonary edema. N Engl J Med. 2008;359:142–51.
2. McMurray JJ, et al. ESC Guidelines for the diagnosis and treatment of acute and chronic heart failure 2012: the Task Force for the Diagnosis and Treatment of Acute and Chronic Heart Failure 2012 of the European Society of Cardiology. Developed in collaboration with the Heart Failure Association (HFA) of the ESC. Eur Heart J. 2012;33:1787–847.
3. Mas A, Masip J. Noninvasive ventilation in acute respiratory failure. Int J Chron Obstruct Pulmon Dis. 2014;9:837–52.

4. Vital FM, Ladeira MT, Atallah AN. Non-invasive positive pressure ventilation (CPAP or bilevel NPPV) for cardiogenic pulmonary oedema. Cochrane Database Syst Rev. 2013;(5):CD005351.
5. Wiesen J, Ornstein M, Tonelli AR, Menon V, Ashton RW. State of the evidence: mechanical ventilation with PEEP in patients with cardiogenic shock. Heart. 2013;99(24):1812–7.
6. Antonelli M, Conti G, Moro ML, Esquinas A, Gonzalez-Diaz G, Confalonieri M, et al. Predictors of failure of noninvasive positive pressure ventilation in patients with acute hypoxemic respiratory failure: a multi-center study. Intensive Care Med. 2001;27(11):1718–28.
7. Barrot-Cortés E, Sánchez-Gómez E. Manual SEPAR de procedimientos. Ventilación mecánica no invasiva. Barcelona: Respira-fundación española del pulmón-SEPAR; 2008.
8. Galeas-López JL, Muñoz-Bono J. Ventilación mecánica no invasiva en procedimientos endoscópicos. In: Esquinas Rodriguez AM, editor. Fundamentos de la organización hospitalaria en ventilación mecáncia no invasiva. 2011. p. 103–6.
9. Ambrosino N, Guarracino F. Unusual applications of noninvasive ventilation. Eur Respir J. 2011;38:440–9.

Practical Approach to the Use of Noninvasive Ventilation in Patients with ACPE

45

Jacobo Bacariza Blanco and Antonio M. Esquinas

Contents

45.1 Introduction

With regard to current noninvasive ventilation (NIV) practice, there are just four key A level indications supported by evidence-based medicine: chronic obstructive pulmonary disease (COPD) exacerbation, pulmonary infiltrates in immunocompromised patients, weaning with COPD, and, finally, cardiogenic pulmonary edema. These are what Nava [1] called "the fabulous four." Acute-on-chronic cardiac failure exacerbation was not among those admitted to this club, but it is the only current indication among the cardiac diseases. The reason for the use of NIV in this clinical situation can be explained by the heart-lung interactions during mechanical ventilation (MV). When, how, and especially where to apply NIV are of major concern in achieving our therapeutic goals. The objective of this chapter is to answer these questions, why and where, based on current data in the literature.

J.B. Blanco (✉)
Department of Critical Care Medicine, Hospital Garcia de Orta, Almada, Portugal
e-mail: jacobobacariza@hotmail.com

A.M. Esquinas
Department of Critical Care Medicine, Hospital Morales Meseguer, Murcia, Spain
e-mail: antmesquinas@gmail.com

A.M. Esquinas (ed.), *Noninvasive Mechanical Ventilation: Theory, Equipment, and Clinical Applications*, DOI 10.1007/978-3-319-21653-9_45

45.2 Heart-Lung Interactions during NIV: Why? (The Essentials)

Heart-lung interactions during MV represent the cornerstone of the patient's hemodynamic effects. These interactions are explained by the relationship between positive pressure ventilation and the cardiovascular system. They are not simple, but understanding them is mandatory when facing a patient who needs ventilatory support. Briefly, heart-lung interactions result from the dynamic response of some physiological factors to balance the metabolic organ demand in a particular clinical situation. These physiological factors are intravascular volume, blood flow, and cardiac function, on the one hand, and autonomic and endocrinologic response with lung volume and transpulmonary pressure (TPP), which is the difference between alveolar pressure and intrathoracic pressure, on the other hand [2]. When ventilated, the lung volume changes due to the positive pressure produce a hemodynamic effect termed by [11] as reverse pulsus paradoxus, which is the increase in systolic arterial pressure during mechanical inspiration (dUp effect) and the decrease during expiration (dDown effect).

In the left heart, transpulmonary pressure increases and is transmitted backward through the left atrial chamber, improving venous return and left ventricle preload. However, this transpulmonary increase leads to another augmentation in the transmural pressure (the distending pressure of a heart chamber), squeezing the heart chambers and helping to discharge them into the blood flow. The results of this dUp effect are an increase in the stroke volume (SV) and, thereby, an improvement in the left systolic outcome [11]. There is also a reduction in the afterload secondary to the decrease into the transmural left ventricle pressure as a response to the intrathoracic elevation. Finally, there is a reduction in heart rate (HR), mean arterial pressure (MAP), and pulse pressure (PP), improving systemic oxygenation and reducing the myocardial oxygen demand. At this point, the positive pressure ventilation effects on stroke volume are highly dependent on the global hemodynamic state, with the reduction effect on the preload being more dominant than the one on the afterload during the hypovolemic states, which means that, in this situation, the MV will lead not to an improvement in the SV but to a remarkable reduction. There are no major concerns regarding the euvolemic or hypervolemic states, where the predominant effect is on afterload reduction, thus increasing the SV. This allows the appropriate volume status in the ventilated patient, which is the turning point of the hemodynamic behavior during MV.

In the right heart, intrathoracic pressure increases the right atrial intravascular pressure, reducing the driving pressure gradient for venous return and also collapsing the superior cava vein, leading to a preload reduction. With the afterload, the effect is an augmentation resulting from the pulmonary vascular resistance increase. As a result, there is a right ventricle SV reduction, and thus a reduction in the vascular congestion and lung edema, once again improving oxygenation and ventilation.

Regarding respiratory effects, direct oxygenation by O_2 administration and alveolar unit recruitment, resulting from the direct positive pressure effect on the airway, improves oxygenation and ventilation and, thereby, the arterial blood gases. MV contributes to a significant reduction in respiratory muscle effort, as does muscular oxygen consumption, and systemic oxygen availability is elevated as a result. The resulting cardiovascular effect is an increase in PaO_2 and mixed venous oxygen (SVO_2) and reduction in respiratory rate (RR) and HR.

Based on the main current published studies, Masip and coworkers [4] concluded in their meta-analysis of 15 selected trials from the period from 1988 to 2005 that NIV, continuous positive airway pressure (CPAP) and bi-level positive airway pressure (BiPAP), significantly reduced the mortality rate by nearly 45 % compared with standard medical therapy (SMT) (RR, 0.55; CI 95 %, 0.40–0.78; $p=0.72$). Moreover, when the techniques were compared (and also the SMT), a relevant reduction in the intubation needs was seen with CPAP (RR, 0.40; 95 % CI, 0.27–0.58; $p=.21$) and with BiPAP (RR, 0.48; 95 % CI, 0.30–0.76; $p=.24$). Furthermore, a meta-analysis by Mariani et al. [5], and more recently Li et al. [6] and Sun et al. [7], concluded that when comparing the effects of CPAP versus BiPAP on acute cardiogenic pulmonary edema (ACPE), there is a relevant decrease in mortality of around 40 % in CPAP and 30 % in BiPAP, without finding once again relevant differences between them in terms of hospital length of stay or acute myocardial infarction (MI) incidence.

In 1997, [12] when comparing CPAP versus BiPAP, detected a higher MI rate in the enrolled BiPAP group patients. Because MI is one of the major concerns when using NIV in acute chronic cardiac patients, several studies have been performed to clarify this issue. Ho et al. [8], in a meta-analysis published in 2006, confirmed the lack of a significant trend toward an increase in new-onset acute MI in patients treated with BiPAP (RR 2.10, 95 % CI 0.91–4.84; $p=0.08$). Later papers [7–10] showed the same results. In conclusion, CPAP is recommended, in addition to SMT, in patients with severe respiratory failure due to cardiogenic pulmonary edema (class IIa recommendation, level of evidence A). CPAP must be considered the first-line intervention in patients with ACPE because it is easier to use than BiPAP and no differences have been shown between then when comparing both techniques.

45.3 NIV in Acute Chronic Cardiac Exacerbations: When, How and Where to Do It?

When facing a situation involving acute chronic cardiac exacerbations, there are some major considerations, including when, where, and how NIV should be used:

1. Where? The location where NIV is used is important because it can determine the success or the failure of the ventilation. The optimal location depends on the previous condition of the patient, the total care investment, and the indication or not for endotracheal intubation (ETI), depending on the patient's comorbidities. Patients with indications for ETI can be treated in a conventional cardiology, respiratory, internal medicine, or even emergency ward, but without the need of an intermediate unit, if available, and, depending on the patient's risk factors, an intensive care unit (ICU). Patients without indications for ETI can be treated in

same wards, but without the need of an intermediate unit. Regarding the intermediate care unit, it should have staff educated in NIV. This staff should include doctors, nurses, and physiotherapists who know the ventilator devices, the masks, proper hospital protocols for NIV, and hemodynamic monitoring in case it is needed. The space should be prepared to perform the proper monitoring and to deal with central venous catheters, arterial lines, and the orotracheal intubation technique. These intermediate units must be directly connected to the ICU, or rapid response teams should be available in case of ETI or the necessity for invasive ventilation and later discharge to the ICU.

2. When? The use of NIV depends on risk factors such as RR >25 bpm, HR >120 bpm, PaO_2/FiO_2 <200, pH <7.35, pCO_2 >45 mmHg, and the activity of the accessory muscles. All the patients must have a Glasgow Coma Scale (GCS) >8 and, depending on their APACHE II score (>29), the ICU should be considered for their medical care.
3. How? Algorithm 45.1 may be useful as a treatment protocol in ACPE.

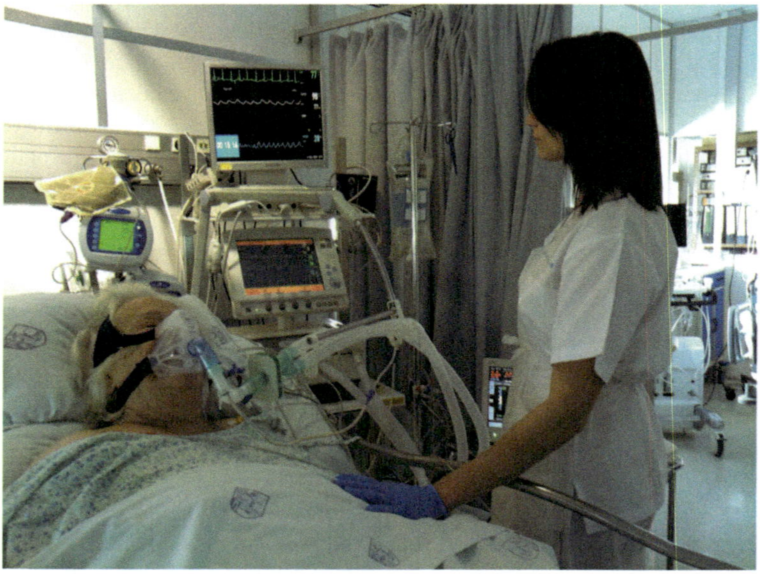

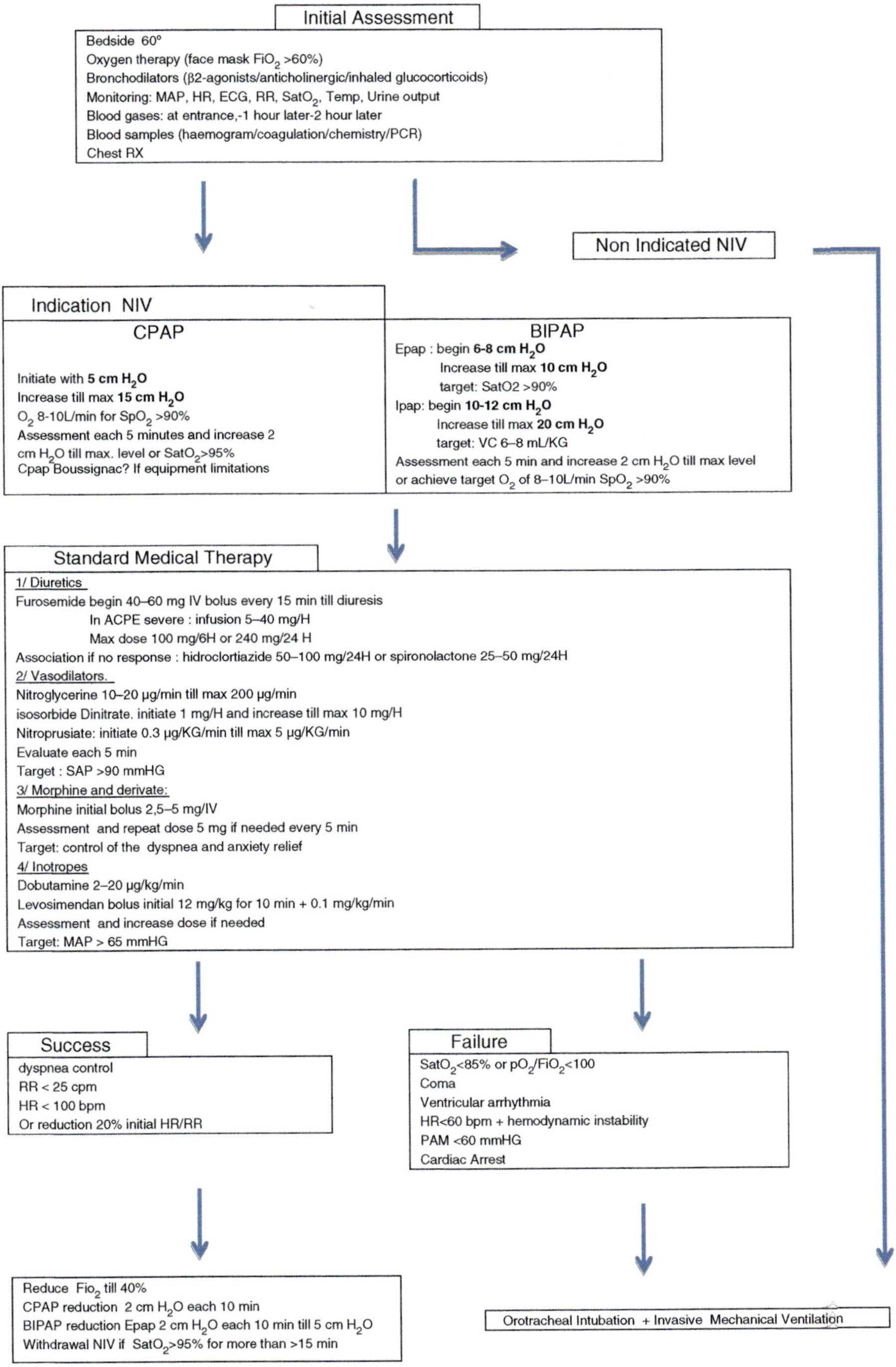

Algorithm 45.1 Practical approach to the use of noninvasive ventilation in patients with ACPE

Key Major Recommendations

- Positive pressure ventilation improves left ventricular stroke volume through the predominant effect on afterload reduction in euvolemic or hypervolemic patients.
- NIV reduces the need for intubation and the mortality rate in patients with acute chronic cardiac exacerbations compared with standard therapy.
- No difference in myocardial infarction risk has been shown between patients treated with CPAP/BiPAP versus standard oxygen therapy.
- No significant differences have been shown when studying CPAP versus BiPAP in terms of hospital mortality or need for intubation. There were no significant differences between the two ventilatory techniques in terms of hospital length of stay or risk of myocardial infarction.
- CPAP is recommended, in addition to SMT, in patients with severe respiratory failure due to cardiogenic pulmonary edema (class IIa recommendation, level of evidence A). CPAP must be considered the first-line intervention in patients with ACPE because it is easier to use than BiPAP and no differences have been shown between them when the two techniques were compared.
- The best location for NIV use depends on the hospital conditions, the indication or lack thereof for orotracheal intubation, and the multidisciplinary team that includes nurses, doctors, and physiotherapists.

References

1. Nava S. Behind a mask: tricks, pitfalls, and prejudices for noninvasive ventilation. Respir Care. 2013;58(8):1367–76.
2. Pinski MR, Polanco PM. Cardiovascular issues in respiratory care. In: Yearbook respiratory care clinics and applied technologies. International Association of Noninvasive Mechanical Ventilation. A.M. Esquinas; Murcia Spain 2008.
3. Vieillard-Baron A. Heart lung interactions in mechanical ventilation. In: Backer D, Cholly BP, Slama M, Vieillard-Baron A, Vignon P, editors. Hemodynamic monitoring using echocardiography in the critically Ill. Philadelphia: Springer; 2011.
4. Masip J, Roque M, Sanchez B, et al. Noninvasive ventilation in acute cardiogenic pulmonary edema: systematic review and meta-analysis. JAMA. 2005;294(24):3124–30.
5. Mariani J, Macchia A, Belziti C, Deabreu M, Gagliardi J, Doval H, Tognoni G, Tajer C. Noninvasive ventilation in acute cardiogenic pulmonary edema: a meta-analysis of randomized controlled trials. J Card Fail. 2011;17(10):850–9.
6. Li H, Hu C, Xia J, Li X, Wei H, Zeng X, Jing X. A comparison of bi-level and continuous positive airway pressure noninvasive ventilation in acute cardiogenic pulmonary edema. Am J Emerg Med. 2013;31(9):1322–7. doi:10.1016/j.ajem.2013.05.043. Epub 2013 Aug 6.
7. Sun T, Wan Y, Kan Q, Yang F, Yao H, Guan F, Zhang J, Li L. Efficacy of noninvasive ventilation on in-hospital mortality in patients with acute cardiogenic pulmonary edema: a meta-analysis. Zhonghua Xin Xue Guan Bing Za Zhi. 2014;42(2):161–8.

8. Ho KM, Wong K. A comparison of continuous and bi-level positive airway pressure non-invasive ventilation in patients with acute cardiogenic pulmonary edema: a meta-analysis. Crit Care. 2006;10:R49. doi:10.1186/cc4861.
9. Rusterholtz T, Bollaert PE, Feissel M, et al. Continuous positive airway pressure vs. proportional assist ventilation for noninvasive ventilation in acute cardiogenic pulmonary edema. Intensive Care Med. 2008;34:840–6.
10. Ferrari G, Olliveri F, De Filippi G, et al. Noninvasive positive airway pressure and risk of myocardial infarction in acute cardiogenic pulmonary edema: continuous positive airway pressure vs. noninvasive positive pressure ventilation. Chest. 2007;132:1804–9.
11. Massumi R, Mason D, Zakauddin V, Zelis R, Otero J, Amsterdam E. Reverse pulsus paradoxus. N Engl J Med. 1976;289:1272–1275
12. Mehta S, Jay GD, Woolard RH, Hipona RA, Connolly EM, Cimini DM, Drinkwine JH, Hill NS. Crit Care Med. 1997;25:620–628

Noninvasive Ventilation in Acute and Chronic Heart Failure: Evidence and Key Topics

46

Simon G. Pearse and Martin R. Cowie

Contents

Abbreviations

ACPE	Acute cardiogenic pulmonary edema
ASV	Adaptive servo-ventilation
BiPAP	Bi-level positive airway pressure
CO_2	Carbon dioxide
CPAP	Continuous positive airway pressure
CRT	Cardiac resynchronization therapy
CSA	Central sleep apnea
HF	Heart failure
HFPEF	Heart failure with preserved ejection fraction

S.G. Pearse, MBChB • M.R. Cowie, MD, FRCP (✉)
Department of Cardiology, National Heart and Lung Institute, Imperial College London and the Royal Brompton Hospital, London, UK
e-mail: s.pearse@rbht.nhs.uk; m.cowie@imperial.ac.uk

A.M. Esquinas (ed.), *Noninvasive Mechanical Ventilation: Theory, Equipment, and Clinical Applications*, DOI 10.1007/978-3-319-21653-9_46

HFREF	Heart failure with reduced ejection fraction
LV	Left ventricle
NIV	Noninvasive ventilation
OMT	Optimal medical therapy
OSA	Obstructive sleep apnea
$PaCO_2$	Arterial partial pressure of carbon dioxide
PEEP	Positive end-expiratory pressure
SDB	Sleep-disordered breathing

46.1 Introduction

Heart failure (HF) can be described as a state in which cardiac output is insufficient for the body's metabolic requirements at rest, or during exercise, despite adequate filling pressures. In clinical practice, HF is defined as a syndrome in which patients have typical symptoms (such as breathlessness, ankle swelling, and fatigue) and signs (including elevated venous pressure, pulmonary crepitations, or displaced apex beat) resulting from an abnormality of cardiac structure or function.

Despite significant advances in therapy, HF continues to be a leading cause of morbidity and mortality. Around 2 % of the adult population of Europe lives with HF, and in those over 85, the prevalence is as high as 10 %. HF is responsible for 5 % of emergency hospital admissions in Europe over the age of 65, and 30–40 % of patients die within 1 year of diagnosis.

HF may occur due to abnormalities of systolic function (HF with reduced ejection fraction – HFREF) or due to impaired filling of the heart in diastole (HF with preserved ejection fraction – HFPEF), although deficiencies in both elements of the cardiac cycle are frequently seen in the same patient. HF typically follows a chronic progressive course with intermittent acute exacerbations caused by identifiable triggers such as arrhythmia, poor compliance, myocardial infarction, or inappropriate medication such as nonsteroidal anti-inflammatory drugs. HF may also present acutely de novo, most frequently in the context of acute coronary syndromes or arrhythmia.

Management of HF can be broadly divided into emergency treatment of acute HF (often with pulmonary edema) and management of chronic stable HF. Medical therapy for acute HF complicated by pulmonary edema, including oxygen and intravenous loop diuretics, is supported by international guidelines. Intravenous nitrates, opioids, and inotropes may also be beneficial, as necessary, in selected patients. Noninvasive ventilation (NIV) has significant theoretical benefits for acute cardiogenic pulmonary edema (ACPE), but there are inconsistencies in the evidence base. In chronic stable HF, there is growing interest in the use of NIV in the management of sleep-disordered breathing (SDB), which is common in chronic HF and associated with a poorer prognosis. This chapter outlines the current evidence for noninvasive respiratory support in acute and chronic HF.

46.2 ACPE: Pathophysiology

In the lung, fluid is constantly exuded from the alveolar capillaries. This exudate passes through the alveolar interstitium and airspace and is reabsorbed by the peribronchial lymphatics across a pressure gradient. The rate of exudation depends upon the hydrostatic pressure within the alveolar capillaries, the permeability of the capillary walls, and the plasma oncotic pressure. A significant rise in pulmonary capillary pressure can be compensated for by increased lymphatic drainage. Left ventricular (LV) failure, systolic or diastolic, results in high end-diastolic pressure which is conducted back to the left atrium. The atrium can expand to accommodate some increase in pressure over time, but if the pressure rises acutely or to a marked degree, pulmonary venous pressure rises. This pressure is in turn passed to the alveolar capillaries and the rate of fluid exudation increases, which may exceed the maximal rate of reabsorption (Fig. 46.1). Fluid first accumulates in the peribronchovascular interstitium before spilling over to the alveolar membranes and flooding the airspaces.

The presence of excess fluid in the alveolar spaces has several effects. It acts as a barrier to gas exchange both between the air and the alveolar membrane and within the edematous membrane cells. It also dilutes the surfactant within the alveolus with the result that surface tension is increased and greater force is required to inspire. The alveoli are thus predisposed to collapse, which further increases the work of inspiration according to Laplace's law (in which the pressure required to inflate a sphere is inversely related to the diameter). Areas of edema in the lungs cause shunting of blood and hypoxemia, which is partially counteracted by relative vasoconstriction in the hypoxic areas. Increased capillary pressure in the lung ultimately leads to rising pulmonary artery pressure and can subsequently cause failure

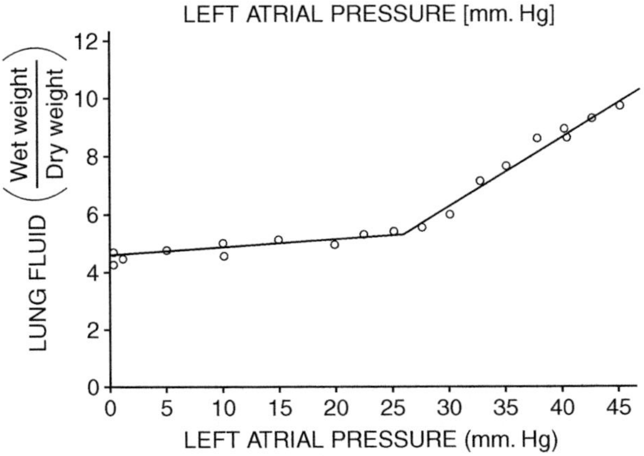

Fig. 46.1 The effect of rising left atrial pressure on the development of pulmonary edema in a canine model (Reproduced from Guyton and Lindsey [1]. With kind permission of Wolters Kluwer Health publishers)

of the right ventricle. This pathophysiological sequence can lead to respiratory failure – impaired gas exchange resulting in hypoxemia (usually defined as PaO_2 <8 kPa) – with or without hypercapnia.

46.3 ACPE: The Role of NIV

46.3.1 Continuous Positive Airway Pressure

Continuous positive airway pressure (CPAP) is the simplest form of respiratory support and has the greatest evidence base in the treatment of ACPE. CPAP provides constant pressure, typically 5–10 cmH_2O, via an airtight facemask, nasal mask, or helmet throughout the respiratory cycle. The resultant positive end-expiratory pressure (PEEP) helps prevent alveolar collapse and recruits alveoli that have collapsed. The alveoli are thus maintained at a greater diameter, lung compliance is increased, and the work of breathing is reduced. Lesser shunting of blood improves oxygenation and the positive intrathoracic pressure reduces venous return, thus reducing cardiac preload. LV transmural pressure is also reduced, with an effective reduction in afterload.

The earliest studies of NIV in ACPE compared CPAP plus optimal medical therapy (OMT) with OMT alone [2–4]. CPAP was administered in the emergency room and/or intensive care unit until respiratory failure resolved, intubation was required, or the patient was unable to tolerate CPAP further. The weight of evidence demonstrated an advantage of CPAP over OMT in terms of both in-hospital mortality and the need for endotracheal intubation. CPAP plus OMT also resulted in more rapid improvement in oxygenation and respiratory rate and was safe and effective in elderly patients. A further study revealed a similar benefit of CPAP for HF with both HFREF and HFPEF [5]. The studies did not, however, demonstrate a survival advantage for CPAP over OMT at 30-day follow up.

Two larger recent studies have shed some doubt on the benefit of a routine strategy of NIV in ACPE. The 3CPO trial is the largest multicenter randomized controlled trial (1,069 patients) comparing CPAP or bi-level positive airway pressure (BiPAP) plus OMT against OMT alone [6]. Although there was a more rapid reduction in respiratory rate, heart rate, hypercapnia, and acidosis in the NIV groups, there was no benefit for NIV at 7 days for the combined endpoint of intubation or mortality (9.5 % vs 9.8 %, $p=0.87$), and no mortality benefit at 30 days (15.2 % vs 16.4 %, $p=0.64$). There was, however, a high frequency of crossover from OMT to NIV on clinical grounds (16 % of OMT patients; presumably those with the most severe respiratory distress) and 9 % of NIV patients crossed into the OMT arm, many of whom are likely to have had less severe respiratory compromise. The mean duration of NIV therapy of approximately 2 h is also shorter than several previous studies. A further trial randomized 124 patients to receive either CPAP plus OMT or OMT alone for ACPE in the pre-hospital setting [7]. This demonstrated no benefit for CPAP over OMT for the primary combined outcome of respiratory rate (<25/min) and oxygen saturation (>90 %) at 1 h (31.7 % vs 35.5 %, $p=0.65$). There was no difference in hospital stay, intubation rates (3.3 % vs 4.8 % $p=0.52$), or mortality (10 % vs 11.3 % at 30 days, $p=0.52$), although the study was not powered for these outcomes.

A meta-analysis of the randomized trials, including the "negative" studies above, concluded there was an overall relative in-hospital mortality advantage for CPAP over OMT of 28 % and a relative reduction in intubation of 45 % [8]. There was no reduction in length of hospital stay.

46.3.2 BiPAP

BiPAP provides background positive pressure in the same manner as CPAP but also gives additional pressure during inspiration (inspiratory positive airway pressure). This reduces the effort required of the inspiratory muscles and may improve ventilation, with particular benefit for patients with hypercapnia and reduced respiratory drive or capability.

The evidence base for BiPAP in ACPE is more limited than for CPAP. Trials show significant heterogeneity, but overall there appears to be a more rapid resolution of hypercapnia, respiratory rate, and hypoxemia with BiPAP than with OMT. Some (but not all) studies showed reduced intubation rates with BiPAP, but a mortality advantage has not been demonstrated. This may be due to small studies in heterogeneous populations [6, 9].

Studies comparing BiPAP to CPAP have produced inconsistent results [9]. Overall, CPAP and BiPAP produce a similar advantage in terms of improved physiological parameters over OMT, but only CPAP has evidence (albeit variable) for improved short-term survival. Improvement in hypercapnia appears to be similar for CPAP and BiPAP.

Early studies found a higher incidence of myocardial infarction in those treated with BiPAP, but subsequent research with adequate power has repudiated this [10].

In practice, CPAP is a simpler and more extensively studied form of respiratory support for ACPE and should be considered for those with persistent respiratory failure not responding to optimal medical therapy. BiPAP should be reserved for those with hypercapnia unresponsive to CPAP, or with underlying lung disease that predisposes to hypercapnia with CPAP (such as advanced chronic obstructive pulmonary disease or obesity hypoventilation syndrome, which may be associated with HFPEF). The evidence does not support the routine use of NIV for all patents presenting with ACPE, and an individualized approach based on clinical findings and arterial blood gas analysis is recommended in European HF guidelines [11].

46.4 SDB in Chronic HF: Epidemiology and Pathophysiology

Around 50 % of patients with HF suffer from SDB. This may comprise obstructive sleep apnea (OSA) or central sleep apnea (CSA), although many patients have a mixed pattern that may change over the sleep period. In OSA, there is loss of pharyngeal muscle tone leading to upper airway collapse and obstruction. This is often associated with obesity and retrognathism, and in HF rostral shift of fluid during sleep leads to edema of the pharynx, exacerbating the tendency to airway collapse. In CSA, there is an abnormality of the regulation of breathing in the respiratory centers of the brainstem. The pathophysiology in HF involves reflex hyperventilation due to activation of pulmonary J receptors by edema and pulmonary congestion, a delayed circulation time between the alveoli and brainstem, and raised chemosensitivity leading to relative hyperventilation in response to rises in arterial carbon dioxide ($PaCO_2$). Hyperventilation leads to falls in $PaCO_2$ to below the apneic threshold, at which point the neural drive to breathe is inadequate to stimulate respiration. The resultant hypopnea or apnea causes the $PaCO_2$ to rise until hyperventilation again occurs and the cycle is repeated. Recurrent cyclical CSA is termed Cheyne-Stokes respiration.

Both forms of SDB are associated with recurrent arousals from sleep, episodes of hypoxemia, and enhanced sympathetic nervous system stimulation with increased catecholamine release. This predisposes to tachycardia, arrhythmia, and – particularly in the case of OSA – hypertension, which may increase the risk of stroke and myocardial infarction [12]. There is an excess of arrhythmia at night in those with OSA and increased rate of therapies from implantable cardioverter-defibrillators [13]. Daytime somnolence is a particular problem for those with OSA, and sufferers are at increased risk of road traffic accidents.

In OSA, the negative intrathoracic pressure generated by respiratory muscles attempting to inspire against a collapsed pharynx increases venous return to the heart and causes a high transcardiac gradient, increasing afterload. The septum shifts leftward and output from the failing LV is compromised. Abnormalities of endothelial function are also found in patients with OSA, including a high expression of the vasoconstrictor endothelin-1 and a blunted response to cholinergic vasodilators [14]. There is an increase in inflammatory markers such as C-reactive protein (known to be associated with vascular events) and prothrombotic factors (leading to enhanced platelet aggregation) [15].

The prevalence of CSA increases with the severity of HF and is a marker of poor prognosis. In a study of patients with moderate to severe LV dysfunction, median survival amongst those with CSA was 45 months versus 90 months for those without – a difference that persisted even when adjusted for several confounding factors [16]. Although this demonstrates association rather than causation, the recurrent hypoxemia, sympathetic stimulation, and changes in pre- and afterload associated with apnea are presumed to accelerate the vicious cycle of HF. Other risk factors associated with the development of CSA include male sex, atrial fibrillation, resting hypocapnia, and age over 60 years.

46.5 SDB in Chronic HF: NIV

46.5.1 OSA

Nocturnal CPAP is an established therapy for symptomatic OSA in the general population, in addition to lifestyle and weight management. CPAP improves daytime somnolence and may have an effect on hypertension and vascular events. In those with HF and OSA, CPAP reduces sympathetic activity and ventricular ectopy and can improve LV and right ventricular function [17]. In one nonrandomized study of 88 patients over a mean of 25 months follow-up, treatment with CPAP was associated with improved survival versus standard medical therapy (Hazard Ratio (HR) for death or hospitalization 2.03 in untreated group vs CPAP, 95 % Confidence Interval (CI) 1.07–3.68, $p=0.03$) [18].

Medical therapy for HF may reduce pharyngeal edema and consequently the severity of OSA, although trial data for this are lacking. Cardiac resynchronization therapy (CRT) improves LV function in selected patents with left bundle branch block and HF. Evidence that CRT improves OSA in HF is contradictory and a meta-analysis concludes no overall improvement [19].

CPAP should therefore be considered for patients with HF and moderate to severe OSA with symptoms of daytime somnolence, alongside optimization of medical therapy and CRT as appropriate. There is no consensus as to whether to recommend CPAP therapy in those with HF and OSA but no daytime somnolence.

46.5.2 CSA

Optimization of medical therapy for HF improves cardiac output, relieves pulmonary congestion, and reduces sympathetic drive. This would be expected to lessen the inappropriate hyperventilation that underpins CSA, although data for this are sparse. There is good evidence that CRT can improve CSA in appropriately selected patients. A recent meta-analysis of 7 trials investigating CRT in HF with SDB showed a significant mean reduction in Apnea-Hypopnea Index (AHI) of 13.5 events/h for those with predominant CSA, but a nonsignificant reduction of 3.3/h for OSA [19].

Experience of CPAP in the management of OSA led to research into CSA. Based on work showing a partial normalization in noradrenaline concentrations and LV ejection fraction in patients with HF and CSA treated with CPAP, as well as a possible reduction in mortality [20], a large randomized study (the CANPAP trial [21]) was performed to evaluate clinical endpoints in this group. Over a mean of 2 years of follow-up of 258 patients, there was no difference in transplant-free survival between the treated and untreated arms. There was, however, a significant reduction in AHI (mean reduction of 21 events/h) in those treated with CPAP, which persisted over 2 years. In addition, post -hoc subgroup analysis showed that those in whom AHI was suppressed to below 15 events per hour had significantly fewer adverse events than controls, suggesting a possible therapeutic role for more efficacious ventilatory techniques [22].

Adaptive servo-ventilation (ASV) is an advanced form of NIV in which the device provides varying levels of inspiratory pressure support depending on the patient's effort and minute ventilation. In addition, the device provides mandatory breaths during apneas and PEEP to maintain airway patency. This has the effect of greatly reducing apneas and hypopneas while moderating episodes of

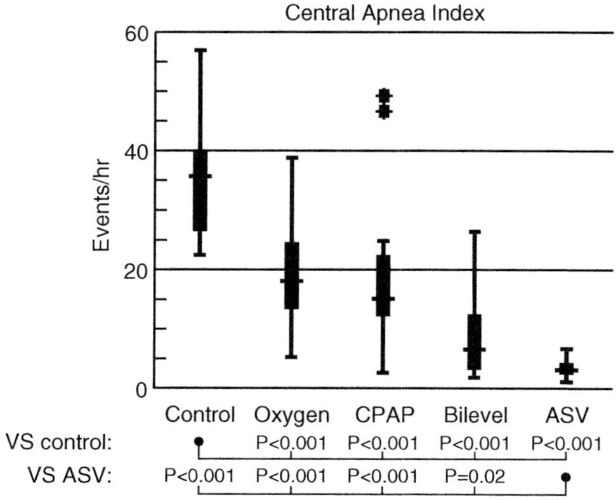

Fig. 46.2 The effect of different modalities of NIV on CSA events in HF (Reproduced from Teschler et al. [25]. Reprinted with permission of the American Thoracic Society. Copyright © 2015 American Thoracic Society. The *American Journal of Respiratory and Critical Care Medicine* is an official journal of the American Thoracic Society)

hyperventilation and is effective in both OSA and CSA. ASV is well tolerated and suppresses CSA more effectively than CPAP [23] (Fig. 46.2). A large randomized trial powered to detect mortality and morbidity endpoints in CSA (SERVE-HF) has recently been published [24]. Surprisingly, this reported no change in the combined mortality-morbidity endpoint with ASV, but a 28 % increase in all-cause mortality (95 % CI 1.06–1.55, p=0.01) and a 34 % increase in cardiovascular mortality (95 % CI 1.09–1.65, p=0.006). The mechanism of this harm remains to be elucidated. A further randomized trial in HF (enrolling patients with either OSA or CSA) is ongoing (ADVENT-HF - NCT01128816).

Conclusions

CPAP may be a useful tool in the management of ACPE in selected patients with respiratory failure. The role of BiPAP in this setting requires further assessment but may be considered for patients intolerant of CPAP or with refractory hypercapnia. Nocturnal CPAP is of significant benefit for those with OSA and daytime somnolence and may have additional cardiovascular benefits. The use of NIV in CSA cannot currently be recommended.

Key Major Recommendations

- In patients with ACPE and respiratory failure, NIV should be initiated early and up-titrated as tolerated.
- Patients with chronic HF and symptoms of sleepiness or fatigue should undergo sleep polygraphy or polysomnography to diagnose SDB.
- Patients with OSA should be referred to a specialist for consideration of nocturnal CPAP.
- Patients with CSA and HF should be established on OMT, including CRT as indicated.

Acknowledgments MRC's salary is supported by the National Institute for Health Research Cardiovascular Biomedical Research Unit at the Royal Brompton Hospital, London. SGP's salary is supported by a research grant from Boston Scientific.

References

1. Guyton AC, Lindsey AW. Effect of elevated left atrial pressure and decreased plasma protein concentration on the development of pulmonary edema. Circ Res. 1959;7:649–57.
2. Ducros L, Logeart D, Vicaut E, et al. CPAP for acute cardiogenic pulmonary oedema from out-of-hospital to cardiac intensive care unit: a randomised multicentre study. Intensive Care Med. 2011;37(9):1501–9.
3. Park M, Sangean MC, Volpe MDS, et al. Randomized, prospective trial of oxygen, continuous positive airway pressure, and bilevel positive airway pressure by face mask in acute cardiogenic pulmonary edema. Crit Care Med. 2004;32(12):2407–15.
4. Räsänen J, Heikkilä J, Downs J, et al. Continuous positive airway pressure by face mask in acute cardiogenic pulmonary edema. Am J Cardiol. 1985;55(4):296–300.
5. Bellone A, Vettorello M, Etteri M, et al. The role of continuous positive airway pressure in acute cardiogenic edema with preserved left ventricular systolic function. Am J Emerg Med (Elsevier Inc). 2009;27(8):986–91.
6. Gray A, Goodacre S, Newby D, et al. Noninvasive ventilation in acute cardiogenic pulmonary edema. N Eng J Med. 2008;359:142–51.
7. Frontin P, Bounes V, Houzé-Cerfon CH, et al. Continuous positive airway pressure for cardiogenic pulmonary edema: a randomized study. Am J Emerg Med. 2011;29(7):775–81.
8. Vital F, Saconato H, Ladeira M. Non-invasive positive pressure ventilation (CPAP or bilevel NPPV) for cardiogenic pulmonary edema. Cochrane Database Syst Rev. 2013;(5):1–201.
9. Weng CL, Zhao YT, Liu QH, et al. Meta-analysis: noninvasive ventilation in acute cardiogenic pulmonary edema. Ann Intern Med. 2010;152(9):590–600.
10. Ferrari G, Olliveri F, De Filippi G, et al. Noninvasive positive airway pressure and risk of myocardial infarction in acute cardiogenic pulmonary edema: continuous positive airway pressure vs noninvasive positive pressure ventilation. Chest. 2007;132(6):1804–9.
11. McMurray JJ, Adamopoulos S, Anker SD, et al. ESC Guidelines for the diagnosis and treatment of acute and chronic heart failure 2012: the Task Force for the Diagnosis and Treatment of Acute and Chronic Heart Failure 2012 of the European Society of Cardiology. Eur Heart J. 2012;33(14):1787–847.
12. Floras JS. Sleep apnea and cardiovascular risk. J Cardiol (Japanese College of Cardiology). 2014;63(1):3–8.

13. Bitter T, Westerheide N, Prinz C, et al. Cheyne-Stokes respiration and obstructive sleep apnoea are independent risk factors for malignant ventricular arrhythmias requiring appropriate cardioverter-defibrillator therapies in patients with congestive heart failure. Eur Heart J. 2011;32(1):61–74.
14. Kato M, Roberts-Thomson P, Phillips BG, et al. Impairment of endothelium-dependent vasodilation of resistance vessels in patients with obstructive sleep apnea. Circulation. 2000;102(21):2607–10.
15. Yokoe T. Elevated levels of C-reactive protein and interleukin-6 in patients with obstructive sleep apnea syndrome are decreased by nasal continuous positive airway pressure. Circulation. 2003;107(8):1129–34.
16. Javaheri S, Shukla R, Zeigler H, et al. Central sleep apnea, right ventricular dysfunction, and low diastolic blood pressure are predictors of mortality in systolic heart failure. J Am Coll Cardiol. 2007;49(20):2028–34.
17. Kaneko Y, Floras JS, Usui K, et al. Cardiovascular effects of continuous positive airway pressure in patients with heart failure and obstructive sleep apnea. N Engl J Med. 2003;348(13):1233–41.
18. Kasai T, Narui K, Dohi T, et al. Prognosis of patients with heart failure and obstructive sleep apnea treated with continuous positive airway pressure. Chest. 2008;133(3):690–6.
19. Lamba J, Simpson CS, Redfearn DP, et al. Cardiac resynchronization therapy for the treatment of sleep apnoea: a meta-analysis. Europace. 2011;13(8):1174–9.
20. Sin DD, Logan AG, Fitzgerald FS, et al. Effects of continuous positive airway pressure on cardiovascular outcomes in heart failure patients with and without Cheyne-Stokes respiration. Circulation. 2000;102(1):61–6.
21. Bradley TD, Logan AG, Kimoff RJ, et al. Continuous positive airway pressure for central sleep apnea and heart failure. N Engl J Med. 2005;353(19):2025–33.
22. Arzt M, Floras JS, Logan AG, et al. Suppression of central sleep apnea by continuous positive airway pressure and transplant-free survival in heart failure: a post hoc analysis of the Canadian Continuous Positive Airway Pressure for Patients with Central Sleep Apnea and Heart Failure Trial. Circulation. 2007;115:3173–80.
23. Hastings PC, Vazir A, Meadows GE, et al. Adaptive servo-ventilation in heart failure patients with sleep apnea: a real world study. Int J Cardiol. 2010;139(1):17–24.
24. Cowie MR, Woehrle H, Wegsheider K, et al. Adaptive Servo-Ventilation for Central Sleep Apnea in Systolic Heart Failure. N Eng J Med. 2015;373(12):1095–105.
25. Teschler H, Döhring J, Wang YM, et al. Adaptive pressure support servo-ventilation: a novel treatment for Cheyne-Stokes respiration in heart failure. Am J Resp Crit Care Med. 2001;164:614–9.

Noninvasive Ventilation in Drug Overdose: Is It a Potentially Safe Application? Key Practical Implications

47

Michalis Agrafiotis, Evangelia Serasli, and Venetia Tsara

Contents

Abbreviations

COPD	Chronic obstructive pulmonary disease
EPAP	Expiratory positive airway pressure
HDU	High dependency unit
ICU	Intensive care unit
NIV	Noninvasive ventilation

47.1 Introduction

Respiratory complications and acute respiratory failure are common following acute drug overdose. Respiratory failure in acute drug overdose can present as respiratory pump failure, a compromise of the gas exchange, or a combination of both.

M. Agrafiotis, MD (✉) • E. Serasli, MD, PhD • V. Tsara, MD, PhD
Department of Pulmonary Medicine, "Georgios Papanikolaou" General Hospital of Thessaloniki, Thessaloniki, Greece
e-mail: m.agrafiotis@gmail.com; serasli@patsialas.gr; bpneumonologiki@yahoo.gr

A.M. Esquinas (ed.), *Noninvasive Mechanical Ventilation: Theory, Equipment, and Clinical Applications*, DOI 10.1007/978-3-319-21653-9_47

These manifestations can be a direct consequence of the drug's pharmacologic action, while other factors such as aspiration syndromes or complications of treatment may also play an important contributory role [1]. In any case, management consists of removal of the drug from the organism, administration of antidote (if available), and supportive measures.

Invasive mechanical ventilation satisfies the need for a secure airway, providing at the same time an effective support of gas exchange, and it is traditionally considered the mainstay of management for severe cases of respiratory failure in drug overdose patients. Noninvasive positive pressure ventilation is alternative method of ventilation that can effect positive pressure breathing via a noninvasive interface and has become a widely accepted method for the management of several common conditions, including the hypercapnic exacerbation of chronic obstructive pulmonary disease (COPD) and cardiogenic pulmonary edema [2].

However, whether noninvasive ventilation (NIV) might also play a role in the supportive management of drug overdose-associated respiratory failure is an issue that remains largely obscure. Interestingly, the use of bi-level ventilation for the management of drug overdose patients was reported as early as 1996 [3]. A more recent cohort reported on the use of NIV in 157 patients with various causes of respiratory failure, including five cases with drug overdose, although specific data on the management and outcome of this subset of patients were not provided [4]. In another study, NIV was applied to 1 out of 29 patients with respiratory complications related to drug overdose, while 12 other patients were intubated [5]. Thus, considering the widespread use and availability of NIV today, it is possible that some experienced departments might regard it as a suitable option for the management of selected cases of respiratory failure caused by drug overdose. Nevertheless, published experience in that field remains largely anecdotal, and several issues pertaining to patient selection, practicalities of management, and outcomes have not yet been clarified.

47.2 Evidence

We searched PubMed and Scopus databases up to October 2014 for papers written in English, using the following key terms: ("non-invasive" OR "noninvasive") AND ("drug overdose" OR "intoxication" OR "poisoning"). Out of 1,161 initially retrieved articles, we identified 11 eligible papers (all of them case reports) providing data on the characteristics, management details, and outcomes of patients who were treated with NIV for drug overdose-associated acute respiratory failure [6–16] (Table 47.1). Opioids were the most common culprit associated with respiratory failure (5 out of 11 cases), whereas ventilatory depression (6/11) and non-cardiogenic pulmonary edema (5/11) were the most common clinical manifestations of drug respiratory toxicity. Extra-respiratory manifestations were invariably present in all patients and included impaired consciousness (7/11), circulatory abnormalities (5/11), and renal failure (4/11). Bi-level ventilation was the preferred noninvasive mode (6 out of 8 cases with available data). In the majority of the patients (10/11),

Table 47.1 Papers reporting the use of NIV in drug overdose-associated respiratory failure

No	First author (year) [Ref.]	Sex/age	Implicated toxin (s)	Type of respiratory involvement	Other complications	Antidote administered	Type of noninvasive ventilatory assistance	Other interventions	Outcome
1	Pichot (2014) [6]	Male/24	Cocaine Opioids	Ventilatory depression NCPE	Supraventricular tachycardia Metabolic acidosis Vomitus	Naloxone	Bi-level	Magnesium Amiodarone Antibiotics	Survived
2	Algren (2014) [7]	Female/54	Acepromazine	Ventilatory depression	CNS depression Hypotension	None	Bi-level	Activated charcoal Fluids Vasopressors	Survived
3	Agrafiotis (2014) [8]	Male/74	Fentanyl (transdermal patch) Tramadol	Ventilatory depression	CNS depression	Naloxone	Bi-level volume assured	None	Survived
4	Naha (2014) [9]	Female/18	Amlodipine Atenolol	NCPE	Metabolic acidosis Renal failure Hypotension	Calcium gluconate	NS	Gastric lavage Fluids Vasopressors	Survived
5	Koncicki (2013) [10]	Female/15	Cochicine	NCPE	Confusion Diarrhea Pancytopenia Renal failure Rhabdomyolysis Transaminasemia	None	NS	Transfusion	Survived

(continued)

Table 47.1 (continued)

No	First author (year) [Ref.]	Sex/age	Implicated toxin (s)	Type of respiratory involvement	Other complications	Antidote administered	Type of noninvasive ventilatory assistance	Other interventions	Outcome
6	Range (2013) [11]	Male/74	Amiodarone	NCPE	Renal failure	None	NS	Corticosteroids Dialysis Extracorporeal oxygenation	Died
7	Gonzva (2013) [12]	Male/20	Methadone Cannabis Alcohol	Ventilatory depression NCPE	CNS depression	Naloxone	Bi-level	Antibiotics	Survived
8	Maraffi (2011) [13]	Male/27	Cocaine Heroin	Ventilatory depression NCPE	Atrial fibrilation CNS depression	Naloxone	CPAP	NS	Survived
9	Klenner (2008) [14]	Female/84	Phenprocoumon	Alveolar hemorrhage	Anemia Coagulopathy	Vitamin K Vitamin K-dependent clot factors	Bi-level	Transfusion	Survived
10	Ridgway (2007) [15]	Male/54	Methadone	Ventilatory depression NCPE	CNS depression	Naloxone	Bi-level	Furosemide Glyceryl trinitrate	Survived
11	Vogt (2006) [16]	Male/42	Amlodipine Chlorothalidone Mefenamic acid Alcohol	Cardiogenic pulmonary edema	CNS depression Left heart failure Vomitus Renal failure	Calcium gluconate	CPAP	Fluids Inotropes Vasopressors Insulin infusion Furosemide	Survived

Abbreviations: CNS central nervous system, *CPAP* continuous positive airway pressure, *NCPE* non-cardiogenic pulmonary edema, *NS* not specified

NIV was successful in the management of drug overdose-associated respiratory failure, with only one patient failing NIV and switched to invasive ventilation; this patient sustained amiodarone-induced pulmonary toxicity and eventually died [11].

47.3 NIV for the Management of Drug Overdose-Associated Respiratory Failure: Advantages and Limitations

The rationale behind the use of NIV for the management of drug overdose-associated respiratory failure stems from the encouraging experience obtained from patients with hypercapnic COPD exacerbation and cardiogenic pulmonary edema. In these instances, NIV has been shown to reduce mortality and length of hospital stay and avert endotracheal intubation, along with its associated complications (e.g., infections) [2]. Additionally, when NIV was directly compared with invasive mechanical ventilation in patients with COPD exacerbation, it was associated with a lower frequency of complications, although the rate of NIV failure was high, and eventually 60 % of the NIV-treated patients required intubation [17]. Nevertheless, controlled clinical studies are needed to explore whether the benefits from NIV application in these categories of patients might also apply to patients with respiratory failure related to drug overdose.

A particular advantage in the use of NIV is that it can be applied early in the course of the disease. In this way, respiratory compromise can be managed at an initial stage and its complications (e.g., hypercapnic coma) can be prevented, while in the same time other measures such as drug removal and antidote administration take immediate effect. Therefore, considering that drug overdose syndromes can be quickly and fully reversed when promptly diagnosed and treated, NIV can become a powerful tool in the early management of these patients. Additionally, the application of expiratory positive airway pressure (EPAP) could also reduce the tendency for atelectasis, minimizing the requirements for oxygen, and improve upper airway patency, averting episodes of obstructive sleep disordered breathing and hypoventilation [18]. The use of NIV could also allow for prolonged periods of ventilatory support, an important advantage for patients with heavy overdose, chronic respiratory disease, or limited physiological reserve. In addition, NIV could also be regarded as an acceptable alternative option for the management of patients with a "do-not-intubate" order, as in the case of terminal stage cancer. These patients are commonly treated with opioids for chronic pain and are particularly prone to their side effects [19].

This approach, however, has several inherent limitations. First, drug overdose patients often present with impaired level of consciousness and inability to protect the airway. In these cases, and unless the condition can be rapidly reversed (e.g., by administering naloxone in the case of opioid intoxication), the requirement for a secure airway takes precedence and endotracheal intubation should be regarded as the management of choice. On the other hand, in a study by Duncan et al. [20] involving 73 patients treated for acute poisoning in a high-dependency unit (HDU), none out of the 12 patients who presented with an impaired level of consciousness (Glasgow Coma Scale score <8) required intubation or exhibited signs of aspiration. Moreover, the presence of moderate to severe encephalopathy in COPD patients who received NIV for the management of acute exacerbation was not associated with higher tracheotomy and mortality rates compared with endotracheal intubation; however, these results should not be readily extrapolated to patients with drug overdose [21]. Of note, a successful combination of NIV and antidote administration in cases of opioid-induced hypercapnic acidosis (with or without non-cardiogenic pulmonary edema) has been reported by several authors. In this setting, early antidote administration can promptly improve respiratory acidosis and restore the level of consciousness, creating a "therapeutic window" that obviates the requirement for invasive airway management and buys time for NIV to control carbon dioxide levels and reverse hypoxemia [6, 8, 12, 13, 15].

An additional shortcoming is related to the common occurrence of gastric distention in patients on NIV, a condition that can impair effective ventilatory support and exacerbate the risk of aspiration. Moreover, the presence of a nasogastric tube can interfere with mask sealing, and the interface itself can compromise effective gastric lavage. Both these conditions can contribute to patient discomfort and increase the risk for NIV failure.

An important consideration also pertains to the frequent occurrence of multiple organ involvement given that complications as severe hemodynamic instability, profound metabolic acidosis, and renal or hepatic failure are common in patients with drug overdose and might compromise the effectiveness of NIV, necessitating the use of invasive ventilation. Finally, caution should be particularly applied in cases with severe hypoxemia due to acute respiratory distress syndrome, as roughly half of these patients respond poorly to NIV and will eventually require invasive ventilatory support [22].

47.4 Practical Issues

The choice of the ventilatory support method should always be made after a careful assessment of the individual risk factors in each case. Therefore, intensive care unit (ICU) ventilators are particularly advantageous for the management of severe hypoxemia because of their high performance capabilities and because they incorporate oxygen blenders that allow exact regulation of the inspired oxygen fraction. A spontaneous/timed bi-level mode should be preferred in patients with impaired level of consciousness and blunted ventilatory response, whereas volume guarantee modes might benefit patients with severe ventilatory depression and poorly controlled hypercapnia. In this regard, measures should also be taken to minimize carbon dioxide rebreathing, ideally by using devices with dual-limb circuits. When single-limb systems are used, either a true expiratory valve or a vented interface with a minimal dynamic dead space should be employed. In the latter case, the implementation of EPAP could also reduce carbon dioxide rebreathing by providing fresh gas flow at the end of expiration [23]. As a general rule, patients with drug overdose-associated respiratory failure should be admitted and monitored in HDUs or ICUs and access to invasive ventilation or advanced life support facilities should be readily available.

Conclusion

There is limited evidence to support the application of NIV for the management of drug overdose-associated respiratory failure, and invasive mechanical ventilation should be regarded as the definite procedure for ensuring oxygenation and ventilation and providing protection against aspiration in severely ill patients with drug overdose. Alternatively, NIV might be an acceptable choice for selected cases of relatively stable patients with a low risk of aspiration and absence of overt signs of multiple organ failure. In these cases, a trial of NIV could be cautiously offered while the patient is being carefully monitored, should an indication for invasive ventilation appear. In addition, NIV might be considered for the management of drug overdose-associated respiratory failure when a "do-not-intubate" decision has been made.

Key Major Recommendations

- NIV is a potentially suitable alternative to invasive ventilation for patients with drug-overdose associated respiratory failure when there is a low risk of aspiration, limited involvement of other organ systems, or when a "do-not-intubate" order is in place.
- Ventilators with oxygen blenders and advanced performance characteristics should be used for the management of severe hypoxemia.
- Spontaneous/timed bi-level modes should be employed for patients with a blunted ventilatory response. Volume guarantee modes should be considered in difficult-to-control respiratory acidosis.
- Intensive monitoring should be provided to all patients with drug overdose who are being treated with NIV.

References

1. Wilson KC, Saukkonen JJ. Acute respiratory failure from abused substances. J Intensive Care Med. 2004;19(4):183–93.
2. Boldrini R, Fasano L, Nava S. Noninvasive mechanical ventilation. Curr Opin Crit Care. 2012;18(1):48–53.
3. Pollack Jr C, Torres MT, Alexander L. Feasibility study of the use of bilevel positive airway pressure for respiratory support in the emergency department. Ann Emerg Med. 1996;27(2):189–92.
4. Bülow HH, Thorsager B, Hoejberg JM. Experiences from introducing non-invasive ventilation in the intensive care unit: a 2-year prospective consecutive cohort study. Acta Anaesthesiol Scand. 2007;51(2):165–70.

5. Jayakrishnan B, Al Asmi A, Al Qassabi A, Nandhagopal R, Mohammed I. Acute drug overdose: clinical profile, etiologic spectrum and determinants of duration of intensive medical treatment. Oman Med J. 2012;27(6):501–4.
6. Pichot C, Petitjeans F, Ghignone M, et al. Swift recovery of severe acute hypoxemic respiratory failure under non-invasive ventilation. Anaesthesiol Intensive Ther. 2015;47(2):138–42.
7. Algren DA, Ashworth A. Acute acepromazine overdose: clinical effects and toxicokinetic evaluation. J Med Toxicol. 2015;11(1):121–3.
8. Agrafiotis M, Tryfon S, Siopi D, et al. Successful management of drug-induced hypercapnic acidosis with naloxone and noninvasive positive pressure ventilation. Am J Emerg Med. 2015;33(2):312.e3–4.
9. Naha K, Suryanarayana J, Aziz RA, et al. Amlodipine poisoning revisited: acidosis, acute kidney injury and acute respiratory distress syndrome. Indian J Crit Care Med. 2014; 18(7):467–9.
10. Koncicki M, Dewan M. A teenager with multiple organ system dysfunction. Pediatr Emerg Care. 2013;29(3):399–401.
11. Range FT, Hilker E, Breithardt G, et al. Amiodarone-induced pulmonary toxicity – a fatal case report and literature review. Cardiovasc Drugs Ther. 2013;27(3):247–54.
12. Gonzva J, Prunet B, Deniel C, et al. Early antidote use associated with noninvasive ventilation in prehospital treatment of methadone intoxication. Am J Emerg Med. 2013;31(2):448.e5–6.
13. Maraffi T, Ruvolo L, Aliberti S, et al. Early application of non-invasive continuous positive airway pressure in acute respiratory distress syndrome due to a drug overdose: a case report. Intern Emerg Med. 2011;6(3):275–6.
14. Klenner AF, Friesecke S, Schäper C, et al. Diffuse alveolar hemorrhage with acute respiratory distress syndrome associated with phenprocoumon therapy. Blood Coagul Fibrinolysis. 2008;19(8):813–5.
15. Ridgway ZA, Pountney AJ. Acute respiratory distress syndrome induced by oral methadone managed with non-invasive ventilation. Emerg Med J. 2007;24(9):681.
16. Vogt S, Mehlig A, Hunziker P, et al. Survival of severe amlodipine intoxication due to medical intensive care. Forensic Sci Int. 2006;161(2–3):216–20.
17. Squadrone E, Frigerio P, Fogliati C, et al. Noninvasive vs invasive ventilation in COPD patients with severe acute respiratory failure deemed to require ventilatory assistance. Intensive Care Med. 2004;30(7):1303–10.
18. Wang D, Teichtahl H. Opioids, sleep architecture and sleep-disordered breathing. Sleep Med Rev. 2007;11(1):35–46.
19. Dahan A, Overdyk F, Smith T, Aarts L, Niesters M. Pharmacovigilance: a review of opioid-induced respiratory depression in chronic pain patients. Pain Physician. 2013;16(2):E85–94.
20. Duncan R, Thakore S. Decreased Glasgow Coma Scale score does not mandate endotracheal intubation in the emergency department. J Emerg Med. 2009;37(4):451–5.
21. Scala R, Nava S, Conti G, et al. Noninvasive versus conventional ventilation to treat hypercapnic encephalopathy in chronic obstructive pulmonary disease. Intensive Care Med. 2007;33(12):2101–8.
22. Antonelli M, Conti G, Esquinas A, et al. A multiple-center survey on the use in clinical practice of noninvasive ventilation as a first-line intervention for acute respiratory distress syndrome. Crit Care Med. 2007;35(1):18–25.
23. Mojoli F, Braschi A. Carbon dioxide rebreathing during noninvasive mechanical ventilation. In: Esquinas AM, editors. Noninvasive mechanical ventilation. Theory, equipment, clinical applications. Berlin Heidelberg: Springer; 2010. p. 77–82.

Atelectasis and Noninvasive Mechanical Ventilation

48

Paulo Matos

Contents

Abbreviations

CPAP	Continuous positive airway pressure
EPAP	Expiratory positive airway pressure
IPAP	Inspiratory positive airway pressure
NIMV	Noninvasive mechanical ventilation

48.1 Introduction

Atelectasis is a common finding in hospitalized patients. It contributes to deterioration of pulmonary function and gas exchange, leading to significant morbidity, mortality, and health-care costs [1]. After thoracic or upper abdominal surgery, the incidence of atelectasis is high, up to 54–92 %. Multiple factors, such as pleural opening, postoperative diaphragmatic dysfunction, pain, immobilization, and bed

P. Matos, MD
Pulmonology Department, Coimbra Hospital and University Centre, Coimbra, Portugal
e-mail: pmsotto@hotmail.com

A.M. Esquinas (ed.), *Noninvasive Mechanical Ventilation: Theory, Equipment, and Clinical Applications*, DOI 10.1007/978-3-319-21653-9_48

rest, in addition to possible preexisting respiratory disease, are involved in the development of atelectasis in this clinical situation [2].

In patients with neuromuscular diseases and in critically ill patients who develop atelectasis, bronchoscopy and respiratory physiotherapy are the techniques of choice for treatment. However, physiotherapy is usually neglected and bronchoscopy is an invasive technique with some contraindications and complications. Some authors have shown a few clinical cases where noninvasive mechanical ventilation (NIMV) was useful in treatment of atelectasis [3]. We will discuss the use of continuous positive airway pressure (CPAP) and NIMV in preventing and treating atelectasis in these two clinical scenarios.

48.2 Discussion

48.2.1 Postoperative Atelectasis and NIMV

Atelectasis occurs regularly during anesthesia induction and persists in the postoperative period. This may contribute to significant morbidity, delay in discharge, and additional health-care costs. It is found in almost 90 % of all patients who are anaesthetized, on average involving 10 % of total lung tissue.

During general anesthesia, lung collapse may be caused by three basic mechanisms: compression atelectasis by loss of diaphragm tone and abdominal pressure; absorption atelectasis, when less gas enters the alveolus than that removed by blood uptake; and by loss of surfactant, with a rise in surface alveolus tension [4].

In the postoperative period, pulmonary function is substantially decreased. In addition to the mechanisms that occur during induction and the intrinsic drug effect, others, such as pain, pleural opening, and diaphragm dysfunction, especially in thoracic or upper abdominal surgery, contribute to ventilation/perfusion mismatch, worsening of hypoxemia, gas exchange, and atelectasis, expressed by a restrictive syndrome (reduced vital capacity, tidal volume, and functional residual capacity) and possibly respiratory failure [5]. Diaphragm dysfunction may last from 7 to 10 days after surgery. Bed rest contributes to this scenario.

One of the most feared postsurgical complications are pulmonary infections, which are predisposed by persistent atelectasis and can cause irreversible loss of functioning parenchyma. The most important risk factors for postsurgical respiratory complications, especially atelectasis, are thoracic or upper abdominal surgery (close to the diaphragm), obesity, chronic obstructive pulmonary disease, and older age.

The prevention of atelectasis has, therefore, always been one of the aims of postoperative rehabilitation. In the 1980s, it was thought that the application of a positive pressure through CPAP would, on the one hand, reduce the work of the respiratory muscles and, on the other, promote early recruitment of poorly aerated regions of the lungs. The first pioneering studies regarding both abdominal and thoracic surgery demonstrated that, following radiologic evidence of postoperative atelectasis, it was possible to reduce or prevent pneumonia and loss of respiratory function and improve gas exchange. More recently, some researchers have focused on the prevention of respiratory complications, starting treatment before the surgery or immediately after the surgical procedure has been completed.

CPAP or NIMV are commonly used in this clinical circumstance with proven benefits. Their use promotes lung recruitment and improves oxygenation, without hemodynamic adverse effects or pleural leaks. The work of breathing is diminished when using NIMV, providing more effective ventilation and oxygen spare. In cardiac or lung resection surgery, NIMV was shown to decrease the need for tracheal intubation and hospital mortality [6]. Many of these benefits are explained by prevention or treatment of preexisting atelectasis.

Kindgen-Milles et al. [7] showed that patients treated prophylactically with CPAP of 10 cmH_2O for 12–24 h after thoracoabdominal surgery (aneurysm of thoracoabdominal aorta) had significantly better oxygenation rates and shorter lengths of intensive care unit and hospital stay. Pasquina et al. [1] reported that when CPAP was applied in patients who developed postoperative atelectasis (based on roentgenographic evidence) following cardiac surgeries, there was considerable improvement of atelectasis, as determined by radiological scores.

Lorut et al. [8] reported a large prospective randomized trial involving seven thoracic surgery departments, investigating postoperative NIMV, and their findings showed no statistically significant differences in reintubation rate, mortality rates, and length of hospital stay. However, the authors point out that the selection of patients, the methodology regarding NIMV, and even the expertise of medical and nonmedical personnel are essential to good outcomes.

Further studies are needed to identify the best protocol for preventive NIMV in at-risk patients or curative NIMV in patients who develop postoperative atelectasis or acute respiratory failure. To our knowledge, the lowest possible pressures should be used to ensure a satisfactory therapeutic level, keeping patient comfort and safety in mind. When using CPAP, pressure up to 10 cmH_2O may be needed. In pressure support ventilation, expiratory positive airway pressure (EPAP) should also be used from 5 to 10 cmH_2O, providing support pressures of 6–15 cmH_2O, without exceeding inspiratory positive airway pressure (IPAP) of 25 cmH_2O.

48.2.2 Atelectasis in Neuromuscular Disorders and Critically Ill Patients

In patients with neuromuscular disorders and in critically ill patients, atelectasis may be prevented with respiratory physiotherapy and mechanical insufflation-exsufflation devices. Nevertheless, respiratory physiotherapy has been largely ignored in hospitalized patients, especially outside the intensive care unit. Bronchoscopy is the end-of-line procedure to treat these patients, many of them with critical diseases and with relative or absolute contraindications to this invasive treatment. NIMV has been shown to be effective in preventing atelectasis in the postoperative period, so we might extrapolate this data to prevent atelectasis in these patients. There are only a few published clinical cases of success treating atelectasis with NIMV in patients with neuromuscular disorders, acute hypercapnic respiratory failure, and with contraindications to bronchoscopy [9], although we lack prospective studies to support this NIMV application. The most suitable ventilation mode in these cases is bi-level pressure support ventilation in spontaneous/timed mode.

Conclusion

NIMV seems to play a major role in preventing and treating atelectasis, and it should not be delayed in patients known to be at risk. Awareness and training of personnel, including doctors, nurses, and respiratory therapists, is essential to NIMV success. Further studies are needed to better identify patients at risk of atelectasis and, furthermore, elaborate more concise NIMV protocols.

Key Recommendations

- Consider NIMV in patients at risk of developing atelectasis.
- Consider NIMV to treat atelectasis in the postoperative period
- Consider NIMV for treating atelectasis in patients with contraindications to bronchoscopy.
- Use CPAP/EPAP pressures up to 10 cmH_2O without exceeding IPAP of 25 cmH_2O in postoperative patients.
- Provide NIMV in an adequate environment and with qualified personnel.

References

1. Pasquina P, Merlai P, Granier JM, Ricou B. Continuous positive airway pressure versus noninvasive pressure support ventilation to treat atelectasis after cardiac surgery. Anesth Analg. 2004;99:1001–8.
2. Vargas FS, Cukier A, Terra-Filho M, et al. Influence of atelectasis on pulmonary function after coronary artery bypass graft. Chest. 1993;104:434–7.
3. Villalona RM, Alises MA, Lobato SD. Resolution of obstructive atelectasis with non-invasive mechanical ventilation. Arch Bronconeumol. 2014;50(10):452–3.
4. Magnusson L, Spahn DR. New concepts of atelectasis during general anaesthesia. Br J Anaesth. 2003;91(1):61–72.
5. Jaber S, Jong A, Castagnoli A, Futier E, et al. Non-invasive ventilation after surgery. Ann Fr Anesth Reanim. 2014;33:487–91.
6. Auriant I, Jallot A, Herve P, Cerrina J, et al. Noninvasive ventilation reduces mortality in acute respiratory failure following lung resection. Am J Respir Crit Care Med. 2001;164:1231–5.
7. Kindgen-Milles D, Müller E, Buhl R, Böhner H, et al. Nasal-continuous positive airway pressure reduces pulmonary morbidity and length of hospital stay following thoracoabdominal aortic surgery. Chest. 2005;128(2):821–8.
8. Lorut C, Lefebvre A, Planquette B, Quinquis L, et al. Early post-operative prophylactic non-invasive ventilation after major lung resection in COPD patients: a randomized controlled trial. Intensive Care Med. 2014;40:220–7.
9. Duncan S, Negrin R, Mihm FG, Guilleminault C, et al. Nasal continuous positive airway pressure in atelectasis. Chest. 1992;92(4):621–4.

Noninvasive Ventilation in Patients with Severe Community-Acquired Pneumonia: What Have We Learned? Key Response Determinants and Practical Implications

49

Michele Carron and Francesco Zarantonello

Contents

Abbreviations

ARDS	Acute respiratory distress syndrome
ARF	Acute respiratory failure
BiPAP	Bi-level positive airway pressure
CAP	Community-acquired pneumonia
COPD	Chronic obstructive pulmonary disease
CPAP	Continuous positive airway pressure
FiO_2	Fraction inspired oxygen
ICU	Intensive care unit
NIV	Noninvasive ventilation
OI	Oxygenation index
OR	Odds ratio
$PaCO_2$	Partial arterial carbon dioxide pressure
PaO_2	Partial arterial oxygen pressure

M. Carron, MD (✉) • F. Zarantonello, MD
Department of Medicine, Anesthesiology and Intensive Care, University of Padova, Padova, Italy
e-mail: michele.carron@unipd.it; fzarantonello@gmail.com

A.M. Esquinas (ed.), *Noninvasive Mechanical Ventilation: Theory, Equipment, and Clinical Applications*, DOI 10.1007/978-3-319-21653-9_49

PEEP	Positive end-expiratory pressure
PSV	Positive inspiratory ventilatory support
RCT	Randomized controlled trial
SaO_2	Arterial oxygen saturation
SAPS	Simplified Acute Physiology Score

49.1 Introduction

In the United States, pneumonia is the most common cause of mortality among infectious diseases and the sixth most common cause of death overall [1]. Pneumonia is an infection of the lung parenchyma, which is referred to as community-acquired pneumonia (CAP) when the infection is acquired outside a hospital or health-care facility [1]. The incidence of CAP varies with age, increasing from 18/1,000 person-years in individuals 65–69 years old to 52/1,000 person-years in individuals 85 years and older. Approximately 20–40 % of individuals with CAP will require hospitalization, 10–20 % of whom will have severe CAP [1]. Severe CAP had been defined as a CAP that requires intensive care unit (ICU) admission. It is associated with mortality rates as high as 50 %, and almost half of the patients will require mechanical ventilation [1]. Antimicrobial therapy is the mainstay of CAP treatment, administered empirically at first and then tailored to culture results when they are available. Oxygen therapy is often necessary to counteract hypoxemia [1]. If patients fail to maintain adequate gas exchange (i.e., PaO_2 >65 mmHg while receiving supplemental oxygen at a FiO_2 of 60 %) and acute respiratory failure (ARF) occurs, tracheal intubation and mechanical ventilation should be considered [1–4].

49.2 Discussion and Analysis

49.2.1 Noninvasive Ventilation Techniques and Devices

Noninvasive ventilation (NIV) refers to the delivery of assisted mechanical ventilation without an invasive airway conduit [1, 2]. This term includes different NIV modalities, such as continuous positive airway pressure (CPAP), pressure support ventilation (PSV), and bi-level positive airway pressure (BiPAP) [2]. CPAP is a method that delivers constant positive airway pressure noninvasively throughout both inspiration and expiration [3]. With PSV, the patient breathes spontaneously, and, when the patient triggers the ventilator, the ventilator delivers a preset additional level of pressure to assist the patient during the inspiration phase. The tidal volume varies from breath to breath during PSV [3]. When CPAP is applied with PSV, it is referred to as positive end-expiratory pressure (PEEP) [3]. BiPAP is a technique that delivers different levels of pressure during inspiration (IPAP) and expiration (EPAP) [3]. BiPAP involves the application of two different levels of positive airway pressure, in contrast to CPAP, which involves the use of only one positive airway pressure [3].

NIV can be delivered via many interfaces (nasal mask, face mask, or helmet), each of which has its own advantages and disadvantages [2]. Appropriate selection and adequate management of the device are crucial for minimizing the risk of complications and failure during NIV [2, 3]. It is important to choose an interface that fits properly and minimizes air leaks, and to help the patient become familiar with the equipment in the first few minutes of NIV [2]. If a patient feels claustrophobic, the use of a different size or type of mask or helmet may enhance comfort [2]. A helmet is usually better tolerated than masks, resulting in longer use and lower NIV failure rates [2, 3] (Fig. 49.1).

49.2.2 Rationale for NIV in ARF

Clinical evidence supports the use of NIV to avoid intubation in patients with ARF due to chronic obstructive pulmonary disease (COPD) exacerbations and acute cardiogenic pulmonary edema [2–4]. Although supporting evidence is less abundant, NIV may also be considered for patients with acute respiratory distress syndrome (ARDS) [2–4]. In patients with hypoxemic ARF, a trial of NIV is justified if patients are carefully selected by highly experienced teams in accordance with the available guidelines, while considering the known risk factors and predictors for NIV failure [2, 3].

Regarding ventilatory strategy, both CPAP and PEEP prevent alveolar collapse, reduce atelectasis by recruiting and stabilizing previously collapsed lung units, and reduce ventilation/perfusion mismatch and shunt fraction, thereby resulting in improved gas exchange. They decrease the work of breathing, counterbalancing the inspiratory threshold load imposed by intrinsic PEEP in some patients (e.g., those with COPD). Furthermore, PEEP and CPAP reduce left ventricular afterload and increase cardiac output. PSV is more effective than CPAP at achieving improved muscle unloading and relief from dyspnea during NIV. PSV plus PEEP improves alveolar ventilation compared with that achieved using CPAP alone [2, 3].

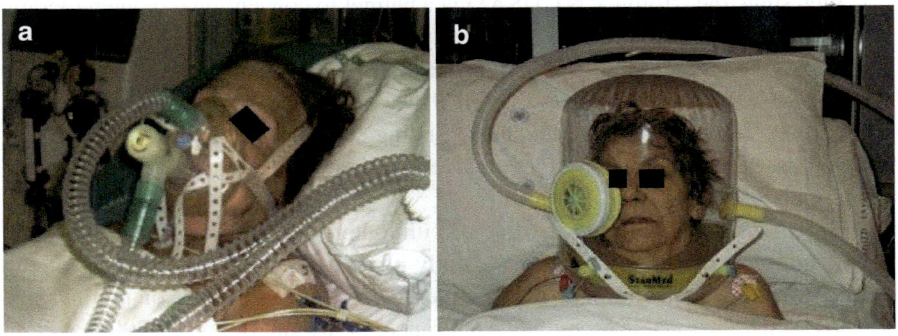

Fig. 49.1 Use of NIV in patients admitted to ICU with severe CAP. The patients received noninvasive mechanical ventilation (PSV with PEEP by Servo Ventilator 300A, MAQUET, Cinisello Balsamo, MI, Italy) through a face mask (**a**) and a helmet (**b**)

49.2.3 Rationale for NIV in CAP

Randomized controlled trials (RCTs) describing whether NIV is beneficial in pneumonia are scarce. Most have considered very heterogeneous populations of patients with varying causes of ARF including, even if a small percentage, pneumonia [3]. Ferrer et al. [4], in a study involving 105 ARF patients, showed that BiPAP (BiPAP Vision, Respironics Inc., Murrysville, PA, USA) produced a faster improvement in oxygenation and dyspnea in patients receiving NIV and reduced the need for intubation from 52 % with conventional oxygen therapy to 25 % with NIV ($p=0.01$). Furthermore, NIV was linked to a decreased incidence of septic shock ($p=0.028$). These benefits were also evident for patients with pneumonia, in whom ICU mortality was reduced from 53 % with conventional therapy to 15 % with NIV ($p=0.03$).

The role of NIV in patients with CAP has been reported in the literature, each with a different response to NIV. To better understand the benefit, the patients should be considered as part of different subgroups [5–9]. They include a "de novo" group, defined as patients with CAP without previous cardiac or pulmonary disease; a "comorbidities" group, defined as CAP in patients with cardiac or pulmonary diseases (i.e., COPD); and an "immunodepressed" group, defined as CAP in patients with an impaired immune system due to a hematologic malignancy or being a transplant recipient [5–9].

Whereas older studies consistently reported that NIV in "de novo" CAP patients was associated with a high likelihood of failure and consequently high intubation rates, some more recent studies have suggested otherwise. Brambilla et al. [5] reported promising results in a RCT conducted in 4 Italian ICUs evaluating 81 patients with no history of COPD or heart failure, who developed severe hypoxemia (PaO_2/FiO_2 <250 mmHg) due to pneumonia. Patients were randomized to receive either CPAP (VitalSigns Inc., Totowa, NJ, USA) by helmet or oxygen therapy by Venturi mask [5]. Compared with those receiving supplemental oxygen therapy, patients in the CPAP group exhibited a faster improvement in PaO_2/FiO_2 ratio, respiratory rate, and dyspnea, and a lower percentage met intubation criteria (15 % vs 63 %, $p<0.001$) [5]. In a multicenter RCT comparing CPAP (high-flow generator, VitalSigns Inc., Totowa, NJ, USA) via a helmet to conventional oxygen therapy in 47 CAP patients with moderate-severe hypoxemia, Cosentini et al. [6] found that NIV was associated with a faster improvement in oxygenation (median 1.5 h vs 48 h, $p<0.001$), but as soon as the CPAP was stopped, oxygenation returned to lower levels in most patients. The latter finding suggests that longer use of CPAP may be needed to recruit the flooded alveoli characteristic of the initial phase of pneumonia [6].

For patients with previous cardiac or pulmonary diseases, the available RCTs report more encouraging results. In a study of 56 patients with CAP randomized to receive either conventional oxygen therapy via Venturi mask or noninvasive PSV (Cesar [Thaema, Antony Cedex, France]; Puritain Bennett 7200 [Puritain Bennett Co., Overland Park, KS, USA]; Vential [Saime, Savigny-le-Temple, France]; Servo 900 C [Siemens Elema, Uppsala, Sweden]) via face mask,

Confalonieri et al. [7] reported a decrease in intubation rate from 50 % with Venturi mask to 21 % with PSV ($p=0.03$) but no reduction in mortality or length of hospital stay. Subgroup analysis found that COPD patients with hypercapnic respiratory failure benefited from NIV and had a reduced mortality rate at 2 months (11 % vs 63 %, $p=0.05$). More recently, Carrillo et al. [8] prospectively followed 250 CAP patients treated with BiPAP (BiPAP ST-D and VISION Ventilator, Respironics, Inc., Murrysville, PA, USA) by means of nasal or face mask in a highly experienced center. They found that NIV success was more frequent in patients with a history of cardiac and pulmonary disease compared with those with "de novo" ARF (74 % vs 54 %, $p=0.007$) [8].

Immunodepressed patients in whom ARF develops often require mechanical ventilatory support. In these patients, NIV has the potential to avoid endotracheal intubation and its complications [2, 3]. In a RCT by Squadrone et al. [9], 40 neutropenic patients with ARF, tachypnea, and pulmonary infiltrates were randomized to early CPAP (WhisperFlow, Caradyne, Ireland) with helmet or conventional oxygen therapy. Among patients admitted to the ICU, oxygenation was better and the intubation rate was lower in the CPAP than in the control group ($p=0.0001$). NIV showed a reduction in the relative risk for intubation to 0.46 (95 % confidence interval [CI], 0.27–0.78) [9]. A systematic review by Zhang et al. [1], which included one RCT involving immunodepressed patients with fever and pulmonary infiltrates, reported that, compared with standard treatment, PSV (Evita, Dräger, Lübeck, Germany) by means of a full face mask decreased the need for endotracheal intubation (odds ratio [OR], 0.26; 95 % CI, 0.08–0.85), shortened the ICU length of stay (mean difference −2; 95 % CI, −3.92 to −0.08), reduced the incidence of complications (OR, 0.24; 95 % CI, 0.07–0.82), and reduced in-hospital mortality (OR 0.24; 95 % CI, 0.07–0.82). However, NIV did not affect the duration of mechanical ventilation [1].

One of the major issues at present is the concern that submitting a patient to an ineffective NIV trial will result in more harm than if invasive ventilation is established immediately [8, 10]. Carrillo et al. [8] demonstrated in "de novo" CAP patients that increased duration of NIV before intubation for NIV failure was associated with decreased in-hospital survival (adjusted OR, 0.978; 95 % CI, 0.962–0.995, $p=0.012$) [8]. Survivors and nonsurvivors had comparable illness severity scores at baseline, thereby suggesting that the increased risk was directly related to postponing intubation after an ineffective NIV trial [8]. Interestingly, delayed intubation in patients with previous cardiac or pulmonary comorbidities did not increase mortality in the same study [8]. Similar results have been found in other studies, providing further evidence suggesting that intubation should not be delayed when patients are not doing well with NIV, because delaying intubation might result in worse outcome [2, 8].

The possibility of being able to predict an individual patient's response to NIV is of great importance to avoiding a delay in intubation after beginning a trial of NIV in patients with a high likelihood of failure. In the study by Carrillo et al. [8], variables independently associated with NIV failure in CAP patients were a worsening radiological infiltrate at 24 h after admission and a higher heart rate, lower PaO_2/FiO_2 ratio, and lower plasmatic level of bicarbonate after 1 h of NIV. In 2010, Carron et al. [10] reported the results of their study investigating various cardiorespiratory parameters as potential predictors of NIV failure. The study included 64 patients with severe CAP treated with PSV (Servo Ventilator 300A, MAQUET, Cinisello Balsamo, MI, Italy) delivered by means of a helmet [10]. Intubation was avoided in 44 % of these patients, and a successful NIV trial was associated with a shorter stay in the ICU and lower ICU and in-hospital mortality rates [10]. The group of patients requiring intubation had a higher Simplified Acute Physiology Score (SAPS) II at ICU admission and a lower arterial pH before starting NIV. After the 1st hour of treatment, patients who later required intubation had a lower arterial pH and PaO_2/FiO_2 ratio and a higher respiratory rate, $PaCO_2$, and oxygenation index (OI; calculated as the mean airway pressure x $FiO_2 \times 100/PaO_2$) [10]. The only variables independently associated with successful of NIV were a post-trial-to-pretrial increase in PaO_2/FiO_2 ratio of >42.2 and decrease of OI of >1.2 [10]. In a review article, Nava et al. [2] noted that the predictors of NIV failure differed in hypercapnic and hypoxemic ARF. In patients with hypercapnic ARF, the predictors were an unchanged or worsening arterial pH, no change or an increase in respiratory rate after 1–2 h of NIV, a higher illness severity at admission (SAPS II >34), and low patient compliance [2]. Predictors for failure in patients with hypoxemic ARF were minimum improvement in PaO_2/FiO_2 ratio after 1–2 h of NIV, age >40 years, higher illness severity at admission, and the presence of ARDS or multiorgan system failure [2].

Conclusion

The goal of using NIV is to overcome the acute illness without the need of endotracheal intubation, thereby leading to a reduction in morbidity and mortality related to invasive mechanical ventilation [3]. The most frequent causes of death in patients with ARF – septic shock and multiple organ failure – have been specifically attributed to complications associated with invasive mechanical ventilation [4].

Although evidence of its effectiveness from clinical studies is still not conclusive, there has been a steady increase in the use of NIV for the treatment of severe CAP in recent years. Whenever NIV is considered beneficial, it is suggested to apply it as soon as possible and after rigorous selection of appropriate patients, timely application of a proper ventilation interface, judicious use of sedation, and continuous monitoring of patients and predictors of NIV failure by a skilled care team (Table 49.1). The immediate availability of a means to perform endotracheal intubation is mandatory to avoid unnecessary and dangerous delays, especially in patients with factors predictive of NIV failure or those who fail to achieve previously chosen targets (i.e., adequate oxygenation, dyspnea relief, and patient comfort).

Table 49.1 Criteria for selection of patients and for management of a trial of NIV in case of severe CAP

Criteria for NIV trial (1–2 h)	Application of NIV	Success/failure predictors of NIV trial
Increased dyspnea at rest	Explain technique to patient	Success
Deterioration of gas exchange (PaO_2/FiO_2 <300, $PaCO_2$ >45 mmHg, pH <7.35)	Choose correct interface	Increase of arterial oxygenation
Respiratory rate >24 breaths per minute	Select the proper ventilatory support (i.e., PS 8–10 mmHg and PEEP 4–5 mmHg in case of PSV)	Decrease in respiratory rate
Increased work of breathing, accessory muscle use, and/or paradoxical abdominal motion	Set FiO_2 aiming for SaO_2 >90 %	Decrease of dyspnea
Absence of contraindication(s) to NIV (respiratory arrest, agitated or uncooperative and/or medically unstable patient, inability to protect airway or excessive secretions not managed by secretion clearance techniques, two or more organ failures).	Optimize patient comfort	Significant increase of PaO_2/FiO_2
	Minimize air leakage	Decrease of OI
	Consider mild sedation if patient is agitated	Absence of contraindication(s) to NIV
	Monitor comfort, dyspnea, respiratory rate, oxygen saturation, indices of NIV success/failure	Failure
		Stable or decrease of arterial oxygenation
		Stable or rise in respiratory rate
		Stable or increase of dyspnea
		Stable or decrease of PaO_2/FiO_2
		Stable or increase of OI
		Presence of contraindication(s) to NIV

NIV noninvasive ventilation, *FiO_2* fraction inspired oxygen, *PaO_2* partial arterial oxygen pressure, *$PaCO_2$* partial arterial carbon dioxide pressure, *PS* pressure support, *PEEP* positive end-expiratory pressure, *PSV* pressure support ventilation, *SaO_2* arterial oxygen saturation, *OI* oxygenation index

Key Major Recommendations

- Invasive mechanical ventilation represents a cornerstone for the treatment of ARF due to severe CAP.
- NIV may be used with caution in selected and strictly monitored patients with severe CAP, particularly in those with a history of cardiac or pulmonary disease or who are immunodepressed.
- Predicting success or failure of NIV may reduce the risks of a delayed intubation in patients with severe CAP.

Conflict of Interest Disclosure The authors have no interests to disclose.

References

1. Zhang Y, Fang C, Dong BR, et al. Oxygen therapy for pneumonia in adults. Cochrane Database Syst Rev. 2012;3:CD006607.
2. Nava S, Hill N. Non-invasive ventilation in acute respiratory failure. Lancet. 2009;374:250–9.
3. Ferrer M, Torres A. Noninvasive ventilation for acute respiratory failure. Curr Opin Crit Care. 2015;21:1–6.
4. Ferrer M, Esquinas A, Leon M, et al. Noninvasive ventilation in severe hypoxemic respiratory failure: a randomized clinical trial. Am J Respir Crit Care Med. 2003;168:1438–44.
5. Brambilla AM, Aliberti S, Prina E, et al. Helmet CPAP vs. oxygen therapy in severe hypoxemic respiratory failure due to pneumonia. Intensive Care Med. 2014;40:942–9.
6. Cosentini R, Brambilla AM, Aliberti S, et al. Helmet continuous positive airway pressure vs oxygen therapy to improve oxygenation in community-acquired pneumonia: a randomized, controlled trial. Chest. 2010;138:114–20.
7. Confalonieri M, Potena A, Carbone G, et al. Acute respiratory failure in patients with severe community-acquired pneumonia. A prospective randomized evaluation of noninvasive ventilation. Am J Respir Crit Care Med. 1999;160:1585–91.
8. Carrillo A, Gonzalez-Diaz G, Ferrer M, et al. Non-invasive ventilation in community-acquired pneumonia and severe acute respiratory failure. Intensive Care Med. 2012;38:458–66.
9. Squadrone V, Massaia M, Bruno B, et al. Early CPAP prevents evolution of acute lung injury in patients with hematologic malignancy. Intensive Care Med. 2010;36:1666–74.
10. Carron M, Freo U, Zorzi M, et al. Predictors of failure of noninvasive ventilation in patients with severe community-acquired pneumonia. J Crit Care. 2010;25:540.e9–14.

Noninvasive Ventilation in Acute Respiratory Distress Syndrome

50

Seval Urkmez and Yalim Dikmen

Contents

Abbreviations

ARDS	Acute respiratory distress syndrome
ARF	Acute respiratory failure
CPAP	Continuous positive airway pressure
EACC	European-American Consensus Conference
NPPV	Noninvasive positive pressure ventilation
PaO_2/FiO_2	Ratio of arterial oxygen tension to fractional inspired oxygen concentration
PEEP	Positive end-expiratory pressure
PSV	Pressure support ventilation

S. Urkmez • Y. Dikmen (✉)
Department of Anesthesiology and Reanimation, Cerrahpasa Medical School, Istanbul University, Istanbul, Turkey
e-mail: sevalurkmez@yahoo.com; ydikmen@istanbul.edu.tr

A.M. Esquinas (ed.), *Noninvasive Mechanical Ventilation: Theory, Equipment, and Clinical Applications*, DOI 10.1007/978-3-319-21653-9_50

50.1 Introduction

Acute respiratory distress syndrome (ARDS) is a syndrome of diffuse lung injury that is characterized by acute dyspnea and tachypnea, severe hypoxemia, bilateral opacities on the chest X-ray, and decreased respiratory compliance. The European-American Consensus Conference (EACC) suggested four clinical criteria for a uniform definition of ARDS. These are acute onset of hypoxemic respiratory failure (hypoxemia was defined as the ratio of arterial oxygen tension to fractional inspired oxygen concentration (PaO_2/FiO_2) below 300 for acute lung injury and below 200 for ARDS), bilateral infiltrations in chest X-ray, pulmonary capillary wedge pressure below 18 mmHg, and the absence of clinical symptoms of left atrial hypertension [1]. In 2011, an expert panel convened to update the EACC definitions of ARDS and the new Berlin definitions were proposed. These definitions make a classification of ARDS in three stages of severity, from mild to severe [2].

Whatever the definition is, the mainstay of treatment of ARDS is mechanical ventilation to improve gas exchange and decrease work of breathing. Moreover, the only evidence-based treatment in ARDS is mechanical ventilation using a lung-protective strategy with high positive end-expiratory pressure (PEEP) and low tidal volumes, which almost always necessitates endotracheal intubation [3]. However, recent efforts have been focused on the use of noninvasive positive pressure ventilation (NPPV) in acute respiratory failure (ARF) to avoid complications associated with intubation. The guidelines suggest use of NPPV in acute exacerbations of chronic obstructive pulmonary disease, cardiogenic pulmonary edema, postoperative patients, and immunosuppressed patients with strong evidence [4]. Use of NPPV in these settings improves outcomes, decreases length of stay in the intensive care unit and hospital, and lowers costs of hospitalization.

50.2 Discussion

The use of NPPV in hypoxemic ARF, especially in ARDS, is somewhat controversial. Early studies, which compared application of NPPV with standard therapy, yielded different success rates in different etiologies. For example, in the work of Antonelli et al. [5], the overall failure rate of NPPV was found to be 30 % in 354 patients, where the highest intubation rate was in ARDS and community-acquired pneumonia (50 and 51 %, respectively). Generally, in these studies, ARDS patients comprised only a small portion of the study patients; in the Antonelli et al. study, only 86 of 354 patients had ARDS. In another randomized controlled study from Ferrer et al. [6], 105 hypoxemic respiratory failure patients were randomized to receive either NIPPV or high-concentration oxygen therapy. In this study, most of the patients had pneumonia or cardiogenic lung edema. Only 7 patients in the NPPV group and 8 patients in high-concentration oxygen group had ARDS when they were recruited. Overall, NPPV decreased the need for endotracheal intubation and rate of septic shock occurrence and decreased mortality in hypoxemic respiratory failure, but the efficacy of NPPV in ARDS subgroup was poor, and ARDS was associated with increased need for endotracheal intubation. In their randomized study, Delclaux et al. [7] observed that use of continuous positive airway pressure (CPAP) was not effective in preventing endotracheal intubation when compared with standard oxygen therapy, although it resulted in a physiological improvement at the early stages.

Actually, there is a strong rationale for the use of NPPV in ARDS. Inflammation and edema in lung tissue collapse alveoli, decrease inflatable lung volume, and cause intrapulmonary shunting. Loss of surfactant function and functional residual capacity cause cyclic opening and closing of alveoli, leading to further lung injury, and increased elastance of the lungs increases work of breathing. Applying positive pressure to the airways increases lung volumes, improves alveolar stability, and decreases work of breathing [8, 9]. All of these may help to stop deterioration in respiratory function and avoid intubation.

On the other hand, in ARDS, the pressure levels needed to overcome alveolar collapse may be very high, which by itself necessitates endotracheal intubation for a firm connection with the ventilator. Indeed, it has been shown that presence of ARDS and inability to improve PaO_2/FiO_2 ratio were independent predictors of NPPV failure [5]. In the Berlin consensus meeting, the experts who evaluated the evidence on ARDS proposed NPPV as a matter of research in mild ARDS patients who have a PaO_2/FiO_2 ratio between 300 and 200 and need low to moderate levels of PEEP along with low tidal volume ventilation [2].

The suggestion from the Berlin meeting may be rather conservative. Given the lack of good-quality evidence, the need for further studies is obvious; however, there are some studies that show a good success rate of NPPV in ARDS patients with lower PaO_2/FiO_2 ratios. For instance, another study from Antonelli et al. [10] showed that endotracheal intubation could be avoided in 54 % of ARDS patients in a multiple center survey. In this study, 174 patients who fulfilled the EACC criteria for ARDS were treated with NPPV as a first-line treatment. These patients had a mean initial PaO_2/FiO_2 ratio below 120. The success rate of this study contradicts the findings in the meta-analysis of Agarwall et al. [11]. In this meta-analysis of three studies, the authors concluded that the addition of NPPV to standard treatment had no effect on avoidance of endotracheal intubation and intensive care unit (ICU) mortality, and the use of NPPV in ARDS could not be suggested. One important fact regarding the trial by Antonelli et al. is that the centers that applied NPPV to the ARDS patients as initial therapy had considerable experience in NPPV applications. In a second meta-analysis, which included 13 studies (540 patients), Agarwal et al. [12] observed that endotracheal intubation could be avoided in 52 % patients, and NPPV could be used with strict caution in ARDS patients.

These examples show that the use of NPPV in ARDS patients is still a controversial issue. Although a success rate of 50 % in this group of patients should be considered as a strong signal for the use of NPPV as an initial treatment, several problems like patient selection, selection of interface and ventilator mode, and signs of the need for intubation should be kept in mind.

Because ARDS is a syndrome that affects heterogeneous patient populations, contraindications of NPPV should be kept in mind [13]. These patients may have other organ failures and/or hemodynamic instability, and delays in intubation may cause excessive mortality, which is why the clinician should be cautious when initiating NPPV treatment. Current knowledge prevents using NPPV in patients with severe ARDS (PaO_2/FiO_2 <100). In moderate ARDS, patients should be monitored carefully and intubated at the first instance when needed. For this reason, admitting patients to the ICU would be appropriate [12].

The aims of NPPV treatment in ARDS are to improve gas exchange (PaO_2/FiO_2 ratio), relieve dyspnea, and decrease work of breathing. These can be achieved by choosing the right interface and ventilator mode for the patient. Unfortunately, no studies have addressed these issues, so the choice should be made depending on limited experience. In most of the studies investigating NPPV in acute hypoxemic respiratory failure, an oronasal mask was used as an interface. This has a physiologic rationale, as this type of interface minimizes leaks and permit use of higher airway pressures. Also, keeping the mouth in the mask increases effectiveness and gives the clinician an opportunity to use modes other than CPAP. In their study, Antonelli et al. [10] reported that they used either oronasal masks or helmets to provide noninvasive pressure support ventilation (PSV) with high PEEP. This can be an important practical approach to increase the success of NPPV. However, it should be kept in mind that helmets may require use of higher tidal volumes because some of the volume is needed to distend the helmet, and they may cause synchronization problems with the ventilator if the pressure or volume changes cannot be sensed by the ventilator.

It has been shown that the use of CPAP is generally ineffective in avoiding intubation in ARDS patients [7]. Although this application may increase PaO_2/FiO_2 ratio at the beginning it is ineffective in relieving dyspnea and decreasing work of breathing. Modes other than PSV of biphasic airway pressure are not studied in the ARDS setting.

Another issue is the choice of ventilator. As with modes of ventilation, there is no study comparing the effectiveness of noninvasive and intensive care ventilators. However, it is logical to use intensive care ventilators because these allow a higher control on FiO_2, better monitoring and alarm capabilities, and a wide range of modes to choose from.

Patients should be monitored carefully after the institution of NPPV for signs of failure and need for intubation. An experienced clinician, whether a nurse, respiratory therapist, or a physician, should be available at the bedside to assess the effectiveness of NPPV. The first hours of therapy are especially critical; it has been shown that a lack of improvement of PaO_2/FiO_2 ratio, dyspnea, and respiratory rate at the first hour predicts NPPV failure [5, 10].

Once started, application of ventilation support should be sustained for several days. Because these patients are severely hypoxemic, loss of lung volumes due to a loss in positive pressure cannot be tolerated. For this reason, leaks around the mask should be minimized at all times. If the patient does not show signs of NPPV failure and gas exchange improves, than NPPV can be applied intermittently. In their survey, Antonelli et al. [10] observed that in the patients who avoided intubation, continuous NPPV was applied for about 48 h. In this study, the patients who needed intubation were intubated within 48 h. The main determinants for intubation were Simplified Acute Physiologic Scale (SAPS) II score above 34 and PaO_2/FiO_2 ratio below 175 after 1 h of noninvasive ventilation.

Conclusion

NPPV can be the first treatment in mild and, to some extent, moderate ARDS. It can be omitted in patients with severe ARDS, where the PaO_2/FiO_2 levels are below 100 and the physiological condition is severe (high Acute Physiologic Score and Chronic Health Evaluation (APACHE) II or SAPS II scores). The clinician has to regard the risks and benefits of NPPV in all ARF, which are, if NPPV is successful, reduced rate of nosocomial infections, lower length of stay in the ICU, and lower mortality; and if NPPV fails is increased mortality, if intubation is delayed. Hypoxemic respiratory failure includes a diverse group of patients with various etiologic factors, and ARDS can be considered the most severe form of this clinical condition.

The evidence supporting use of NPPV in ARDS is quite weak, and it can be suggested that it is contraindicated in these patients. But, considering the benefits of NPPV, it should be tried early and as the first-line treatment at least in mild ARDS patients. The selection of interface and ventilator mode should aim to improve gas exchange by applying high airway pressures, and to alleviate dyspnea by application of pressure support during inspiration. During NPPV application, patients should be monitored closely for worsening gas exchange and physiologic status and gas leaks around the mask. When there is no improvement in patients during the first hours of NPPV, the clinician should not hesitate to intubate the patient. When NPPV is considered successful, it should be applied continuously for at least 24 h. The airway pressures should be titrated upwards by 2–3 cmH_2O increments in PEEP and pressure support level, and kept at the highest levels, which provide the best gas exchange and lowest leakage around the mask.

Key Points

- NPPV can be used in patients with mild and mild-to-moderate ARDS, but it should be employed in ICUs, where prompt endotracheal intubation and invasive mechanical ventilation are feasible.
- Patient selection is of the utmost importance in the success of NPPV in patients with ARDS.
- Patients with multiple organ failure, high severity scores, severe metabolic acidosis, or in shock should be intubated for invasive ventilation.
- Patients should be closely monitored for the signs of failure of NPPV in the first hours; patients with hemodynamic instability, without improvement in gas exchange or dyspnea, or who cannot tolerate NPPV through a mask should be intubated promptly.

References

1. Bernard GR, Artigas A, Brigham KL, et al. Report of the American-European Consensus Conference on ARDS: definitions, mechanism, relevant outcomes and clinical trial coordination. The Consensus Committee. Intensive Care Med. 1994;20:225–32.
2. Ferguson ND, Fan E, Camporota L, et al. The Berlin definition of ARDS: an expanded rationale, justification, and supplementary material. Intensive Care Med. 2012;38:1573–82.
3. Ventilation with lower tidal volumes as compared with traditional tidal volumes for acute lung injury and the acute respiratory distress syndrome. The Acute Respiratory Distress Syndrome Network. N Engl J Med. 2000;342:1301–8.
4. Keenan SP, Sinuff T, Burns KE, et al. Clinical practice guidelines for the use of noninvasive positive-pressure ventilation and noninvasive continuous positive airway pressure in the acute care setting. CMAJ. 2011;83:E195–214.
5. Antonelli M, Conti G, Moro ML, et al. Predictors of failure of noninvasive positive pressure ventilation in patients with acute hypoxemic respiratory failure: a multi-center study. Intensive Care Med. 2001;27:1718–28.
6. Ferrer M, Esquinas A, Leon M, et al. Noninvasive ventilation in severe hypoxemic respiratory failure: a randomized clinical trial. Am J Respir Crit Care Med. 2003;168:1438–44.
7. Delclaux C, L'Her E, Alberti C, et al. Treatment of acute hypoxemic nonhypercapnic respiratory insufficiency with continuous positive airway pressure delivered by a face mask: a randomized controlled trial. JAMA. 2000;284:2352–60.
8. L'Her E, Deye N, Lellouche F, et al. Physiologic effects of noninvasive ventilation during acute lung injury. Am J Respir Crit Care Med. 2005;172:1112–8.
9. Katz JA, Marks JD. Inspiratory work with and without continuous positive airway pressure in patients with acute respiratory failure. Anesthesiology. 1985;63:598–607.
10. Antonelli M, Conti G, Esquinas A, et al. A multiple-center survey on the use in clinical practice of noninvasive ventilation as a first-line intervention for acute respiratory distress syndrome. Crit Care Med. 2007;35:18–25.
11. Agarwal R, Reddy C, Aggarwal AN, Gupta D. Is there a role for noninvasive ventilation in acute respiratory distress syndrome? A meta-analysis. Respir Med. 2006;100:2235–8.
12. Agarwal R, Aggarwal AN, Gupta D. Role of noninvasive ventilation in acute lung injury/acute respiratory distress syndrome: a proportion meta-analysis. Respir Care. 2010;55:1653–60.
13. Organized jointly by the American Thoracic Society, the European Respiratory Society, the European Society of Intensive Care Medicine, and the Société de Réanimation de Langue Française, and approved by ATS Board of Directors, December 2000. International Consensus Conferences in Intensive Care Medicine: noninvasive positive pressure ventilation in acute Respiratory failure. Am J Respir Crit Care Med. 2001;163:283–91.

Noninvasive Mechanical Ventilation in Transfusion-Related Acute Lung Injury

51

Sami Alsolamy, Hasan M. Al-Dorzi, and Yaseen M. Arabi

Contents

Abbreviations

ALI	Acute lung injury
APACHE II	Acute Physiology and Chronic Health Evaluation II
ARDS	Acute respiratory distress syndrome
CPAP	Continuous positive airway pressure

S. Alsolamy, MD, MPH
Department of Emergency Medicine and Intensive Care Department, King Saud Bin Abdulaziz University for Health Sciences, Riyadh, Saudi Arabia
e-mail: SolamyS@ngha.med.sa

H.M. Al-Dorzi, MD
Intensive Care Department, King Saud Bin Abdulaziz University for Health Sciences, Riyadh, Saudi Arabia
e-mail: aldorzih@yahoo.com

Y.M. Arabi, MD, FCCP, FCCM (✉)
Intensive Care Department, College of Medicine, King Saud bin Abdulaziz University for Health Sciences, PO Box 22490, Mail code 1425, Riyadh 11426, Saudi Arabia
e-mail: yaseenarabi@yahoo.com

A.M. Esquinas (ed.), *Noninvasive Mechanical Ventilation: Theory, Equipment, and Clinical Applications*, DOI 10.1007/978-3-319-21653-9_51

FiO_2	Fraction of inspired oxygen
ICU	Intensive care unit
NIV	Noninvasive ventilation
PaO_2	Partial pressure of arterial oxygen
PEEP	Positive end-expiratory pressure
PSV	Pressure-support ventilation
SpO_2	Oxygen saturation
TACO	Transfusion-associated circulatory overload
TRALI	Transfusion-related acute lung injury

51.1 Introduction

Transfusion-related acute lung injury (TRALI) is a clinical syndrome associated with the transfusion of blood products. A rare and potentially fatal complication, it is reported to have a prevalence of 1 in 1,323–5,000 transfused units [1]. It is generally agreed that TRALI is underdiagnosed and underreported, meaning that its true incidence is unknown [2]. With growing awareness of the syndrome, however, reports of TRALI are increasing. TRALI occurs at similar rates in both sexes and in all age groups [3]. TRALI is estimated to occur in up to 8 % of critically ill patients who undergo blood transfusion [4].

51.2 Pathogenesis of TRALI

Although the pathogenesis of TRALI is not yet completely understood, a two-hit mechanism is the currently accepted theory. The first hit is the patient's condition, which causes neutrophil sequestration and priming in the lung microvasculature and an increase in the number of neutrophils within the pulmonary capillary vasculature [5, 6]. The second hit is related to trigger factors in transfused blood that activate neutrophils, resulting in damage to the pulmonary capillary endothelium [5].

51.3 Risk Factors

Risk factors for TRALI can be categorized as patient-specific or transfusion-specific (Table 51.1). Patient-specific risk factors include shock, chronic alcohol abuse, volume overload, smoking, mechanical ventilation with a high peak airway pressure, high interleukin-8 levels, liver transplantation, a high Acute Physiology and Chronic Health Evaluation (APACHE) II score, hematologic malignancy, sepsis, massive transfusion, and emergency coronary artery bypass grafting [4, 7]. Transfusion-specific risk factors include plasma from female donors or whole blood, increased quantities of cognate anti-human leukocyte antigen class II, and volume of anti-human neutrophil antigen in the blood [7]. In addition, increased numbers of transfusions are associated with increased risk of TRALI [4].

Table 51.1 Risk factors for TRALI

Patient-specific risk factors	Transfusion-specific risk factors
Shock	Plasma from female donors
Chronic alcohol abuse	Whole blood transfusion
Volume overload	High quantities of cognate anti-human leukocyte antigen class II
Smoking	High quantities of anti-human neutrophil antigen
High peak airway pressure in mechanically ventilated patients	Massive transfusion
High interleukin-8 levels	FFP or platelets
Liver transplantation	
High Acute Physiology and Chronic Health Evaluation (APACHE) II score	
Hematologic malignancy	
Sever sepsis	

FFP fresh-frozen plasma

51.4 Diagnosis and Clinical Manifestations

The clinical presentation of TRALI is variable. Symptoms and signs may include dyspnea, hypoxia, tachycardia, hypotension, fever, and pulmonary edema [8]. Chest radiography may show bilateral infiltrates. TRALI may occur during transfusion or within 6 h of transfusion [9]. TRALI can be classified as mild, moderate, or severe, depending on the immediacy of onset, the duration, and the degree of patient disability.

Large multinational collaborations, such as the National Heart Lung and Blood Institute Working Group on TRALI and the Canadian Consensus Conference on TRALI, have developed the following diagnostic criteria [8, 9]:

- New acute lung injury (ALI) during or within 6 h of transfusion.
- Hypoxemia defined as partial pressure of arterial oxygen (PaO_2)/fraction of inspired oxygen (FiO_2) $\leq$300 or oxygen saturation (SpO_2) <90 % of room air.
- No evidence of cardiogenic pulmonary edema.
- No preexisting ALI or acute respiratory distress syndrome (ARDS) before transfusion.

TRALI has been reported to occur later than 6 h after transfusion [10]. This has led other agencies and authors to extend the window for diagnosis to up to 24–72 h after transfusion [11]. Despite the presence of these diagnostic criteria, TRALI is frequently classified as possible, probable, or definite, depending on the temporal relationship to blood transfusion or coexisting alternative risk factors for ALI [8]. Additionally, it is sometimes difficult make a distinction between TRALI and transfusion-associated circulatory overload (TACO). TACO is a second type of lung injury related to blood transfusion. It is characterized by the rapid accumulation of fluid within the interstitial tissue of the lung, resulting from increased intravascular volume and increased hydrostatic pressure after blood transfusion [12]. The clinical presentation of TACO is similar to that of TRALI. However, patients with TACO show symptoms of venous overload, such as an elevated jugular venous pulse, hypertension, and elevated levels of B-type natriuretic peptide, which are not seen with TRALI [12].

51.5 Management

TRALI is a self-limited condition that generally lasts for 48–96 h and has a good prognosis [13]. Its treatment is usually supportive, including oxygen supplementation, but it frequently requires intensive care unit (ICU) admission [11]. The reported rates of requirement for mechanical ventilation are variable. In a study from Canada, Silliman et al. [1] found that only 3 % of TRALI patients required mechanical ventilation, whereas a surveillance program in the United Kingdom reported that 45 % of TRALI patients required mechanical ventilation [11]. In a series of 37 patients with TRALI, all patients required oxygen supplementation and 72 % required mechanical ventilation [14]. In a study of ICU patients who developed TRALI, 78 % of patients were treated with mechanical ventilation, the median duration of support being 3.6 days (interquartile range, 1.6–7.1 days) [1, 2].

51.6 Physiological Basis for Noninvasive Ventilation in TRALI

TRALI frequently results in acute hypoxemic respiratory failure. Noninvasive ventilation (NIV) has been established as a treatment modality for respiratory failure, with variable rates of success depending on the cause, severity, and patient characteristics. The beneficial physiological effects of NIV include reduced work of breathing, decreased inspiratory effort, increased dynamic lung compliance, increased tidal volume, improved pulmonary gas exchange, and improved arterial blood gas content [2–6].

51.7 Evidence for NIV Use in TRALI

The use of NIV in ARDS is controversial, as large and specific randomized controlled trials on this topic are lacking. Ferrer et al. randomized 105 patients with severe hypoxemic respiratory failure, 15 of whom had ARDS, to NIV or high O_2 [7, 8, 15]. NIV prevented intubation and was associated with better survival. However, in another study of 123 patients with acute hypoxemic respiratory failure, 102 had ARDS, NIV did not reduce intubation or mortality [7, 9]. A meta-analysis of six randomized controlled trials involving 227 patients concluded that early use of NIV can decrease the endotracheal intubation rate in patients with ALI, but does not change the mortality of these patients [2, 10, 12]. A more recent systematic review and meta-analysis evaluating the efficacy of NIV in non-chronic obstructive pulmonary disease and non-trauma patients with acute hypoxemic respiratory failure concluded that using NIV as adjunctive therapy in patients with heterogeneous causes of acute hypoxemic respiratory failure decreases the need for intubation, ICU length of stay, and mortality rate [10, 13]. However, the use of NIV in ARDS is associated with a failure rate as high as 83 %. In fact, ALI and ARDS have been found to be independent risk factors for NIV failure in patients with acute hypoxemic respiratory failure, together with age >40 years, a Simplified Acute Physiology Score II of > 35, and $PaO_2/FiO_2 < 146$ after 1 h of NIV [2, 11, 14, 16, 17].

Nevertheless, because TRALI usually represents a milder, self-limited form of ARDS and most patients recover within 48–96 h with supportive care [14, 16, 18], the outcome of TRALI patients with the use of NIV is expected to be different than the outcome of those who have ARDS from other causes. No clinical trials have yet investigated the role of NIV in TRALI. In a prospective cohort study investigating transfusion risk factors, of 74 patients who developed TRALI, 58 were treated with mechanical ventilation and 10 with NIV [2, 19]. In addition, a case of severe TRALI associated with myocardial stunning in a 14-year-old girl treated with NIV has been reported [20, 21]. The use of NIV in TACO has a potentially greater effect than it does in TRALI because of the similarity of TACO to cardiogenic pulmonary edema, in which NIV is the preferable initial mode of assisted ventilation. This is supported by evidence from meta-analyses reporting that NIV decreases in-hospital mortality in patients with cardiogenic pulmonary edema [16, 22].

The ventilation modes of NIV that are used in ALI include continuous positive airway pressure (CPAP) and pressure-support ventilation (PSV) combined with positive end-expiratory pressure (PEEP). Clinical data show that, compared with CPAP alone, PSV with PEEP performs better for inspiratory muscle unloading and improved dyspnea [6, 23].

Conclusions

The key to TRALI management is ventilation and oxygenation support. If NIV is applied early and restricted to selected patients with mild to moderate severity in whom the criteria for immediate intubation are absent, it can be safe for TRALI patients and can improve oxygenation and reduce invasive ventilation morbidity. Because clinical studies for the use of NIV in patients with TRALI are lacking, its routine use in these patients has not been clearly established.

Key Major Recommendations

- Transfusion-related ALI is a rare and potentially fatal complication associated with the transfusion of blood products.
- Ventilation and oxygenation support is key to TRALI management.
- The role of noninvasive ventilation in TRALI is not yet been established and is controversial.

References

1. Silliman CC, Boshkov LK, Mehdizadehkashi Z, et al. Transfusion-related acute lung injury: epidemiology and a prospective analysis of etiologic factors. Blood. 2003;101:454–62.
2. Gajic O, Rana R, Winters JL, et al. Transfusion-related acute lung injury in the critically ill: prospective nested case-control study. Am J Respir Crit Care Med. 2007;176:886–91.
3. Kopko PM, Marshall CS, MacKenzie MR, et al. Transfusion-related acute lung injury: report of a clinical look-back investigation. JAMA. 2002;287:1968–71.
4. Kallet RH, Diaz JV. The physiologic effects of noninvasive ventilation. Respir Care. 2009;54:102–15.
5. Holness L, Knippen MA, Simmons L, et al. Fatalities caused by TRALI. Transfus Med Rev. 2004;18:184–8.
6. L'Her E, Deye N, Lellouche F, et al. Physiologic effects of noninvasive ventilation during acute lung injury. Am J Respir Crit Care Med. 2005;172:1112–8.
7. Bux J, Sachs UJH. The pathogenesis of transfusion-related acute lung injury (TRALI). Br J Haematol. 2007;136:788–99.
8. Fung YL, Silliman CC. The role of neutrophils in the pathogenesis of transfusion-related acute lung injury. Transfus Med Rev. 2009;23:266–83.
9. Girou E, Schortgen F, Delclaux C, et al. Association of noninvasive ventilation with nosocomial infections and survival in critically ill patients. JAMA. 2000;284:2361–7.
10. Toy P, Gajic O, Bacchetti P, et al. Transfusion-related acute lung injury: incidence and risk factors. Blood. 2011;119:1757–67.
11. Antonelli M, Conti G, Moro M, et al. Predictors of failure of noninvasive positive pressure ventilation in patients with acute hypoxemic respiratory failure: a multi-center study. Intensive Care Med. 2001;27:1718–28.
12. Luo J, Wang M-Y, Zhu H, et al. Can non-invasive positive pressure ventilation prevent endotracheal intubation in acute lung injury/acute respiratory distress syndrome? A meta-analysis. Respirology. 2014;19:1149–57.
13. AlYami MA, AlAhmari MD, Alotaibi H, et al. Evaluation of efficacy of non-invasive ventilation in Non-COPD and non-trauma patients with acute hypoxemic respiratory failure: a systematic review and meta-analysis. Ann Thorac Med. 2015;10(1):16–24.
14. Toy P, Lowell C. TRALI – definition, mechanisms, incidence and clinical relevance. Best Pract Res Clin Anaesthesiol. 2007;21:183–93.
15. Ferrer M, Esquinas A, Leon M, et al. Noninvasive ventilation in severe hypoxemic respiratory failure: a randomized clinical trial. Am J Respir Crit Care Med. 2003;168:1438–44.
16. Kleinman S, Caulfield T, Chan P, et al. Toward an understanding of transfusion-related acute lung injury: statement of a consensus panel. Transfusion. 2004;44:1774–89.
17. Rana S, Jenad H, Gay PC, et al. Failure of non-invasive ventilation in patients with acute lung injury: observational cohort study. Crit Care. 2006;10:R79.
18. Barrett NA, Kam PCA. Transfusion-related acute lung injury: a literature review. Anaesthesia. 2006;61:777–85.
19. Moore SB. Transfusion-related acute lung injury (TRALI): clinical presentation, treatment, and prognosis. Crit Care Med. 2006;34:S114–7.
20. Chapman CE, Stainsby D, Jones H, et al. Ten years of hemovigilance reports of transfusion-related acute lung injury in the United Kingdom and the impact of preferential use of male donor plasma. Transfusion. 2009;49:440–52.
21. Piastra M, Luca E, Stival E, et al. Non-invasive ventilation for severe TRALI and myocardial stunning: report and literature review. Int J Hematol. 2012;96:390–4.
22. Weng C-L, Zhao Y-T, Liu Q-H, et al. Meta-analysis: noninvasive ventilation in acute cardiogenic pulmonary edema. Ann Intern Med. 2010;152:590–600.
23. Gajic O, Gropper MA, Hubmayr RD. Pulmonary edema after transfusion: how to differentiate transfusion-associated circulatory overload from transfusion-related acute lung injury. Crit Care Med. 2006;34:S109–13.

Noninvasive Ventilation in Patients with Blunt Chest Trauma: What Have We Learned? Key Response Determinants and Practical Implications

52

Abhijit Duggal and Tasnim Sinuff

Contents

Abbreviations

ARDS	Acute respiratory distress syndrome
COPD	Chronic obstructive pulmonary disease
CPAP	Continuous positive airway pressure
FiO_2	Fraction of inhaled oxygen
GCS	Glasgow Coma Scale

A. Duggal, MD, MPH, FACP (✉)
Department of Pulmonary, Allergy and Critical Care, Cleveland Clinic, Cleveland, OH, USA
e-mail: Duggala2@ccf.org

T. Sinuff, MD, PhD, FRCPC
Department of Critical Care Medicine, Sunnybrook Research Institute, Sunnybrook Health Sciences Centre, and Interdepartmental Division of Critical Care, University of Toronto, Toronto, ON, Canada
e-mail: taz.sinuff@sunnybrook.ca

A.M. Esquinas (ed.), *Noninvasive Mechanical Ventilation: Theory, Equipment, and Clinical Applications*, DOI 10.1007/978-3-319-21653-9_52

ICU	Intensive care unit
ISS	Injury severity score
NIV	Noninvasive ventilation
NPPV	Noninvasive positive pressure ventilation
PaO_2	Partial pressure of oxygen
PCA	Patient-controlled analgesia

52.1 Introduction

Chest trauma is associated with significant morbidity and is second to only head and spinal-cord injuries as a reason for trauma-associated mortality [1]. Outcomes are worse in the elderly and in patients with existing lung pathology [1, 2]. The most common injuries associated with chest trauma are rib fractures, flail chest (fracture of three or more ribs in two places or multiple rib fractures associated with sternal fracture), pulmonary contusions, pneumothorax, and hemothorax. Pulmonary contusions have been reported to be present in nearly 20 % of patients with multiple traumas [1–4].

Chest trauma causes parenchymal damage with direct lung injury and may also cause hemorrhage into the lung tissue. This causes significant dysfunction of the alveolar capillary barrier and increases the influx of extravascular lung water [3, 4]. Patients with chest trauma also have significant pain, excessive bronchial secretions, and a diminished cough reflex [5]. All of these factors can result in atelectasis and ventilation perfusion mismatch, resulting in significant hypoxemia [3, 5]. If this disruption of the alveolar–capillary barrier is not controlled, 20–30 % of patients with chest trauma will develop acute respiratory distress syndrome (ARDS) [5, 6]. The risk is highest within the first 72 h of the injury [3, 6]. ARDS in trauma patients is associated with significant mortality (16–29 %) and morbidity (increased intensive care and hospital lengths of stay) [3–6].

In modern medicine, trauma victims are evaluated using a multidisciplinary approach with management decisions made according to the mechanism of injury, anatomic involvement, and staging of the injury. The clinical significance of blunt chest trauma varies, depending on the size and location of the injury and the extent of the underlying lung contusion. Clinical management of less severely injured patients employs multimodal therapy but focuses primarily on the stabilization of fractures, pulmonary toilet, effective physiotherapy, and early and adequate pain control [4, 5, 7]. Patients with significant injuries, hemodynamic collapse, closed head injuries, significant flail chest or lung contusions, or those in immediate need for surgery undergo intubation and mechanical ventilation [3, 4].

The use of noninvasive ventilation (NIV) in blunt chest trauma is still controversial [4, 5, 7]. This is reflected in the "low grade recommendation" for the use of NIV in trauma patients by the British Thoracic Society guidelines compared with the "no recommendation" by the Canadian Critical Care Trials Group/Canadian Critical Care Society Noninvasive Ventilation Guidelines Group due to a lack of sufficient evidence [3, 5, 7]. Despite the lack of strong evidence to support the use of NIV in patients with blunt chest trauma, it has gained more prominence in the management of these patients. This may be attributed to its potential benefits versus harm, compared with mechanical ventilation.

In this chapter, we review the current evidence regarding the use of NIV for patients with blunt chest trauma and identify the patients who would benefit the most from this therapeutic modality. We also discuss the most appropriate time to implement NIV and the safety of its use for patients with blunt chest trauma.

52.2 Discussion

52.2.1 Pathophysiology of Lung Injury in Blunt Chest Trauma

The lung is exquisitely sensitive to compressive or concussive forces [1, 3, 4]. A sudden application of such forces results in parenchymal lacerations and damage to pulmonary alveolar blood vessels. Three mechanisms have been recognized in the etiology of pulmonary contusions: (i) the stripping of alveolar tissues from the hilum because of differential acceleration of the tissues, (ii) damage to the alveoli at the alveolar-arterial interface, and (iii) a direct concussive injury to the alveoli, associated with blunt chest trauma [3–5]. This mechanical injury to the lung results in intraparenchymal hemorrhage and significant edema formation. The direct mechanical damage to the lung parenchyma as well as additional indirect lung injury due to an inflammatory cascade results in the development of ARDS in these patients.

Animal studies have shown that, early in the course of blunt chest trauma, polymorphonuclear cells infiltrate lung tissue and release numerous cytotoxic products and further damage the alveolocapillary barrier [3, 4, 7]. This in turn results in increased permeability and accumulation of protein-rich alveolar and interstitial edema. Due to this inflammatory cascade and loss of alveolar surfactant, the airspaces are destabilized. This process is further complicated by the development of posttraumatic atelectasis, which results in significant ventilation-perfusion mismatch and hypoxemia refractory to supplemental oxygen. Atelectasis also interferes with the clearance of bacteria. The resultant lack of adequate clearance of these secretions associated with atelectrauma explains why patients with substantial chest injuries worsen 48–72 h after presentation [3, 5, 7].

52.2.2 Potential Benefits of Early Application of NIV

The benefits of *early* use of NIV in patients with blunt chest trauma are due to the avoidance of intubation and mechanical ventilation and its associated complications. Early identification of at-risk patients with prompt institution of NIV in appropriate patients may allow for the greatest benefit. Early initiation of NIV may offer the benefit of a wider and earlier use of ventilator support outside the intensive care unit (ICU), thereby limiting the development of atelectrauma and minimizing the risk of pneumonia [3–5]. NIV may also significantly lower the risk of ARDS because of its role in lung recruitment (i.e., limiting lung collapse).

Early use of NIV, through chest stabilization and lung recruitment, prevents the failure of spontaneous breathing and avoids the need for intubation. The use of NIV in chest trauma is associated with a significant and rapid improvement in the oxygenation and other physiologic variables. The improvement is more pronounced if the therapy is instituted earlier in the course of the disease, before the onset of respiratory failure [3, 7]. NIV increases the transpulmonary pressure, thus recruiting poorly ventilated atelectatic regions of the lung, decreases work of breathing, and improves gas exchange. These finding are similar to studies evaluating the use of NIV in acute cardiogenic pulmonary edema, acute exacerbation of chronic obstructive pulmonary disease (COPD), and acute respiratory failure [5–7].

The rate of failure of NIV in patients with blunt chest trauma who developed acute respiratory distress and respiratory failure is similar to the rates reported for any cause of acute hypoxemic respiratory failure [8]. In a prospective multicenter cohort study of hypoxemic patients after pulmonary contusion, the intubation rate was 18 %, which is significantly lower than the rates reported in patients with community-acquired pneumonia (50 %) and acute respiratory distress syndrome (51 %) [8].

52.2.3 Safety of the Use of NIV in Chest Trauma: Overview of the Literature

Four studies have compared the use of NIV with endotracheal intubation in patients with chest trauma [5, 7]. Three of these studies used continuous positive airway pressure (CPAP), and one study used noninvasive positive pressure ventilation (NPPV). Only two were randomized controlled trials [7]. Unfortunately, all these studies compared patients with less severe injuries who were treated with NIV, with those who suffered severe injuries or had decreased levels of consciousness requiring mechanical ventilation [7, 9, 10]. The differences in transfusion requirements of blood products were also not mentioned in any of the studies [7]. Bolliger et al. [9] developed the first randomized controlled trial to evaluate the use of CPAP compared with intubation and mechanical ventilation. Patients with significant chest trauma were randomly allocated to receive CPAP with either epidural or intercostal nerve for pain control or an endotracheal intubation with systemic analgesia. The NIV group had a shorter length of stay in the ICU and hospital. However, there were significant methodological flaws with the study, and the patients in the endotracheal intubation group had a higher incidence of major abdominal trauma and higher injury severity scores (ISS). Gunduz et al. [10] published the other trial and also reported no need for intubation in patients undergoing NIV and, more importantly, a lower mortality with the use of CPAP compared with endotracheal intubation in a randomized controlled trial (18 % vs 48 %, $p=0.001$). Although this is encouraging, the results have to be analyzed carefully as the researchers excluded patients undergoing emergent intubation after randomization for the study.

Hernandez et al. [11] randomized patients with chest trauma related hypoxemia to a high-flow oxygen mask or NIV. This trial included patients requiring oxygen by high-flow mask within the first 48 h after thoracic trauma with PaO_2/FiO_2 ratio ≤200 for ≥8 h. The utilization of co-interventions, such as epidurals and patient-controlled analgesia (PCA) for pain control, early chest physiotherapy, and need for surgical intervention, was also similar in both groups. The authors evaluated the need for intubation as their primary objective, and survival and length of hospital stay were secondary objectives. The use of NIV resulted in a significant difference in the rates of intubation ($P=0.02$) [11].

Endotracheal intubation in patients initially managed with NIV has been associated with decreased survival. Length of stay in ICU was lower in patients with NIV use compared with invasive mechanical ventilation [5, 7]. These results need to be assessed carefully as the trials were performed before the era of spontaneous breathing and awakening trials. Additionally, in all studies, ventilated patients received continuous sedation, whereas the NIV group received either epidural anesthesia or PCA (Table 52.1).

52.2.4 Approach to the Use of NIV in Chest Trauma

Given the available evidence, a reasonable approach would be to use NIV judiciously in patients with blunt chest trauma. The use of NIV can slow the progression of lung injury and prevent the need for intubation in select patients. This means appropriate selection of patients who may benefit, and a trial early in the course of

Table 52.1 Summary of randomized control trials on the use of NIV in blunt chest trauma

Study	Inclusion criteria	Control intervention	Pain control	Outcomes reported
Hernandez (2010) [11]	PaO_2/FiO_2 <200 for >8 h while receiving oxygen by high-flow mask	High-flow oxygen	Epidural analgesia (bupivacaine and fentanyl) Remifentanil infusion	Rates of intubation, mortality, length of stay in ICU and hospital, complications
Gunduz (2005) [10]	Flail chest; PaO_2/FiO_2 <300; Acute respiratory distress	Mechanical ventilation	Morphine patient Controlled analgesia	ICU mortality, ICU and hospital length of stay, infections
Bollinger (1990) [9]	Chest trauma with >3 rib fractures Insufficient cough mechanism	Mechanical ventilation	Lumbar epidural analgesia (buprenorphine) Intercostal nerve blocks	ICU mortality, length of stay in hospital and ICU, complications, and infections, ICU

PaO2 partial pressure of oxygen, *FiO2* fraction of inhaled oxygen, *ICU* intensive care unit

Table 52.2 Indications and contraindications to the use of NIV in chest trauma

Key indications for NIV in chest trauma
Hypoxemia (PaO_2/FiO_2 ratio 200–300)
Flail chest
Significant pulmonary contusion
Presence of underlying lung disease (e.g., COPD)
Contraindications to NIV in chest trauma
Absolute
Inability to protect airway
Significant facial trauma
Upper airway obstruction
Hemodynamic instability
Cardiac arrest
Need for major surgery
GCS <8
High risk for aspiration
ARDS (PaO_2/FiO_2 ratio <100)
Relative
Major multiorgan trauma
Encephalopathy (GCS 8–10)
Cardiac arrhythmias (if stabilized)
Pneumothorax (if chest tube already inserted)
Moderate ARDS (PaO_2/FiO_2 ratio 150–200)

PaO2 partial pressure of oxygen, *FiO2* fraction of inhaled oxygen, *GCS* Glasgow Coma Scale, *ARDS* acute respiratory distress syndrome, *COPD* chronic obstructive pulmonary disease

the injury and respiratory distress, prior to the development of ARDS and overt respiratory failure. The identification of patients for whom a trial of NIV would be appropriate is challenging, partly because there are few reliable selection criteria (Table 52.2). Because there is no clear threshold of severity for hypoxemia beyond which NIV is contraindicated, these decisions need to be made on an individual basis. Patients for whom a trial of NIV is initiated require close monitoring in the ICU, where endotracheal intubation is promptly available if they deteriorate any further. Although the optimal duration of the initial NIV trial remains uncertain, a reasonable expectation would be a response within 1–4 h of initiation. Patients who are failing an NIV trial should be promptly intubated and mechanically ventilated, as any delays in endotracheal intubation in patients managed with NIV have been associated with decreased survival [3–5, 7].

NIV should be avoided in patients with severe and worsening hypoxemia. It has been shown that many patients with blunt chest trauma deteriorate rapidly on the second or third posttraumatic day, and thus intubation and mechanical ventilation become necessary to ensure adequate oxygenation. In studies that compared the use of NIV with invasive mechanical ventilation, mortality was higher in patients undergoing invasive mechanical ventilation compared with NIV, but, of note, most patients died as a result of non-thoracic injuries rather than a direct result of respiratory failure [5, 7]. Hence, we need to acknowledge that the progression of respiratory failure may also be dependent on non- thoracic injuries and other factors such as transfusion-associated reactions. This reaffirms the need for proper patient selection and continuous close monitoring of patients being treated with NIV. Moreover, because these patients can deteriorate quickly, their respiratory and overall clinical status should be reassessed every 2–4 h when they are undergoing treatment with NIV. Although the use of NIV in patients with blunt chest trauma has a vital role in patients with significant injuries, its use should be limited to those patients who are relatively hemodynamically stable.

52.2.5 Late Application of NIV Does Not Benefit Patients

Failure of NIV has been reported primarily following the period after the initial stabilization of patients. Most of the safety data on the use of NIV derived from observational studies refers to its use within the first 48–72 h after trauma. Patients who develop hypoxemic failure *later* in the course of their hospitalization likely have other factors present, such as progression of lung contusions or the development of pneumonia or ARDS, which result in severe hypoxemia and respiratory distress. In trauma patients, the risk for intubation depends not only on the severity of the gas exchange impairment but also on the severity of trauma on the extension of lung contusion and on the hemodynamic status. Thus, for patients who do not respond to an early trial of NIV, NIV should be discontinued as soon as possible within the first 24 h and endotracheal intubation should be considered early to mitigate the potential for harm [3, 7].

52.2.6 Pain Management as an Important Adjunct to the Use of NIV

A major component of care for patients with blunt chest trauma is the need for adequate pain control. Unfortunately, this aspect of care for these patients is often overlooked. A close working relationship with the Anesthesia and Pain Control Service might improve the institution of NIV when a patient with blunt chest trauma is being evaluated. There is convincing evidence that the use of early epidurals, nerve blocks, or PCA pumps is associated with better outcomes in these patients [3, 7]. Judicious use of epidurals with good pain control, along with the use of NIV, prevents the progression of lung injury and ensures earlier discharge from ICU for these patients. In situations where epidurals are contraindicated or not possible, analgesia with nerve blocks and PCA should be considered [3, 4, 7].

52.2.7 Outcomes of Patients Managed with NIV

No significant morbidity has been associated with the appropriate use of NIV in patients with blunt chest trauma. Rates of nosocomial pneumonia range from 20 to 40 % of the patients, but these rates are comparable to all patients with significant lung contusions and blunt chest trauma [5, 7]. Prolonged use of NIV and a higher PEEP have been identified as risk factors for the development of nosocomial pneumonia, but these might be a surrogate marker for the severity of the lung contusion rather than the use of NIV itself [3, 5]. In most individuals with significant lung contusions, there is a higher risk of development of pneumothoraces, so there is a fear that the use of positive pressure ventilation has potential to cause or worsen pneumothorax [5, 7]. There were no differences in the rates of pneumothorax in patients undergoing NIV compared with patients who underwent standard medical management. Due to a lower physiological risk of barotrauma with the use of CPAP, it might be considered first in the treatment of patients with severe chest trauma [3, 5].

Conclusion

Ventilatory management in the trauma population is more challenging because of the difficulty in achieving a balance between the avoidance of further harm to the lungs and sufficient ventilation. Hence, selection of appropriate patients is crucial for optimizing NIV success rates and resource utilization. The *early* use of NIV is an effective and safe option for patients with blunt chest trauma who are neurologically intact, hemodynamically stable, and not in respiratory distress. NIV facilitates chest stabilization and promotes alveolar recruitment, significantly reducing the need for the intubation and progression of lung injury. But NIV is only effective if it is used in the appropriate population and integrated with other medical and/or surgical therapies. There is no apparent benefit of NIV in the prevention of intubation in patients with respiratory decompensation. In fact, delaying intubation in these patients leads to harm.

The use of NIV can be associated with a significant reduction in the incidence of overall complications, endotracheal intubation rate, length of intensive care unit stay, and mortality. Therefore, the role of NIV in managing respiratory insufficiency associated with trauma may become significant if applied to the properly selected patient at an earlier stage of lung injury by appropriately trained and experienced personnel. More research is required to determine the optimal role of NIV in blunt chest trauma. Future studies evaluating the use of NIV in blunt chest trauma need to be methodologically rigorous and identify patients early in the course of the disease.

Key Recommendations

- Noninvasive mechanical ventilation for blunt chest trauma should only be considered in patients who are neurologically intact, hemodynamically stable, and not in respiratory distress.
- The benefit of NIV is early in the course of blunt chest trauma, prior to the development of overt respiratory failure.
- There is no apparent benefit of NIV in the prevention of intubation in patients with respiratory decompensation. Late application of NIV does not benefit patients.
- Appropriate and early pain management is an important adjunct to the use of NIV in chest trauma.

References

1. Wanek S, Mayberry JC. Blunt thoracic trauma: flail chest, pulmonary contusion, and blast injury. Crit Care Clin. 2004;20:71–81.
2. Johnson JA, Cogbill TH, Winga ER. Determinants of outcome after pulmonary contusion. J Trauma. 1986;26:695–7.
3. Karcz MK, Papadakos PJ. Noninvasive ventilation in trauma. World J Crit Care Med. 2015;4(1):47–54.
4. Karmy-Jones R, Jurkovich GJ, Shatz DV. Management of traumatic lung injury: a Western Trauma Association Multicenter review. J Trauma. 2001;51:1049–53.
5. Chiumello D, Coppola S, Froio S, et al. Noninvasive ventilation in chest trauma: systematic review and meta-analysis. Intensive Care Med. 2013;39:1171–80.
6. Treggiari MM, Hudson LD, Martin DP, et al. Effect of acute lung injury and acute respiratory distress syndrome on outcome in critically ill trauma patients. Crit Care Med. 2004;32:327–31.
7. Duggal A, Perez P, Golan E, et al. Safety and efficacy of noninvasive ventilation in patients with blunt chest trauma: a systematic review. Crit Care. 2013;17:R142.
8. Antonelli M, Conti G, Moro ML, et al. Predictors of failure of noninvasive positive pressure ventilation in patients with acute hypoxemic respiratory failure: a multicenter study. Intensive Care Med. 2001;27:1718–28.
9. Bolliger CT, Van Eeden SF. Treatment of multiple rib fractures. Randomized controlled trial comparing ventilatory with nonventilatory management. Chest. 1990;97:943–8. doi:10.1378/chest.97.4.943. PMID:2182301.
10. Gunduz M, Unlugenc H, Ozalevli M, et al. A comparative study of continuous positive airway pressure (CPAP) and intermittent positive pressure ventilation (IPPV) in patients with flail chest. Emerg Med J. 2005;22:325–9. doi:10.1136/emj.2004.019786. PMID: 15843697.
11. Hernandez G, Fernandez R, Lopez-Reina P, et al. Noninvasive ventilation reduces intubation in chest trauma-related hypoxemia: a randomized clinical trial. Chest. 2010;137:74–80. doi:10.1378/chest.09-1114. PMID: 19749006.

Noninvasive Ventilation in Acute Respiratory Failure and Severe Neurological Deterioration

53

Andrés Carrillo, Antonia Lopez, and Pablo Bayoumy

Contents

53.1 Introduction

Both respiratory and central nervous systems are intimately interconnected through a delicate balance. Any disorder in this equilibrium can translate to devastating consequences for a patient. Respiratory dysfunction, either acute or chronic, can cause neurologic impairment [1], and the signs and symptoms observed in these patients can be caused by hypoxia and/or hypercapnia. The effects of hypoxia depend on factors such as severity, duration, and speed of onset. The hypoventilatory processes that produce retention of carbonic anhydride can cause alteration in mental status; nevertheless, patients who are able to

A. Carrillo (✉) • A. Lopez • P. Bayoumy
Intensive Care Medicine, Morales Meseguer Hospital, Avda. Marques de los Velez s/n. 30008, Murcia, Spain
e-mail: andres.carrillo@carm.es; almdosmiltres@gmail.com

A.M. Esquinas (ed.), *Noninvasive Mechanical Ventilation: Theory, Equipment, and Clinical Applications*, DOI 10.1007/978-3-319-21653-9_53

maintain a correct oxygenation, showing slight elevations in the partial pressure of CO_2, may not manifest signs and symptoms of neurological dysfunction. The clinical spectrum of neurologic impairment secondary to respiratory failure is known as hypercapnic encephalopathy syndrome [2], where patients with a wide variability of neuropsychiatric symptomatology are grouped. The point of maximum severity is the hypercapnic hypoxic coma, defined as the presence of coma, with a Glasgow Coma Score (GCS) of 8 or less, pH <7.20, and $PaCO_2$ >80 mmHg in an arterial gas analysis [3]. From the pathophysiological point of view, hypercapnic encephalopathy syndrome is a complex process, where respiratory alterations are combined (tissular hypoxia, a state of acidosis in the brain tissue, and cerebrospinal fluid increased by extreme CO_2 diffusion), but extrapulmonary processes also are involved (hemodynamic and renal) and even external factors such as inadequate oxygen therapy or use of depressant drugs of the central nervous system [2].

53.2 Neurological Dysfunction in Acute Respiratory Failure

The prevalence of neurological dysfunction in acute respiratory failure (ARF) is not well known. On an epidemiologic study, Carlucci et al. [4] found that the necessity for mechanical ventilation is produced by hypoxemic ARF in 48 % of cases, 15 % for acute-on-chronic respiratory failure (ACRF), 7 % for cardiac failure, and 30 % for coma. However, these authors did not specify the type of coma, and many cases were likely the result of organic or metabolic rather than respiratory causes. Corrado et al. [3] found 150 patients with hypercapnic coma out of a total of 1430 patients with acute-on-chronic respiratory failure, which is a prevalence of 10.4 %. In our intensive care unit between 1996 and 2013, we treated 3962 episodes of severe ARF with noninvasive ventilation (NIV); 988 (24.9 %) showed some degree of neurological impairment (GCS <15 points) and 256 patients (6.4 %) presented hypercapnic coma. More recently, we also found a decrease in the number of patients arriving at the hospital with impaired mental status. In fact, improved care of extra-hospital emergency services with the availability of NIV devices has improved the care of patients with respiratory failure significantly (no published data). Neurological impairment can occur with any etiology of respiratory failure, being more frequent in patients with ACRF, particularly in patients with chronic obstructive pulmonary disease (COPD) and obesity hypoventilation syndrome [5].

53.3 Assessment of Neurological Function in Patients with ARF

In numerous published articles, one of the variables analyzed in patients with ARF is their neurological situation at the onset of therapy or during it. Three scales have been mainly used for assessment of neurological status: the GCS [6], the

Kelly-Matthay scale [7], and the encephalopathy scale proposed by Brochard et al. [8]. In each paper, the authors use their own preferred scale, the Kelly-Matthay scale being the most used because of its simplicity and the ease of detecting small changes in mental status of mechanically ventilated patients. The Kelly-Matthay scale has also shown prognostic value in patients with neurological impairment treated with NIV [9]. However, none of these scales have been validated for measuring neurological changes induced by hypoxia-hypercapnia in patients with respiratory failure treated with NIV. The use of these tools is advised because some studies show that neurological impairment at the onset of the therapy is a predictive factor for ventilatory support failure, and mainly because evolution of neurological impairment during the first hours of NIV application predicts much better the success or failure of therapy [5].

53.4 Which Is the Treatment of Choice for Patients with ARF and Neurological Impairment?

Classically, the treatment of ARF has been based on the utilization of oxygen therapy and the etiological treatment of the respiratory process. When this initial approach fails or the patient is in a severe situation, ventilatory support is started. More recently, NIV has been positioned as a first-line therapy in ARF, having shown its efficacy for decreasing endotracheal intubation and mortality in different types of patients with ARF [10].

Although severe encephalopathy (GCS <8–10 or a Kelly Mathay score >4 points) has been proposed as a possible contraindication to the use of NIV [11], some articles have shown its effectiveness in patients with altered state of consciousness or even coma secondary to respiratory failure. This discussion has been motivated by a number of reasons that have never been analyzed in *well-designed* studies. Controversy exists regarding the use of noninvasive mechanical ventilation in patients with severe alteration in level of consciousness, with arguments for and against its use. The main argument against the utilization of NIV is the impossibility of isolation and protection of the airway, which for years has been considered an indication for endotracheal intubation [12], to prevent a possible pneumonitis for gastric fluid aspiration, which at the same time is favored by the existence of positive pressure in an airway not isolated from the digestive tract. Furthermore, a deteriorating level of consciousness decreases the effectiveness of cough and respiratory secretions removal, worsening suitable airway clearance. Finally, it has also been argued that patients with altered mental status due to respiratory failure cannot properly cooperate and the application of NIV is therefore more likely to fail. For proponents of these arguments, the presence of impaired consciousness at baseline and during early hours of NIV therapy is a risk factor for failure [13]. However, other studies do not show this relationship, or, because of their focus on complications do not detect improvements [14] and conclude that the risk of complications related to a low level of consciousness is overestimated in patients with NIV.

53.5 Effectiveness of NIV in Treatment of ARF with Severe Neurological Dysfunction

The controversy about the use of NIV in patients with severe neurological impairment due to ARF has been ongoing for years. Different case series or case-control methodology studies have attempted to clarify this issue.

53.5.1 Cases Series

The first major *series* of patients with neurological impairment secondary to ARF treated with NIV was published by Benhamou et al. [15]. This is a study of 30 elderly patients with ACRF treated with NIV by nasal mask. Six patients had a normal neurological status, 5 were agitated, 4 were confused, 12 experienced drowsiness, and 3 patients were in coma. Patients with normal consciousness had a failure rate of 33.3 %, 25 % failure was observed in patients with drowsiness, 33.3 % in comatose patients, 80 % in agitated patients, and 50 % in confused patients. NIV-related complications were common, 5 patients had conjunctivitis, 5 had intolerance, 3 had skin lesions, and 3 experienced atelectasis.

A few years later, a retrospective series of 15 patients with neuromuscular disease and acute respiratory failure, secondary to respiratory infection or heart failure, was published [16]. All of the patients presented hypoxia and hypercapnia at admission. The mean score on the GCS was 10.7 ± 3.6 points. Five patients (33.3 %) had hypercapnic-hypoxic coma (GCS 6.4 ± 2.1 points) and 5 others obnubilation (GCS 11.8 ± 0.4 points). All patients were treated with NIV with negative pressure. Therapy was effective in 12 of 15 patients (80 %).

Corrado et al. [3] retrospectively analyzed 150 patients in hypercapnic coma, with different ACRF etiologies in hypoxic hypercapnic coma treated by "iron lung." A nasogastric tube and an oropharyngeal airway were placed in all patients. NIV failure was defined as the need for endotracheal intubation or death in the hospital. The mean arterial pH was 7.13 ± 0.3 and the $PaCO_2$ was 112 ± 21 mmHg. The median duration of NIV was 27 h, with rapid recovery of consciousness (median of 4 h). The treatment was successful in 105 patients (70 %), clearly relating NIV failure with consciousness level, between 100 % failure of NIV in patients with GCS 3 points, and 15 % of failure in patients with GCS 8 points. With regard to NIV-related complications, 5 patients (3.3 %) developed clinical and radiological findings suggesting aspiration pneumonia, but all were successfully treated without requiring intubation. Using multivariate analysis, the presence of GCS ≤6 and age ≥70 years were the only two variables associated with NIV failure.

Dueñas et al. [17] published a series of 13 patients with do-not-intubate orders, admitted to a conventional ward once ICU admission was ruled out, with severe hypercapnic encephalopathy (GCS ≤7). The mean age was 81 years and 10 patients were diagnosed with COPD. On admission, the mean arterial pH was 7.18 ± 0.11 and $PaCO_2$ was 92 ± 35 mmHg. Ventilatory therapy was applied by conventional ventilators, and the mean NIV length was 74 ± 19 h. The evolution showed a coma recovery in 78 % of patients within 48 h and 9 patients survived. Complications such as skin ulcerations on the bridge of the nose were recorded in the 23 % of cases and transient psychomotor agitation in 30 %, without the need to discontinue ventilatory therapy in any case.

Both positive and negative pressure noninvasive ventilation have been used in the same patients to minimize complications [18]. In a series of 152 patients with different ACRF etiologies, the initial treatment was performed with negative pressure NIV, switching the mode to positive pressure NIV in the presence of intolerance or complication. In this series of patients, 13 had hypercapnic coma, 11 of whom had an adequate response to the "iron lung," and they were discharged alive.

In a prospective series of 95 patients with hypercapnic coma of diverse etiology [5] treated with NIV, the success rate was 80 %, even slightly higher than patients with a higher level of consciousness (70 %). This apparent contradiction can be related to the prevalence of ACRF in the group of patients in coma. At the beginning of ventilatory therapy, the arterial pH value was 7.13 ± 0.06 and $PaCO_2$ was 99 ± 19. With the application of NIV, all physiological parameters, with the exception of respiratory frequency and systolic blood pressure, improved. The improvement of consciousness status after 1 h with NIV therapy is an independent predictor of NIV success, and this has repercussions for hospital survival [5]. Complications related to NIV in coma patients were skin and ocular lesions, 5 cases of abdominal distension, 3 cases of vomiting, and 1 pulmonary aspiration.

53.5.2 Case-Control Studies

Several studies with a case-control methodology have been published, which attempt to analyze the impact of positive pressure NIV in patients with neurological impairment secondary to respiratory failure.

Scala et al. [19] reported a study where patients with severe COPD were analyzed to assess the effectiveness of NIV according to different degrees of neurological involvement. Cases were patients with COPD exacerbation with neurological impairment, assessed by the Kelly-Matthay scale, divided into three groups: group I with slight neurological involvement (2 points on the Kelly-Matthay scale), group II with moderate neurological involvement (3 points), and group III with severe neurological involvement (>3 points). Controls were patients with 1 point on Kelly-Matthay scale. Variables used for matching cases and controls were age, gender, etiology of the COPD exacerbation, serum bicarbonate, severity of respiratory process, and the patient's number of comorbidities. At the NIV onset, pH was 7.31 in the control group, 7.28 in group I, 7.26 in group II, and 7.22 in group III. Median GCS score in these four groups had the values 15, 13, 11, and 7 respectively; the median duration of NIV was 55, 34, 34, and 41 h. The need for intubation was 15 % for the control group, 25 % for group I, 30 % for group II, and 45 % for group III. The number of patients with gastric distension was 1, 3, 4, and 7, respectively, and in all cases was completely reversible. There were no cases of gastric aspiration or nosocomial pneumonia, even though not all patients had a nasogastric tube.

Two years later, the same author published a new case-control study comparing patients with neurological impairment secondary to COPD acute exacerbation treated with NIV or conventional ventilation [20]. The cases were 20 patients with diagnosis of COPD exacerbation or who were decompensated by community-acquired pneumonia, with a score on the Kelly-Matthay scale between 3 and 5, treated with NIV. Controls were patients with a similar diagnosis admitted during the same period to the ICU, but treated with endotracheal intubation and conventional ventilation. Patients were matched by age, PaO_2/FiO_2, $PaCO_2$, basal pH, and Simplified Acute Physiology Score II (SAPS II). Arterial pH and mean $PaCO_2$ in NIV patients were 7.22 ± 0.02 and 88 ± 15 mmHg and in controls were 7.22 ± 0.05 and 90 ± 10 mmHg. Oxygen ratio and Kelly-Matthay score were similar in both groups. Consciousness level improved in NIV patients, after 2 h of therapy going from a mean of 3.4 ± 0.6 to 2.1 ± 0.8 points, and 1.6 ± 1.0 at 24 h. Length of NIV was 55.1 ± 81 h, and failed in 7 patients (35 %). The placement of a nasogastric tube was necessary in 3 patients due to gastric distension, and skin lesions were observed in 4 patients. No patient in the NIV group presented gastric aspiration or developed nosocomial pneumonia. Hospital mortality was 25 % in both groups.

More recently, Zhu et al. [21] reported a study of 43 patients with COPD and ACRF requiring NIV. Patients were divided into two groups according to the presence (22 patients) or absence (21 patients) of encephalopathy, defined as a GCS <10 points. Patients were matched by age, gender, smoking, evolution years of COPD, and previous hospitalization. A nasogastric tube was placed in patients with encephalopathy and in those controls in whom gastric distension was objectified. Arterial pH in both groups clearly differed: 7.18 ± 0.06 and 7.28 ± 0.07, respectively. NIV success and hospital mortality in the encephalopathy group were 72.7 and 13.6 %, whereas in the control group they were 68.2 and 14.3 %. Complications related to NIV were minor: 5 patients in the encephalopathy group and 4 in control group had gastric distension, with one bronchoaspiration in the first group that led to endotracheal intubation.

Briones et al. [22] published a study with 24 patients, 12 with severe COPD exacerbation who came to the emergency room with pH ≤7.25 and neurological impairment (GCS <8 points). The control group was selected among COPD patients requiring conventional mechanical ventilation. Patients were matched by Acute Physiology and Chronic Health Evaluation (APACHE) II, age, arterial pH, and GCS. The mean GCS score was 6.3 ± 1.5 points in the NIV group and 5.6 ± 1.3 in controls. Two patients with NIV required orotracheal intubation (16.6 %). Mortality was 33.3 % in the conventional ventilation group and 16.7 % in patients with NIV ($p = 0.01$). The only complications associated with NIV were nasal irritation in one patient and gastric distension in another.

Scala et al. [23] compared 15 patients with COPD decompensated by pneumonia with profuse respiratory secretions and encephalopathy. In all patients it was necessary to perform a bronchoscopy for bronchial toilet and they were treated with NIV or conventional mechanical ventilation. Patients were matched by blood gases, APACHE III, Kelly-Mathey scale, and severity of pneumonia. The mean arterial pH of patients was 7.27 in both groups, and the mean $PaCO_2$ was 76 and 78 mmHg in the noninvasive and invasive groups. Mean Kelly-Mathey scale scores were 3.4 and 3.2, respectively. Intubation avoidance was achieved in 80 % of NIV patients, and related complications were four cases of mild facial erythema (26.6 %) and no cases of pulmonary aspiration.

Finally, Briones et al. [24] designed a study comparing 11 patients with COPD and altered consciousness (GCS <10 points) treated with NIV in volume assured pressure support (AVAPS) mode with 11 other patients with exacerbated COPD treated with bi-level positive airway pressure. The AVAPS group had a faster improvement of consciousness level and arterial gas analysis.

Final conclusions of these studies were similar. From authors point of view, hypercapnic encephalopathy is not a contraindication for use of NIV, although it is expected an increase of failures in most severe forms. On the other hand, despite the commonly accepted, complications from noninvasive support are neither frequent nor severe. However, most published series have been submitted by teams with extensive experience in this ventilatory support, and it is difficult to know whether these results can be extrapolated to other groups with less experience.

53.6 Security of NIV in the Treatment of ARF with Severe Neurological Dysfunction

NIV security, applied to patients in hypercapnic coma, refers to the inherent risks of this ventilatory therapy, which may be exacerbated in patients with consciousness impairment. In fact, this is why hypercapnic coma has been considered as a contraindication for NIV use. However, when referring to complications related to the technique, the most important and those that can lead to a worsening of ARF (gastric distension, vomiting, aspiration, pneumothorax, pulmonary superinfection, and intolerance) are rare. The low number of severe complications arising from NIV could be related to the rapid improvement of consciousness of patients, which could give rise to a recovery of lung defense mechanisms. Moreover, a decrease in pressures used as the respiratory improvement occurs could minimize the risk of gastric distention, vomiting, bronchoaspiration, and respiratory nosocomial infection. Among patients in hypercapnic coma where NIV is applied successfully, mean recovery time of 15 points on the Glasgow Coma Scale was 4 h [5]. Scala et al. [20] showed an improvement in neurological status of more than 1 point on the a Kelly-Matthey scale in patients with severely impaired consciousness within 2 h of NIV onset. This rapid recovery when ventilation is effective explains the low number of complications in these patients.

Some measures have been proposed to reduce the risk of complications in these patients. Although some authors advocate the routine use of a nasogastric tube in an attempt to reduce gastric distension in comatose patients [21], others do not consider it necessary, because of the low prevalence of serious complications and the risk of increasing leaks and encouraging ventilator-patient asynchrony [5]. Although hypercapnic coma patients are not more difficult to treat than a conscious patient, some less severe forms of neurological dysfunction may hinder the application of ventilatory support. Agitation and lack of initial collaboration, or when the patient gradually recovers consciousness, are sometimes additional problems that may influence patient prognosis. Our initial recommendation is always to treat these problems with non-pharmacological measures: a caring nurse may ease patient distress, helping the patient to gain strength and motivation to tolerate NIV. In the same way, we advise applying different interfaces to minimize claustrophobia and discomfort, and likewise lower pressures, helping with patient collaboration and improving the probability of success. However, sometimes it is necessary to resort to pharmacological treatment to improve patient tolerance, although, traditionally, physicians have been reluctant to treat with medication that is potentially a depressant of consciousness in patients with NIV. We advocate its use in selected cases. In this sense, we prefer use opioids or benzodiazepines in punctual bolus, even though we also use, often successfully, continuous infusion of these drugs or other anesthetics such as propofol or dexmedetomidine at low doses, to achieve conscious sedation, which favors patient cooperation without increasing the risk of complications.

53.7 How to Ventilate a Patient with ARF and Severe Neurologic Dysfunction

Different studies published about NIV use in the treatment of the most severe forms of ARF show a wide variability in utilization protocols. There is near unanimity, however, regarding the use of a ventilation mode based on pressure support, using pressure support plus positive end-expiratory pressure (PEEP), or ventilation with a double level of pressure. Support pressure between 10 and 12 cm H_2O on a 5–6 cm H_2O PEEP seems an appropriate approach for ventilatory therapy onset. The clinical response, respiratory as well as neurological, and blood gas controls between 1 and 2 h mark the changes in respiratory parameters. Series that have addressed this issue show that levels of pressure support, or maximum inspiratory positive airway pressure (IPAP), required by coma patients are usually higher than those of patients with a better situation of consciousness. It is not recommended to exceed 25 cm H_2O pressure support or 30 cm H_2O IPAP. The rescue frequency on the ventilator is usually set between 12 and 16 breaths per minute, with a short rise time. It is advisable to continue with high pressures while the patient has not fully regained consciousness and does not present discomfort secondary to pressure/airflow. Once pH is normalized or nearly normalized, one can begin to reduce the pressure support of the ventilator. We suggest maintaining continuous NIV during the first 12–24 h of treatment. The weaning of NIV should be performed with a progressive decrease in IPAP or pressure support levels, especially if they had achieved high pressures for $PaCO_2$ normalization.

Conclusions

Application of NIV in patients with impaired consciousness and ARF should be restricted to sufficiently trained teams in these kinds of therapies, in a hospital area capable of close monitoring. The medical staff should be aware that the patient may suffer a sudden deterioration of respiratory status, requiring immediate endotracheal intubation. Only in patients with a do-not-intubate order can ventilatory therapy be used in a conventional ward; all other patients must be admitted to an intensive care or high-dependency unit. Regardless of treatment, a patient whose neurological status does not improve in the first 1–2 h with ventilatory therapy and medical treatment should be intubated to avoid unnecessary delays that could lead to increased patient risk.

Key Recommendations

- Patients with ARF with impaired consciousness can be treated with NIV.
- Severe complications such as abdominal distension, vomiting, and aspiration related to ventilatory support are rare.
- Treatment of patients with hypoxic hypercapnic coma must be performed by well-trained teams with extensive experience in NIV, as well as in hospital areas that allow close monitoring of patients.

References

1. Kirsch DB, Józefowicz RF. Neurologic complications of respiratory disease. Neurol Clin. 2002;20:247–64.
2. Scala R. Noninvasive ventilation in acute respiratory failure with altered consciousness syndrome: a bargain or an hazard? Minerva Anestesiol. 2013;79:1291–9.
3. Corrado A, De Paola E, Gorini M, et al. Intermittent negative pressure ventilation in the treatment of hypoxic hypercapnic coma in chronic respiratory insufficiency. Thorax. 1996;51:1077–82.
4. Carlucci A, Richard JC, Wysocki M, et al. Noninvasive versus conventional mechanical ventilation an epidemiologic survey. Am J Respir Crit Care Med. 2001;163:874–80.
5. Diaz GG, Alcaraz AC, Talavera JC, et al. Noninvasive positive-pressure ventilation to treat hypercapnic coma secondary to respiratory failure. Chest. 2005;127:952–60.
6. Teasdale G, Jennet B. Assessment of coma and impaired consciousness: a practical scale. Lancet. 1974;2:81–4.
7. Kelly BJ, Matthay HD. Prevalence and severity of neurological dysfunction in critically ill patients. Influence on need for continued mechanical ventilation. Chest. 1993;104:1818–24.
8. Brochard L, Mancebo J, Wysocki M, et al. Noninvasive ventilation for acute exacerbations of chronic obstructive pulmonary disease. N Engl J Med. 1995;333:817–22.
9. Scala R, Naldi M, Coniglio G, et al. Neurological evaluation in hypercapnic encephalopathy treated with non-invasive ventilation: comparison of two scores. Eur Respir J. 200; 30:262S–63S.
10. Cabrini L, Landoni G, Oriani A, et al. Noninvasive ventilation and survival in acute care settings: a comprehensive systematic review and metaanalysis of randomized controlled trials. Crit Care Med. 2015;43:880–8.
11. American Thoracic Society, European Respiratory Society, European Society of Intensive Care Medicine, Societè de Reanimation de Langue Francaise. International Consensus Conference in Intensive Care Medicine: noninvasive positive pressure ventilation in acute respiratory failure. Approved by the ATS Board of Directors, December 2000. Am J Respir Crit Care Med. 2001;163:283–91.
12. Pierson D. Indications for mechanical ventilation in adults with acute respiratory failure. Respir Care. 2002;47:249–62.

13. Lightowler JV, Elliott MW. Predicting the outcome from NIV for acute exacerbations of COPD. Thorax. 2000;55:815–6.
14. Honrubia T, García López FJ, Franco N, et al. Noninvasive vs conventional mechanical ventilation in acute respiratory failure: a multicenter, randomized controlled trial. Chest. 2005;128:3916–24.
15. Benhamou D, Girault C, Faure C, et al. Nasal mask ventilation in acute respiratory failure. Experience in elderly patients. Chest. 1992;102:912–7.
16. Corrado A, Gorini M, De Paola E. Alternative techniques for managing acute neuromuscular respiratory failure. Sem Neurol. 1995;15:84–9.
17. Dueñas-Pareja Y, López-Martín S, García-García J, et al. Ventilación no invasiva en pacientes con encefalopatía hipercápnica grave en una sala de hospitalización convencional. Arch Bronconeumol. 2002;38:372–5.
18. Todisco T, Baglioni S, Eslami A, et al. Treatment of acute exacerbations of chronic respiratory failure. Integrated use of negative pressure ventilation and noninvasive positive pressure ventilation. Chest. 2004;125:2217–23.
19. Scala R, Naldi M, Archinucci I, et al. Noninvasive positive pressure ventilation in patients with acute exacerbations of COPD and varying levels of consciousness. Chest. 2005; 128:1657–66.
20. Scala R, Nava S, Conti G, et al. Noninvasive versus conventional ventilation to treat hypercapnic encephalopathy in chronic obstructive pulmonary disease. Intensive Care Med. 2007; 33:2101–8.
21. Zhu GF, Zhang W, Zong H, et al. Effectiveness and safety of noninvasive positive-pressure ventilation for severe hypercapnic encephalopathy due to acute exacerbation of chronic obstructive pulmonary disease: a prospective case-control study. Chin Med J. 2007;120:2204–9.
22. Briones Claudet KH, Briones Claudet MH, Chung Sang Wong MA, et al. Noninvasive mechanical ventilation in patients with chronic obstructive pulmonary disease and severe hypercapnic neurological deterioration in the emergency room. Eur J Emerg Medicine. 2008;15:127–33.
23. Scala R, Naldi M, Maccari U. Early fiberoptic bronchoscopy during non-invasive ventilation in patients with decompensated chronic obstructive pulmonary disease due to community-acquired-pneumonia. Critical Care. 2010;14:R80.
24. Briones Claudett KH, Briones Claudett M, Chung Sang Wong M, et al. Noninvasive mechanical ventilation with average volume assured pressure support (AVAPS) in patients with chronic obstructive pulmonary disease and hypercapnic encephalopathy. BMC Pulm Med. 2013;13:12.

Noninvasive Ventilation in Cord Paralysis Diseases: Is It a Possible Safe Indication?

54

Sven Stieglitz

Contents

Abbreviations

COPD	Chronic obstructive pulmonary disease
FRC	Functional residual capacity
FVC	Forced vital capacity
NM	Nasal mask
OHS	Obesity hypoventilation syndrome
PEEP	Positive end-expiratory pressure
Pimax	Maximal inspiratory pressure
RV	Residual volume
VC	Vital capacity

S. Stieglitz, MD
Department of Pneumology and Cardiology, Petrus Hospital Wuppertal, Academic Teaching Hospital of the University of Duesseldorf, Carnaper Str. 48, Wuppertal 42283, Germany
e-mail: sven.stieglitz@cellitinnen.de

A.M. Esquinas (ed.), *Noninvasive Mechanical Ventilation: Theory, Equipment, and Clinical Applications*, DOI 10.1007/978-3-319-21653-9_54

54.1 Introduction

About three-quarters of the cases of patients with seriously impaired spinal cord function result from traumatic injuries. Epidural abscesses, tumors or metastatic lesions, vascular incidents, or syringomyelia are less common. Therefore, the onset of paralysis is usually sudden, whereas it may be subacute in the other circumstances [1]. A spinal cord injury leads to multiple nonrespiratory (severe depression; immobility; bradycardia; loss of bowel, bladder, and sexual function; decubiti; and infections) and respiratory diseases (respiratory muscle paralysis, impaired speaking and coughing).

The impairment depends on the level of injury. Traumatic spinal cord injury of the cervical spine and also of the upper thoracic spine can lead to respiratory insufficiency, often due to concomitant thorax trauma or lung contusion. The respiratory failure is often transient if the trauma is below C4. Nevertheless, injuries above C3 lead to nearly complete respiratory muscle paralysis. In this case, patients recruit the trapezius, platysma, mylohyoid, and sternohyoid muscles to assist the sternomastoid muscles with respiration [1]. The situation is further complicated when additional central alveolar hypoventilation occurs. The automatic control of breathing is disturbed by disrupting the reticulospinal pathways of the upper cervical cord (lesions ventrally located). Lesions located laterally preserve the automatic control but impair voluntary ventilation [1]. Studies examining the control of breathing inconsistently report a normal ventilatory response to carbon dioxide [2].

Above C6, the sympathetic innervation of the heart is interrupted, which leads to an increased vagal tone with bradycardia. This may lead to cardiac arrest during suction in intubated patients and sometimes a transient pacemaker is necessary. Depending on the level of spinal cord injury, peripheral paralysis of the arms, legs, or both will occur, followed later by spasticity.

In about 5 % of the cases, a syringomyelia above or below the initial lesion occurs within 6 months or after many years. This can result in a worsening of the neurological impairment [3].

The symptoms of upper spinal cord injury are dyspnea, which may be aggravated in the sitting position, due to paralysis of respiratory muscles. This also impairs coughing because the inspiratory phase of cough consists of a deep inspiration. Additionally, the expiratory muscles that contribute to cough are also paralyzed. Consequently, secretion plugging and development of atelectasis develop. For similar reasons, speech is impaired and patients speak in a low voice.

54.2 Discussion and Analysis

The respiratory mechanics of upper spinal cord injury may be regarded as a prototype of a neuromuscular disorder. Lung function shows a restrictive pattern with reduced vital capacity (VC) and total lung capacity (TLC). Patients typically develop rapid shallow breathing. There are limited data on lung function of spinal cord injuries above C4, but VC values of about 20 % of predicted normal may be measured. The absent tone of the chest wall muscles results in a reduction of the chest wall recoil pressure. If compliance is measured by esophageal catheter, the typical findings are a normal or even increased compliance but a markedly reduced transpulmonary pressure at TLC (Pel 100). C4-7 injury leads to a forced vital capacity (FVC) of 52 % and a maximal inspiratory pressure (Pimax) of 64 % predicted normal, whereas T3-12 injuries lead to a FVC of 69 % and a Pimax 79 % of predicted normal [1]. The body position has a considerably stronger influence on lung function compared with healthy subjects. Unlike normal subjects, patients with cervical cord transection have an increase in VC and Pimax and a decrease of RV and FRC when changing from the seated to the supine posture. In the sitting position, the diaphragm is pulled down by the abdomen, whereas in the supine position, the abdomen pushes the diaphragm upward [4]. Furthermore, the loss of the intercostal muscle function may move the upper rib cage paradoxically inwards during inspiration [5]. Spinal cord injuries between C3 and C8 usually do not lead to ventilatory failure. But respiratory failure may develop more often with comorbidities (e.g., chronic obstructive pulmonary disease (COPD), obesity, sleep apnea).

Patients suffering from acute respiratory insufficiency due to acute spinal trauma are usually intubated, followed by tracheostomy. Nevertheless, VC and the periods of spontaneously breathing may be reduced by tracheostomy due to diaphragm deconditioning, tube-induced airway secretions, hyperventilation causing hypocapnia, impaired ability to cough, and loss of glottis valving [6]. Furthermore, there are data indicating that patients who underwent tracheostomy after an acute spinal injury have an increased risk of airway complications compared with those who were intubated for 3–4 weeks with subsequent NIV after extubation [7]. An increase of VC after decannulation can be observed.

Nevertheless, a common long-term treatment for high-level quadriplegic patients with chronic respiratory failure is tracheostomy and invasive out-of-hospital ventilation. Long-term invasive ventilation has numerous complications that apply to the tracheostomy itself (e.g., tracheomalacia, tracheal stenosis, stomal enlargement with air leakage and tube migration, hemorrhage, and granulation formation) [8] as well to critical incidents due to the invasive ventilation (e.g., accidental disconnection and mucous plugging) [9]. This contributes to a mortality rate of 37 % in 3 years for spinal cord injured patients on tracheostomy [10].

Some aspects of spinal cord injury are important with regard to NIV. If the spinal injury leads to a paralysis of the hands and arms, the patient will not be able to apply the interface for NIV autonomously. Once NIV is started and the mask is fit to the face, the patient will be neither able to remove the mask nor to activate the nurse call system. Patients under these conditions require special attention by the treating doctors and nurses and modified nurse call systems are required. In this context, the use of a nasal mask is preferred because of the ability to allow some (and sometimes improved) speech, thereby enabling the patient to shout for help during critical incidents.

The impairment of the respiratory muscles is due to paralysis and not an increased load as in COPD or obesity hypoventilation syndrome (OHS). The time on NIV is often longer compared with other diseases and can exceed 20 h and even more. On the other hand, due to the reduced chest wall recoil pressure, patients with spinal cord injury do not require high inspiratory pressures. On the contrary, patients are often hyperventilated, which results in hypocapnia and electrolyte disturbance. The latter problem is even marked in invasive ventilation. Therefore, a more careful setting of the initial NIV parameters and monitoring of the patient are important in spinal cord injury.

The extensive time on NIV sometimes requires interfaces other than full face mask, and the use of a mouthpiece or a combination of different interfaces is common practice [8]. Using a mouthpiece usually requires NIV without PEEP and a volume-controlled mode. The alarm on the ventilator must be switched off. It must be ensured that the ventilator used does not turn off in a standby mode. Ventilators that fulfill these requirements usually require non-vented masks, which have to be considered when a dual mode is used. Establishing a daytime mode using a mouthpiece and a volume-controlled mode without PEEP (frequency set at zero) followed by a nighttime mode using a nasal mask with a pressure-controlled mode with PEEP is one possible way to establish NIV in spinal cord paralysis. Such a complex ventilator setting is facilitated by ventilators that allow the setting of two different modes that can be activated alternatively (Fig. 54.1).

Another serious problem with high-level quadriplegia is reduced effectiveness of coughing, which requires elimination techniques of bronchial secretions such as mechanically assisted coughing. This problem is not solved by intubation and invasive ventilation, and simple tracheal sucking does not avoid the occurrence of atelectasis. In this regard, NIV is superior to invasive ventilation, especially when using specialized techniques like "air stacking." Air stacking permits volitional sighing, shouting, and assisted coughing.

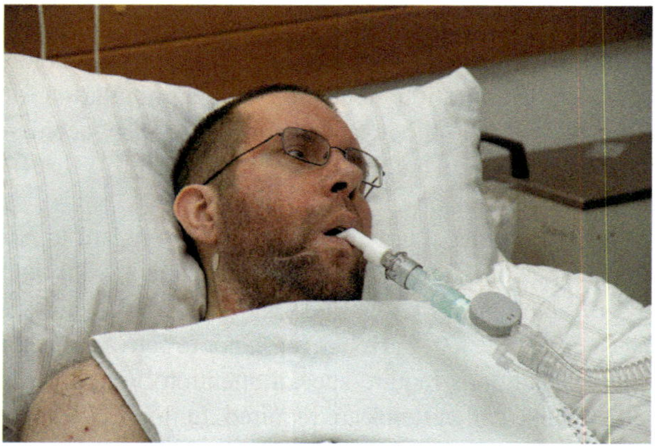

Fig. 54.1 Patient with tetraplegia using a mouthpiece during the day (volume-controlled ventilation with volume set at 500 ml, frequency 0, expiratory trigger off, inspiratory pressure sensitive) and a nasal mask (NM) during the night. The mouthpiece has an angle and a small rill so that the patient may hold the mouthpiece by their incisors. Compared with NM, the patient prefers the mouthpiece

An alternative treatment approach consists of electrophrenic nerve stimulation. For patients with no ventilator-free breathing ability or ability to grab a mouthpiece for noninvasive ventilation, electrophrenic pacing may be an alternative ventilator approach or may simplify decannulation [11]. Decannulation and establishing subsequent NIV is usually possible with patients who have a functioning bulbar musculature [12]. The ability of neck rotation may also be a decision-making aid in establishing NIV, because it simplifies the use of a mouthpiece for ventilation.

Compared with invasive ventilation, NIV improves quality of life, decreases nursing requirements and costs, improves the quality of speech [13], is more effective in coughing, and facilitates transition to the community. NIV also permits the ability of glossopharyngeal breathing, which is a safeguard in the event of ventilatory equipment failure.

Conclusion

Is NIV safe in spinal cord paralysis? There is clear evidence that NIV can be used in a safe manner in spinal cord paralysis. Actually, when neck rotation is possible and bulbar musculature is intact, NIV is superior compared with invasive ventilation concerning quality of life, nursing requirements and costs, effectiveness of coughing, and speech. The preferred devices for NIV adaptation are the nasal mask, nasal pillows, and the mouthpiece, whereas full face and total face masks should be avoided. Compared with other diseases leading to chronic hypercapnic failure (e.g., COPD, OHS), patients with spinal cord injury require longer time periods on NIV but a lower inspiratory pressure. Because hyperventilation is common, a more intensive monitoring after initiation and during the course of treatment is required. Additional problems of spinal cord paralysis, such as hypophonia and reduced effectiveness of coughing, may also be improved with NIV.

Key Major Recommendations

- NIV is the preferred approach to ventilation in patients with spinal cord injury.
- Special care has to be taken because of the patients' limb paralysis, which affects self-management of NIV and requires interfaces such as a mouthpiece.
- NIV in patients with spinal cord injury is characterized by long periods on NIV (often ≥20 h) but with low pressure settings due to the reduced elastic recoil of the chest wall.
- Because hyperventilation is common, special awareness of hypocapnia and electrolyte disturbance is necessary.
- Problems such as hypophonia and reduced effectiveness of coughing require solutions like secrete elimination techniques that have to be established alongside initiation of NIV.

References

1. Thomas K. Aldrich, Raymond Tso. The lungs and neuromuscular diseases. In: Mason JR, Courtney Broaddus V, Murray JF, Nadel JA, editors. Murray and Nadel's textbook of respiratory medicine, vol. 2. 4th ed. Philadelphia: Elsevier Saunders; 2000. p. 2283–310.
2. Stone DJ, Keltz H. The effect of respiratory muscle dysfunction on pulmonary function. Studies in patients with spinal cord injuries. Am Rev Respir Dis. 1963;88:621–9.
3. Biyani A, el Masry WS. Post-traumatic syringomyelia: a review of the literature. Paraplegia. 1994;32(11):723–31. doi:10.1038/sc.1994.117.
4. Estenne M, Ketelbant P, Primo G, Yernault JC. Human heart-lung transplantation: physiologic aspects of the denervated lung and post-transplant obliterative bronchiolitis. Am Rev Respir Dis. 1987;135(4):976–8.
5. Estenne M, De Troyer A. Relationship between respiratory muscle electromyogram and rib cage motion in tetraplegia. Am Rev Respir Dis. 1985;132(1):53–9.
6. Bach JR. Inappropriate weaning and late onset ventilatory failure of individuals with traumatic spinal cord injury. Paraplegia. 1993;31(7):430–8. doi:10.1038/sc.1993.72.
7. Fishburn MJ, Marino RJ, Ditunno Jr JF. Atelectasis and pneumonia in acute spinal cord injury. Arch Phys Med Rehabil. 1990;71(3):197–200.
8. Bach JR, Alba AS. Noninvasive options for ventilatory support of the traumatic high level quadriplegic patient. Chest. 1990;98(3):613–9.
9. Stieglitz S, George S, Priegnitz C, Hagmeyer L, Randerath W. Frequency and management of respiratory incidents in invasive home ventilation. Chron Respir Dis. 2013;10(3):135–40. doi:10.1177/1479972313493099.
10. Splaingard ML, Frates Jr RC, Harrison GM, Carter RE, Jefferson LS. Home positive-pressure ventilation. Twenty years' experience. Chest. 1983;84(4):376–82.
11. Bolikal P, Bach JR, Goncalves M. Electrophrenic pacing and decannulation for high-level spinal cord injury: a case series. J Spinal Cord Med. 2012;35(3):170–4. doi:10.1179/2045772311Y.0000000056.
12. Bach JR, Goncalves MR, Hamdani I, Winck JC. Extubation of patients with neuromuscular weakness: a new management paradigm. Chest. 2010;137(5):1033–9. doi:10.1378/chest.09-2144.
13. Toki A, Hanayama K, Ishikawa Y. Resolution of tracheostomy complications by decannulation and conversion to noninvasive management for a patient with high-level tetraplegia. Top Spinal Cord Inj Rehabil. 2012;18(2):193–6. doi:10.1310/sci1802-193.

Noninvasive Mechanical Ventilation in Older Patients

55

Cuneyt Salturk, Zuhal Karakurt, and Huriye Berk Takir

Contents

Abbreviations

ARF	Acute respiratory failure
COPD	Chronic obstructive pulmonary disease
CPAP	Continuous positive airway pressure
CRF	Chronic respiratory failure
DNI	Do-not-intubate order
ICU	Intensive care unit
NIMV	Noninvasive mechanical ventilation

C. Salturk, MD (✉) • Z. Karakurt, MD • H.B. Takir, MD
Respiratory Intensive Care Unit Clinic, Sureyyapasa Chest Diseases and Thoracic Surgery Teaching and Research Hospital, Istanbul 34732, Turkey
e-mail: csalturk@yahoo.com; zuhalkarakurt@hotmail.com; huriyeberk@yahoo.com

A.M. Esquinas (ed.), *Noninvasive Mechanical Ventilation: Theory, Equipment, and Clinical Applications*, DOI 10.1007/978-3-319-21653-9_55

55.1 Introduction

Prolonged human life has led to an increase in intensive care unit (ICU) admissions of older patients (>65 years). Older patients constitute 42–52 % of ICU admissions and 60 % of ICU days [1]. With limited ICU beds and an ever-increasing elderly population, physicians need to be aware of the differences in treatment and diagnoses of these patients, to provide the best care.

The incidence of acute respiratory failure (ARF) increases significantly with age [2]. Aggressive treatment of ARF, such as invasive mechanical ventilation, should be limited in these patients, especially those over 80, due to their low survival rate. Thus, noninvasive mechanical ventilation (NIMV) plays a crucial role in the treatment of ARF in these patients. As with the younger population, NIMV also decreases intubation and mortality rates in these patients with exacerbations of chronic obstructive pulmonary disease (COPD) and acute pulmonary edema. It also prevents post-extubation ARF [3]. In addition, NIMV is frequently recommended for the respiratory support of patients with a do-not-intubate (DNI) order as comfort palliative treatment [4].

The aim of this chapter is to define and elaborate the particular circumstances related to NIMV treatment indications, methods, recommendations, and outcomes in older patients.

55.2 Pathophysiology

Aging is a process that leads to a decrease in physiological reserves in the respiratory system, as well as in other organ systems. Loss of function in the respiratory system is due to changes, both in the chest wall and the lung [5]. Increased stiffness and consequent decreased compliance of the thoracic cage is caused by cartilage calcification, kyphosis, and vertebral collapse [5]. Reduction in respiratory muscle strength may cause a reduction in the strength of the diaphragm and accessory respiratory muscles, resulting in decreased maximal inspiratory and expiratory pressures [5]. Decreased elasticity with age causes the loss of supporting tissues around the small airways with a resulting increased tendency for airway closure at small volumes [5]. Thus, the smaller airways lead to less ventilation and ultimately a ventilation-perfusion mismatch. The ventilatory response to hypoxia and hypercapnia also decreases in the older population [5]. Decreased mucociliary clearance in older patients can also be a handicap for NIMV treatment [5].

NIMV improves many of the above-mentioned adverse changes. For instance, it corrects collapsed alveoli and ventilation-perfusion mismatch, and it facilitates reduction in work of breathing by applying positive end-expiratory pressure [6]. It also reduces the afterload in patients with acute cardiogenic pulmonary edema by increasing intrathoracic pressure. NIMV resets decreased carbon dioxide sensitivity of the ventilatory center [6]. It raises lung volume, improves lung compliance, and reduces dead space [6].

55.3 NIMV and Acute Respiratory Failure

The incidence of ARF increases with each decade until the age of 85 years [7]. In addition to physiological changes in the respiratory system with aging, comorbidities (cardiac, neurological, and infectious), the presence of acute illness (malnutrition, delirium), and prior respiratory disease may all predispose older patients to ARF [7]. Non-pulmonary causes of ARF are more common in older patients and these added complexities in the etiology lead to diagnostic difficulties. Nonspecific presentations and atypical manifestations also contribute to difficulties in diagnosis.

Ray et al. [8] prospectively evaluated 514 patients (mean age of 80 years) who presented with ARF to the emergency department. Congestive heart failure (43 %), pneumonia (35 %), COPD exacerbation (32 %), and acute pulmonary embolism (18 %) were the primary causes, whereas pneumothorax, lung cancer, severe sepsis, and acute asthma were less frequent (<5 %). The authors postulated that almost half of the patients admitted to the emergency department with ARF had a multiple diagnosis.

Age is one of the prognostic factors for ICU patients, however, it should not be considered as a criterion for the selection of patients in intensive care alone. Comorbidities, previous health, and the patient's functional status are more important when determining treatment options [9]. In older patients with ARF, NIMV should be considered the first choice of ventilatory support. It is more comfortable, has fewer complications, and has better short-term results compared with invasive mechanical ventilation [4].

After excluding upper airway obstruction, physicians should determine whether the respiratory failure is acute or subacute. If there is a subacute history of respiratory failure, NIMV treatment should be the first and consistent choice of treatment. If there is no subacute history of respiratory failure, the prior clinical status of the patient should be assessed. In the presence of a poor previous clinical status, palliative NIMV should be considered. In cases with good prior clinical status, treatment should focus on determining the etiology. Invasive mechanical ventilation may be the treatment of choice only when the etiology is known and after discussion with family or relatives.

The incidence of COPD increases with age, and, in addition, acute exacerbations become more frequent [9]. NIV is well tolerated and has a high success rate in older patients, even when disabilities or dementia are present. NIMV decreases the rate of endotracheal intubation, ventilator days, and ICU length of stay [10].

Chronic heart failure (CHF) is the most frequent cause of hospitalization in patients aged >65 years [11]. These patients usually present with acute pulmonary edema and ARF. In patients with CHF, continuous positive airway pressure (CPAP) reduces afterload and improves left ventricular function. It is considered the first line of care (at 0.98–1.23 kPa) in patients with acute pulmonary edema, but should be used with caution in patients with myocardial infarction [11]. NIMV may be used in cases of CPAP treatment failure or significant hypercapnia. Mehta et al. [12] compared CPAP and NIMV and found a speedier improvement in respiratory rate, hypercapnia, and dyspnea scores with NIMV, but also a higher rate of myocardial infarction. Studies conducted in recent years have shown that CPAP decreases mortality in patients with acute cardiogenic pulmonary edema [13].

The higher incidence of pneumonia in older patients is associated with the presence of COPD. The effect of NIMV treatment in patients with ARF caused by pneumonia is controversial. In a randomized clinical study, NIMV was associated with a decrease in respiratory rate and only those patients with ARF caused by pneumonia with preexisting COPD required intubation [14]. On the other hand, another study showed a >60 % intubation rate in patients with ARF secondary to pneumonia, without COPD [15]. NIMV should be considered in patients with adequate secretion control, and with the presence of COPD.

55.4 NIMV and Chronic Respiratory Failure

The success of NIMV has been proven in the long-term treatment of chronic respiratory failure (CRF) caused by chest wall disorders, neuromuscular diseases, and morbid obesity. It improves daytime gas exchange, quality of life, and length of hospital stay (16). On the other hand, results with the use of long-term NIMV therapy for obstructive diseases, mainly COPD, are controversial.

In older patients, chest wall disorders are the most frequent cause of restrictive CRF. Obesity, which is increasingly prevalent in all ages, is another important etiology. In elderly subjects with associated parenchymal diseases such as tuberculous sequelae, bronchiectasis is usually present. Age is not a restriction for long-term NIMV and indications for long-term NIV treatment for elderly patients do not differ from their younger counterparts.

Data on domiciliary NIMV in elderly patients are limited. Farrero et al. (17) studied 43 patients with chronic hypercapnic respiratory failure who began domiciliary ventilation at age 75 or above. The distribution of these patients according to their diagnosis was as follows: 11 (25%) had kyphoscoliosis, 14 (33 %) had post-tuberculosis sequelae, 9 (21 %) had neuromuscular disease, 8 (19 %) were hypoventilatory, and 1 (2 %) had bronchiectasis plus kyphosis. Their results showed the efficacy of NIMV in the elderly in terms of improved arterial blood gases and nocturnal desaturations, and a decrease in hospital admissions. Compliance was also good in this elderly population, that is, 8.3 (3.1) h/day, comparable to the general population.

Therefore, domiciliary NIMV treatment should be recommended in all patients who successfully pass the initial trial period, regardless of age.

55.5 Technical Aspects

A decrease in elastic recoil in elderly lungs causes an increased risk for barotrauma. Therefore, methods that preserve spontaneous ventilation are preferred in older patients with ARF. Pressure support ventilation is usually the first choice, but pressure controlled assisted ventilation may also be used. Facial masks covering the nose and mouth are the most efficient for NIMV due to ARF due to less leakage.

In the chronic setting, a ventilator should be easy to use, contain a battery, and be light and portable. Although there is no study showing clinical superiority, pressure preset ventilators are preferred to volume preset ventilators. Nasal masks are preferred for domiciliary NIMV, however, nasal pillows may sometimes be used for better local skin tolerance.

55.6 Palliative Use of NIMV

Management of ARF in very old patients (>80 years) may comprise lesser use of invasive ventilation and less admission to ICU due to their low survival rate compared with "younger" elderly patients (age < 80 years). Patients in this age group may be candidates for a DNI order. Refusing ICU admission is common among older patients, especially those with chronic respiratory disorders and cancer. Palliative use of NIMV in patients with a DNI order was first studied by Benhamou et al. [14]. They found that NIMV was successful in 60 % of these patients and well tolerated in 75 %. In another prospective study including 114 patients (aged > 63 years) with DNI orders, survival after hospital discharge was 72 % in the case of acute pulmonary edema, 52 % in COPD, and worse in patients with pneumonia or cancer [15]. The prognosis was heavily influenced by the underlying cause of respiratory failure, efficiency of cough, and mental status, and again by the initial selection of patients. Palliative NIMV is regularly performed in the ICU as well as in the medical wards and the emergency department. Indeed, because of the chronic shortage of ICU beds, NIMV may be better implemented outside ICU. Some hospitals have created special units to perform NIMV treatment. Vargas and colleagues [3] studied elderly DNI patients with ARF. They treated these patients with NIMV in a half-open geriatric ward with trained physicians and nurses. After 12 h of NIMV in the geriatric ward, 75 % of these patients were able to be discharged. Hospital mortality was related to the admission diagnosis and was especially high in cases of active end-stage cancer or hypoxemic respiratory failure.

Dyspnea is a common symptom in patients with terminal disease, and if the cause is irreversible it is called terminal dyspnea. NIMV is used to relieve dyspnea near the end of life. However, pharmacological treatment of dyspnea and anxiety should be at a maximum dose, both before and during the course of therapy. Note that realistic expectations about the purpose and effectiveness of treatment should be given to the relatives of the patient.

Conclusion

An increase in the elderly population has led to an increased frequency of admissions to hospitals and ICUs of older patients with respiratory failure. Avoiding invasive ventilation in these patients increases the frequency of NIMV treatment. In the acute setting, NIMV is preferred in the majority of cases, and the decision is based on the previous status of the patient and the level of comorbidities. CRF patients with restrictive respiratory failure are the most responsive to NIMV, although this is controversial when there is concomitant obstructive disease. NIMV is used for palliative therapy of ARF in patients with a DNI order as well as the palliative treatment of dyspnea.

Key Major Recommendations

- NIMV is well tolerated and has a high success rate in older patients with ARF resulting from COPD.
- Age is not a restriction for long-term NIMV, and domiciliary NIMV treatment should be recommended in all patients who successfully pass the initial trial period.
- Palliative use of NIMV in patients with a DNI order is recommended and the prognosis is heavily influenced by the underlying cause of respiratory failure.

References

1. Marik PE. Management of the critically ill geriatric patient. Crit Care Med. 2006;34(Suppl):176–82. Review.
2. Behrendt CE. Acute respiratory failure in the United States: incidence and 31-day survival. Chest. 2000;118(4):1100–5.
3. Vargas N, Vargas M, Galluccio V, et al. Non-invasive ventilation for very old patients with limitations to respiratory care in half-open geriatric ward: experience on a consecutive cohort of patients. Aging Clin Exp Res. 2014;26(6):615–23.
4. Nava S, Grassi M, Fanfulla F, et al. Non-invasive ventilation in elderly patients with acute hypercapnic respiratory failure: a randomized controlled trial. Age Ageing. 2011;40:444–50.
5. Rossi A, Ganassini A, Tantucci C, et al. Aging and the respiratory system. Aging. 1996;8:143–61.
6. Gay P, Patel A, Viggiano R, et al. Nocturnal nasal ventilation for treatment of patients with hypercapnic respiratory failure. Mayo Clin Proc. 1991;66:695–703.
7. Delerme S, Ray P. Acute respiratory failure in the elderly: diagnosis and prognosis. Age Ageing. 2008;37:251–7.
8. Ray P, Birolleau S, Lefort Y, et al. Acute respiratory failure in the elderly: etiology, emergency diagnosis and prognosis. Crit Care. 2006;10:R82.
9. Muir JF, Benhamou D, Molano C, et al. Noninvasive ventilation: a remedy for geriatric patients. ERS Monograph 43. 2009;19:286–306.
10. El Solh AA, Ramadan FH. Overview of respiratory failure in older adults. J Intensive Care Med. 2006;21:345–51.
11. Rasanen J, Heikkila J, Downs J, et al. Continuous positive airway pressure by face in acute cardiogenic pulmonary oedema. Am J Cardiol. 1985;55:296–300.
12. Mehta S, Jay G, Woolard RH, et al. Randomised, prospective trial of bilevel versus continuous airway pressure in acute pulmonary oedema. Crit Care Med. 1997;25:620–8.
13. Crane SD, Elliott MW, Gilligan P, et al. Randomized controlled comparison of continuous positive airways pressure, bilevel noninvasive ventilation, and standard treatment in emergency department patients with acute cardiogenic pulmonary oedema. Emerg Med J. 2004;21:155–61.
14. Benhamou D, Girault C, Faure C, et al. Nasal mask ventilation in acute respiratory failure. Experience in elderly patients. Chest. 1992;102:912–7.
15. Levy M, Tanios MA, Nelson D, et al. Outcomes of patients with do not intubate orders treated with noninvasive ventilation. Crit Care Med. 2004;32:2002–7.

Role of Noninvasive Mechanical Ventilation in Difficult Weaning

56

Inderpaul Singh Sehgal, Sahajal Dhooria, Ashutosh N. Aggarwal, and Ritesh Agarwal

Contents

I.S. Sehgal, MD, DM • S. Dhooria, MD, DM • A.N. Aggarwal, MD, DM, FCCP •
R. Agarwal, MD, DM, FCCP (✉)
Department of Pulmonary Medicine, Postgraduate Institute of Medical Education and Research, Chandigarh, India
e-mail: agarwal.ritesh@outlook.in

A.M. Esquinas (ed.), *Noninvasive Mechanical Ventilation: Theory, Equipment, and Clinical Applications*, DOI 10.1007/978-3-319-21653-9_56

56.1 Introduction

Mechanical ventilation is an essential part of the management of critically ill patients. It involves provision of positive pressure, either using invasive (endotracheal tube, tracheostomy) or noninvasive (oronasal or face mask) methods. The use of invasive mechanical ventilation is associated with several complications, both infectious (ventilator-associated pneumonia) and noninfectious (volutrauma, barotrauma, ventilator-induced diaphragmatic dysfunction, and others). Hence, in several situations, especially acute exacerbations of chronic obstructive pulmonary disease (COPD) and cardiogenic pulmonary edema, a trial of noninvasive ventilation (NIV) is preferred prior to intubation [1–6]. However, in some clinical circumstances, endotracheal intubation is inevitable [7–10]. Once the underlying respiratory illness starts recovering, the patient is ready to be weaned off the mechanical ventilatory support. Weaning is defined as a process that involves liberation of a person from mechanical ventilation and from the endotracheal/tracheostomy tube [11].

The management of a patient with respiratory failure comprises of a continuum of six steps [11]: (1) treatment of acute respiratory failure; (2) diagnosis of the probability of weaning; (3) assessment for weaning; (4) determination of the ability of a patient to breathe spontaneously through a spontaneous breathing trial (SBT); (5) removal of the endotracheal tube (extubation); and (6) reintubation, if the patient is unable to breathe spontaneously. Failure in identification of stage 2 and assessment of readiness to wean (stage 3) is considered the most important factor responsible for delay in weaning. Delay in weaning or prolonged mechanical ventilation has several adverse outcomes, including increased risk of ventilator-associated complications, and adds to the cost of management [12–14]. In this chapter, we review the role of NIV in weaning patients from invasive ventilation in critical care. We specifically look at the role of NIV in facilitating extubation in patients who fail SBT, without discussing the role of NIV in established post-extubation respiratory failure or the role of NIV in preventing reintubation in those with planned extubation (as a preemptive strategy for preventing reintubation) [15].

56.2 Definitions

56.2.1 Weaning Failure

Weaning failure is defined as either failure of SBT or need for reintubation or death within 48 h of extubation [11]. Failure of SBT is characterized by a combination of objective (respiratory rate >30 breaths/min, heart rate of >110 beats/min, hypotension, cardiac arrhythmias, hypoxemia, or acidosis) and subjective (agitation, altered mental status, diaphoresis, labored breathing, and others) parameters [7–9, 16–19].

56.2.2 Weaning in Progress

Weaning in progress is a term used to define an intermediate category of weaning process wherein the patient is liberated from invasive mechanical ventilation but needs the support of NIV to facilitate weaning [11]. Patients with difficult weaning have high morbidity and mortality up to 40 %. Patients with prolonged weaning usually require long-term ventilatory support, with only 50 % alive at 5 years [11].

56.2.3 Classification of Weaning

Weaning is classified into three categories [11]: (1) simple weaning is a condition in which the patient proceeds from initiation of weaning to successful extubation on the first attempt without difficulty; (2) difficult weaning is a condition in which the patient fails initial weaning and requires up to three SBTs or as many as 7 days from the first SBT to achieve successful weaning; (3) prolonged weaning is a condition in which the patient fails at least four weaning attempts or requires >7 days of weaning after the first SBT.

56.2.4 Criteria for Weaning

The decision to initiate the weaning process is a clinical art and requires a combination of certain criteria (Table 56.1) that need to be accomplished before applying weaning assessment methods.

56.3 Pathophysiology of Weaning Failure

Patients who face weaning difficulties usually develop rapid shallow breathing on liberation from positive pressure ventilation. This results in dynamic hyperinflation and development of intrinsic positive end-expiratory pressure (iPEEP) [6, 20, 21]. The iPEEP, along with high ventilatory demand, leads to an increase in the respiratory work of breathing and causes respiratory muscle fatigue, thus causing weaning failure. The increase in respiratory work of breathing is further compounded by cardiovascular responses associated with removal of positive pressure ventilation, leading to an increase in the venous return along with escalation in resistance to left ventricular outflow [22]. An inappropriate cardiovascular response, especially in those with compromised left ventricular function, further increases the load on already-burdened respiratory muscles [23].

Table 56.1 Criteria for readiness for weaning (combination of one or more of the following)

Subjective parameters
Resolution of the disease for which the patient needed ventilatory support
Good effective cough/ability to clear secretions
Absent or minimal tracheobronchial secretions
Clear sensorium/ no delirium
Absent or minimal neuromuscular weakness
Objective parameters
Respiratory rate ≤35/min
Heart rate ≤140/min
Resolution of hypotension or minimal need of vasopressors
SpO_2 >89 % on ≤ FiO_2 0.4 (or Pa_{O_2} / Fi_{O_2} ≥150mmHg)
PEEP ≤8 cmH_2O
Pa_{CO_2} ≤ 45mmHg
MIP ≤ −20 to −25 cmH_2O
V_T >5 ml/kg
RSBI <105 breaths/min/l

MIP maximum inspiratory pressure, *PEEP* positive end expiratory pressure, *RSBI* rapid shallow breathing index, *VT* tidal volume

56.4 Assessment Tools for Weaning

A weaning assessment tool should ideally be able to correctly identify all the individuals who can be safely liberated from the ventilator. Patients who meet the weaning criteria should be screened with one of the weaning assessment tools. The various weaning assessment tools include respiratory frequency-to-tidal volume ratio, maximum inspiratory pressure, integrative weaning index, diaphragm ultrasound, and others. The currently available methods for weaning assessment are far from perfect, thus creating a need for an ideal assessment tool.

56.4.1 Respiratory Frequency-to-Tidal Volume Ratio (f/V_T)

Also known as rapid shallow breathing index (RSBI), the f/V_T is measured during spontaneous breathing for 1 min. During spontaneous breathing, the ventilator is set at a pressure support of 0 cm of H_2O or continuous positive airway pressure (CPAP) of 0 cm H_2O. A RSBI of 100 discriminates between successful weaning and failure, with a value of <100 suggesting a successful weaning trial with a sensitivity of 0.97 and a specificity of 0.65 [24].

56.4.2 Diaphragm Ultrasonography

Mechanical ventilation can lead to rapidly progressive diaphragmatic weakness and may hinder weaning from ventilation [25]. Bedside ultrasound is a useful modality to assess the diaphragm function. In a single-center study involving mechanically ventilated patients, diaphragm dysfunction (excursion of <10 mm on M-mode) could be identified in 29 % patients by using bedside ultrasound. Presence of diaphragmatic dysfunction on ultrasound assessment was associated with prolonged weaning time (17 vs 4 days, $p<0.01$) and a longer time spent on mechanical ventilation (24 vs 9 days, $p<0.01$) [26].

56.4.3 Integrative Weaning Index

A prospective study assessed a combination of several factors (respiratory system compliance x arterial oxygen saturation/f/V_T ratio) to predict the weaning from mechanical ventilation. The Integrative Weaning Index (IWI) performed better than several other parameters, including RSBI, tidal volume (V_t), tracheal airway occlusion pressure in the first 0.1 s (P 0.1), the product of P 0.1 and f/V_t ($P\ 0.1 \times f/V_t$), respiratory rate (f), static compliance of the respiratory system (Cst), and ratio of arterial oxygen tension to fraction of inspired oxygen (PaO_2/FiO_2) with an area under the receiver-operating characteristic (ROC) curve of 0.96 [27].

56.5 Weaning Trials

Once the patient is assessed for weaning and is considered suitable for weaning, a weaning trial is instituted before extubation. An ideal weaning trial should be able to identify all the individuals who will successfully tolerate extubation. The weaning techniques that are used include SBT, automated tube compensation, pressure support ventilation (PSV), and synchronized intermittent mechanical ventilation (SIMV).

56.5.1 Spontaneous Breathing Trial

SBT is the oldest and most commonly employed method used for weaning [16]. It involves removing the patient from the ventilator and providing supplemental oxygen by using a T-piece or T-tube device or a pressure support of 5–8 cm of H_2O in adults [19, 28–30]. A pooled analysis of nine randomized trials comparing PSV SBT versus T-piece trial SBT did not find any difference between the methods or the pressure used in weaning success, intensive care unit (ICU) mortality, reintubation rate, length of stay in ICU or long-term weaning unit, and pneumonia [30]. However, PSV was more effective in predicting successful

SBT in patients with simple weaning compared with T-piece trial [19, 30]. A few studies have also used CPAP of 5 cm H_2O for SBT [30]. It is reasoned that provision of CPAP maintains functional residual capacity at a level similar to that following extubation. Further, CPAP also helps maintain the patency of small airways, especially in patients with COPD [31]. However, in patients with poor left ventricular function, provision of CPAP may falsely predict successful extubation [23].

56.5.2 Pressure Support Ventilation

PSV is another commonly used method for weaning. With PSV, all the breaths are patient triggered, flow cycled, and provide ventilatory support that is gradually reduced over time until patient is successfully liberated from mechanical ventilation. Both inspiratory positive airway pressure (IPAP) or pressure support and expiratory positive airway pressure (EPAP) or CPAP are reduced gradually by 1–2 cm of H_2O until an acceptable IPAP of 5–7 cm of H_2O and EPAP of 0–5 cm of H_2O is reached [19].

56.5.3 Synchronized Intermittent Mandatory Ventilation

With SIMV, ventilation is assisted intermittently either as mandatory or as spontaneous breaths. During the spontaneous mode there is no support to the respiratory muscle, which have an additional burden to overcome dead space due to ventilatory circuit [5, 32]. This increased burden leads to fatigue of respiratory muscles and hence weaning failure and increased need for invasive mechanical ventilation. Therefore, the use of SIMV as a mode for weaning is discouraged. SIMV can also be combined with PSV, where the spontaneous breaths are assisted by pressure support. However, even this mode is inferior as the respiratory center and respiratory muscles have to alter their output in anticipation of the next breath, which may either be mandatory or spontaneous. Moreover, it does not does not allow partitioning of the work of breathing performed by either the ventilator or the patient [5, 32–35].

56.6 Role of NIV in Weaning

Noninvasive ventilation has been used in three different scenarios for weaning: (i) advancing extubation in patients with difficult or prolonged weaning (weaning strategy); (ii) avoidance of reintubation after extubation in patients with post-extubation respiratory failure (management strategy); and (iii) to prevent development of post extubation respiratory failure (prophylactic strategy). Herein, we discuss only the weaning strategy.

56.6.1 Rationale of NIV in Weaning Failure

By reducing the work of breathing and preventing the development of the rapid shallow breathing pattern, NIV may be useful where weaning has failed. Further, EPAP akin to positive end-expiratory pressure acts as an external splint and helps in avoiding dynamic hyperinflation seen in patients with COPD. NIV by its favorable cardiovascular effects may also facilitate weaning [3, 4, 6, 15, 36, 37].

56.7 Role of NIV in Difficult/Prolonged Weaning (Weaning Strategy)

NIV has been tried in the management of acute respiratory failure as a strategy to shorten the weaning process and facilitate liberation from invasive mechanical ventilation, especially in patients with COPD [38–40]. The trial design in most studies involved patients who failed SBT; they were subsequently randomized to continued invasive ventilation or extubated and initiated on NIV. The results of nine randomized controlled trials (RCTs) evaluating the role of NIV in augmenting extubation are summarized in Tables 56.2 and 56.3. Of the nine studies identified, three studies included patients with acute exacerbation of COPD (AECOPD) [38–40], while three studies encompassed patients with acute respiratory failure due to heterogeneous etiology (COPD, heart failure, pneumonia, thoracic trauma, and chest wall deformity) [41–43]. One study comprised patients with acute hypoxemic respiratory failure [44], and two studies involved patients with acute-on-chronic respiratory failure (COPD, persistent asthma, bronchiectasis, obesity hypoventilation syndrome, restrictive lung diseases, and others) [45, 46]. The most common weaning assessment tool applied in all the studies was SBT with duration ranging between 5 min and 2 h. Weaning success, as defined by the lack of need of reintubation within 48–72 h of extubation or hospital survival, was reported in eight studies. Other parameters reported included duration of invasive mechanical ventilation, length of ICU/hospital stay, hospital mortality, and complications associated with invasive mechanical ventilation and weaning.

56.7.1 NIV in Weaning Patients with AECOPD

Three randomized trials involving 120 patients of acute exacerbation of COPD have assessed the role of NIV in weaning patients with AECOPD [38–40]. Weaning success (avoidance of re-intubation) was reported in two studies. The use of NIV was associated with successful weaning in 86 % (39/45) of the patients, whereas the use of conventional methods led to successful weaning in 71 % (32/45). In comparison with invasive mechanical ventilation, the use of NIV was associated with a comparable improvement in arterial blood gas and clinical parameters such as respiratory rate and sensorium, and a lesser incidence of

Table 56.2 Summary of studies describing use of noninvasive pressure ventilation (NIV) in difficult weaning

Author/year of study	Type of study	No. of patients	Comparator strategy (*n*)	Cause of respiratory failure	Weaning trial given	Weaning success (*p* value)
Nava et al. (1998) [38]	RCT	50	NIV vs PSV (25 vs 25)	AECOPD	T-piece trial	22/25 vs 17/25 (0.002)
Girault et al. (1999) [46]	RCT	33	NIV vs PSV (17 vs 16)	AECOPD, restrictive lung disease, mixed lung disease	2 h T-piece trial	13/17 vs 12/16 (>0.05)
Ferrer et al. (2003) [41]	RCT	43	NIV vs conventional weaning strategy (21 vs 22)	AECOPD, heart failure, pneumonia, thoracic trauma, post-operative	T-piece trial	18/21 vs 16/22 (>0.05)
Trevisan at al. (2008) [43]	RCT	65	NIV vs IMV (28 vs 37)	AECOPD, heart failure, pneumonia, thoracic trauma, post-operative	30 min T-piece trial	15/28 vs 15/37 (NA)
Prasad et al. (2009) [40]	RCT	30	NIV vs PSV (15 vs 15)	AECOPD	2 h T-piece trial	NA
Girault et al. (2011) [45]	RCT	208	NIV vs PSV vs oxygen therapy (69 vs 69 vs 70)	Chronic hypercapnic respiratory failure due to COPD, persistent asthma, bronchiectasis, obesity-hypoventilation syndrome, chest wall deformity, sequelae of pulmonary tuberculosis	5 mins-2 h T-piece trial	46 vs 32 vs 20 (<0.001)
Vaschetto et al. (2012) [44]	RCT	20	NIV vs PSV (10 vs 10)	Acute hypoxemic respiratory failure	30 min SBT	9/10 vs 5/10
Tawfeek et al. (2012) [42]	RCT	42	NIV vs SIMV (21 vs 21)	AECOPD, heart failure, pneumonia, thoracic trauma, post-operative, neuromuscular disease	2 h SBT	18/21 vs 11/21 (<0.05)
El-Shimy et al. (2013) [39]	RCT	40	NIV vs SIMV (20 vs 20)	AECOPD	0.5–2 h SBT	17/20 vs 15/20 (0.049)

AECOPD acute exacerbation of COPD, *COPD* chronic obstructive pulmonary disease, *IMV* invasive mechanical ventilation, *PSV* pressure support ventilation, *RCT* randomized control trial, *SBT* spontaneous breathing trial, *SIMV* synchronized intermittent mandatory ventilation

Table 56.3 Outcome parameters in studies describing noninvasive ventilation as a weaning strategy

Author/year	Total duration of IMV, in days	Total duration of ventilatory support (both NIV and IMV), in days	Length of ICU stay, in days	Length of hospital stay, in days	In hospital deaths (*n*)	Complication related to IMV and weaning (*n*)
Nava et al. (1998) [38]	10.2 ± 6.8 vs 16.6 ± 11.8	NA	15.1 ± 5.4 vs 24 ± 13.7	NA	2 vs 7	NA
Girault et al. (1999) [46]	4.56 ± 1.85 vs 7.69 ± 3.79	11.54 ± 5.24 vs 3.46 ± 1.42	12.35 ± 6.82 vs 14.06 ± 7.54	27.12 ± 14.33 vs 27.69 ± 13.09	0 vs 2	6 vs 9
Ferrer et al. (2003) [41]	9.5 ± 8.3 vs 20.1 ± 13.1	11.4 ± 8 vs 20.1 ± 13.1	14.1 ± 9.2 vs 25 ± 12.5	27.8 ± 14.6 vs 40.8 ± 21.4	2 vs 9	5 vs 16
Trevisan et al. (2008) [43]	7.5 ± 7.8 vs 10 ± 9.1	14.9 ± 9.9 vs 17.3 ± 10.5	18.9 ± 11.3 vs 20.8 ± 10.9	34.5 ± 20.6 vs 42.4 ± 24.5	9 vs 10	8 vs 28
Prasad et al. (2009) [40]	6.20 ± 5.20 vs 7.47 ± 6.38	NA	8.47 ± 4.79 vs 10.80 ± 5.28	NA	5 vs 9	6 vs 5
Girault et al. (2011) [45]			7.5 [4.5–15.5] vs 7.5 [4.5–14.5] vs 7.5 [4.5–17.5][a]	17.5 [9.5–28] vs 7.5 [4.5–14.5] vs 7.5 [4.5–17.5][a]	16 vs 9 vs 9	33 vs 35 vs 43
Vaschetto et al. (2012) [44]	8 vs 15	NA	15 ± 11 vs 21 ± 13	NA	2 vs 3	3 vs 5
Tawfeek et al. (2012) [42]	12.8 ± 8.3 vs 22.3 ± 13.3	NA	NA	NA	2 vs 6	4 vs 19
El-Shimy et al. (2013) [39]	35 ± 1.63 vs 47 ± 2.25	NA	9.50 ± 3.2 vs 11.4 ± 2.70	NA	5 vs 9	0 vs 16

All values are expressed as mean ± SD unless otherwise stated
IMV invasive mechanical ventilation, *NA* not available
[a]Median with interquartile range

nosocomial pneumonia. The use of NIV was not without complications, which included dryness of mouth, abrasion of nasal skin, claustrophobia, gastric distension, poor quality of sleep, and others.

The first RCT included 50 patients with severe COPD [38], with 35 of these patients receiving long-term oxygen therapy. Most patients (approximately 50 %) had comorbid illnesses, including rhythm disturbances, hypertension, diabetes mellitus, heart failure, and others. The application of NIV for weaning significantly reduced the need for invasive ventilation and ICU stay; it was associated with a higher 60-day survival. The other two trials did not mention the severity of underlying COPD and comorbid conditions [39, 40]. In the two trials reporting the weaning time, the NIV group had shorter weaning times in comparison with the control arm (invasive mechanical ventilation) [39, 40]. Further, the mean IPAP and EPAP (15.07 ± 1.27 and 6.21 ± 0.43 cm of H_2O, respectively) in the NIV arm and the mean pressures in the invasive arm (18.21 ± 1.1 cm of H_2O above PEEP of 5 cm of H_2O) were similar in the two groups [40].

Thus, in carefully selected patients with AECOPD who fail initial weaning trials, the use of NIV may be associated with a reduction in weaning time, less need for invasive mechanical ventilation, lower incidence of nosocomial pneumonia, better survival rates, and superior weaning rates.

56.7.2 NIV in Weaning Patients of Acute Hypoxemic Respiratory Failure

Only one single-center feasibility study has described the use of NIV as a weaning strategy in patients with acute hypoxemic respiratory failure [44]. Ten patients each were randomized to undergo either a NIV-based strategy or a conventional (invasive PSV) strategy for weaning from invasive mechanical ventilation. The etiology of ARDS included both direct (thoracic trauma, aspiration pneumonia, pneumonia) and indirect (sepsis, pancreatitis, blood transfusion related) causes, with baseline Acute Physiology and Chronic Health Evaluation (APACHE) II scores ranging from 8 to 13. Extubation failure was defined as an inability to sustain spontaneous unassisted breathing for 48 consecutive hours without the need for invasive or noninvasive ventilation. The use of NIV resulted in weaning success in 90 % of the patients compared with 50 % in the conventional arm. There were three ICU deaths in the conventional arm and only one death in the NIV arm. Three patients in the invasive PSV arm required tracheostomy, whereas none needed tracheostomy in the NIV arm. The most common cause of death was multiorgan failure. One additional patient in the NIV arm succumbed to underlying comorbid illness (chronic kidney disease and diabetes mellitus) after discharge from the ICU. Although NIV resulted in a significantly shorter duration of invasive ventilation, overall 28-day ventilation-free days (invasive and NIV) and weaning time were similar in the two groups.

There is sparse evidence on the role of NIV in facilitating extubation in patients recovering from acute hypoxemic respiratory failure. Thus, NIV should not be used in weaning this group of patients. More evidence is required regarding the use of NIV in weaning patients with acute hypoxemic respiratory failure.

56.7.3 NIV in Weaning Patients with Acute-on-Chronic Respiratory Illness

Two trials have addressed the role of NIV in acute-on-chronic respiratory diseases [45, 46]. Both trials included patients ($n = 241$) with chronic respiratory disorders such as COPD, persistent asthma, bronchiectasis, restrictive lung disorders, and others. In the first trial, 33 patients were randomized to either NIV ($n = 17$) or the conventional mode of weaning ($n = 16$) [46]. Weaning failure was defined as inability to sustain unassisted ventilation for at least 5 days or death or reintubation. Most of the included patients had severe underlying disease as defined by previous history of intubation ($n = 12$) or need for long-term oxygen therapy (LTOT) ($n = 10$). Although the NIV group had fewer days on invasive mechanical ventilation, there was no difference in weaning success, mortality, or complications. A subsequent larger multi-center study randomized patients ($n = 208$) into three groups (NIV group, invasive PSV, and oxygen therapy group) [45]. Patients in the non-NIV group were allowed NIV trial prior to reintubation, after extubation failure. Weaning failure was defined as an inability to sustain unassisted ventilation for at least 7 days or death or reintubation. The duration of 7 days was included to account for late NIV failure. In this study also, apart from a decline in the duration of invasive mechanical ventilation, no difference was seen in the weaning success rate, hospital mortality, or complications. The lack of difference in this study could be explained by the use of NIV prior to reintubation in both the non-NIV arms.

Thus, current evidence supports judicious use of NIV as a weaning strategy in patients with chronic respiratory diseases, as NIV may improve weaning results in these patients by shortening the duration of intubation and reducing the risk of post-extubation acute respiratory failure.

56.7.4 NIV in Weaning Patients with Acute Respiratory Failure of Heterogeneous Causes

Three trials have addressed the role of NIV in weaning from invasive mechanical ventilation in acute respiratory failure due various causes such as acute exacerbation of COPD, asthma, heart failure, postoperative respiratory failure, thoracic trauma, post-tuberculosis sequelae, pneumonia, and others [41–43]. The initial trial randomized 43 consecutive patients with acute respiratory failure in two arms using either NIV or the conventional approach (invasive PSV) as a weaning strategy [41]. Patients who failed SBT for 3 consecutive days and were considered difficult to wean were enrolled in the study. Successful weaning was defined as ability to sustain spontaneous breathing at least for 3 consecutive days and extubation failure was defined as the need for reintubation within 72 h of extubation. The use of NIV resulted in significant reduction in duration of total and invasive mechanical ventilation and ICU and hospital stay, better hospital survival, fewer complications, and need for tracheostomy. There was no difference in the reintubation rate in the two study arms, although the patients in the conventional arm were allowed a trial of NIV before attempting reintubation. Use of the conventional weaning approach (odds ratio (OR), 6.6; 95 % confidence interval (CI), 1.1–38.8) and age >70 years (OR, 5.1; 95 % CI, 1.7–15) had higher odds of death in the study population on multivariate analysis [41]. In another trial of 65 patients with a similar study population, the use of NIV resulted in less risk of complications and a trend toward shorter ICU and hospital stay. The patients in this study were sicker at baseline compared with the previous study and had multiple comorbidities [43]. A study of 42 patients compared NIV using proportional assist ventilation (PAV) with conventional weaning using SIMV with pressure support (SIMV-PS); PAV-NIV resulted in significantly higher weaning success with shorter duration of mechanical ventilation and fewer complications (ventilator-associated pneumonia, pneumothorax, sepsis, and others) [42]. There was no difference in the 60-day survival. However, the positive results in this study could also be the result of the use of the SIMV mode for weaning in the comparator arm that has been associated with poor outcomes [18].

Thus, the current evidence suggests a possible role of NIV in reducing the duration of invasive mechanical ventilation in weaning patients with heterogeneous causes of respiratory failure. However, variable results in the three studies do not provide conclusive evidence in support of NIV in reducing mortality or ICU and hospital stay and improving weaning success.

Conclusion

The use of NIV in difficult weaning should be restricted in patients with COPD and other hypercapnic respiratory failure states such as bronchiectasis and chronic asthma. In our ICU, we use NIV as a tool for weaning patients with the aforementioned conditions who fail two attempts at weaning using the SBT strategy (Table 56.4). Importantly, a strict vigil needs to be maintained to identify NIV failure and intubate the patients at the earliest sign of failure.

Table 56.4 Practical approach to the use of NIV in difficult weaning

Underlying conditions	Chronic obstructive pulmonary disease
	Long standing asthma
	Bronchiectasis
Weaning readiness	Significant improvement in the underlying condition
	Respiratory rate <32 breaths/min
	Fi_{O_2} requirement less than 0.4
	PEEP ≤5 cm H_2O
	Good cough reflex
	Normal in mental status
	Minimal airway secretions
	Hemodynamically stable
Spontaneous breathing trial failure	At least on two occasions defined by one or more of the following:
	Increase in respiratory rate ≥40 breaths/min (or >25 % of baseline)
	$Sp_{O_2} < 85\%$ despite Fi_{O_2} of 0.5
	$Pa_{CO_2} > 55 mmHg$ (or >20 % of baseline) and pH <7.3
	Heart rate >140 beats/min or <50 beats/min (or increase or decrease by >25 % of baseline)
	Alteration in mental status or agitation associated with diaphoresis
	Hypotension (systolic BP <90 mmHg) or hypertension (systolic BP >180 mmHg)
	Cardiac arrhythmia
NIV application	Full face mask
	Start with IPAP of 8 cm H_20 and EPAP of 4 cm H_20
	Titrate to clinical endpoints of respiratory rate <30 breaths/min; $Sp_{O_2} \geq 90\%$ with $Fi_{O_2} < 0.4; Pa_{CO_2} < 50 mmHg$ with pH between 7.3 and 7.4
NIV failure (defined at 30 min and 1 h)	Increase in respiratory rate ≥40 breaths/min (or >25 % of baseline)
	$Sp_{O_2} < 85\%$ despite Fi_{O_2} of 0.5
	$Pa_{CO_2} > 55 mmHg$ (or >20 % of baseline) and pH <7.3
	Heart rate >140 beats/min or <50 beats/min (or increase or decrease by >25 % of baseline)
	Alteration in mental status or agitation associated with diaphoresis
	Hypotension (systolic BP <90 mmHg) or hypertension (systolic BP >180 mmHg)
	Cardiac arrhythmia
	Pooling of secretions
	Gasping respiration

BP blood pressure, *PEEP* positive end expiratory pressure

References

1. Agarwal R. Noninvasive ventilation in acute lung injury/acute respiratory distress syndrome. In: Esquinas AM, editor. Noninvasive mechanical ventilation: theory, equipment, and clinical applications. Berlin: Springer; 2010. p. 241–8.
2. Agarwal R, Aggarwal AN, Gupta D. Non-invasive ventilation in acute asthma. Int J Tuberc Lung Dis. 2006;10(10):1182–3.
3. Agarwal R, Aggarwal AN, Gupta D. Role of noninvasive ventilation in acute lung injury/acute respiratory distress syndrome: a proportion meta-analysis. Respir Care. 2010; 55(12):1653–60.
4. Agarwal R, Aggarwal AN, Gupta D, Jindal SK. Non-invasive ventilation in acute cardiogenic pulmonary oedema. Postgrad Med J. 2005;81(960):637–43.
5. Sassoon CS, Del Rosario N, Fei R, Rheeman CH, Gruer SE, Mahutte CK. Influence of pressure- and flow-triggered synchronous intermittent mandatory ventilation on inspiratory muscle work. Crit Care Med. 1994;22(12):1933–41.
6. Agarwal R, Gupta R, Aggarwal AN, Gupta D. Noninvasive positive pressure ventilation in acute respiratory failure due to COPD vs. other causes: effectiveness and predictors of failure in a respiratory ICU in North India. Int J Chron Obstruct Pulmon Dis. 2008;3(4):737–43.
7. Agarwal R, Handa A, Aggarwal AN, Gupta D, Behera D. Outcomes of noninvasive ventilation in acute hypoxemic respiratory failure in a respiratory intensive care unit in north India. Respir Care. 2009;54(12):1679–87.
8. Gupta D, Nath A, Agarwal R, Behera D. A prospective randomized controlled trial on the efficacy of noninvasive ventilation in severe acute asthma. Respir Care. 2010;55(5):536–43.
9. Sharma S, Agarwal R, Aggarwal AN, Gupta D, Jindal SK. A survey of noninvasive ventilation practices in a respiratory ICU of North India. Respir Care. 2012;57(7):1145–53.
10. Agarwal R, Reddy C, Aggarwal AN, Gupta D. Is there a role for noninvasive ventilation in acute respiratory distress syndrome? Respir Med. 2006;100(12):2235–8.
11. Boles JM, Bion J, Connors A, et al. Weaning from mechanical ventilation. Eur Respir J. 2007;29(5):1033–56.
12. Esteban A, Alia I, Ibanez J, Benito S, Tobin MJ. Modes of mechanical ventilation and weaning. A national survey of Spanish hospitals The Spanish Lung Failure Collaborative Group. Chest. 1994;106(4):1188–93.
13. Ely EW, Baker AM, Dunagan DP, et al. Effect on the duration of mechanical ventilation of identifying patients capable of breathing spontaneously. N Engl J Med. 1996; 335(25):1864–9.
14. Wagner DP. Economics of prolonged mechanical ventilation. Am Rev Respir Dis. 1989;140 (2 Pt 2):S14–8.
15. Agarwal R, Aggarwal AN, Gupta D, Jindal SK. Role of noninvasive positive-pressure ventilation in postextubation respiratory failure: a meta-analysis. Respir Care. 2007;52(11):1472–9.
16. Esteban A, Frutos F, Tobin MJ, et al. A comparison of four methods of weaning patients from mechanical ventilation. Spanish Lung Failure Collaborative Group. N Engl J Med. 1995;332(6):345–50.
17. Vallverdu I, Calaf N, Subirana M, Net A, Benito S, Mancebo J. Clinical characteristics, respiratory functional parameters, and outcome of a two-hour T-piece trial in patients weaning from mechanical ventilation. Am J Respir Crit Care Med. 1998;158(6):1855–62.
18. Brochard L, Rauss A, Benito S, et al. Comparison of three methods of gradual withdrawal from ventilatory support during weaning from mechanical ventilation. Am J Respir Crit Care Med. 1994;150(4):896–903.
19. Gnanapandithan K, Agarwal R, Aggarwal AN, Gupta D. Weaning by gradual pressure support (PS) reduction without an initial spontaneous breathing trial (SBT) versus PS-supported SBT: a pilot study. Rev Port Pneumol. 2011;17(6):244–52.
20. Jubran A, Tobin MJ. Passive mechanics of lung and chest wall in patients who failed or succeeded in trials of weaning. Am J Respir Crit Care Med. 1997;155(3):916–21.

21. Jubran A, Tobin MJ. Pathophysiologic basis of acute respiratory distress in patients who fail a trial of weaning from mechanical ventilation. Am J Respir Crit Care Med. 1997;155(3):906–15.
22. Pinsky MR. Cardiovascular issues in respiratory care. Chest. 2005;128(5 Suppl 2):592s–7.
23. Lemaire F, Teboul JL, Cinotti L, et al. Acute left ventricular dysfunction during unsuccessful weaning from mechanical ventilation. Anesthesiology. 1988;69(2):171–9.
24. Yang KL, Tobin MJ. A prospective study of indexes predicting the outcome of trials of weaning from mechanical ventilation. N Engl J Med. 1991;324(21):1445–50.
25. Jaber S, Petrof BJ, Jung B, et al. Rapidly progressive diaphragmatic weakness and injury during mechanical ventilation in humans. Am J Respir Crit Care Med. 2011;183(3):364–71.
26. Kim WY, Suh HJ, Hong SB, Koh Y, Lim CM. Diaphragm dysfunction assessed by ultrasonography: influence on weaning from mechanical ventilation. Crit Care Med. 2011;39(12):2627–30.
27. Nemer SN, Barbas CS, Caldeira JB, et al. A new integrative weaning index of discontinuation from mechanical ventilation. Crit Care. 2009;13(5):R152.
28. Kollef MH, Shapiro SD, Silver P, et al. A randomized, controlled trial of protocol-directed versus physician-directed weaning from mechanical ventilation. Crit Care Med. 1997; 25(4):567–74.
29. Matic I, Majeric-Kogler V. Comparison of pressure support and T-tube weaning from mechanical ventilation: randomized prospective study. Croat Med J. 2004;45(2):162–6.
30. Ladeira MT, Vital FM, Andriolo RB, Andriolo BN, Atallah AN, Peccin MS. Pressure support versus T-tube for weaning from mechanical ventilation in adults. Cochrane Database Syst Rev. 2014;5:Cd006056.
31. Hess D. Ventilator modes used in weaning. Chest. 2001;120(6 Suppl):474s–6.
32. Marini JJ, Smith TC, Lamb VJ. External work output and force generation during synchronized intermittent mechanical ventilation. Effect of machine assistance on breathing effort. Am Rev Respir Dis. 1988;138(5):1169–79.
33. Imsand C, Feihl F, Perret C, Fitting JW. Regulation of inspiratory neuromuscular output during synchronized intermittent mechanical ventilation. Anesthesiology. 1994;80(1):13–22.
34. Leung P, Jubran A, Tobin MJ. Comparison of assisted ventilator modes on triggering, patient effort, and dyspnea. Am J Respir Crit Care Med. 1997;155(6):1940–8.
35. Hess DR. Ventilator modes: where have we come from and where are we going? Chest. 2010;137(6):1256–8.
36. Agarwal R. Noninvasive ventilation in in post-extubation respiratory failure. In: Esquinas AM, editor. Noninvasive mechanical ventilation: theory, equipment, and clinical applications. Berlin: Springer; 2010. p. 305–14.
37. Agarwal R, Gupta D. What is the role of noninvasive ventilation in diastolic heart failure? Intensive Care Med. 2005;31(10):1451; author reply 1452.
38. Nava S, Ambrosino N, Clini E, et al. Noninvasive mechanical ventilation in the weaning of patients with respiratory failure due to chronic obstructive pulmonary disease. A randomized, controlled trial. Ann Intern Med. 1998;128(9):721–8.
39. El-Shimy WS, Barima MA, Abo El-Magd GH, Mansour SA. Non invasive ventilation versus synchronized intermittent mandatory ventilation with pressure support in weaning of COPD patients: comparative study. Egyp J Chest Dis Tuberculosis. 2013;62(1):159–66.
40. Prasad SB, Chaudhry D, Khanna R. Role of noninvasive ventilation in weaning from mechanical ventilation in patients of chronic obstructive pulmonary disease: an Indian experience. Indian J Crit Care Med. 2009;13(4):207–12.
41. Ferrer M, Esquinas A, Arancibia F, et al. Noninvasive ventilation during persistent weaning failure: a randomized controlled trial. Am J Respir Crit Care Med. 2003;168(1):70–6.
42. Tawfeek MM, Ali Elnabtity AM. Noninvasive proportional assist ventilation may be useful in weaning patients who failed spontaneous breathing trial. Egyp J Anaesthes. 2012; 28(1):89–94.
43. Trevisan CE, Vieira SR. Noninvasive mechanical ventilation may be useful in treating patients who fail weaning from invasive mechanical ventilation: a randomized clinical trial. Crit Care. 2008;12(2):R51.

44. Vaschetto R, Turucz E, Dellapiazza F, et al. Noninvasive ventilation after early extubation in patients recovering from hypoxemic acute respiratory failure: a single-centre feasibility study. Intensive Care Med. 2012;38(10):1599–606.
45. Girault C, Bubenheim M, Abroug F, et al. Noninvasive ventilation and weaning in patients with chronic hypercapnic respiratory failure: a randomized multicenter trial. Am J Respir Crit Care Med. 2011;184(6):672–9.
46. Girault C, Daudenthun I, Chevron V, Tamion F, Leroy J, Bonmarchand G. Noninvasive ventilation as a systematic extubation and weaning technique in acute-on-chronic respiratory failure: a prospective, randomized controlled study. Am J Respir Crit Care Med. 1999;160(1):86–92.

Psychological Factors as Determinants of Noninvasive Continuous Positive Airway Pressure Response: Key Practical Aspects and Topics

57

Alex H. Gifford

Contents

Abbreviations

ALS	Amyotrophic lateral sclerosis
ARF	Acute respiratory failure
CRF	Chronic respiratory failure
HRQOL	Health-related quality of life
ICU	Intensive care unit
IMV	Invasive mechanical ventilation
NIPPV	Noninvasive positive pressure ventilation
RRT	Renal replacement therapy

A.H. Gifford, MD
Section of Pulmonary and Critical Care Medicine, Dartmouth-Hitchcock Medical Center, Lebanon, NH, USA
e-mail: Alex.H.Gifford@hitchcock.org

A.M. Esquinas (ed.), *Noninvasive Mechanical Ventilation: Theory, Equipment, and Clinical Applications*, DOI 10.1007/978-3-319-21653-9_57

57.1 Introduction

Surprisingly little has been published about the ways in which psychological factors influence acceptance and tolerance of noninvasive positive pressure ventilation (NIPPV) by patients with acute and chronic respiratory insufficiency. Much of what has been written pertains to the latter circumstance when the natural history of the underlying condition, usually a progressive neuromuscular disease, permits a measure of forethought by the patient and caregivers about how NIPPV stands to impact health-related quality of life (HRQOL) and what lifestyle adjustments need to be made before it can be initiated. The proposition of long-term NIPPV has been shown to elicit distinct cognitive and behavioral perspectives within patients and their families that have been categorized by some authors using semi-structured interviewing and interpretive phenomenological techniques. Patients whose acute respiratory failure (ARF) is treated with NIPPV are often anxious and scared by the experience of dyspnea. These responses may be heightened and sustained, however, by underlying psychiatric disorders of which clinicians may or may not be aware and which may inform the need to titrate sedating medications and/or offer close emotional support to improve NIPPV tolerance. In an isolated report, NIPPV actually mitigated agitation in an older male patient, but this provides only anecdotal support for its utility in this context [1].

57.2 Current Gaps in General Knowledge

The literature review performed for this chapter has revealed several deficiencies in our knowledge about psychological factors associated with responses to NIPPV. First, a dearth of information exists regarding how anxiety, depression, or even psychosis, affect NIPPV tolerance in ARF. Evidence from several case series [2–4] suggests that the alpha-2-adrenergic receptor agonist dexmedetomidine facilitates NIPPV tolerance during ARF by inducing anxiolysis without insulting central ventilatory drive. These reports are limited by small numbers of patients, a focus on the pharmacodynamics of the drug, and lack of a systematic appraisal of the psychological status of the patients. Second, data on children are conspicuously limited. A single descriptive study of young children with chronic respiratory failure (CRF) has determined that alternative NIPPV interfaces must be found in approximately 20 % of patients, mostly due to facial discomfort, but any contributions of psychological factors to this requirement were not given [5]. Third, practice guidelines for the initiation and maintenance of NIPPV in patients with affective and/or behavioral disorders are currently unavailable. Lastly, novel strategies to enhance the acceptance of NIPPV, like meditation, hypnosis, and acupuncture, are appealing but unsubstantiated.

57.3 The Psychology of Decision-Making About NIPPV in Amyotrophic Lateral Sclerosis

A number of psychological and illness severity factors inform decision-making about NIPPV in patients with amyotrophic lateral sclerosis (ALS). In recently published work, Martin et al. [6] provide a detailed appraisal of the physical, cognitive, and psychological characteristics of 32 ALS patients who had been diagnosed at least 6 months earlier and who made one or more decisions regarding NIPPV and/or gastrostomy tube placement during the 3-month follow-up interval. In the subset of patients who died during the observation period, NIPPV decisions were made closer to the end of life (mean: 2.7 ± 2.2 months) than gastrostomy tube placement decisions (mean: 6.1 ± 4.2 months). The authors had such limited post-NIPPV refusal data that NIPPV and gastrostomy tube placement decisions (acceptance or refusal) were analyzed together, an important caveat in the interpretation of their findings. Not surprisingly, a greater burden of physical ailments was associated with decisions made within the observation period. Patients who felt that they understood their illness less well, those with a proactive attitude about decision-making, and those with fewer depressive symptoms were more likely to refuse either intervention.

The study of Martin et al. [6] highlights the potential for knowledge limitation and apathy to complicate decision-making about NIPPV in ALS and refutes the argument that depressed patients are more likely to refuse this intervention out of a sense of relegation and/or deference to input from their caregivers. The authors concluded that ALS patients who have a more passive approach to interventions and fewer years of education, in contrast to those who were better informed about the disease and had clear opinions about interventions, may benefit from assistance to make informed decisions. Often, though, the benefits of NIPPV on HRQOL in ALS motivate patients to continue using it and have led some to view it as being worth the effort [2]. Patients who have refused NIPPV have expressed that it undermines their sense of identity, dignity, and/or autonomy [3]. Some of these patients have cited concerns about claustrophobia, loss of control, and vomiting while wearing the mask as reasons for declining NIPPV [3]. That some patients with ALS readily accept this intervention while others promptly refuse it underscores the need for clinicians to explore the psychological forces that drive the decision-making process for each patient (Table 57.1).

57.4 How the Clinician Influences NIPPV Acceptance by the Patient

The extent to which clinicians are compassionate, receptive, and circumspect in their counseling about NIPPV can significantly influence a patient's perspective about therapy. In the report by Ando et al. [3], some ALS patients felt that their

Table 57.1 Psychological influences on acceptance and tolerance of NIPPV

Amyotrophic lateral sclerosis (ALS)
Perceptions of choice and control [9]
Acceptance and need [9]
Aspects of fear [9, 13]
Active coping styles [14]
Preservation of the self [15]
Acute exacerbation of chronic obstructive pulmonary disease (AECOPD)
Experience of anxiety, panic, and loss of control [8]
Experience of mobilizing willpower [8]
Respiratory failure (multiple etiologies)
Anticipatory anxiety [11]
Home versus institutional environment [12]
Claustrophobia [16]
Perception of compassion by caregivers (especially upon initiation of treatment) [7]
Ability to maintain positive outlook about treatment despite its strenuousness [7]
Reduced sensory abilities (older patients) [10]
Reduced satisfaction with achievements in life and expectations for future (older patients) [10]

clinicians were forcing NIPPV on them. This perception was associated with a generalized disdain for hospitals and a sense of threatened autonomy. The focus of clinicians can easily drift to alarms on ventilatory equipment and physiological parameters like oxyhemoglobin saturation and away from the psychological needs of patients. This can unintentionally lead patients to question the efficacy of treatment and feel subjugated to technology; moreover, family members can feel guilty about asking clinicians to explain the rationale for NIPPV in the care of their loved one [7]. Tolerance of NIPPV can be improved when patients trust that their clinicians will be attentive to their emotional and physical needs and when continuity of care by the same clinicians is maintained [8]. Patients are also quite cognizant of the expertise that their clinicians have with NIPPV and/or the underlying disease for which it is being used [9]. More research is needed to elucidate the attitudes and practices that clinicians should foster to best help patients and their families cope with NIPPV.

57.5 NIPPV Acceptance by Older Patients

Life experiences and concerns about HRQOL are factors that shape the preferences of older patients for NIPPV. In the ETHICA study [10], investigators questioned whether octogenarians who had either been admitted to hospital for treatment of a chronic disease or who lived in a nursing home or assisted-living facility would agree to intensive care unit (ICU) admission for a future hypothetical illness requiring the use of NIPPV and/or renal replacement therapy (RRT). Of note, the authors excluded patients with cognitive impairment and included those with reasonably good functional status. They found that refusal rates for NIPPV, invasive mechanical ventilation (IMV), and RRT (after IMV) were 27 %, 43 %, and 63 %, respectively. Married patients were nearly three times more likely than those who were unmarried to refuse NIPPV (RR 2.9, 95 % 1.5–5.8, $p=0.002$). Patients with lower scores on an inventory that measured the integrity of sensory faculties and satisfaction with achievements in life and expectations for the future were also more likely to refuse NIPPV. The authors point out that in emergency situations, clinicians are often not privy to information about HRQOL, and in the absence of a surrogate decision maker and/or an advanced directive, they may render life-sustaining services out of sheer necessity. This scenario highlights the importance of earnest and timely communication among clinicians, patients, and their family members about goals and values.

57.6 NIPPV Acceptance by Children

Because children often cannot intellectualize the experience of being treated with NIPPV, they are susceptible to considerable anticipatory anxiety, which can evolve into a formidable barrier to therapy. In an intriguing pilot study, Delord et al. [11] performed medical hypnosis in nine children with CRF with the objective of acclimatizing them to NIPPV. In the youngest patient, a technique based on distraction was used, whereas in the older children, indirect or direct hypnotic suggestions were employed to progressively induce psychocorporeal relaxation. These authors found that a median of three sessions were needed to achieve acceptance of NIPPV for 6 or more hours per night. After 6 months of sustained hypnotherapy, median objective compliance with NIPPV was 7.5 h per night in eight of the nine patients. The parents of one patient were instructed in the hypnotherapy technique and performed it at home. Interestingly, the investigators noted that anxiety was also reduced in the parents of treated children and concluded that this fact alone could have promoted successful NIPPV use.

A 1997 survey of long-term ventilation in children throughout the United Kingdom identified 136 cases with sufficient descriptive information [12]. Of the 93 children who received long-term ventilation at home, 52 (56 %) used NIPPV delivered by face or nasal masks, reflecting the preponderance of neuromuscular diseases in this subset of patients. Forty-three (53 %) of the 81 school-age children requiring NIPPV attended mainstream educational institutions. The authors of this study advanced the position that providing NIPPV at home is the "best option for meeting the child's psychological needs and enhancing quality of life." Although this statement is probably correct, their work and others like it did not glean from the patients themselves specific data about emotional well-being as it relates to supported ventilation. Additional studies are needed to flesh out the many psychological determinants of NIPPV tolerance in children.

Conclusion

In summary, most of the research about the psychological determinants of NIPPV outcomes has been conducted in patients with ALS or other neuromuscular diseases. Significantly less inquiry has been undertaken in children and older patients and in patients of all ages with ARF. Clinicians are sometimes unaware of the extent to which patients with emotional and/or behavioral difficulties need close support and guidance, regardless of whether these difficulties arise from or are unassociated with the use of NIPPV.

Key Recommendations

- Discuss the anticipated benefits of NIPPV on HRQOL and potential drawbacks of treatment, such as lifestyle adjustments, with patients at an early stage of illness.
- Empower patients to have some degree of control over the apparatus and settings as they become acclimatized to NIPPV.
- Elicit patient concerns about NIPPV using an empathetic tone and language that is compatible with the level of education and comprehension of the patient.
- Life experiences and future plans in older patients and anticipatory anxiety in children play important roles in NIPPV acceptance and/or tolerance.

References

1. Yamamoto N, Fukuda Y, Shiba H, et al. Noninvasive positive pressure ventilation improved refractory behavioral and psychological symptoms of dementia in an elderly adult with type 2 respiratory failure. J Am Geriatr Soc. 2012;60:1576–8.
2. Demuro JP, Mongelli MN, Hanna AF. Use of dexmedetomidine to facilitate non-invasive ventilation. Int J Crit Illn Inj Sci. 2013;3:274–5.
3. Akada S, Takeda S, Yoshida Y, et al. The efficacy of dexmedetomidine in patients with noninvasive ventilation: a preliminary study. Anesth Analg. 2008;107:167–70.
4. Takasaki Y, Kido T, Semba K. Dexmedetomidine facilitates induction of noninvasive positive pressure ventilation for acute respiratory failure in patients with severe asthma. J Anesth. 2009;23:147–50.
5. Ramirez A, Delord V, Khirani S, et al. Interfaces for long-term noninvasive positive pressure ventilation in children. Intensive Care Med. 2012;38:655–62.
6. Martin NH, Landau S, Janssen A, et al. Psychological as well as illness factors influence acceptance of non-invasive ventilation (NIV) and gastrostomy in amyotrophic lateral sclerosis (ALS): a prospective population study. Amyotroph Lateral Scler Frontotemporal Degener. 2014;15:376–87.
7. Ingadottir TS, Jonsdottir H. Technological dependency–the experience of using home ventilators and long-term oxygen therapy: patients' and families' perspective. Scand J Caring Sci. 2006;20:18–25.
8. Torheim H, Gjengedal E. How to cope with the mask? Experiences of mask treatment in patients with acute chronic obstructive pulmonary disease-exacerbations. Scand J Caring Sci. 2010;24:499–506.

9. Greenaway LP, Martin NH, Lawrence V, et al. Accepting or declining non-invasive ventilation or gastrostomy in amyotrophic lateral sclerosis: patients' perspectives. J Neurol. 2015; 262(4):1002–13.
10. Philippart F, Vesin A, Bruel C, et al. The ETHICA study (part I): elderly's thoughts about intensive care unit admission for life-sustaining treatments. Intensive Care Med. 2013; 39:1565–73.
11. Delord V, Khirani S, Ramirez A, et al. Medical hypnosis as a tool to acclimatize children to noninvasive positive pressure ventilation: a pilot study. Chest. 2013;144:87–91.
12. Jardine E, O'Toole M, Paton JY, et al. Current status of long term ventilation of children in the United Kingdom: questionnaire survey. BMJ. 1999;318:295–9.
13. Lemoignan J, Ells C. Amyotrophic lateral sclerosis and assisted ventilation: how patients decide. Palliat Support Care. 2010;8:207–13.
14. Ando H, Chakrabarti B, Angus RM, et al. Experience of long-term use of non-invasive ventilation in motor neuron disease: an interpretative phenomenological analysis. BMJ Support Palliat Care. 2014;4:50–6.
15. Ando H, Williams C, Angus RM, et al. Why don't they accept non-invasive ventilation?: insight into the interpersonal perspectives of patients with motor neurone disease. Br J Health Psychol. 2015;20(2):341–59.
16. Gay PC, Hess DR, Hill NS. Noninvasive proportional assist ventilation for acute respiratory insufficiency. Comparison with pressure support ventilation. Am J Respir Crit Care Med. 2001;164:1606–11.

Part VI

Hospital Critical Care Applications: Critical Care Postoperative

Preoperative Noninvasive Ventilation: Key Practical Recommendations and Evidence

58

R. Zaimi, J. Bardet, and Patrick Bagan

Contents

Abbreviations

COPD	Chronic obstructive pulmonary disease
FEV1	Forced expiratory volume on first second
NIV	Noninvasive ventilation
VC	Vital capacity

58.1 Introduction

The risk factors of postoperative respiratory complications can be dependent on the patient, the anesthesia, or the surgery. Prevention therefore targets each of these factors when possible. Despite the efficacy of different prevention methods, pulmonary outcomes after surgery still cause a high rate of postoperative morbidity and mortality.

Noninvasive ventilation (NIV) has been used in the preoperative period and studies show its potential benefits in the preoperative prevention of pulmonary

R. Zaimi, MD • J. Bardet, MD • P. Bagan, MD (✉)
Thoracic and Vascular Department, Victor Dupouy Hospital, Argenteuil, France
e-mail: rymzaimi@hotmail.fr; Jeremy.bardet@me.com; Patrick.bagan@ch-argenteuil.fr

A.M. Esquinas (ed.), *Noninvasive Mechanical Ventilation: Theory, Equipment, and Clinical Applications*, DOI 10.1007/978-3-319-21653-9_58

complications. Therefore, further studies need to be performed to provide more precision of NIV use before surgery, elucidate the selection criteria of the patients, and prove its efficacy in a large cohort of patients.

58.2 Discussion and Analysis Main Topic

Pulmonary complications are the most frequent causes of postoperative morbidity and mortality. The principal risk factors are age, smoking, lung diseases, location of surgery, and hospital stay [1]. Several methods of prevention and treatment of these complications have been used over the years and have proven their efficacy, including oxygen therapy, aerosols, physiotherapy, and NIV. Usually, respiratory care has been used in the postoperative period, in patients with asthma, and chronic obstructive pulmonary diseases.

Preoperative prevention of respiratory complications is crucial in decreasing respiratory morbidity, especially in high risk patients. Patients requiring respiratory rehabilitation can be selected by preoperative evaluation. Smokers should have a smoking cessation program, as it is known that reducing smoking to 50 % or stopping it decreases risk of bronchospasm and postoperative pneumonia when the program is in effect at least 6–8 weeks before surgery [2].

Bronchodilator medication in chronic obstructive pulmonary disease (COPD) patients increases forced expiratory volume in 1 second (FEV1) and vital capacity (VC) and reduces airway resistance by 24 h, which is essential when surgery has to be performed in short delays [2]. Chest physiotherapy performed 2–4 weeks before surgery facilitates dealing with exercise in the postoperative period and reduces risks of postoperative atelectasis and pneumonia. These methods are currently used and can be associated with NIV in the preoperative period to improve the prevention of respiratory postoperative morbidity.

Several studies have observed that NIV reduces infectious problems of invasive ventilation and enhances comfort of the patient [3]. Its efficacy in acute respiratory failure in obstructive diseases such as asthma and COPD and in acute cardiogenic pulmonary edema is proven [3]. Its use has been extended to surgical fields by studying its benefits in patients who develop respiratory failure after surgery.

Most reports of postoperative NIV were concerned with thoracic and upper abdominal surgery, specialties with high rates of pulmonary complications. Major changes in respiratory function occur when the site of surgery is closer to the diaphragm. In this case, the surgical site associated with anesthesia and postoperative pain causes a diaphragmatic dysfunction and lung volumes decrease, leading to postoperative hypoxemia and acute respiratory failure [1].

Several other studies have demonstrated the efficacy of NIV in various types of surgery: it reduces extravascular lung water after cardiac surgery [3], improves lung mechanics and oxygenation after coronary artery bypass surgery [3], decreases pulmonary dysfunction following gastroplasty [3], reduces atelectasis, improves oxygenation, and decreases infectious risk in patients with postoperative hypoxemia after abdominal surgery [4, 5].

In parallel to the postoperative period, benefits of NIV were studied in preoperative prevention of respiratory morbidity and mortality. Postoperative pulmonary complications are related to surgery and anesthesia, and they consist principally of atelectasis, pneumonia, respiratory failure, and exacerbation of chronic lung diseases [6, 7]. The identification of the risk factors for postoperative pulmonary complications is crucial in defining the prevention modalities in the preoperative period. Smetana et al. [6], in their systematic review, found that age, American Society of Anesthesiologists (ASA) class II or greater, functional dependence, COPD, congestive heart failure, surgical site, emergency surgery, prolonged surgery, and a low serum albumin level were high risk factors of pulmonary postoperative complications. This may help to define the group of patients who would benefit the most from preoperative NIV.

Few authors have studied prophylactic use of NIV. The selection criteria were different; Bagan et al. [7] reported the contribution of preoperative rehabilitation and NIV in patients with stage I and II lung cancer; inclusion criteria were FEV1, diffusing capacity of the lungs for carbon monoxide (DLCO), and maximal oxygen consumption (VO_2 max) below the lower threshold or patients with high risk of cardiac morbidity. Perrin et al. [8], in their study of preoperative noninvasive ventilation in patients undergoing lobectomy for lung cancer, fixed a FEV1 below 70 % as an inclusion criterion. Benefits of the rehabilitation program were studied according to respiratory criteria in both studies. Paleiron et al. [9], in their protocol of preoperative noninvasive ventilation in pulmonary resection surgery, fixed respiratory parameters as inclusion criteria (FEV1/VC<70 %, FEV1<80 %, VC<80 %, CPT<80 %), cardiac failure, and obesity.

With patients, FEV1 seemed significantly improved after a NIV program [7, 8], and even allowed pulmonary resection in patients who had limited respiratory functions [7]. For the same type of surgery (lung resection), modality of application of preoperative NIV varied from one center to another; it was performed 2 weeks prior surgery, for 1 h, 3 times a day in the Bagan et al. report [7], whereas in the series by Perrin et al., NIV was performed 1 week prior to surgery, in at least five 1-h periods per day [8]. In both reports, postoperative application of NIV was systematic. For Paleiron et al. [9], NIV was required 1–2 weeks prior to surgery, twice a day for a 3-h period, and postoperative application was performed only in case of complications.

Despite the differences in the manner of application of NIV in the perioperative period, authors noted its benefits on the postoperative outcomes, such as decreasing atelectasis and pneumonia [7] and reducing hypoxemia and pulmonary function impairment [8]. In addition to its benefits on prophylactic perioperative application in pulmonary resection, NIV use was also reported in prevention of pulmonary complications in aortic aneurysm surgery in patients who were smokers (>40 packets per year) with COPD. In another report of Bagan et al. [10], preoperative NIV was performed 2 weeks prior to surgery, 3 times a day, for a 30-min period, and, comparatively, the rate of pulmonary complications and the mean hospital length of stay in the intensive care unit were significantly lower in the NIV group. It was also observed that postoperative application of NIV was made easier when patients were prepared for it in the preoperative period, in fact, observance rate was higher after surgery.

In general, NIV seems to be efficient the in perioperative period. First performed after thoracic and upper abdominal surgery, many authors demonstrated its benefits in the postoperative period in various other surgeries. More recently, its indication was extended to the preoperative period, especially in lung resection, and the few reports show its efficacy. NIV is safe and well tolerated when applied correctly in specific selected patients. Failure is usually due to side effects and also to intolerance related to patient discomfort or claustrophobia. To optimize the use of NIV, clinicians can adapt the adequate inflation pressure by making frequent readjustments. Patient coaching and encouragement can also contribute to a reduction in the failure rate [3].

Conclusion

The aim of NIV in the perioperative period is not to replace the other measures of prevention of pulmonary risk factors; all methods of prevention should be used in association to reduce pulmonary complications and improve postoperative lung function. Smoking cessation, evaluation and equilibration of chronic lung disease, congestive heart failure, and other comorbidities, and nutrition care for patients with low serum albumin level should be always performed prior to an operation, but this must not delay the surgery.

Although perioperative NIV was considered by several authors to have effective benefits, its value in the preoperative period still needs to be demonstrated. To date, few reports have evaluated preoperative NIV, and the cohort of patients was not sufficient to prove with good evidence the positive impact of NIV. Furthermore, selection criteria and modalities of application were different, depending on the study and the local conditions of the different centers. A multicenter, standardized study with a large cohort is required to assess the impact of preoperative NIV and to precise to which group of patients it should be performed. In the future, the report of Paleiron and colleagues about the evaluation of preoperative NIV prior to pulmonary resection will perhaps provide more answers to the question of the efficacy of preoperative NIV, as the study (PréOVNI GFPC 12–01) is controlled, randomized, and multicentric.

The advances in research on preoperative NIV may decrease postoperative pulmonary complications and also permit improvement of respiratory status in patients who initially could not support a surgical treatment.

Key Major Recommendations

- We recommend preoperative NIV in patients undergoing abdominal and thoracic surgery, with limited respiratory function (FEV1 <80 %).
- NIV should be performed at least 1 week before surgery, twice a day for a 1-h period. Postoperative NIV can be completed in case of respiratory complications.
- Patients having preoperative NIV should be included in prospective trials to set international parameters for its indication and application.

References

1. Kenneth G, Torrington MD, Henderson C. Perioperative respiratory therapy (PORT). A program of preoperative risk assessment and individualized postoperative care. Chest. 1988;93:946–51.
2. Delay JM, Jaber S. Préparation respiratoire des patients insuffisants respiratoires chroniques. Presse Med. 2012;41:225–33.
3. Mehta S, Hill SN. Noninvasive ventilation. Am J Respir Crit Care Med. 2001;163:540–77.
4. Squadrone V, Coha M, Cerutti E, et al. Continuous positive airway pressure for treatment of postoperative hypoxemia. JAMA. 2005;293:589–95.
5. Kindgen-Milles D, Buhl R, Gabriel A, et al. Nasal continuous positive airway pressure. A method to avoid endotracheal reintubation in post operative high-risk patients with severe nonhypercapnic oxygenation failure. Chest. 2000;117:1106–11.
6. Smetana GW, Lawrence VA, Cornell JE. Preoperative pulmonary risk stratification for noncardiothoracic surgery: systematic review for the American College of Physicians. Ann Intern Med. 2006;144:581–95.
7. Bagan P, Ben Abdesselam A, Dakhil B, et al. Réhabilitation et VNI avant exérèse pulmonaire chez les patients à haut risque opératoire. Rev Mal Respir. 2013;30:414–9.
8. Perrin C, Jullien V, Vénissac N, et al. Prophylactic use of noninvasive ventilation in patients undergoing lung resectional surgery. Respir Med. 2007;101:1572–8.
9. Paleiron N, André M, Grassin F, et al. Evaluation de la ventilation non invasive préopératoire avant chirurgie de résection pulmonaire. Etude pré OVNI GFPC 12–01. Rev Mal Respir. 2013;30:231–7.
10. Bagan P, Bouayad M, Benabdesselam A, et al. Prevention of pulmonary complications after aortic surgery: evaluation of prophylactic noninvasive perioperative ventilation. Ann Vasc Surg. 2011;1–3. doi:10.1016/j.avsg.2010.10.020.

Intraoperative Noninvasive Ventilation: Key Technical and Practical Recommendations

59

Luca Cabrini, Giovanni Landoni, and Alberto Zangrillo

Contents

Abbreviations

ARF Acute respiratory failure
COPD Chronic obstructive pulmonary disease
CPAP Continuous positive airway pressure
FOB Fiber-optic bronchoscopy
NIV Noninvasive ventilation
NPPV Noninvasive positive pressure ventilation

L. Cabrini, MD (✉) • G. Landoni • A. Zangrillo
Department of Anesthesia and Intensive Care, IRCCS San Raffaele Hospital, Vita-Salute University, Via Olgettina 60, Milan 20132, Italy
e-mail: cabrini.luca@hsr.it; landoni.giovanni@hsr.it; zangrillo.alberto@hsr.it

A.M. Esquinas (ed.), *Noninvasive Mechanical Ventilation: Theory, Equipment, and Clinical Applications*, DOI 10.1007/978-3-319-21653-9_59

59.1 Introduction

Noninvasive ventilation (NIV) has traditionally been applied to treat acute respiratory failure (ARF) in pulmonary wards, intensive care units, and emergency departments [1]. New indications (such as prevention of ARF) and new settings (pre-hospital and ordinary wards) have been proposed and evaluated. In particular, NIV has been evaluated in the perioperative period to prevent or to treat postoperative pulmonary complications and ARF. NIV proved effective in improving relevant outcomes in surgical patients, especially when applied in high-risk patients in the postoperative period [2].

Furthermore, a growing number of studies have reported the application of NIV in the operating theatre. During surgery, NIV could be of help at least in four conditions: to prevent ARF in patients in whom tracheal intubation must be avoided or was refused, to treat ARF in the same patients, to improve ventilation in sedated patients, or as an aid for tracheal intubation/airway management [3–6]. In the following section, the main indications and available evidence are reported. Relevant technical and practical aspects will be addressed.

59.2 Discussion and Analysis

59.2.1 NIV to Prevent ARF During Surgery in Patients with Respiratory Diseases

In patients with a very labile respiratory function, postoperative weaning from mechanical ventilation and tracheal extubation can be difficult or even impossible. On the other hand, avoiding intraoperative curarization and tracheal intubation when feasible could prevent the risk of ARF and emergent tracheal intubation during surgery, mainly due to the surgery itself, the anesthetic strategy (especially if it includes sedation or spinal/epidural anesthesia), and the position (e.g., supine decubitus in orthopnoic patients). As a consequence, when the risk of causing a permanent dependency from mechanical ventilation is considered too high, an otherwise indicated surgery can be denied by the surgeon or the anesthetist; similarly, the patient can refuse to undergo surgery when facing this risk.

Noninvasive ventilation can be a logical solution when curarization is not absolutely required. NIV can support the respiratory function, allowing maintenance of the correct position. Moreover, NIV can counterbalance the respiratory depression associated to sedative and local anesthetic agents.

So far, at least 16 papers, including 24 patients with severe respiratory limitation (7 already on chronic NIV treatment), have reported the application of NIV to prevent ARF during surgery [4, 5]. The procedures included ophthalmic, urologic, thoracic, orthopedic, neurosurgical, and cardiac interventions. ARF was prevented in all cases. Face mask and nasal mask use was reported. NIV was mainly applied as noninvasive positive pressure ventilation (NPPV), but continuous positive airway pressure (CPAP) was also used.

59.2.2 NIV to Treat ARF During Surgery

At least six papers described the application of NIV in 86 patients undergoing NIV during different kinds of surgery for an established ARF [4, 5]. In most cases, general anesthesia tracheal intubation had been previously excluded due to the poor patient conditions, including severe chronic obstructive pulmonary disease (COPD) or neuromuscular diseases. Surgery was successfully completed in all cases. Moreover, five cases of vaginal delivery and six cases of caesarean section in which NIV was used to treat ARF have been published. All cases were completed uneventfully, although one mother (affected by cystic fibrosis) died 10 days after the caesarean section due to pneumonia. NPPV was almost always the applied NIV modality; most patients were already on domiciliary NIV.

59.2.3 NIV to Improve Ventilation in Healthy, Sedated Patients During Surgery

Deep sedation is frequently used in patients undergoing surgery without general anesthesia. Respiratory depression and inability to keep the airway open may ensue even in healthy patients if sedated [7]. NIV could help in improving spontaneous ventilation and in keeping the airway open, similar to manual ventilation with an oropharyngeal cannula in place. Four Japanese papers including more than 500 patients reported NIV use in the operating theatre with this aim, mainly during orthopedic or gynecologic surgery under spinal/epidural anesthesia plus sedation [4, 5]. Nasal mask and NPPV were always applied. In two cases, NIV failed to maintain the airway open, so other tools were required. All other cases were successful and no major complications were observed.

59.2.4 NIV to Facilitate Tracheal Intubation

Tracheal intubation in patients with difficult airway management can be challenging; the same is true in patients with an augmented risk of hypoxemia during the procedure, for example, morbidly obese patients and patients with lung disease. In these cases, NIV can improve pre-oxygenation as compared with manual ventilation before tracheal intubation [8–10]. Moreover, fiber-optic bronchoscopy (FOB)-guided tracheal intubation through the nasal or oral route can be performed during NIV to minimize the risk of hypoxemia. Different technical solutions have been tested, but dedicated interfaces are also available. At least 10 studies including almost 300 patients evaluated NIV use with this aim, although some studies were performed in the intensive care unit [3, 5]. Only one failure was recorded, without any other complications. Two randomized controlled trials compared NIV with laryngeal mask and oxygen therapy, and NIV was safer in both studies.

59.2.5 Practical Recommendations

Application of NIV in these risky settings requires accurate preoperative planning [4, 5]. Patients should be informed and, whenever possible, trained to tolerate NIV. Ethical aspects can be complex and must be addressed and documented before surgery. All staff must be aware of the scope and limits of NIV, and cooperation from the surgeon is required. Strict patient monitoring must be in place. If tracheal intubation is an available option, all the equipment to perform it immediately must be present. Preoperative patient preparation should be carefully optimized, if possible, to maximize ventilator function during surgery. Many sizes and models of masks should be available to allow the patient to tolerate NIV for the entire procedure. When NIV-aided tracheal intubation is performed, dedicated masks might be the safest choice.

Finally, but most relevant, the staff must be highly expert in crucial aspects of NIV, such as the choice of interface and the ventilatory setting. Patient's tolerance and NIV efficacy and safety strongly depend on the competence and experience of the anesthesiologist. NIV use in this setting can be dangerous in untrained hands.

Conclusions

In surgical patients, a growing number of studies have suggested that NIV could help to prevent ARF in patients in whom tracheal intubation must be avoided or was refused, to treat ARF in the same patients, to improve ventilation in sedated patients, or as an aid for tracheal intubation/airway management. In expert hands, NIV proved effective and safe, with a very low failure rate and no complications. Careful monitoring and cooperation among the staff are key elements. However, so far, evidence came almost entirely from case series or observational studies. Randomized controlled trials are required to better assess efficacy and safety of NIV in the operating theatre.

Key Major Recommendations

- In the operating theatre, NIV help to prevent ARF in patients in which tracheal intubation must be avoided or was refused, to treat ARF, to improve ventilation in sedated patients, or as an aid for tracheal intubation/airway management.
- NIV application in the operating room requires an expert and cooperative team, careful patient preparation, strict monitoring, and a full array of equipment.
- So far, few data of low quality are available on these novel indications. Despite the promising results, more studies are required to assess NIV efficacy and safety in the operating theatre.

References

1. Nava S, Hill N. Non-invasive ventilation in acute respiratory failure. Lancet. 2009;374:250–9.
2. Jaber S, Chanques G, Jung B. Postoperative noninvasive ventilation. Anesthesiology. 2010;112(2):453–61.
3. Cabrini L, Nobile L, Cama E, et al. Non-invasive ventilation during upper endoscopies in adult patients. A systematic review. Minerva Anestesiol. 2013;79:683–94.
4. Cabrini L, Nobile L, Plumari VP, et al. Intraoperative prophylactic and therapeutic non-invasive ventilation: a systematic review. Br J Anaesth. 2014;112:638–47.
5. Esquinas AM, Jover JL, Úbeda A, et al. Non-invasive mechanical ventilation in the pre- and intraoperative period and difficult airway. en nombre del Grupo de Trabajo Internacional de Ventilación Mecánica No Invasiva Anestesiología y Críticos. Rev Esp Anestesiol Reanim. 2015; pii: S0034-9356(15)00016-X doi:10.1016/j.redar.2015.01.007. Epub ahead of print on pubmed.
6. Esquinas A, Zuil M, Scala R, et al. Bronchoscopy during non-invasive mechanical ventilation: a review of techniques and procedures. Arch Bronconeumol. 2013;49:105–12.
7. Tobias JD, Leder M. Procedural sedation: a review of sedative agents, monitoring, and management of complications. Saudi J Anaesth. 2011;5:395–410.
8. Baillard C, Fosse JP, Sebbane M, et al. Noninvasive ventilation improves preoxygenation before intubation of hypoxic patients. Am J Respir Crit Care Med. 2006;174:171–7.
9. Delay JM, Sebbane M, Jung B, et al. The effectiveness of noninvasive positive pressure ventilation to enhance preoxygenation in morbidly obese patients: a randomized controlled study. Anesth Analg. 2008;107:1707–13.
10. Baumann HJ, Klose H, Simon M, et al. Fiber optic bronchoscopy in patients with acute hypoxemic respiratory failure requiring noninvasive ventilation – a feasibility study. Crit Care. 2011;15:R179.

Use of NIMV in the Early Postoperative Period: Key Practical Aspects and Clinical Evidence

60

Emre Erbabacan

Contents

Abbreviations

BIPAP	Bi-level positive airway pressure
CPAP	Continuous positive airway pressure
EPAP	Expiratory positive airway pressure
FiO_2	Fraction of inspired oxygen
ICU	Intensive care unit
IPAP	Inspiratory positive airway pressure
NIMV	Noninvasive mechanical ventilation
PARF	Postoperative acute respiratory failure
PEEP	Positive end-expiratory pressure
PSV	Pressure support ventilation

E. Erbabacan, MD
Department of Anesthesiology and Reanimation, Istanbul University, Cerrahpasa Medical School, Istanbul, Turkey
e-mail: emreerbabacan@hotmail.com

A.M. Esquinas (ed.), *Noninvasive Mechanical Ventilation: Theory, Equipment, and Clinical Applications*, DOI 10.1007/978-3-319-21653-9_60

60.1 Introduction

Although the surgical and anesthesia techniques have advanced vastly in the past decades, postoperative respiratory complications such as atelectasis formation, related pneumonia, decrease in pulmonary volumes, diaphragm dysfunction, and postoperative acute respiratory failure (PARF) are still major problems, especially in high-risk patients. PARF is observed in 5–10 % of patients undergoing major thoracic or abdominal surgery and is closely associated with outcome [1].

Anesthesia decreases muscle tone; surgery affects the thoracoabdominal muscles and diaphragm. As the functional residual capacity decreases and closing capacity is unaffected, atelectasis occurs. In addition, pain related to the surgical incision can cause hypoventilation. All these factors lead to hypoxemia. [2]. Although noninvasive mechanical ventilation (NIMV) is used mainly in the intensive care units (ICU), use of NIMV during the early postoperative period in the recovery room has also become widespread to help reduce the prevalence of PARF [3]. NIMV reduces the work of breathing, increases ventilation, and prevents atelectasis formation. Preventing the occurrence of PARF can also prevent endotracheal reintubation, hemodynamic impairment, longer hospital stay durations, increased costs, and, most importantly, higher morbidity and mortality [4].

NIMV treatment should be considered in the early postoperative period when dyspnea, respiratory rates over 25/min, and use of accessory muscles are observed and when $PaCO_2$ is above 45 mmHg, pHa is below 7.35, and PiO_2/FiO_2 values are below 250. However, it should not be initiated in patients with hemodynamic instability, facial surgery, poor cooperation or Glasgow Coma Scale below nine, and unstable arrhythmias.

60.2 Discussion and Analysis Main Topic

NIMV can be used in high-risk patients as a prophylactic measure and it also can be used for curative purposes in patients with PARF to avoid intubation. Different studies support the efficiency of prophylactic and curative NIMV in different types of surgeries.

60.2.1 Cardiac Surgery

Zarback et al. [5] used either continuous prophylactic nasal continuous positive airway pressure (CPAP) for 6 h following extubation or standard postoperative oxygen support in 500 patients undergoing cardiac surgery and showed that continuous CPAP increased arterial oxygenation and reduced pulmonary complications and the rate of ICU admission. Olper et al. [6] showed that postoperative bi-level positive airway pressure (BIPAP) and CPAP are effective treatments in patients with developed respiratory failure following cardiac surgery.

60.2.2 Thoracic Surgery

Thoracic surgery carries a higher risk for PARF compared with cardiac surgery. In their randomized clinical trial, Perrin et al. [7] administered prophylactic preoperative and postoperative NIMV treatment to patients with severe obstructions undergoing lung resection. They found that oxygenation and lung volumes improved, whereas hospital stay duration decreased compared with patients who received standard postoperative treatment. In a study by Lefebvre et al. [8], 89 patients with both hypercapnic and hypoxemic PARF following lung resection surgery were administered early curative NIMV in the ICU, and the overall success rate of NIMV was 85.3 %, confirming the feasibility and efficacy of NIMV in PARF following lung resection.

60.2.3 Abdominal Surgery

Abdominal surgery can result in diaphragm dysfunction, which can lead to PARF. As the incision approaches the diaphragm, the dysfunction may worsen. Kindgen-Milles et al. [4] showed that prophylactic use of CPAP with a pressure of 10 cmH_2O for 12–24 h improved oxygenation and shortened the ICU stay in patients undergoing thoracoabdominal aortic surgery. In patients with PARF who underwent abdominal surgery, Conti et al. [9] administered NIMV with helmet in one group and with face mask in the other group and showed that NIVM improves PiO_2/FiO_2 and is an alternative method to conventional ventilation.

60.2.4 General Considerations

As also noted in the studies mentioned above, use of NIMV in the early postoperative period is effective in both preventing and treating PARF. It improves arterial oxygenation and decreases intubation rate compared with standard medical therapy. An issue that needs further debate is when, how, and how long to use it. In patients with severe PARF where deep hypoxia ($PiO_2/FiO_2 < 120$), metabolic acidosis with base excess higher than −5 mEq/L, or shock is present, and patient is not able to protect the airways or clear the secretions, early endotracheal intubation should be considered instead of curative NIV therapy. On occasion, delaying endotracheal intubation can also be life threatening. Instead of giving specific targets, patients' preoperative arterial blood gas samples and previous respiratory and cardiac state should be taken into account in deciding the intubation need and ending NIMV therapy. However, an uncooperative patient with values <150 even after 4 h of effective NIMV should be considered as a candidate for invasive mechanical ventilation.

Although noninvasive ventilators, which administer CPAP or BIPAP modes, are common in recovery rooms, some anesthesiologists and respiratory therapists also prefer to use ICU ventilators in postoperative care units. The most common ventilation modes are CPAP, BIPAP, assisted spontaneous breathing, or pressure support ventilation (PSV) [10]. Some practitioners also consider CPAP with high-flow generators as an effective option. PSV mode has some advantages, mainly in patients with nasogastric tubes because indented tidal volumes can be reached against the leak.

The aim should be the lowest inspiratory pressures or volumes that will improve the oxygenation, decrease the respiratory rate, and not impair patient comfort. In our practice, we use CPAP with high-flow generators and CPAP, BIPAP, and PSV with different types of ventilators in the recovery room and postoperative care unit. When using CPAP, we prefer starting with a pressure level of 5 cmH_2O and increase up to 10 cmH_2O according to patient need and comfort. When using BIPAP, we start with expiratory positive airway pressure (EPAP) values of 5 cmH_2O and inspiratory positive airway pressure (IPAP) values of 12 cmH_2O. In PSV mode, we start with a positive end-expiratory pressure (PEEP) level of 5 cmH_2O and increase inspiratory pressure 2 cmH_2O above PEEP progressively to a maximum 15–20 cmH_2O to reach the desired tidal volumes of 6–8 ml/kg. PEEP is increased to a maximum value of 10 cmH_2O if needed. but with the condition of preventing the increase of maximum inspiratory pressure above 25 cmH_2O, mainly in patients with anastomosis in the upper digestive tract. The initial FiO_2 level we use is 40 %. We increase FiO_2 levels up to 60 % to keep SpO_2 levels above 95 % (90 % in patients with a severe chronic obstructive pulmonary disease). If the NIMV administration is prophylactic, an administration of 60 min is usually enough following extubation in the recovery room. Arterial blood gas samples should be checked at 2-h intervals, and, if the need occurs, NIMV treatment should be started again. If PARF is suspected or occurs, NIMV for curative purposes should be started with the same settings and therapy should be directed according to the response of the patient. In curative treatment, we prefer using NIMV for 4 h initially and then for 60 min at 3-h intervals. Between the NIMV treatments, patients breathe through a Venturi mask or nasal oxygen is used. The length of the treatment is shortened when possible, aiming for an improved oxygenation and metabolic state and comfort without NIMV. Our recommendations are based on our clinical experience rather than a randomized clinical trial.

NIMV practitioners must share the justified concern of surgeons about damage to a recent surgical anastomosis. Mainly in surgeries with upper gastrointestinal tract, there is a higher risk related to indigested air and high peak inspiratory pressures. Hence, extra care must be taken in these types of patients (mainly in patients undergoing esophagus and gastric resections and bariatric surgery). Although a peak inspiratory pressure above 25 cmH_2O is not recommended in using NIMV for PARF, 20 cmH_2O should be chosen as a limit in these patients to prevent PARF and protect the anastomosis. Use of nasogastric tubes should be used to monitor the air accumulation in the gastrointestinal tract as an alarm to change the ventilator settings.

Different types of interfaces may be used during postoperative NIMV. The most suitable choice usually depends both on the characteristics of the patient and the surgery as no advantage has been shown between the different types of masks [10]. Interface that minimizes the leak and is the one that the patient is most comfortable with may be used. However, in patients who have undergone facial surgery or have facial anomalies, use of a helmet can be more effective and enable the use of NIMV. An important aspect of NIMV with helmets is to use higher inspiration pressures compared with face masks.

Conclusion

Abdominal, thoracic, and cardiac surgeries have negative effects on respiratory function during the postoperative period. NIMV can be helpful in overcoming these negative issues. In addition to its curative effect on postoperative respiratory failure, NIMV in the early postoperative period can also be used as a prophylactic treatment in high-risk patients in recovery rooms and decrease ICU admission.

Key Major Recommendations

- NIV can be used in high-risk patients as a prophylactic measure, and it also can be used for curative purposes in patients with PARF to avoid intubation
- The aim should be the lowest inspiratory pressures or volumes that will improve oxygenation, decrease respiratory rate, and not impair patient comfort.
- The NIV practitioners must share the justified concern of surgeons about damage to a recent surgical anastomosis. A peak inspiratory pressure of 20 cmH_2O should be chosen as a limit in these patients to prevent PARF and protect the anastomosis.
- The most suitable choice of interface, mask or helmet, usually depends both on the characteristics of the patient and the surgery.

References

1. Warner DO. Preventing postoperative pulmonary complications: the role of the anesthesiologist. Anesthesiology. 2000;92(5):1467–72.
2. Jaber S, De Jong A, Castagnoli A, et al. Non-invasive ventilation after surgery. Ann Fr Anesth Reanim. 2014;33:487–91.
3. Glossop AJ, Shephard N, Bryden DC, et al. Non-invasive ventilation for weaning, avoiding reintubation after extubation and in the postoperative period: a meta-analysis. Br J Anaesth. 2012;109:305–14.
4. Kindgen-Milles D, Müller E, Buhl R, et al. Nasal-continuous positive airway pressure reduces pulmonary morbidity and length of hospital stay following thoracoabdominal aortic surgery. Chest. 2005;128(2):821–8.
5. Zarbock A, Mueller E, Netzer S, et al. Prophylactic nasal continuous positive airway pressure following cardiac surgery protects from postoperative pulmonary complications: a prospective, randomized, controlled trial in 500 patients. Chest. 2009;135:1252–9. doi:10.1378/chest.08-1602.
6. Olper L, Cabrini L, Landoni G, et al. Non-invasive ventilation after cardiac surgery outside the intensive care unit. Minerva Anestesiol. 2011;77:40–5.
7. Perrin C, Jullien V, Vénissac N, et al. Prophylactic use of noninvasive ventilation in patients undergoing lung resectional surgery. Respir Med. 2007;101:1572–8.
8. Lefebvre A, Lorut C, Alifano M, et al. Noninvasive ventilation for acute respiratory failure after lung resection: an observational study. Intensive Care Med. 2009;35:663–70.

9. Conti G, Cavaliere F, Costa R, et al. Noninvasive positive-pressure ventilation with different interfaces in patients with respiratory failure after abdominal surgery: a matched-control study. Respir Care. 2007;52:1463–71.
10. Mathai AS. Non-invasive ventilation in the postoperative period: is there a role? Indian J Anaesth. 2011;55:325–33.

61 Noninvasive Mechanical Ventilation After Cardiac Surgery

Gökhan İnangil and Ahmet Ertürk Yedekçi

Contents

Abbreviations

ARDS	Acute respiratory distress syndrome
ARF	Acute respiratory failure
CO	Cardiac output
COPD	Chronic obstructive pulmonary disease
CPAP	Continuous positive airway pressure
CPB	Cardiopulmonary bypass
FRC	Functional residual capacity
ICU	Intensive care unit
LV	Left ventricle
NIV	Noninvasive ventilation

G. İnangil, MD (✉)
Department of Anesthesiology and Reanimation, GATA Haydarpasa Training Hospital, Istanbul 34668, Turkey
e-mail: ginangil2@gmail.com; ginangil@gata.edu.tr

A.E. Yedekçi, MD
Department of Anesthesiology and Reanimation, Girne Military Hospital, Girne, Turkish Republic of North Cyprus
e-mail: aeyedekci@gata.edu.tr

A.M. Esquinas (ed.), *Noninvasive Mechanical Ventilation: Theory, Equipment, and Clinical Applications*, DOI 10.1007/978-3-319-21653-9_61

PEEP	Positive end-expiratory pressure
PPV	Positive pressure ventilation
PVR	Pulmonary vascular resistance
RV	Right ventricle
VC	Vital capacity

61.1 Introduction

Major changes in respiratory function occur in all patients after cardiac surgery, which has a relatively high incidence of postoperative acute respiratory failure. Noninvasive ventilation (NIV) is used clinically in the treatment of cardiogenic pulmonary edema, decompensated chronic obstructive pulmonary disease (COPD), and hypoxemic respiratory failure. It is also used in the postoperative period to improve gas exchange, decrease work of breathing, and reduce atelectasis, both as preventive therapy and as a curative tool to avoid reintubation [1]. The aim of this chapter is to review the effects of cardiac surgery and cardiopulmonary bypass (CPB) on postoperative lung dysfunction and postoperative use of NIV after cardiac surgery and discuss physiology and clinical practice with recommendations.

61.2 Cardiac Surgery and Acute Respiratory Failure

Patients undergoing cardiac surgery experience physiologic stresses from general anesthesia, thoracotomy, CPB, surgical manipulation, diaphragm dysfunction, sternotomy, postoperative pain, fluid overload, and massive transfusion. Each of these in itself may lead to pulmonary dysfunction, and acute respiratory failure (ARF) may develop. These effects may worsen clinical prognosis in the presence of preexisting risk factors including severe COPD and congestive heart failure [2–4].

Almost all patients undergoing cardiac surgery have some degree of postoperative lung dysfunction, with an incidence of about 25 %. While patients with adequate pulmonary reserve can tolerate this dysfunction well, 2–5 % of patients are at risk of developing severe lung dysfunction leading to increased morbidity, mortality, and prolonged hospitalization. Postoperative pulmonary complications such as pleural effusion (27–95 %), atelectasis (16.6–88 %), and acute respiratory distress syndrome (ARDS) (0.5–1.7 %) may occur after cardiac surgery, as cardiac surgery causes systemic inflammatory response, which causes lung injury. There are several factors affecting pathogenesis of postoperative pulmonary dysfunction after cardiac surgery and that are also related to the patient's preoperative pulmonary status and the degree of procedural stress [2, 5].

Factors related to general anesthesia include supine position, neuromuscular block, altered chest wall compliance, acute functional residual capacity (FRC), and vital capacity (VC) reduction, which results in ventilation-perfusion mismatch and abnormal pulmonary shunt fraction. Opioids used commonly in cardiac anesthesia practice reduce hypoxic and hypercapnic ventilatory response postoperatively. As a result, a reduction of VC and FRC of lungs can lead to the onset of hypoxemia and atelectasis with increased work of breathing, which increases oxygen consumption and myocardial work [3, 5].

Postoperative ARF risk is also increased in cardiac surgery when the internal mammary artery used for grafting. Topical and systemic cooling, use of CPB, and surgical manipulations during surgery are risk factors specific to cardiac surgery. The CPB procedure allows extracorporeal maintenance of both circulation and respiration during a non-beating heart at hypothermic temperatures. It is the most likely factor for causing ARF, with two different mechanisms. Whereas interruption of ventilation results in collapsed lungs, causing atelectasis, interruption of pulmonary circulation results in pulmonary ischemia, causing release of inflammatory mediators. Systemic inflammatory response induces intrapulmonary aggregation of leukocytes and platelets, causing further impairment of gas exchange, atelectasis, and increased pulmonary shunt fraction. Because anticoagulation with heparin is essential for CPB after termination of CPB, protamine is used for reversal. Administration of protamine is also associated with systemic reactions and pulmonary hypertension. These many interrelated factors cause ARF after CPB, especially with CPB time exceeding 120 min and massive transfusion, and additional risk factors of prolonged ventilation and extubation failure postoperatively are reported. Furthermore studies report that off-pump cardiac surgery is associated with lower postoperative pulmonary complication rates [5].

Postoperative respiratory complications may be expected in the majority of patients undergoing cardiac surgery, especially if CPB is performed, for the reasons mentioned above.

61.3 NIMV in the Postoperative Period

After cardiac surgery, patients are transferred to the intensive care unit (ICU) under anesthesia with ventilation support with an endotracheal tube. In this period, most patients are under the effects of both anesthesia and curarization, and ventilatory support plays important role because the operated heart and affected lungs work by interacting with each other to supply oxygen demands of tissues. After arriving in the ICU, the patient is warmed, allowed to awaken, and observed for hemodynamic instability and surgical complications.

In recent experience, fast-track cardiac anesthesia has become the standard of care, allowing rapid recovery and early tracheal extubation in many centers. About 25 % of cardiac surgical patients were extubated within 4 h of ICU arrival, and about half within 8 h of ICU arrival. Hemodynamically stable patients with normal left ventricular (LV) function preoperatively, with adequate rewarming and postoperative analgesia, may be considered for early extubation. About 8 % of patients need prolonged mechanical ventilation, which is defined as >72 h following ICU arrival, and about 7 % required reintubation after extubation [3].

Although cardiac function was improved with valve repair or replacement and myocardial oxygen delivery improved with revascularization, cardiac performance may be lower than the preoperative status for a period of time after CPB. This ventricular dysfunction is usually a temporary state of contractile impairment and is usually treated with positive inotropic agents. Generally, coronary revascularization procedures are mostly performed with CPB, which is associated with myocardial damage. It is difficult to predict the response of the heart to the altered loading conditions after valve repair surgery. This critical period starts with the termination of CPB and continues in the ICU. Patients with normal preoperative LV function are expected to recover 90 % of baseline LV function by 4 h postoperatively in the presence of an uncomplicated intraoperative course for revascularization procedures [3].

During invasive ventilation postoperatively, FRC is maintained by positive end-expiratory pressure (PEEP), but, after extubation, FRC and oxygen transfer decrease and derecruitment of alveolar units occurs with poor coughing, lack of respiratory exercise, and pleural effusions. Thus, following extubation, it is essential to prevent atelectasis and development of pulmonary complications and to maintain oxygenation [5, 6].

In the last 20 years, postoperative NIV has been evaluated as a preventive and curative tool to avoid reintubation. NIV can be applied as continuous positive airway pressure (CPAP), a fixed level of positive airway pressure during whole respiratory cycle in spontaneously breathing patients, and as positive pressure ventilation (PPV) whereby the ventilator supports the inspiratory effort of patient. This technique improves gas exchange, decreases work of breathing, and reduces atelectasis while increasing patient comfort, allowing coughing and communication, and reducing need for sedation. It also reduces costs and workload [1, 7, 8].

The available evidence suggests that CPAP and NIV could be effectively used to improve oxygenation and reduce the incidence of complications such as pneumonia, atelectasis, and the need for endotracheal intubation after abdominal and thoracic surgery, which results in greater length of stay, morbidity, and mortality. Both conventional ventilators and portable ventilators can be used for this purpose [1, 8].

Cardiac surgery patients can benefit from NIV, restoring lung volumes and reducing the work of breathing. Both PPV NIV and CPAP are frequently used in clinical practice to prevent development of atelectasis and improve gas exchange postoperatively after extubation. Studies have shown that the use of NIV may increase lung aeration, increase FRC, and prevent collapse of alveolar units during the postoperative period of abdominal surgery with radiologic imaging [1, 7].

Prophylactic nasal CPAP with pressures of 10 cmH_2O following cardiac surgery has also been shown to improve arterial oxygenation, reduce incidence of pulmonary complications and reintubation rates, and reduce readmission rate to the ICU, with better patient tolerance when used outside the ICU. It is also simple and inexpensive, as PEEP is generated by a PEEP valve and high-flow gas source, thus not requiring a ventilator [6].

However, interventions to support the respiratory function may have both beneficial and undesirable side effects inasmuch as pulmonary physiology and cardiac function vary in spontaneously breathing and mechanically ventilated patients. ARF may also develop as a result of the use of an improper ventilatory strategy, with high volumes causing mechanical stress and biotrauma or inadequate PEEP levels that lead to atelectasis and impairment of lung function. Atelectasis and the loss of functional alveolar units has been accepted as the main pathophysiological mechanism of postoperative hypoxemia and intrapulmonary shunt [5, 6].

PPV causes intrathoracic pressure changes, which can affect preload, afterload, heart rate, and myocardial contractility because respiration and circulation are interdependent physiological processes. The use of mechanical ventilation in affected lungs and an operated heart increases the complexity of this interaction. Ventilatory strategies should be used with care because the tendency to cardiovascular instability may occur easily in the early post-bypass patient [9].

Increased intrathoracic pressure during mechanical ventilation is also transmitted to the heart chambers, pericardium, and to the vascular structures. PPV increases both intrathoracic and right atrial pressures during inspiration, reduces venous return, right ventricular (RV) preload, and cardiac output (CO). In the presence of PEEP, these pressures remain above the atmospheric pressure throughout both inspiration and expiration, and usually 8–10 cm H_2O is enough to reduce CO throughout the respiratory cycle [8].

Patients with LV failure and pulmonary edema are associated with an increased preload and afterload. By limiting venous return and lowering LV afterload, PPV or PEEP application can improve the CO. PEEP also provides alveolar patency against alveolar edema and reduces risk of atelectasis. Consequently, an increase in intrathoracic pressure can increase CO in patients with LV dysfunction and reduced ventricular compliance [9].

Because RV physiology is inadequate, tolerating afterload increases the effect of PPV in patients with RV dysfunction can be inconvenient. Pulmonary vascular resistance (PVR) is affected mainly by lung volumes and depends on the balance between the vascular tone of alveolar and parenchymal vessels. Increases in PEEP or lung inflation above FRC impair RV function by increasing PVR. As lung volume falls from FRC toward residual volume, PVR increases again with terminal airway collapse, leading to pulmonary hypoxic vasoconstriction. Thus, both PEEP application and the cautious delivery of conservative tidal volumes should be considered for preventing excessive increase in PVR and unfavorable circulatory effects, especially in patients with postoperative RV failure or hypovolemia [8, 9].

Patients with asthma have increased resistance in the airways and hyperinflated lungs. Special care should be taken to avoid excessive gas trapping. Mechanical ventilation with smaller volumes and adequate expiratory time to reduce auto-PEEP is essential [9, 10].

Before initiating NIV, possible surgical complications such as anastomosis leakage, hemorrhage, pneumothorax, and cardiac tamponade should be excluded. Sufficient communication must be established with the patient so that the procedure is well understood, as patient cooperation is essential. It is useful to describe this procedure to patients with preoperative risk factors for postoperative ARF prior to the operation. Preoperative prophylactic inspiratory muscle training is also advised to improve respiratory muscle function and gas exchange. It is reported that training has reduced the need for prolonged ventilatory support (>24 h) from 26 to 5 % [3].

Ventilator settings should be set at the lowest inspiratory pressures possible for patient comfort while providing effective gas exchange. This may be achieved by starting with only 3–5 cmH_2O PEEP. After starting 3–5 cmH_2O pressure support, slightly increase the pressure support by 2–3 cmH_2O, allowing patient to adapt the mask and the ventilator until adequate expiratory tidal volume is achieved with acceptable respiratory rate and arterial oxygenation. The PEEP could be increased as needed to improve oxygenation without adverse hemodynamic effects up to

7–10 cmH_2O with cautious monitoring. It is recommended not to exceed an insufflation pressure (PPV + PEEP) of 20–25 cmH_2O. Duration of NIV should be 30–45 min at 2–4 h intervals according to the patient's clinical status to avoid facial skin lacerations [1].

The Society of National Adult Cardiac Surgery Database Thoracic Surgeons offers a customized model to predict prolonged ventilation. Factors assessing risk status include age, gender, body surface area, presence of diabetes or renal failure, chronic lung disease, cerebrovascular and peripheral vascular disease, and emergency or unstable status preoperatively. Mild to moderate COPD was not assessed as a major risk for postoperative morbidity and mortality as expected but rated as a factor in many models. COPD patients, especially with age more than 75 years and receiving steroids, have higher rates of pulmonary complications, atrial fibrillation, and death. Obesity is indicated not to increase ARF postoperatively [3].

Conclusion

Pulmonary complications are frequent after cardiac surgery because many complex mechanisms involve both surgical stress and systemic inflammatory processes. Thus, protective ventilation strategies during surgery and CPB are essential for preventing postoperative respiratory complications. Postoperative NIV requires an experienced and trained team and continuous hemodynamic monitoring. The effects of PEEP and PPV on the hemodynamic system should be carefully monitored so that tailored management of both the respiratory and cardiovascular system can be obtained. Although NIV is shown to be effective in preventing postoperative ARF, it remains controversial in the treatment of ARF. Further randomized controlled studies should be performed to better identify the patients who may benefit from NIV after cardiac surgery, and clinical guidelines and protocols should be established [8, 11].

Key Major Recommendations

- Before initiating NIV, possible surgical complications such as anastomosis leakage, hemorrhage, pneumothorax, and cardiac tamponade should be excluded. Sufficient communication must be established with the patient so that the procedure is well understood, as patient cooperation is essential.
- Ventilator settings should be set at the lowest inspiratory pressures possible for patient comfort while providing effective gas exchange. It is recommended not to exceed insufflation pressure (PPV + PEEP) of 20–25 cmH_2O.
- Patients should be monitored for ventilator asynchrony, mask intolerance, gastric distension, and facial skin lacerations.
- Postoperative NIV requires an experienced and trained team and continuous hemodynamic monitoring in critical patients. The effects of PEEP and PPV on the hemodynamic system should be carefully monitored so that tailored management of both the respiratory and cardiovascular systems can be achieved.

References

1. Jaber S, Chanques G, Jung B. Postoperative noninvasive ventilation. Anesthesiology. 2010;112:453–61.
2. Schreiber JU, Lancé MD, de Korte M, et al. The effect of different lung-protective strategies in patients during cardiopulmonary bypass: a meta-analysis and semiquantitative review of randomized trials. J Cardiothorac Vasc Anesth. 2012;26:448–54.
3. Higgins TL, Yared JP. Postoperative respiratory care. In: Kaplan JA, editor. Kaplan's cardiac anesthesia. Philadelphia: Saunders Elsevier; 2006. p. 1087–102.
4. Cabrini L, Plumari VP, Nobile L, et al. Non-invasive ventilation in cardiac surgery: a concise review. Heart Lung Vessel. 2013;5:137–41.
5. Badenes R, Lozano A, Belda FJ. Postoperative pulmonary dysfunction and mechanical ventilation in cardiac surgery. Crit Care Res Pract. 2015;2015:420513.
6. Zarbock A, Mueller E, Netzer S, et al. Prophylactic nasal continuous positive airway pressure following cardiac surgery protects from postoperative pulmonary complications: a prospective, randomized, controlled trial in 500 patients. Chest. 2009;135:1252–9.
7. Landoni G, Zangrillo A, Cabrini L. Noninvasive ventilation after cardiac and thoracic surgery in adult patients: a review. J Cardiothorac Vasc Anesth. 2012;26:917–22.
8. Guarracino F, Ambrosino N. Non invasive ventilation in cardio-surgical patients. Minerva Anestesiol. 2011;77:734–41.
9. Shekerdemian L, Bohn D. Cardiovascular effects of mechanical ventilation. Arch Dis Child. 1999;80:475–80.
10. Tonković T, Baronica R, Pavlović DB, et al. Effects of the mechanical ventilation on the cardiovascular system. Signa Vita. 2014;9(Supp l):41–4.
11. Esteban A, Frutos-Vivar F, Ferguson ND, et al. Noninvasive positive-pressure ventilation for respiratory failure after extubation. N Engl J Med. 2004;350:2452–60.

Noninvasive Ventilation in the Post-extubation Period: What Have We Learned? Evidence and Key Practical Recommendations

62

Christophe Girault, Gaëtan Beduneau, and Dorothée Carpentier

Contents

Abbreviations

ARF	Acute respiratory failure
COPD	Chronic obstructive pulmonary disease
CPAP	Continuous positive airway pressure
CRF	Chronic respiratory failure
ICU	Intensive care unit

C. Girault, MD (✉) • G. Beduneau, MD
Department of Medical Intensive Care Medicine, Charles Nicolle University Hospital, Rouen University, 1, rue de Germont, Rouen 76031, France

UPRES EA 3830-IRIB, Institute for Biomedical Research, Rouen University, Rouen, France
e-mail: Christophe.Girault@chu-rouen.fr

D. Carpentier, MD
Department of Medical Intensive Care Medicine, Charles Nicolle University Hospital, Rouen University, 1, rue de Germont, Rouen 76031, France

A.M. Esquinas (ed.), *Noninvasive Mechanical Ventilation: Theory, Equipment, and Clinical Applications*, DOI 10.1007/978-3-319-21653-9_62

MV Mechanical ventilation
NIV Noninvasive ventilation
PSV Pressure support ventilation
RCT Randomized controlled trial
SBT Spontaneous breathing trial

62.1 Introduction

Invasive endotracheal mechanical ventilation (MV) can lead to an excess of morbidity and even mortality in intensive care unit (ICU) patients [1]. In this context, noninvasive ventilation (NIV) has been developed for the management of the post-extubation period, including weaning/extubation from MV and management of post-extubation acute respiratory failure (ARF) [2, 3] (Fig. 62.1). Its results should be distinguished according to the strategy used and populations involved.

62.2 Concerns with Weaning/Extubation from MV

62.2.1 Definitions

Weaning from MV is the entire process that allows passing more or less quickly from MV to spontaneous breathing, or "de-ventilation," leading to extubation. Weaning failure is classically defined as failure of a spontaneous breathing trial (SBT), whereas extubation failure is defined as the need for early reintubation

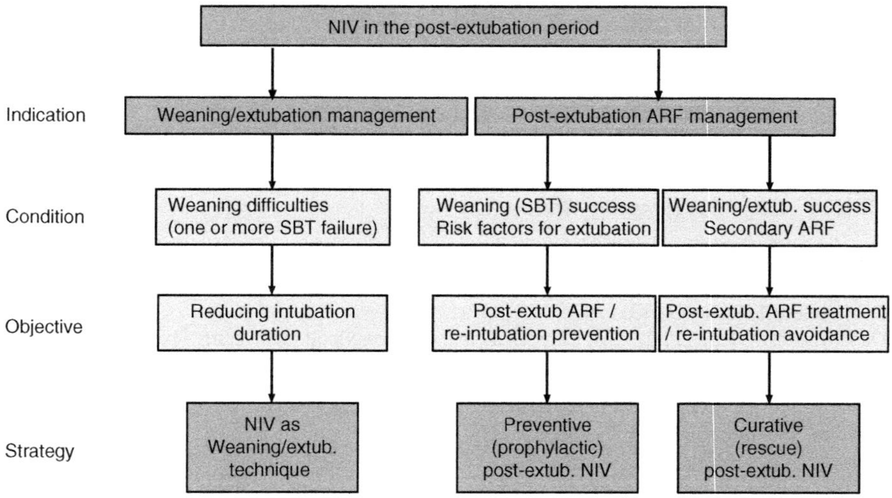

Fig. 62.1 Strategies for using NIV in the post-extubation period (*NIV* noninvasive ventilation, *ARF* acute respiratory failure, *SBT* spontaneous breathing trial, *post-extub.* post-extubation

(48–72 h) after a planned extubation [1, 3]. Nevertheless, the definition of weaning success or failure should also now consider the development of post-extubation NIV, described as "weaning in progress" [1]. In this situation, the time needed to assess weaning/extubation failure should probably be longer, possibly up to 7 days [4].

62.2.2 Epidemiology and Impact of Weaning/Extubation Difficulties

MV can lead to many complications, including prolonged MV due to weaning/extubation difficulties, delaying the extubation time, as well as risk of reintubation and its own complications; all these situations may increase the patient's morbidity-mortality. Weaning/extubation difficulties may also be related to the underlying disease, and chronic obstructive pulmonary disease (COPD) patients represent one of the main high-risk populations [1, 3]. Hence, the ICU clinician should consider the feasibility and potential issue of the weaning/extubation process as soon as possible, according to the underlying status, to optimize the weaning/extubation conditions, limit the MV duration, and eventually propose alternative techniques to conventional weaning.

62.3 Role of NIV in the Post-extubation Period

62.3.1 Definitions and Objectives

When applying NIV in the post-extubation period, the ICU clinician should consider three different indications according to their respective objectives and reported results in the literature [5] (Fig. 62.1). The objective of NIV used as a weaning/extubation technique (to facilitate early liberation from MV) is to reduce MV duration (intubation) in patients exhibiting weaning difficulties (one or more SBT failures). The objective of NIV used for the management of post-extubation ARF is to avoid reintubation according to two strategies: either to prevent the occurrence of post-extubation ARF in patients at risk of extubation failure (i.e., preventive or prophylactic NIV strategy) (Table 62.1), or to treat the occurrence of post-extubation ARF following an extubation (24–48 h) that most often is scheduled (i.e., curative or rescue strategy).

62.3.2 Physiopathological Rationale to Apply NIV in the Post-extubation Period

Despite the absence of endotracheal prosthesis, NIV can meet the physiological objectives of any type of mechanical ventilation (decrease in the work of breathing, improvement in the breathing pattern, gas exchange, and dyspnea) with a good hemodynamic tolerance [2, 6]. Therefore, NIV application in the post-extubation period should consider the following main objectives: to counteract the different physiopathological factors involved in the weaning/extubation failure, to help

Table 62.1 Risk factors for extubation failure based on selection criteria of randomized controlled trials [21–25]

Age ≥ 65 years
APACHE II score > 12 (day of extubation)
Chronic respiratory disease (COPD)
Heart failure
More than one comorbidity (other than heart failure)
More than one consecutive SBT failure
$PaCO_2$ > 45 mmHg during SBT or following extubation
Inefficient cough
Post-extubation stridor
Morbid obesity (BMI ≥ 35 kg/m^2)

COPD chronic obstructive pulmonary disease, *SBT* spontaneous breathing trial, *BMI* body mass index

physicians with difficulties in predicting results of the weaning/extubation process, and, finally, to treat or prevent the occurrence of a post-extubation ARF, sometimes not foreseeable. Finally, it should be kept in mind that NIV is as efficient and beneficial when there is an underlying hypercapnia ($PaCO_2$ > 45 mmHg), a frequent situation in cases of weaning/extubation failure [1, 3].

62.3.3 Clinical Rationale to Apply NIV in the Post-extubation Period

Weaning/extubation from MV should be considered as a true challenge for the ICU clinician. The clinical basis to apply NIV in the post-extubation period is closely related to the epidemiological and physiopathological data involved in weaning/extubation difficulties and failure, as mentioned above. In addition, efficacy and clinical benefit of NIV in morbidity and mortality (avoiding intubation, reducing nosocomial infections, and survival improvement) for the initial management of hypercapnic ARF, leading to routine practice in severe acute exacerbation in COPD patients [7], also represents a strong argument for using NIV in the post-extubation period. In fact, the ICU clinician must find the optimal compromise between the risks of unduly prolonged intubation and those of a too early weaning and extubation process [5]. Therefore, any strategy with the aim of reducing morbidity and mortality of prolonged MV or reintubation appears relevant and should be developed to improve patient prognosis, particularly in those at high risk of weaning/extubation failure [1, 3].

62.3.4 Results of NIV Use in the Post-extubation Period

62.3.4.1 NIV as a Weaning/Extubation Technique from Mechanical Ventilation

Two noncontrolled clinical studies have previously suggested the feasibility of NIV in this indication [8, 9]. Thereafter, six randomized controlled trials (RCTs) that compared weaning with NIV to conventional weaning were conducted

[1, 10–14] (Table 62.2). The results were in favor of NIV in five of the studies [4, 10–13] (Table 62.2). These RCTs have also been included in four systematic reviews or meta-analyses [5, 15–17]. The large Cochrane systematic review (994 patients, 16 RCTs including the six previous English RCTs) stratified its results according to the underlying respiratory disease (COPD or mixed chronic

Table 62.2 Characteristics of the main randomized controlled trials applying NIV in the post-extubation period

Indications/ studies [ref.]	Study type	Population characteristics	NIV modalities/ control group	NIV experience	Main results
Weaning/extubation (control group: invasive conventional weaning or oxygen therapy)					
Nava et al. [10]	Multicentric (3 centers)	Selected CRF, COPD $n=50$	PSV, FM, Cont, ICUv/PSV	≥5 years	Favor NIV
Girault et al. [11]	Monocentric	Selected CRF, mixed (COPD=51 %) $n=33$	PSV or ACV, FM or N, Int. ICUv/ PSV	≥5 years	Favor NIV
Ferrer et al. [12]	Multicentric (3 centers)	Selected CRF, mixed (COPD=44 %) $n=43$	BiPAP, FM or N, Cont., SPEv/PSV or ACV	≥5 years	Favor NIV
Wang et al. [13]	Multicentric (11 centers)	Selected CRF, COPD $n=90$	BiPAP, FM, Int., SPEv/PSV or IMV	–	Favor NIV
Prasad et al. [14]	Monocentric	Selected CRF, COPD $n=30$	BiPAP, FM, Cont., SPEv/PSV	–	Similar
Girault et al. [4]	Multicentric (13 centers)	Selected CRF, mixed (COPD=69 %) $n=208$	PSV or BiPAP, FM, Cont., ICUv or SPEv/PSV or T tube/O_2 #:	≥10 years	Favor NIV
Post-extubation ARF prevention (control group: standard oxygen therapy)					
Nava et al. [21]	Multicentric (3 centers)	Heterogenous (CRF/ COPD=33 %) at risk of extubation failure $n=97$	PSV or BiPAP, FM or N, Int., ICUv. or SPEv/O_2	≥10 years	Favor NIV
Ferrer et al. [22]	Multicentric (2 centers)	Heterogenous (CRF/ COPD=51 %) at risk of extubation failure $n=162$	BiPAP, FM, Cont, SPEv/O_2	≥10 years	Favor NIV
Ferrer et al. [23]	Multicentric (3 centers)	selected CRF (COPD=70 %) at risk of extubation failure $n=106$	BiPAP, FM, Cont, SPEv/O_2	≥10 years	Favor NIV

NIV noninvasive ventilation, *COPD* chronic obstructive pulmonary disease, *CRF* chronic respiratory failure, *PSV* pressure support ventilation ± positive end-expiratory pressure, *ACV* assist control ventilation, *IMV* intermittent mandatory ventilation, O_2 standard oxygen therapy, *BiPAP* bi-level positive airway pressure, *T tube* weaning with spontaneous breathing trials on T piece, *FM or N* mask or nasal mask, *Cont./Int.* NIV applied continuously or intermittently, *ICUv/SPEv* NIV applied with an ICU or specific dedicated ventilator, *#:* 3 groups of randomization = NIV versus conventional weaning versus standard oxygen therapy respiratory failure (CRF)) [17]. Finally, available data show that NIV used as an early weaning/extubation technique in medical populations, mainly COPD or CRF patients, permits a significant decrease in the following outcome parameters: weaning failure, risk of reintubation, duration of MV not related to weaning, ICU and in-hospital length of stay, MV complications (nosocomial pneumonia, tracheostomy), and mortality. Furthermore, the benefit with regard to survival may be more important, as there is an underlying COPD and hypercapnia ($PaCO_2 > 45$ mmHg) during the SBT. Early extubation relayed with NIV appears, therefore, to be a reliable, safe, and beneficial weaning technique in difficult-to-wean medical patients, mainly those with COPD.

Except for CRF patients, few clinical data are currently available for weaning/extubation from MV with NIV. To our knowledge, only two older noncontrolled studies have suggested the potential role of NIV in early extubation of surgical [18] or trauma [19] patients. More recently, in a pilot study, an experienced team has shown that NIV could also be useful in the early extubation of hypoxemic ARF patients [20].

62.3.4.2 NIV and Management of Post-extubation ARF

Preventive Post-extubation NIV

Prior to the occurrence of post-extubation ARF, NIV should be considered earlier after extubation, particularly in patients at risk for extubation failure, that is, for reintubation (Table 62.1). Three large, prospective RCTs compared the use of preventive post-extubation NIV to standard oxygen therapy in mixed CRF or COPD patients having passed a successful SBT but being considered at risk for extubation failure [21–23] (Table 62.2). One other underpowered RCT included only 40 patients with severe COPD [24], and preventive post-extubation NIV has also been applied in a case-control study conducted in obese patients [25]. Only the first two RCTs [21, 22] have been pooled in a meta-analysis [26]. Overall, the findings show that NIV, applied early following scheduled extubation in patients considered at risk of reintubation, prevents the occurrence of post-extubation ARF, decreases the reintubation risk, and may, therefore, improve the morbidity and mortality of patients. Moreover, the benefit regarding mortality appears more relevant as there is an underlying hypercapnia ($PaCO_2 > 45$ mmHg) during or following the SBT. Therefore, this hypercapnia may be considered as a simple objective and useful criteria for clinicians to consider preventive post-extubation NIV, particularly in cases of underlying COPD.

In this indication, however, it is essential to research risk factors for extubation failure, as preventive post-extubation NIV cannot be routinely applied to all intubated patients. Indeed, several studies have shown that systematic use of preventive NIV in nonselected populations could be only slightly [27] or not beneficial [28], and even potentially deleterious [29], compared with standard oxygen therapy.

In surgical patients, interesting physiological results (oxygenation, diaphragmatic dysfunction, atelectasis) have been obtained with preventive post-extubation NIV [30–32], but outcome results appear discordant in terms of benefit and the risk of post-extubation ARF and reintubation, length of stay, and survival, even in surgical patients with COPD [33]. Of note, most of these studies used continuous positive airway pressure (CPAP) rather than pressure support ventilation (PSV) mode.

Curative Post-extubation NIV

Two observational clinical studies have suggested the feasibility and benefit of NIV in this indication [34, 35]. Thereafter, two prospective RCTs comparing curative NIV with standard oxygen therapy in a nonselected medical population with post-extubation ARF were found negative [36, 37], the second even suggesting that NIV could be deleterious in this indication, with an increase in ICU mortality by delaying the reintubation time [37]. Consequently, these negative results have dramatically limited the clinical research and, currently, no RCT is available in this field, particularly in hypercapnic post-extubation ARF. Nevertheless, there are some arguments that promising results could probably be still considered with "curative NIV" in more selected population like patients with COPD: (1) the benefit of NIV in the initial management of hypercapnic ARF in these patients; (2) the increased use of NIV in the post-extubation period in epidemiological study, in part in this particular indication [38]; and (3) the success rates of NIV used as a "rescue" strategy in studies assessing NIV as a weaning/extubation technique (45 and 58 %) [4], in those evaluating preventive post-extubation NIV (63 %) [23], and in the negative RCT by Esteban et al. (75 %) [37]. Therefore, further well-conducted RCTs are still warranted in this indication. For instance, current results should prompt clinicians to be cautious in using curative NIV routinely in the management of post-extubation ARF in medical ICU patients so as not to delay reintubation.

More studies have been conducted in surgical ICU patients in this indication. In the post-operative period, curative post-extubation NIV has been shown to improve oxygenation and decrease atelectasis, reintubation risk, pneumonia, length of stay, and even mortality, according to the studies, after abdominal, cardiothoracic, and solid organ transplantation surgery [15, 39].

62.4 Limits of NIV Application in the Post-extubation Period

To date, outside of the post-operative setting, all studies that have suggested or demonstrated a benefit of post-extubation NIV have involved selected medical populations suffering from underlying chronic respiratory disease, mainly COPD [1, 10–14, 22, 23, 34, 35]. Current available data in this field suggest that NIV use in the post-extubation period first requires knowledge of the principles of weaning/extubation from MV and also NIV techniques and surveillance. The risk factors for weaning/extubation failure must be known and underlying hypercapnia ($PaCO_2$>45 mmHg) during the weaning/extubation period should be looked for. Finally, patients must be able to be reintubated without delay and at any time if needed.

Conclusion

Since the last consensus conferences on weaning and NIV [1, 2], the management of weaning/extubation and post-extubation ARF with NIV can now be considered in ICU patients. Provided a sufficient acquired experience with NIV, current data should prompt ICU physicians to apply post-extubation NIV in selected medical populations, such as COPD patients, in cases of weaning difficulties, or to prevent post-extubation ARF in high-risk patients. Hypercapnia during or following SBT appears to be a useful criteria for decision-making in these indications. Regarding curative post-extubation NIV, despite the lack of formal current evidence, it can be used with cautious in some surgical populations and should probably be tested before reintubation in COPD patients. In all cases, the clinician should keep in mind that post-extubation NIV needs rigorous analysis of the risk/benefit ratio for the patient so as not to unnecessarily delay reintubation.

Key Practical Recommendations

- When applying NIV in the post-extubation period, the ICU clinician should consider three different strategies: NIV as a weaning/extubation technique in difficult to wean patients (one or more SBT failure), NIV to prevent post-extubation ARF in high-risk patients of extubation failure (preventive or prophylactic NIV strategy), and NIV to treat the occurrence of post-extubation ARF within 24–48 h of an extubation (curative or rescue strategy).
- Post-extubation NIV should be reserved to centers with expertise in NIV techniques.
- NIV can be used as a weaning/extubation technique in difficult-to-wean CRF patients, mainly those with COPD.
- Preventive post-extubation NIV can be used after planned extubation in patients considered at risk for extubation failure.
- Because of the lack of evidence, curative post-extubation NIV should not be routinely used in the nonselected population. However, it could probably be applied in some surgical populations and patients with COPD.

References

1. Boles JM, Bion J, Connors A, et al. Weaning from mechanical ventilation. Statement of the sixth international consensus conference on intensive care medicine. Eur Respir J. 2007;29:1033–56.
2. Robert R, Bengler C, Beuret P, et al. Non invasive ventilation in acute respiratory failure (newborn excluded). Consensus Conference from SFAR, SPLF, and SRLF. Réanimation. 2006;13:5–12.
3. Thille AW, Cortes-Puch I, Esteban A. Weaning from the ventilator and extubation in ICU. Curr Opin Crit Care. 2013;19:57–64.

4. Girault C, Bubenheim M, Abroug F, et al. Noninvasive ventilation and weaning in patients with chronic hypercapnic respiratory failure: a randomized multicenter trial. Am J Respir Crit Care Med. 2011;184:672–9.
5. Hess DR. The role of noninvasive ventilation in the ventilator discontinuation process. Resp Care. 2012;57:1619–25.
6. Nava S, Hill N. Non invasive ventilation in acute respiratory failure. Lancet. 2009;374:250–9.
7. Keenan SP, Sinuff T, Burns KEA, et al. Clinical practice guidelines for the use of non-invasive positive-pressure ventilation and noninvasive continuous positive airway pressure in the acute care setting. CMAJ. 2011;183:E195–214.
8. Udwadia ZF, Santis GK, Steven MH, et al. Nasal ventilation to facilitate weaning in patients with chronic respiratory insufficiency. Thorax. 1992;47:715–8.
9. Restrick LJ, Scott AD, Ward EM, et al. Nasal intermittent positive-pressure ventilation in weaning intubated patients with chronic respiratory disease from assisted positive-pressure ventilation. Respir Med. 1993;87:199–204.
10. Nava S, Ambrosino N, Clini E, et al. Noninvasive mechanical ventilation in the weaning of patients with respiratory failure due to chronic obstructive pulmonary disease. Ann Intern Med. 1998;128:721–8.
11. Girault C, Daudenthun I, Chevron V, et al. Noninvasive ventilation as a systematic extubation and weaning technique in acute on chronic respiratory failure. A prospective randomized controlled study. Am J Respir Crit Care Med. 1999;160:86–92.
12. Ferrer M, Esquinas A, Arancibia F, et al. Non-invasive ventilation during persistent weaning failure. A randomised-controlled trial. Am J Respir Crit Care Med. 2003;168:70–6.
13. Wang C, Collaborating Research Group for Noninvasive Mechanical Ventilation of the Chinese Respiratory Society. Pulmonary infection control window in the treatment of severe respiratory failure of chronic obstructive pulmonary diseases: a prospective, randomized controlled, multi-centre study. Chin Med J (Engl). 2005;118:1589–94.
14. Prasad SB, Chaudhry D, Khanna R. Role of noninvasive ventilation in weaning from mechanical ventilation in patients of chronic obstructive pulmonary disease: an Indian experience. Indian J Crit Care Med. 2009;13:207–12.
15. Glossop AJ, Shepherd N, Bryden DC, et al. Non-invasive ventilation for weaning, avoiding reintubation after extubation and in the postoperative period: a meta-analysis. Br J Anaesth. 2012;109:305–14.
16. Zhu F, Liu ZL, Long X, et al. Effect of noninvasive positive pressure ventilation on weaning success in patients receiving invasive mechanical ventilation: a meta-analysis. Chin Med J (Engl). 2013;126:1337–43.
17. Burns KE, Meade MO, Premji A, et al. Noninvasive ventilation as a weaning strategy for mechanical ventilation in adults with respiratory failure: a Cochrane systematic review. CMAJ. 2014;186:E112–22.
18. Kilger E, Briegel J, Haller M, et al. Effects of noninvasive positive pressure ventilation support in non-COPD patients with acute respiratory insufficiency after early extubation. Intensive Care Med. 1999;25:1374–80.
19. Gregoretti C, Beltrame F, Lucangelo U, et al. Physiologic evaluation of noninvasive pressure support ventilation in trauma patients with acute respiratory failure. Intensive Care Med. 1998;24:785–90.
20. Vaschetto R, Turucz E, Dellapiazza F, et al. Noninvasive ventilation after early extubation in patients recovering from hypoxemic acute respiratory failure: a single-centre feasibility study. Intensive Care Med. 2012;38:1599–606.
21. Nava S, Gregoretti C, Fanfulla F, et al. Noninvasive ventilation to prevent respiratory failure after extubation in high risk patients. Crit Care Med. 2005;33:2465–70.
22. Ferrer M, Valencia M, Nicolas JM, et al. Early noninvasive ventilation averts extubation failure in patients at risk: a randomized trial. Am J Respir Crit Care Med. 2006;173:164–70.
23. Ferrer M, Sellarés J, Valencia M, et al. Non-invasive ventilation after extubation in hypercapnic patients with chronic respiratory disorders: randomised controlled trial. Lancet. 2009;374:1082–8.

24. Khilnani GC, Galle AD, Hadda V, et al. Non-invasive ventilation after extubation in patients with chronic obstructive airways disease: a randomised controlled trial. Anaesth Intensive Care. 2011;39:217–22.
25. El Solh AA, Aquilina A, Pineda L, et al. Noninvasive ventilation for prevention of postextubation respiratory failure in obese patients. Eur Respir J. 2006;28:588–95.
26. Agarwal R, Aggarwal AN, Gupta D, et al. Role of noninvasive positive-pressure ventilation in postextubation respiratory failure: a meta-analysis. Respir Care. 2007;52:1472–9.
27. Ornico SR, Lobo SM, Sanches HS, et al. Noninvasive ventilation immediately after extubation improves weaning outcome after acute respiratory failure: a randomized controlled trial. Crit Care. 2013;17:R39.
28. Su CL, Chiang LL, Yang SH, et al. Preventive use of noninvasive ventilation after extubation: a prospective, multicenter randomized controlled trial. Respir Care. 2012;57:204–10.
29. Jiang JS, Kao SJ, Wang SN. Effect of early application of biphasic positive airway pressure on the outcome of extubation in ventilator weaning. Respirology. 1999;4:161–5.
30. Kindgen-Milles D, Muller E, Buhl R, et al. Nasal-continuous positive airway pressure reduces pulmonary morbidity and length of hospital stay following thoracoabdominal aortic surgery. Chest. 2005;128:821–8.
31. Perrin C, Jullien V, Vénissac N, et al. Prophylactic use of noninvasive ventilation in patients undergoing lung resectional surgery. Respir Med. 2007;101:1572–8.
32. Liao G, Chen R, He J. Prophylactic use of noninvasive positive pressure ventilation in post-thoracic surgery patients: a prospective randomized control study. J Thorac Dis. 2010;2:205–9.
33. Lorut C, Lefebvre A, Planquette B, et al. Early postoperative prophylactic noninvasive ventilation after major lung resection in COPD patients: a randomized controlled trial. Intensive Care Med. 2014;40:220–7.
34. Meduri GU, Abou-Shala N, Fox RC, et al. Noninvasive face mask mechanical ventilation in patients with acute hypercapnic respiratory failure. Chest. 1991;100:445–54.
35. Hilbert G, Gruson D, Portel L, et al. Noninvasive pressure support ventilation in COPD patients with postextubation hypercapnic respiratory insufficiency. Eur Respir J. 1998;11:1349–53.
36. Keenan SP, Powers C, McCormack DG, et al. Noninvasive positive-pressure ventilation for post-extubation respiratory distress. A randomized controlled trial. JAMA. 2002;287:3238–44.
37. Esteban A, Frutos-Vivar F, Ferguson ND, et al. Noninvasive positive-pressure ventilation for respiratory failure after extubation. N Engl J Med. 2004;350:2452–60.
38. Penuelas O, Frutos-Vivar F, Fernandez C, et al. Characteristics and outcomes of ventilated patients according to time to liberation from mechanical ventilation. Am J Respir Crit Care Med. 2011;184:430–7.
39. Chiumello D, Chevallard G, Gregoretti C. Non-invasive ventilation in postoperative patients: a systematic review. Intensive Care Med. 2011;37:918–29.

Perioperative Adverse Events in Obstructive Sleep Apnea and Use of Noninvasive Mechanical Ventilation: Key Topics and Clinical Implications

63

C. Gregoretti, A. Braghiroli, G. Insalaco, A. Cortegiani, and R. Corso

Contents

C. Gregoretti (✉)
Critical Care Medicine Department, "Città della salute e della scienza" Hospital, Torino, Italy
e-mail: c.gregoretti@gmail.com

A. Braghiroli
"S. Maugeri" Foundation, IRCCS, Dept Pulmonary Rehabilitation, Scientific Institute of Veruno (NO), Veruno, Italy

G. Insalaco
National Research Council of Italy, Institute of Biomedicine and Molecular Immunology "A. Monroy", Palermo, Italy

A. Cortegiani
Department of Biopathology and Medical Biotechnologies (DIBIMED), Section of Anesthesiology, Analgesia, Emergency and Intensive Care, Policlinico "P. Giaccone," University of Palermo, Palermo, Italy

R. Corso
Emergency Department, Anesthesia and Intensive Care Unit, "G.B. Morgagni" Hospital, Forlì, Italy

A.M. Esquinas (ed.), *Noninvasive Mechanical Ventilation: Theory, Equipment, and Clinical Applications*, DOI 10.1007/978-3-319-21653-9_63

63.1 Introduction

Obstructive sleep apnea (OSA) is a condition occurring in a portion of the general population, unpredicted until a few years ago [1–3], and has been implicated as a comorbid factor in various clinical conditions. OSA is the result of a complex overlap of several features that compromise the ability of the upper airways to maintain patency during sleep [4–6]. Although abnormalities of airway structures – such as enlarged tonsils and uvula, micrognatia, and wide neck circumference linked to obesity – can be a facilitating factor, passive characteristics of the upper airways, which compromise the ability of pharyngeal dilators to maintain upper airway patency, can be blamed from less than a third of the total burden [4]. A partial (hypopnea) or total (apnea) obstruction of airflow leads to the same consequence: local reflex, hypercapnia, acidosis, hypoventilation, and hypoxia stimulate arousal centers, leading to the resumption of wakefulness muscular tone. These changes and an increased ventilatory effort overcome the obstruction, and ventilation resumes [7]. This repetitive collapse of the upper airways may happen cyclically many times per night. The arousals cause sleep fragmentation and sympathetic activation, leading to peripheral vasoconstriction, increased systolic and diastolic blood pressure, and a rise in heart rate, even as the cardiac output continues to fall after the reopening of the airway [8]. The associated intermittent hypoxia causes systemic inflammation with a mechanism very similar to ischemia/reperfusion damage [9], causing cardiovascular consequences, decreased cerebral blood flow and oxygenation [10, 11], and alteration of electric conduction (e.g., supraventricular and ventricular ectopy, sinoatrial and atrioventricular block, atrial fibrillation) [12, 13]. Although obesity has been considered a classic risk factor for OSA, today it is clear that the majority of OSA patients are non-obese and the figures are so high that OSA is now considered more common than asthma among adults.

A few studies have used polysomnography (PSG) to determine the frequency of OSA in the surgical population [14–17]. In most instances, the frequency of OSA was higher than the prevalence in the general population and varies with the type of surgical intervention. For instance, bariatric surgery, which is addressed mainly to super-obese patients, is burdened with a prevalence as high as 70 % [18], presumably due to the high percentage of fat tissue in the neck. Finkel et al. [19] found that 24 % of surgical patients were at high risk based on a screening tool, but almost 4 out of 5 patients (81 %) had not been previously diagnosed with OSA.

Chronic untreated OSA is an independent risk factor for increased mortality in the general population [20], but in the perioperative management it determines an additional treatment due to upper airway collapsibility and associated comorbidities. Memtsoudis et al. [21] found a higher risk of pulmonary complications (PPCs) in OSA patients after non-cardiac surgery. Flink et al. [22] reported a 53 % incidence of postoperative delirium in OSA patients versus 20 % in non-OSA patients. A meta-analysis concluded that patients with OSA undergoing non-cardiac surgery have a higher incidence of postoperative O_2 desaturation, respiratory failure, cardiac events, and ICU transfers than those without OSA [23].

It is possible that the repetitive episodes of hypoxia occurring every night make these patients less fragile according to the mechanism called "pre-conditioning" [9, 24], compensating for the higher incidence with a lower mortality. Indeed, one study found that neither an OSA diagnosis nor suspected OSA were associated with an increased 30-day or 1-year postoperative mortality [25]. These data were confirmed by Mokhlesi et al. [26, 27] in two cohorts of surgical patients who showed an increased number of complications but failed to demonstrate an increase in mortality.

As a matter of fact, this body of evidence associating OSA with adverse perioperative outcomes calls to implement perioperative strategies aimed at improving safety. Various authors have suggested guidelines or clinical algorithms to improve the perioperative care of these patients [28–30]. The aim of this chapter is to determine the effects of perioperative sedatives and anesthetics in surgical patients with OSA, to suggest a diagnostic and therapeutic path, and to define the role of noninvasive ventilation to prevent/treat the respiratory events.

63.2 Preoperative Evaluation

We can summarize the possible scenario the clinician has to face before surgery as follows [31]:

1. Patients with a diagnosis of OSA who are receiving treatment.
2. Patients with OSA already diagnosed who are not receiving treatment yet, are noncompliant with treatment, or with unsuccessful treatment.
3. Patients without a diagnosis of OSA who show an unexplained hypoxemia, polycythemia, hypercapnia, pulmonary hypertension, or right- side heart failure.

These patients could have an undiagnosed, and often severe, OSA and represent a large proportion of those who undergo surgery [32]. They often have the typical symptoms of OSA, such as heavy snoring, witnessed apneas, unrefreshed sleep, excessive daytime sleepiness and/or sleepiness at the examination, obesity, short thick neck, tonsillar hypertrophy, and retrognathia. Although these clinical features are suggestive of OSA, they are not reliable predictors of the presence or severity of the disease [31], since only nocturnal monitoring allows a firm diagnosis and staging (Fig. 63.1). Obviously, the extended use of PSG or ambulatory monitoring for preoperative screening is not feasible, but given the high prevalence of this condition and the high number of undiagnosed OSA patients, all surgical patients should be screened for OSA. As a result, several tools have been developed to meet this need for simple, economic, and sensitive bedside screening tests for the detection of patients with suspected OSA [30, 33, 34]. The quickest and the simplest to use seems to be the STOP Questionnaire [35], further implemented including questions about additional risk factors for OSA such as body mass index (B), age (A), neck circumference (N), and gender (G); the modified tool is called the STOP-BANG Questionnaire (Fig. 63.2). The STOP-BANG questionnaire was originally

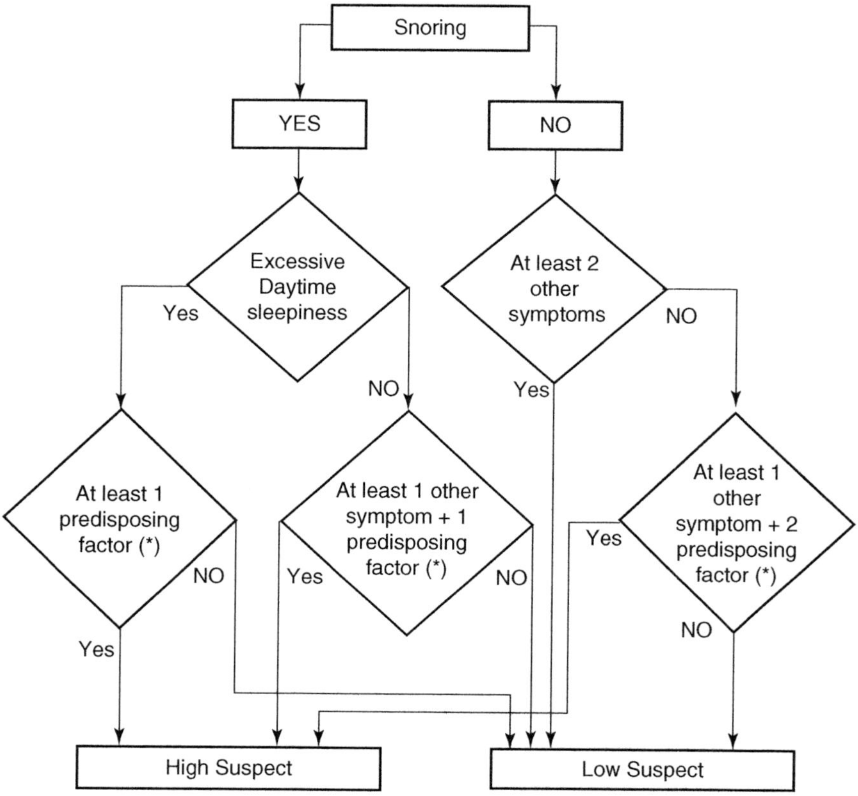

PREDISPOSING FACTORS	Upper airway soft tissue hypertrophy craniofacial abnormalities BMI >25
SYMPTOMS	Snoring Observed apneas Excessive daytime sleepiness (Ess >10) Choking/Gasping Nocturia Depression Irritability Headache on awakening Neurocognitive disorders Erectile dysfunction Decreased libido Gastroesophageal reflux

Fig. 63.1 Diagnostic flow chart in patients with symptoms and clinical signs suggesting a sleep-related obstructive sleep apnea. *BMI* body mass index, *ESS* Epworth Sleepiness Scale

***S.* Snoring** (observed during sleep)		
Do you *s*nore loudly (louder than talking or loud enough to be heard through closed doors)?	Yes	No
***T.* Tiredness** (in the daytime)		
Do you often feel tired, fatigued or sleepy during daytime?	Yes	No
***O.* Observed apnea**		
Has anyone *o*bserved you stop breathing during your sleep?	Yes	No
***P.* Blood Pressure**		
Do you have or are you being treated for high blood pressure?	Yes	No
***B.* Body Mass Index**		
BMI more than 35 kg/m^2?	Yes	No
***A.* Age**		
Age over 50 yr old?	Yes	No
***N.* Neck circumference**		
Neck circumference greater than 40 cm?	Yes	No
***G.* Gender**		
Gender male?	Yes	No

Fig. 63.2 The STOP-BANG Questionnaire. A high risk of sleep apnea is defined as a score of 3 or more; low risk of sleep apnea, a score of less than 3

developed in the surgical population but has been validated in various patient populations [36–38]. Patients with STOP-BANG scores 0–2 may be considered at low risk, 3–4 at intermediate risk, and 5–8 at high risk of OSA [37]. Corso et al. [38] showed that STOP-BANG scores indicative of a high risk of OSA confer a heightened risk of postoperative complications in patients undergoing elective surgery, confirming its value to predict OSA severity and triage patients in the perioperative period.

63.3 Intraoperative Management

Although patients with severe OSA seem to be at higher risk of perioperative complications [39], careful observation and early intervention should be recommended for patients with all grades of severity of sleep-disordered breathing [31, 40]. Various strategies can be employed to reduce the risks and avoid adverse outcomes. Preoperatively, the use of anxiolytic premedication is not recommended [41]. There is evidence that regional anesthesia (RA) is preferable over general anesthesia (GA) whenever possible [42]. Regional anesthesia minimally affects respiratory drive, it avoids the side effect of anesthetic agents, particularly on the arousal responses during apneic episodes. Regional anesthesia may also avoid or reduce the need for sedative drugs and opioids during the entire perioperative period. It has been well established that the presence of OSA may lead to difficulties in airway management both in terms of difficult mask ventilation and tracheal intubation [43–46]. Although these findings do not imply that awake intubation is necessary in all patients with OSA, prudence dictates that clinicians should have immediate access to alternative techniques to secure the airway and ventilate the patient. There is evidence that many anesthetic agents cause exaggerated responses in patients with sleep apnea. Drugs such as thiopentone, propofol, opioids, benzodiazepines, and nitrous oxide may blunt the tone of the pharyngeal musculature that acts to maintain airway patency. The choice of induction and maintenance agents is probably not important, although it would seem reasonable to avoid large doses of long-acting drugs. This is true with both neuromuscular blocking agents and benzodiazepines. As a matter of fact, anesthesia techniques using short half-life agents should be advised to avoid any residual drugs in the respiratory system [47, 48]. Whenever the patient is extubated, whether early in the operating room or later in the recovery room or in the ICU, the patient should be fully awake [49]. Full recovery from neuromuscular blockade should be proven by a neuromuscular blockade monitor. In the case of difficult airways, guidelines for safe extubation should be followed [50].

63.4 Postoperative Management

The postoperative disposition of the OSA patient will depend on three main components: invasiveness of the surgery, severity (known or predicted) of OSA, and requirement for postoperative opioids. The American Society of Anesthesiologists (ASA) guidelines suggest that all patients with known or suspected OSA who have received general anesthesia should be monitored in the PACU (post-anesthesia care unit). However, there are currently no evidence-based guidelines addressing the optimal length of monitoring required in the PACU and the ASA recommendations are difficult to adhere to, especially in the context of a community hospital [50].

63.4.1 Role of Noninvasive Ventilation

All patients with OSA or at high risk of having OSA are at possible risk of worsening to acute respiratory failure (ARF). In that case, the patient becomes incapable of maintaining his/her normal value of arterial blood gases due to an acute lung and/or respiratory pump failure. As mentioned above, a potential cause of immediate postoperative hypoxia is upper airway obstruction causing apnea [51]. However, symptoms of OSAs can be exacerbated during the postoperative period as a result of deterioration of the airway condition and rapid eye movement (REM) sleep rebound caused by opioids predisposing to PPCs and adverse outcomes [51, 52]. Patients with OSA after surgery are at high risk of PPCs, not only for adverse effects linked to their underlying disease but also because of pulmonary complications – that is, formation of atelectasis – which increase significantly the risk for pneumonia and ARF [53]. The risk of respiratory events and PPC could be related to the type of surgery [31], with the higher risk being related to upper airway surgery, for the consequent edema of the pharyngeal district [54, 55], and thorax and upper abdomen surgery, for consequent respiratory muscle impairment [56, 57]. Surgery of any type can be burdened by a higher risk of complications in OSA patients [40, 58].

Noninvasive ventilation (NIV), as widely described in the chapters of the present book, refers to the noninvasive delivery via an external interface through the patient's native airways (mouth, nose, or both) of intermittent positive pressure ventilation (NPPV) or continuous positive airway pressure (CPAP). NIV may improve gas exchange and reduce patient's effort as invasive mechanical ventilation (IMV) delivered via endotracheal tube or tracheostomy, but differently from IMV, NIV does not interfere with patient native upper airways and, in particular, with glottis function [59–62]. The aims of NIV are to partially compensate for the decreased respiratory function by reducing the work of breathing; to improve alveolar recruitment with better gas exchange (oxygenation and ventilation); and to reduce left ventricular afterload, increasing cardiac output and improving hemodynamics. So it may be an important tool to prevent (prophylactic treatment) or to treat (curative treatment) acute respiratory failure avoiding intubation [53].

CPAP and NPPV have different physiological effects on a patient's respiratory system and hemodynamics that need some clarifications. Applying noninvasive positive pressure without bypassing the upper airways (oronasal cavities, the pharynx, the larynx including the epiglottis, glottis and subglottis, and upper esophageal sphincter) introduces to the original equation of motion a new variable, namely the pressure needed to overcome upper airway resistances [63]. The glottis, vocal cords, and genioglossus change their activation and function in phase with inspiration and expiration [64, 65]. This explains the results of Parreira et al. [66] demonstrating closure of the glottis at increasing levels of assist pressure, causing a reduction of the effective ventilation. Moreau-Bussière et al. [67] demonstrated that the activation of the thyroarytenoid muscle (a glottal constrictor) at high levels of noninvasive pressure delivery impeded ventilation. As a matter of fact, the equation of motion should be slightly modified from the original equation: $P_{app} = \mathrm{Pel} + \mathrm{Pres} + $ intrinsic positive end expiratory pressure (PEEPi), where Pel is the pressure needed to overcome the elastic recoil of the lung (P_L) and the chest wall (P_{CW}) and Pres is the pressure needed to overcome the lower airways resistances. During NIV, Pres is the pressure needed to overcome both resistances of the lower (P_{LA}) and the upper airways (P_{UO}), so $\mathrm{Pres} = (P_{UO} + P_{LA})$.

63.5 Role of CPAP in the Perioperative Period

Unlike NPPV, during CPAP the pressure applied to the respiratory system is only generated by the patient's respiratory muscles ($P_{app} = P_{Musc}$). In this case, transpulmonary pressure, which is generated by the respiratory muscles, has to overcome the upper airway resistances, which means that in patients with OSA CPAP is effective on the lower airways only if it opens the upper airways [68, 69]. CPAP maintains a constant pressure in the upper airways during inspiration and expiration that acts as a pneumatic splint, allowing patency of the upper airway throughout the respiratory cycle [70–72]. Beyond this, CPAP is aimed at improving arterial blood gases and at decreasing work of breathing by:

1. Increasing functional residual capacity;
2. Stabilizing the chest wall distortion;
3. Improving left ventricular performance in chronic heart failure
4. Offsetting PEEPi (in patients with COPD).

CPAP is aimed at improving oxygenation through an amelioration of ventilation-perfusion mismatch by promoting alveolar recruitment [73] and by maintaining the alveoli open and by counteracting PEEPi alone in association with NPPV [74–76].

Although "genuine" CPAP is commonly used for mild hypoxemic ARF without clear signs of respiratory muscle fatigue, the level of evidence of CPAP effectiveness as a single mode of ventilation support in manifested ARF without cardiopulmonary edema (CPE) is still low [77]. CPAP is also aimed at improving left ventricular performance in chronic heart failure and is considered as a first-line therapy in CPE [78–81. To understand the mechanism of CPAP in patients with OSA it is necessary to focus on the complex mechanisms of heart-lung interaction (Fig. 63.3). With each obstructive event and the associated hypoxemia and hypercapnia, there is a generation of a deep subatmospheric intrathoracic pressure (ITP) due to the occluded airway with associated left ventricular afterload, increased pulmonary artery pressures, decreased left ventricular compliance, and increased myocardial oxygen demand [68]. The heart and lungs share a common intrathoracic

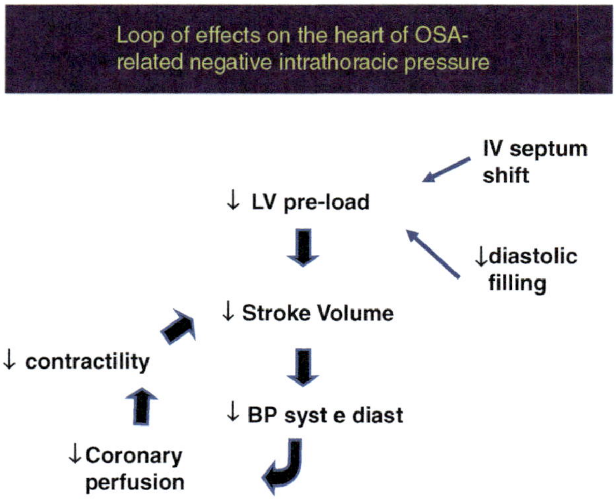

Fig. 63.3 Loop of effects on the heart of OSA-related negative intrathoracic pressure. *BP* blood pressure, *IV* inter-ventricular, *LV* left ventricle, *OSA* obstructive sleep apnea

compartment. The heart feels as a "container" the modification of ITP generated during changes of transpulmonary pressure during tidal breathing and accordingly modifies both venous return to the heart and left ventricular (LV) ejection pressure [82]. ITP decreases with inspiratory efforts and reducing right atrial pressure will augment venous return and its pressure gradient. In turn, the increase in right ventricular (RV) filling increases RV output, but dilating the right ventricle may theoretically cause the shift of intraventricular septum into the left ventricle, decreasing its diastolic compliance and arterial pulse pressure (*pulsus paradoxus*) [82]. With sustained decreases in ITP, as may occur with inspiration against an occluded airway (Mueller maneuver), this transient increase in venous return declines with the increased blood flow to the left ventricle and the intraventricular septum returns to its neutral position [83]. However, the decreasing ITP also increases LV afterload because LV ejection occurs into an arterial circuit in which the surrounding pressure is atmospheric pressure, not ITP [82]. LV afterload reflects the maximal wall stress on the left ventricle during ejection. According to the Laplace theorem, LV wall stress is a function of the product of the transmural pressure and the radius of curvature of the left ventricle [82]. This increased afterload explains the development of acute pulmonary edema in patients with severe airways obstruction or with OSA with repetitive negative swings during deep sleep. The increasing wall stress causes subendocardial ischemia and impairs LV systolic performance for a while, even after the strain phase of the increases ITP is over.

The oxygen desaturation leads to an increase in pulmonary vascular resistance due to hypoxic pulmonary vasoconstriction. In OSA patients, CPAP improves cardiovascular performance and decreases heart failure by reducing the incidence of both negative swings in ITP and arterial desaturation [84]. Interestingly, patients with chronic heart failure (CHF) have a prolonged depression in LV performance following ITP, even in the absence of hypoxemia [85]. Patients with CHF have increased circulating blood volume. Thus, negative swings in ITP will induce a greater increase in venous return than in healthy volunteers, suggesting that RV dilation is the primary cause of depressed LV performance [82]. Theoretically, measures aimed at reducing circulating blood volume, but also aimed to decrease LV afterload, would limit LV depression during OSA events [82].

Interestingly, Kaw et al. [86], in a study reporting the perioperative outcomes in a large cohort of patients undergoing cardiac surgery, comparing those with and without pulmonary hypertension (PH), found that 27 patients encountered significant postoperative complications. Patient characteristics significantly associated with postoperative mortality and morbidity on univariate analysis were affected by diabetes mellitus (DM), OSA, and chronic renal insufficiency (CRI). CPAP, by reducing the obstructive events, should also reduce the risk of increasing LV afterload.

CPAP is usually provided by a flow generator that delivers constant positive pressure or by ventilators [53, 87–90]. Although the intrathoracic pressure delivered by high-flow CPAP used in intensive care units cannot be compared to the unpredictable levels obtained with the devices commonly used for home treatment of OSA, they are all able to maintain the upper airways open, preventing the occurrence of obstructive events.

When CPAP is delivered by a bi-level turbine-driven ventilator, equal levels of inspiratory positive airway pressure (IPAP) and expiratory positive airway pressure (EPAP)/positive end-expiratory pressure (PEEP) generate CPAP.

63.5.1 Indication for Perioperative CPAP Use

As mentioned above, CPAP remains the most effective therapy for OSA, acting as a pneumatic splint to maintain upper airway patency. It appears that the consistent use of CPAP therapy prior to surgery and immediately after surgery holds the best potential for decreasing postoperative complications. However, CPAP does not provide adequate protection against central apnea, associated with the deterioration of airway condition caused by opioids. Although there are no studies addressing this topic, the use of NPPV with a back-up respiratory rate (i.e., spontaneous timed (ST) mode or assisted pressure controlled ventilation (APCV)) may be advisable [91].

63.5.2 Possible Recommendations

- If possible, patients with OSA should be treated with at least 4–6 weeks of CPAP before surgery, because an increase in pharyngeal size and a decrease in tongue volume have been noted on magnetic resonance imaging after 4–6 weeks of nasal CPAP therapy [92, 93].
- During induction of anesthesia, CPAP may be indicated to maintain upper airways patency. Eastwood et al. [94] studied 25 patients undergoing minor surgery on their limbs, and they found that patients who needed positive pressure to maintain airway patency had more severe sleep-disordered breathing.
- During regional anesthesia, sleep-disordered breathing can occur after even minor surgical procedures on the limbs [94].
- After extubation of the surgical patient. Extubation should be performed only when the patient is sufficiently awake, showing an adequate muscle tone in the upper airway, and should be monitored carefully to ensure that the upper airway remains unobstructed. In patients with known OSA, nasal CPAP in the preoperative setting should be started after extubation. Nasal or facial CPAP should be applied if airway obstruction is persistent even after the correct positioning of the patient. The CPAP pressure may need to be adjusted to obtain optimal efficacy. Patients who are unable to sustain spontaneous breathing through an obstructed airway may need NPPV or to undergo reintubation. In one investigation, patients with OSA who received nasal CPAP before surgery and thereafter on an almost continuous basis for 24–48 h for all sleep periods did not experience major complications [95]. Rennotte et al. [95] found that CPAP, started before surgery and resumed immediately after extubation, enabled the safe management of a variety of surgical procedures in patients with OSA, as well as the use of sedative, analgesic, and anesthetic drugs without major complications. Those who conducted the study recommended that every effort

should be made to identify patients with OSA and to perform CPAP therapy before surgery. Monitoring may need to be continued in an intermediate care setting for a longer period than that required in patients who do not have OSA. Nursing the patient in the lateral position may be helpful for patients whose airway obstruction is worse in the supine posture. Morbidly obese patients are at elevated risk of perioperative pulmonary complications, including airway obstruction and atelectasis. CPAP may improve postoperative lung mechanics and reduce postoperative complications in patients undergoing abdominal surgery. Neligan et al. [90] found that in 40 morbidly obese patients with OSA undergoing laparoscopic bariatric surgery with standard anesthesia care who were randomly assigned to receive CPAP via the Boussignac system immediately or 30 min after extubation (Boussignac group) or supplemental oxygen (standard care group), the administration of CPAP immediately after extubation maintains spirometric lung function at 24 h after laparoscopic bariatric surgery better than CPAP started in the PACU.

63.5.3 Indication for Perioperative NPPV Use

Different from CPAP, the pressure applied to the respiratory system (P_{app}) may be generated completely by the ventilator ($P_{app} = P_{Vent}$) or to a variable degree (depending from the operator setting) by the ventilator and the respiratory muscles ($P_{app} = P_{Musc} + P_{vent}$). NPPV is usually applied in the acute settings in pressure-controlled mode both time cycled (APCV) or flow cycled (PSV).

PSV increases tidal volume while unloading the inspiratory muscles [73, 96, 97]. Furthermore, EPAP/PEEP added to PSV may counteract the effects of intrinsic positive end-expiratory pressure (PEEPi) in COPD patients, further improving dyspnea, gas exchange, and inspiratory muscle effort. The majority of NIV studies in ARF use PSV, and it is the most often used mode in COPD exacerbation [76].

There is a paucity of literature regarding the use of NPPV in the perioperative patients.

63.5.4 Possible Indications for NPPV

- Patients with overlap syndrome
- During induction of anesthesia in difficult-to-ventilate patients. The combination of PEEP plus NPPV may allow ventilation [90, 94].
- Patients undergoing upper airway surgery where postoperative swelling in the upper airways may worsen OSA [54, 55]
- Nonrestricted postoperative opioid analgesia when CPAP become ineffective in maintaining airway patency and alveolar ventilation
- All other indications for NPPV after surgery [31, 53, 91]

In patients with OSA with an overlap syndrome, as in other diseases, there could be a rationale behind expiratory trigger adjustability (see cycling variable) to cope with different respiratory mechanics and thus improve patient-ventilator synchrony; the higher the value (i.e., 50 %), the lower the inspiratory time and vice versa. Usually, COPD patients benefit from a value around 40 %, whereas restrictive conditions benefit from lower values (i.e., 5–25 %) [98–100].

Pressure rise time (PRT) setting can also interfere as the expiratory trigger in mechanical inspiratory time [101, 102]. Restrictive conditions usually benefit from medium-range PRT and vice versa in obstructive conditions such as COPD [99, 101–105].

The set-up level of positive inspiratory pressure can be above (usually labeled as PSV) or below the EPAP/PEEP level (usually labeled as IPAP), according to the manufacturer. Some ventilators allow one to preset the set-up mode (above or below PEEP/EPAP) before use, according to the operator's choice [106]. In addition, some turbine-driven ventilators allow one to set a back-up rate (the so-called ST mode).

APCV is an assisted-controlled, pressure-controlled, time-cycled mode where the operator sets a preset respiratory rate and inspiratory time. Its use during NIV may find a rationale in the presence of a large amount of leaks hindering expiratory cycling in pressure-controlled, flow-cycled mode [107, 108], in very restrictive conditions not supporting a flow-cycled breath, or when a back-up rate is needed.

Conclusion

Perioperative management of OSA is characterized by a variety of problems requiring the joint effort of anesthesiologists, surgeons, and sleep experts. Anesthesiologists have the opportunity to closely observe patients in the PACU and can provide important information on where "the patient is going." Appropriate perioperative protocols are the best way to avoid perioperative complications associated with this common syndrome. Last but not least, in daily practice, anesthesiologists need simple solutions to avoid "choking" the PACU and overcrowding the critical care environments [40]. However, well-designed studies on the postoperative effect of CPAP and NIPPV in surgical patients with OSA are required to determine its role in the postoperative management of these patients.

References

1. Young T, Palta M, Dempsey J, Skatrud J, Weber S, Badr S. The occurrence of sleep-disordered breathing among middle-aged adults. N Engl J Med. 1993;328:1230–5.
2. Young T, Peppard PE, Gottlieb DJ. Epidemiology of obstructive sleep apnea: a population health perspective. Am J Respir Crit Care Med. 2002;165:1217–39.
3. Peppard PE, Young T, Barnet JH, Palta M, Hagen EW, Hla KM. Increased prevalence of sleep-disordered breathing in adults. Am J Epidemiol. 2013;177:1006–14.
4. Wellman A, Eckert DJ, Jordan AS, Edwards BA, Passaglia CL, Jackson AC, Gautam S, Owens RL, Malhotra A, White DP. A method for measuring and modeling the physiological traits causing obstructive sleep apnea. J Appl Physiol. 2011;110:1627–37.
5. Ryan CM, Bradley TD. Pathogenesis of obstructive sleep apnea. J Appl Physiol. 2005;99:2440–50.

6. White DP. Pathogenesis of obstructive and central sleep apnea. Am J Respir Crit Care Med. 2005;172:1363–70.
7. Gleeson K, Zwillich CW, White DP. The influence of increasing ventilatory effort on arousal from sleep. Am Rev Respir Dis. 1990;142:295–300.
8. Garpestad E, Katayama H, Parker JA, Ringler J, Lilly J, Yasuda T, Moore RH, Strauss HW, Weiss JW. Stroke volume and cardiac output decrease at termination of obstructive apneas. J Appl Physiol. 1992;73:1743–8.
9. Lavie L. Oxidative stress in obstructive sleep apnea and intermittent hypoxia – revisited – The bad ugly and good: implications to the heart and brain. Sleep Med Rev. 2015;20:27–45.
10. Balfors EM, Franklin KA. Impairment of cerebral perfusion during obstructive sleep apneas. Am J Respir Crit Care Med. 1994;150:1587–91.
11. Hayakawa T, Terashima M, Kayukawa Y, Ohta T, Okada T. Changes in cerebral oxygenation and hemodynamics during obstructive sleep apneas. Chest. 1996;109:916–21.
12. Mehra R, Benjamin EJ, Shahar E, Gottlieb DJ, Nawabit R, Kirchner HL, Sahadevan J, Redline S, Sleep Heart Health Study. Association of nocturnal arrhythmias with sleep-disordered breathing. The Sleep Heart Health Study. Am J Respir Crit Care Med. 2006;173:910–6.
13. Mehra R, Stone KL, Varosy PD, Hoffman AR, Marcus GM, Blackwell T, Ibrahim OA, Salem R, Redline S. Nocturnal arrhythmias across a spectrum of obstructive and central sleep-disordered breathing in older men: outcomes of sleep disorders in older men (MrOS sleep) study. Arch Intern Med. 2009;169:1147–55.
14. Frey WC, Pilcher J. Obstructive sleep-related breathing disorders in patients evaluated for bariatric surgery. Obes Surg. 2003;13:676–83.
15. Malow BA, Levy K, Maturen K, Bowes R. Obstructive sleep apnea is common in medically refractory epilepsy patients. Neurology. 2000;55:1002–7.
16. Pollak L, Shpirer I, Rabey JM, Klein C, Schiffer J. Polysomnography in patients with intracranial tumors before and after operation. Acta Neurol Scand. 2004;109:56–60.
17. Fidan H, Fidan F, Unlu M, Ela Y, Ibis A, Tetik L. Prevalence of sleep apnoea in patients undergoing operation. Sleep Breath. 2006;10:161–5.
18. Lopez PP, Stefan B, Schulman CI, Byers PM. Prevalence of sleep apnea in morbidly obese patients who presented for weight loss surgery evaluation: more evidence for routine screening for obstructive sleep apnea before weight loss surgery. Am Surg. 2008;74:834–8.
19. Finkel KJ, Searleman AC, Tymkew H, Tanaka CY, Saager L, Safer-Zadeh E, Bottros M, Selvidge JA, Jacobsohn E, Pulley D, Duntley S, Becker C, Avidan MS. Prevalence of undiagnosed obstructive sleep apnea among adult surgical patients in an academic medical center. Sleep Med. 2009;10(7):753–8.
20. Young T, Finn L, Peppard PE, Szklo-Coxe M, Austin D, Nieto FJ, Stubbs R, Hla KM. Sleep disordered breathing and mortality: eighteen-year follow-up of the Wisconsin sleep cohort. Sleep. 2008;31:1071–8.
21. Memtsoudis S, Liu SS, Ma Y, Chiu YL, Walz JM, Gaber-Baylis LK, Mazumdar M. Perioperative pulmonary outcomes in patients with sleep apnea after noncardiac surgery. Anesth Analg. 2011;112:113–21.
22. Flink BJ, Rivelli SK, Cox EA, White WD, Falcone G, Vail TP, Young CC, Bolognesi MP, Krystal AD, Trzepacz PT, Moon RE, Kwatra MM. Obstructive sleep apnea and incidence of postoperative delirium after elective knee replacement in the nondemented elderly. Anesthesiology. 2012;116:788–96.
23. Kaw R, Chung F, Pasupuleti V, Mehta J, Gay PC, Hernandez AV. Meta-analysis of the association between obstructive sleep apnoea and postoperative outcome. Br J Anaesth. 2012;109(6):897–906.
24. Jackman KA, Zhou P, Faraco G, Peixoto PM, Coleman C, Voss HU, Pickel V, Manfredi G, Iadecola C. Dichotomous effects of chronic intermittent hypoxia on focal cerebral ischemic injury. Stroke. 2014;45:1460–7.
25. Lockhart EM, Willingham MD, Abdallah AB, Helsten DL, Bedair BA, Thomas J, Duntley S, Avidan MS. Obstructive sleep apnea screening and postoperative mortality in a large surgical cohort. Sleep Med. 2013;14:407–15.

26. Mokhlesi B, Hovda MD, Vekhter B, Arora VM, Chung F, Meltzer DO. Sleep-disordered breathing and postoperative outcomes after elective surgery: analysis of the nationwide inpatient sample. Chest. 2013;144:903–14.
27. Mokhlesi B, Hovda MD, Vekhter B, Arora VM, Chung F, Meltzer DO. Sleep-disordered breathing and postoperative outcomes after bariatric surgery: analysis of the nationwide inpatient sample. Obes Surg. 2013;23:1842–51.
28. Seet E, Chung F. Management of sleep apnea in adults – functional algorithms for the perioperative period: continuing professional development. Can J Anaesth. 2010;57:849–64.
29. Adesanya AO, Lee W, Greilich NB, Joshi GP. Perioperative management of obstructive sleep apnea. Chest. 2010;138:1489–98.
30. American Society of Anesthesiologists Task Force on Perioperative Management of patients with obstructive sleep apnea. Practice guidelines for the perioperative management of patients with obstructive sleep apnea: an updated report by the American Society of Anesthesiologists Task Force on Perioperative Management of patients with obstructive sleep apnea. Anesthesiology. 2014;120:268–86.
31. Jain S, Dhand R. Perioperative treatment of patients with obstructive sleep apnea. Curr Opin Pulm Med. 2004;10:482–8.
32. Young T, Evans L, Finn L, Palta M. Estimation of the clinically diagnosed proportion of sleep apnea syndrome in middle aged men and women. Sleep. 1997;20:705–6.
33. Netzer NC, Hoegel JJ, Loube D, Netzer CM, Hay B, Alvarez-Sala R, Strohl KP. Sleep in Primary Care International Study Group. Prevalence of symptoms and risk of sleep apnea in primary care. Chest. 2003;124:1406–14.
34. Ramachandran SK, Kheterpal S, Consens F, Shanks A, Doherty TM, Morris M, Tremper KK. Derivation and validation of a simple perioperative sleep apnea prediction score. Anesth Analg. 2010;110:1007–15.
35. Chung F, Yegneswaran B, Liao P, Chung SA, Vairavanathan S, Islam S, Khajehdehi A, Shapiro CM. STOP Questionnaire: a tool to screen patients for obstructive sleep apnea. Anesthesiology. 2008;108:812–21.
36. Farney RJ, Walker BS, Farney RM, Snow GL, Walker JM. The STOP-Bang equivalent model and prediction of severity of obstructive sleep apnea: relation to polysomnographic measurements of the apnea/hypopnea index. J Clin Sleep Med. 2011;7:459–65.
37. Chung F, Subramanyam R, Liao P, Sasaki E, Shapiro C, Sun Y. High STOP-Bang score indicates a high probability of obstructive sleep apnoea. Br J Anaesth. 2012;108:768–75.
38. Corso RM, Petrini F, Buccioli M, Nanni O, Carretta E, Trolio A, De Nuzzo D, Pigna A, Di Giacinto I, Agnoletti V, Gambale G. Clinical utility of preoperative screening with STOP-Bang questionnaire in elective surgery. Minerva Anestesiol. 2014;80:877–84.
39. Riley RW, Powell NB, Guilleminault C, Pelayo R, Troell RJ, Li KK. Obstructive sleep apnea surgery: risk management and complications. Otolaryngol Head Neck Surg. 1997;117:648–52.
40. Gupta RM, Parvizi J, Hanssen AD, Gay PC. Postoperative complications in patients with obstructive sleep apnea undergoing hip or knee replacement: a case control study. Mayo Clin Proc. 2001;76:897–905.
41. Chung SA, Yuan H, Chung F. A systemic review of obstructive sleep apnea and its implications for anesthesiologists. Anesth Analg. 2008;107:1543–63.
42. Memtsoudis SG, Stundner O, Rasul R, Sun X, Chiu YL, Fleischut P, Danninger T, Mazumdar M. Sleep apnea and total joint arthroplasty under various types of anesthesia: a population-based study of perioperative outcomes. Reg Anesth Pain Med. 2013;38:274–81.
43. Siyam MA, Benhamou D. Difficult endotracheal intubation in patients with sleep apnea syndrome. Anesth Analg. 2002;95:1098–102.
44. Kim JA, Lee JJ. Preoperative predictors of difficult intubation in patients with obstructive sleep apnea syndrome. Can J Anaesth. 2006;53:393–7.
45. Corso RM, Piraccini E, Calli M, Berger M, Gorini MC, Agnoletti V, Gambale G, Vicini C. Obstructive sleep apnea is a risk factor for difficult endotracheal intubation. Minerva Anestesiol. 2011;77:99–100.

46. Plunkett AR, McLean BC, Brooks D, Plunkett MT, Mikita JA. Does difficult mask ventilation predict obstructive sleep apnea? A prospective pilot study to identify the prevalence of OSA in patients with difficult mask ventilation under general anesthesia. J Clin Sleep Med. 2011;7:473–7.
47. Payen JF, Jaber S, Levy P, Pepin JL, Fischler M. Obstructive sleep-apnoea syndrome in adult and its perioperative management. Ann Fr Anesth Reanim. 2010;29:787–92.
48. Ankichetty S, Wong J, Chung F. A systematic review of the effects of sedatives and anesthetics in patients with obstructive sleep apnea. J Anaesthesiol Clin Pharmacol. 2011;27:447–58.
49. Cooper RM, O'Sullivan E, Popat M, Behringer E, Hagberg CA. Difficult Airway Society guidelines for the management of tracheal extubation. Anaesthesia. 2013;68:217.
50. Sundar E, Chang J, Smetana GW. Perioperative screening for and management of patients with obstructive sleep apnea. JCOM. 2011;18:399–411.
51. Kaw R, Golish J, Ghamande S, Burgess R, Foldvary N, Walker E. Incremental risk of obstructive sleep apnea on cardiac surgical outcomes. J Cardiovasc Surg (Torino). 2006;47:683–9.
52. Ireland CJ, Chapman TM, Mathew SF, Herbison GP, Zacharias M. Continuous positive airway pressure (CPAP) during the postoperative period for prevention of postoperative morbidity and mortality following major abdominal surgery. Cochrane Database Syst Rev. 2014;8, CD008930.
53. Pelosi P, Jaber S. Noninvasive respiratory support in the perioperative period. Curr Opin Anesthesiol. 2010;23:233–8.
54. Burgess LP, Derderian SS, Morin GV, Gonzalez C, Zajtchuk JT. Postoperative risk following uvulopalatopharyngoplasty for obstructive sleep apnea. Otolaryngol Head Neck Surg. 1992;106:81–6.
55. Kravath RE, Pollak CP, Borowiecki B, Weitzman ED. Obstructive sleep apnea and death associated with surgical correction of velopharyngeal incompetence. J Pediatr. 1980;96:645–8.
56. Knudsen J. Duration of hypoxemia after uncomplicated upper abdominal and thoraco-abdominal operations. Anaesthesia. 1970;25:372–7.
57. Entwistle MD, Roe PG, Sapsford DJ, Berrisford RG, Jones JG. Patterns of oxygenation after thoracotomy. Br J Anaesth. 1991;67:704–11.
58. Reeder MK, Goldman MD, Loh L, Muir AD, Casey KR, Lehane JR. Late postoperative nocturnal dips in oxygen saturation in patients undergoing major abdominal vascular surgery. Predictive value of pre-operative overnight pulse oximetry. Anaesthesia. 1992;47:110–5.
59. Brochard L, Mancebo J, Wysocki M, Lofaso F, Conti G, Rauss A, Simonneau G, Benito S, Gasparetto A, Lemaire F, et al. Noninvasive ventilation for acute exacerbations of chronic obstructive pulmonary disease. N Engl J Med. 1995;333:817–22.
60. Nava S, Hill N. Noninvasive ventilation in acute respiratory failure. Lancet. 2009;374: 250–9.
61. Stauffer JL, Olson DE, Petty TL. Complications and consequences of endotracheal intubation and tracheotomy. A prospective study of 150 critically ill adult patients. Am J Med. 1981;70:65–76.
62. Sinuff T, Muscedere J, Cook DJ, Dodek PM, Anderson W, Keenan SP, Wood G, Tan R, Haupt MT, Miletin M, Bouali R, Jiang X, Day AG, Overvelde J, Heyland DK, Canadian Critical Care Trials Group. Implementation of clinical practice guidelines for ventilator-associated pneumonia: a multicenter prospective study. Crit Care. 2013;41:15–23.
63. Sinderby C, Beck J. Neurally adjusted ventilatory assist in non-invasive ventilation. Minerva Anestesiol. 2013;79:915–25.
64. Suzuki M, Kirchner JA. The posterior cricoarytenoid as an inspiratory muscle. Ann Otol Rhinol Laryngol. 1969;78:849.
65. Butler JE, Gandevia SC. The output from human inspiratory motoneurone pools. J Physiol. 2008;586:1257–64.
66. Parreira VF, Jounieaux V, Aubert G, Dury M, Delguste PE, Rodenstein DO. Nasal two-level positive-pressure ventilation in normal subjects. Effects of the glottis and ventilation. Am J Respir Crit Care Med. 1996;153:1616–23.

67. Moreau-Bussière F, Samson N, St-Hilaire M, Reix P, Lafond JR, Nsegbe E, Praud JP. Laryngeal response to nasal ventilation in nonsedated newborn lambs. J Appl Physiol. 2007;102:2149–57.
68. Basner R. Continuous positive airway pressure for obstructive sleep apnea. N Engl J Med. 2007;356:1751–8.
69. Navalesi P, Maggiore SM. Positive end-expiratory pressure. In: Tobin MJ, editor. Principles and practice of mechanical ventilation. 3rd ed. New York: The McGraw-Hill Companies; 2012. p. 253–304.
70. Sanders MH, Kern N. Obstructive sleep apnea treated by independently adjusted inspiratory and expiratory positive airway pressures via nasal mask: physiologic and clinical implications. Chest. 1990;98:317–24.
71. Strohl KP, Redline S. Nasal CPAP therapy, upper airway muscle activation, and obstructive sleep apnea. Am Rev Respir Dis. 1986;134:555–8.
72. Sullivan CE, Issa FG, Berthon-Jones M, Eves L. Reversal of obstructive sleep apnoea by continuous positive airway pres- sure applied through the nares. Lancet. 1981;1:862–5.
73. L'Her E, Deye N, Lellouche F, Taille S, Demoule A, Fraticelli A, Mancebo J, Brochard L. Physiologic effects of noninvasive ventilation during acute lung injury. Am J Respir Crit Care Med. 2005;172:1112–8.
74. Coussa ML, Guerin C, Eissa NT, Corbeil C, Chasse M, Braidy J, Matar N, Milic-Emili J. Partitioning of work of breathing in mechanically ventilated COPD patients. J Appl Physiol (1985). 1993;75:1711–9.
75. Goldberg P, Reissmann H, Maltais F, Ranieri M, Gottfried S. Efficacy of noninvasive CPAP in COPD with acute respiratory failure. Eur Respir J. 1995;8:1894–900.
76. Appendini L, Patessio A, Zanaboni S, Carone M, Gukov B, Donner CF, Rossi A. Physiologic effects of positive end-expiratory pressure and mask pressure support during exacerbations of chronic obstructive pulmonary disease. Am J Respir Crit Care Med. 1994;149:1069–7.
77. Squadrone V, Coha M, Cerutti E, Schellino MM, Biolino P, Occella P, Belloni G, Vilianis G, Fiore G, Cavallo F. Ranieri VM; Piedmont Intensive Care Units Network (PICUN). Continuous positive airway pressure for treatment of postoperative hypoxemia: a randomized controlled trial. JAMA. 2005;293:589–95.
78. Masip J, Roque M, Sanchez B, Fernandez R, Subirana M, Exposito JA. Noninvasive ventilation in acute cardiogenic pulmonary edema: systematic review and meta-analysis. JAMA. 2005;294:3124–30.
79. Winck JC, Azevedo LF, Costa-Pereira A, Antonelli M, Wyatt JC. Efficacy and safety of non-invasive ventilation in the treatment of acute cardiogenic pulmonary edema–a systematic review and meta-analysis. Crit Care. 2006;10:R69.
80. Vital FM, Ladeira MT, Atallah AN. Non-invasive positive pressure ventilation (CPAP or bilevel NPPV) for cardiogenic pulmonary oedema. Cochrane Database Syst Rev. 2013;5, CD005351.
81. Collins SP, Mielniczuk LM, Whittingham HA, Boseley ME, Schramm DR, Storrow AB. The use of noninvasive ventilation in emergency department patients with acute cardiogenic pulmonary edema: a systematic review. Ann Emerg Med. 2006;48:260–9. 269.e261–264.
82. Pinsky MR. Sleeping with the enemy: the heart in obstructive sleep apnea. Chest. 2002;121:1022–4.
83. Buda AJ, Pinsky MR, Ingels Jr NB, Daughters 2nd GT, Stinson EB, Alderman EL. Effect of intrathoracic pressure on left ventricular performance. N Engl J Med. 1979;301:453–9.
84. Tkacova R, Rankin F, Fitzgerald FS, Floras JS, Bradley TD. Effects of continuous positive airway pressure on obstructive sleep apnea and left ventricular afterload in patients with heart failure. Circulation. 1998;96:2269–75.
85. Bradley TD, Hall MJ, Ando S, Floras JS. Hemodynamic effects of simulated obstructive apneas in humans with and without heart failure. Chest. 2001;119:1827–35.
86. Kaw R, Pasupuleti V, Deshpande A, Hamieh T, Walker E, Minai OA. Pulmonary hypertension: an important predictor of outcomes in patients undergoing non-cardiac surgery. Respir Med. 2011;105:619–24.

87. Fu C, Caruso P, Lucatto JJ, de Paula Schettino GP, de Souza R, Carvalho CR. Comparison of two flow generators with a noninvasive ventilator to deliver continuous positive airway pressure: a test lung study. Intensive Care Med. 2005;31:1587–91.
88. Takeuchi M, Williams P, Hess D, Kacmarek RM. Continuous positive airway pressure in new-generation mechanical ventilators: a lung model study. Anesthesiology. 2002;96:162–72.
89. Racca F, Appendini L, Gregoretti C, Varese I, Berta G, Vittone F, Ferreyra G, Stra E, Ranieri VM. Helmet ventilation and carbon dioxide rebreathing: effects of adding a leak at the helmet ports. Intensive Care Med. 2008;34:1461–8.
90. Neligan PJ, Malhotra G, Fraser M, Williams N, Greenblatt EP, Cereda M, Ochroch EA. Continuous positive airway pressure via the Boussignac system immediately after extubation improves lung function in morbidly obese patients with obstructive sleep apnea undergoing laparoscopic bariatric surgery. Anesthesiology. 2009;110:878–84.
91. Pelosi P, Gregoretti C. Perioperative management of obese patients. Best Pract Res Clin Anaesthesiol. 2010;24:211–25.
92. Mehta Y, Manikappa S, Juneja R, Trehan N. Obstructive sleep apnea syndrome: anesthetic implications in the cardiac surgical patient. J Cardiothorac Vasc Anesth. 2000;14:449–53.
93. Ryan CF, Lowe AA, Li D, Fleetham JA. Magnetic resonance imaging of the upper airway in obstructive sleep apnea before and after chronic nasal continuous positive airway pressure therapy. Am Rev Respir Dis. 1991;144:939–44.
94. Eastwood PR, Szollosi I, Platt PR, Hillman DR. Comparison of upper airway collapse during general anaesthesia and sleep. Lancet. 2002;359:1207–9.
95. Rennotte MT, Baele P, Aubert G, Rodenstein DO. Nasal continuous positive airway pressure in the perioperative management of patients with obstructive sleep apnea submitted to surgery. Chest. 1995;107:367–74.
96. Tokioka H, Saito S, Kosaka F. Comparison of pressure support ventilation and assist control ventilation in patients with acute respiratory failure. Intensive Care Med. 1989;15:364–7.
97. Aliverti A, Carlesso E, Dellacà R, Pelosi P, Chiumello D, Pedotti A, Gattinoni L. Chest wall mechanics during pressure support ventilation. Crit Care. 2006;10:R54.
98. Bonmarchand G, Chevron V, Chopin C, Jusserand D, Girault C, Moritz F, Leroy J, Pasquis P. Increased initial flow rate reduces inspiratory work of breathing during pressure support ventilation in patients with exacerbation of chronic obstructive pulmonary disease. Intensive Care Med. 1996;22:1147–54.
99. Stell IM, Paul G, Lee KC, Ponte J, Moxham J. Noninvasive ventilator triggering in chronic obstructive pulmonary disease. A test lung comparison. Am J Respir Crit Care Med. 2001;164:2092–7.
100. Tokioka H, Tanaka T, Ishizu T, Fukushima T, Iwaki T, Nakamura Y, Kosogabe Y. The effect of breath termination criterion on breathing patterns and the work of breathing during pressure support ventilation. Anesth Analg. 2001;92(1):161–5.
101. Bonmarchand G, Chevron V, Ménard JF, Girault C, Moritz-Berthelot F, Pasquis P, Leroy J. Effects of pressure support ramp slope values on the work of breathing during pressure support ventilation in restrictive patients. Crit Care Med. 1999;27:715–22.
102. Gregoretti C, Ranieri VM, Squadrone V. Patient-ventilator interaction. In: Vincent J et al., editors. Textbook of critical care. 6th ed. Philadelphia: Elsevier; 2011. p. 335–41.
103. Chiumello D, Pelosi P, Croci M, Bigatello LM, Gattinoni L. The effects of pressurization rate on breathing pattern, work of breathing, gas exchange and patient comfort in pressure support ventilation. Eur Respir J. 2001;18:107–14.
104. Chatmongkolchart S, Williams P, Hess DR, Kacmarek RM. Evaluation of inspiratory rise time and inspiration termination criteria in new-generation mechanical ventilators: a lung model study. Respir Care. 2001;46:666–77.
105. Chiumello D, Pelosi P, Taccone P, Slutsky A, Gattinoni L. Effect of different inspiratory rise time and cycling off criteria during pressure support ventilation in patients recovering from acute lung injury. Crit Care Med. 2003;31:2604–10.

106. Gregoretti C, Navalesi P, Ghannadian S, Carlucci A, Pelosi P. Choosing a ventilator for home mechanical ventilation. Breathe. 2013;10:395–408.
107. Calderini E, Confalonieri M, Puccio PG, Francavilla N, Stella L, Gregoretti C. Patient- ventilator asynchrony during noninvasive ventilation: the role of expiratory trigger. Intensive Care Med. 1999;25:662–7.
108. Gregoretti C, Foti G, Beltrame F, Giugiaro PM, Biolino P, Burbi L, Turello M, Agostini F, Berardino M, Musto P. Pressure control ventilation and minitracheotomy in treating severe flail chest trauma. Intensive Care Med. 1995;21:1054–6.

Part VII

Hospital Critical Care Applications: Non Invasive Ventilation in Critically Cancer

Respiratory Failure and Noninvasive Mechanical Ventilation in Cancer Patients: Global Overview

64

S. Egbert Pravinkumar and Antonio M. Esquinas

Contents

64.1 Introduction

Acute respiratory failure (ARF) is a common occurrence in cancer patients and is associated with a high mortality rate. The role of NPPV in immunosuppressed, hematological malignancies and solid tumors is an area that interests researchers and clinicians alike. Several randomized controlled trials and systematic reviews have confirmed the benefits of noninvasive positive pressure ventilation (NPPV) in patients with exacerbation of chronic obstructive pulmonary disease (COPD). Benefits achieved from NPPV in patients with COPD are largely a result of the avoidance of invasive mechanical ventilation (IMV) and its complications, including worsening of preexisting infections, morbidity and mortality, ventilator-associated pneumonia (VAP), ventilator-associated lung injury, increased need for

S.E. Pravinkumar, MD, FRCP (✉)
Department of Critical Care, Unit 112, UT-M.D. Anderson Cancer Center, Houston, TX, 77030, USA
e-mail: epravink@mdanderson.org

A.M. Esquinas, MD, PhD, FCCP
Intensive Care and Noninvasive Ventilatory Unit, Hospital Morales Meseguer, Murcia, Spain

A.M. Esquinas (ed.), *Noninvasive Mechanical Ventilation: Theory, Equipment, and Clinical Applications*, DOI 10.1007/978-3-319-21653-9_64

sedation resulting in prolonged ventilation, ventilator dependence, and upper airway complications related to endotracheal tube [1]. The use of NPPV in COPD with hypercapnic ARF is no longer debated and is now considered as first-line intervention before considering endotracheal intubation (ETI) and IMV.

The role of NPPV has been most recently studied in hypoxemic ARF. In this group of patients, several studies have shown that NPPV not only reduced mechanical ventilation and length of intensive care unit (ICU) stay but was associated with fewer complications [2]. Inasmuch as one of the major benefits of NPPV is the reduction of nosocomial infection, patients who are at high risk, such as those who are immunosuppressed, have hematological malignancies or chemotherapy-induced neutropenia, or have undergone organ transplantation, may be particularly likely to benefit from NPPV. Guidelines published by the American Thoracic Society and the Infectious Diseases Society of America in the management of nosocomial infections have provided high-grade evidence-based recommendations on the prevention of nosocomial infections. The guidelines recommend the use of NPPV whenever appropriate in the management of ARF and the avoidance of ETI and IMV whenever possible [3].

64.2 Epidemiology of Hypoxemic ARF

Hypoxemic ARF is the most common reason for ICU admission and ventilatory support. An epidemiological prospective survey of 42 ICUs in Europe (26 university and 16 non-university hospitals) looked at 1,337 admissions over a period of 3 weeks; 689 patients required ventilatory support [4]. ETI and IMV was the mode of treatment in 581 patients (84 %) and NPPV was used as first-line treatment in 108 patients (16 %). The conditions precipitating ARF were hypoxemic ARF, including acute cardiogenic pulmonary edema (55 %), coma (30 %), and hypercapnic ARF (15 %). In this epidemiological study of patients who needed ETI and IMV, mortality rates were much higher in the hypoxemic ARF group than in hypercapnic ARF (47 % vs 27 %). The 28-day hospital mortality was 41 % in those who needed ETI and IMV, compared with 22 % in those who received NPPV ($p<0.001$). The incidence of VAP was 2 % in those who were successfully managed with NPPV compared with 19 % in those who needed IMV ($p<0.002$).

64.3 NPPV in Hypoxemic ARF

Studies in hypoxemic ARF using NPPV have shown varied results, and the outcome is dependent on population selection. An increasing number of trials are emerging, looking at the benefits of NPPV in selected groups with hypoxemic ARF. A systematic review of randomized controlled trials (RCTs) of NPPV use in hypoxemic ARF shows convincing evidence that NPPV decreased the need for ETI and IMV [5]. NPPV also decreased the ICU length of stay and mortality. However, unlike hypercapnic ARF, hypoxemic ARF encompasses several diagnoses and comprises a heterogeneous population. This heterogeneity was observed in multiple studies. Hence, it would be misleading to conclude that NPPV is beneficial for all patients with hypoxemic ARF. Notably, NPPV has had limited success in patients with acute respiratory distress syndrome (ARDS) and lobar consolidation. Further study of specific patient groups with hypoxemic ARF will provide insights into the management of ARF using NPPV [5].

A well-conducted systematic review assessed the effects of NPPV in patients with hypoxemic ARF not due to CPE [1]. The study looked at eight RCTs from six countries that compared NPPV plus standard therapy versus standard therapy alone in 366 patients. The study results are as follows: NPPV was associated with a significantly lower rate of ETI and IMV (RR 0.23, 95% CI: 0.10, 0.35), reduction in length of ICU stay of 1.9 days (95% CI: 1, 2.9), reduced ICU mortality of 17 % (95% CI: 8, 26) and no statistically significant effect on hospital mortality. Based on currently available evidence, routine use of NPPV for hypoxemic ARF is not recommended. However, based on a selected population analysis, NPPV should be strongly considered for immunosuppressed and post-thoracotomy patients, and its use in other groups should be carefully monitored to ensure beneficial effect.

A recent systematic review and meta-analysis of NPPV in an acute setting shows favorable results in a wide variety of conditions [6]. NPPV was associated with a reduction in mortality, especially when applied early in patients with COPD, pulmonary edema, ARF of mixed etiology, and in postoperative ARF. NPPV also has a favorable outcome in a selected patient population when used for prevention of post-extubation ARF and for weaning from IMV. However, the benefits are noted when NPPV is used earlier in the course of ARF.

64.4 ARF in Immunosuppressed and Cancer Patients

Hypoxemic ARF is a common occurrence in immunocompromised patients and in those with malignancies, both hematological malignancies and solid tumors. It is often a dreaded condition in cancer patients due to the high mortality related to ETI and IMV. New types and modalities of chemotherapy and radiation therapy, circulating pluripotent hematopoietic cell grafts, and bone marrow transplantation have contributed to the increase in successful treatment of solid and hematologic malignancies. However, these regimens may predispose patients to various life-threatening complications, such as infection, hemorrhage, capillary leak syndrome, radiation toxicity, and drug-related toxicity. The lung is the target organ most frequently involved in these complications.

Inasmuch as most cancer patients have muscle fatigue, diffuse pulmonary infiltrates, and depressed organ function and reserve as a result of treatment, they are more vulnerable to rapid clinical deterioration and developing ARF. The most common type of respiratory failure in this group of patients is "lung" failure, although it is not uncommon to see "ventilatory pump" failure as the cause of ARF. Several studies have looked at the outcome of patients with acute myelogenous leukemia and recipients of bone marrow transplantation who needed ETI and IMV [7]. Only two variables have been shown to be independently associated with mortality of cancer patients in the ICU, and neither the type of cancer (i.e., solid or hematologic malignancy) nor the presence or absence of neutropenia was independently associated with mortality. The first independent predictor of ICU mortality is the severity of the patient's clinical condition on admission, as recorded by various scores, such as the Simplified Acute Physiologic Score (SAPS I and SAPS II) and the Acute Physiologic and Chronic Health Evaluation (APACHE II and APACHE III). The second and "stronger" independent predictive factor of mortality is the need for ETI and IMV, inasmuch as VAP and worsening of a preexisting infection are significant complications in intubated patients.

64.5 NPPV in Cancer Patients

In a retrospective study of patients with solid or hematologic cancer admitted to the ICU for ARF, the survival rate for cancer patients ($n = 105$) in the period 1996–1998 was significantly higher than those ($n = 132$) admitted between 1990 and 1995 (39 % vs 18 %, respectively; $p = 0.0003$). Multivariate analysis showed that the use of NPPV in the later period was associated with a marked improvement in survival [8]. Other studies using NPPV in cancer patients are summarized in Table 64.1.

Table 64.1 NPPV in cancer patients with hypoxemic ARF [7]

Study	Patient population and intervention	Outcome
Tognet 1994	Hematological malignancies (HM)	ICU mortality: IMV vs NPPV: 100 % vs 55 % significantly lower mortality in NPPV group
Meduri 1994	Cancer patients with do-not-intubate orders Solid tumor (ST) and HM	Improved survival and hospital discharge in NPPV group
Conti 1998	Immunosuppressed and HM	Improvement in blood gases and respiratory rate <1 h of NPPV – 68 % survived to discharge
Hilbert 2000	Fever, neutropenia, AHReF, HM Intermittent CPAP	CPAP avoided ETI in 25 % CPAP success: all survived
Hilbert 2001	RCT, NPPV vs standard care (SC), fever, pulmonary infiltrate, immunosuppressed, HM $n = 52$	Reduced ETI, complications, ICU death, and hospital death in NPPV group
Principi 2004	Pulmonary infiltrate, HM, mask vs helmet NPPV	NPPV intolerance: helmet NPPV (0 %) vs mask NPPV (50 %)
Rocco 2004	Helmet NPPV vs mask NPPV, fever, immunosuppressed, organ transplant, pulmonary infiltrates, HM	Helmet NPPV vs mask NPPV ETI: 36 % vs 63 % ICU mortality: (31 %) vs (47 %) Hospital mortality: 37 % vs 53 %
Meert 2003	Solid tumors and HM, NPPV for hypoxemic ARF	ICU survival: 57 % ETI: 25 %

64.6 Indications and Contraindications

The immediate goals of NPPV therapy should be aimed at relieving patient symptoms and reducing the work of breathing. The intermediate goals should be to improve and stabilize gas exchange and optimize patient ventilator comfort and synchrony; the ultimate goal is avoidance of ETI and IMV. The success of therapy depends on a highly motivated, committed, and knowledgeable team and careful patient selection with the help of a well-structured NPPV guideline (Table 64.2). Application of NPPV early in the process of ARF, along with careful and rigorous

Table 64.2 NPPV for cancer patients (©The University of Texas M.D. Anderson Cancer Center NPPV guideline)

Eligibility criteria	Contraindications
Clinical (all)	Absolute (any)
Acute respiratory failure	Cardiopulmonary arrest
Dyspnea	pH <7.25
Accessory resp. muscle use	Upper airway obstruction
Paradoxical abdominal movement	Facial trauma
RR >25	Uncontrolled arrhythmia
Adequate airway protection	Untreated SBP ≤ 90 mmHg
Adequate secretion clearance	GCS ≤ 8
	Undrained pneumothorax
Gas exchange criteria (any)	Relative
$FiO_2 \geq 0.60$	Copious secretions
$PaO_2 \leq 60$ mmHg on room air	Confusion/agitation
$PaO_2 \leq 75$ mmHg on any FiO_2	GCS 9–13
PaO_2:$FiO_2 < 200$	Two or more organ failures
$PaCO_2 \geq 50$	Focal consolidation on CXR
pH >7.30	
Radiological criteria (any)	Bowel obstruction
Pulmonary Infiltrates	Recent facial/ upper airway/GI surgery
No pneumothorax	Pregnancy
	Thoracic surgery <6 weeks

Blood gases 1 and 4 h post NPPV	Blood gases 1 and 4 h Post NPPV
NPPV success	NPPV failure
Clinical criteria (two or more)	Clinical criteria (any)
Patient tolerates NPPV	Patient intolerant to NPPV
Tolerates periods "off" NPPV	Persistent dyspnea
Dyspnea reduced (score)	RR ≥ 35
RR ≤ 35	Urgent need for ETI
Awake and alert	Development of contraindications
	GCS ≤ 8 (worsening mental status)
Gas exchange criteria (2 or more)	Gas exchange criteria (any)
Improvement in ABG	Failure of ABG improvement
$FiO_2 \leq 0.7$ and $SpO_2 > 92$	$FiO_2 \geq 0.7$ and $SpO_2 \leq 92$
$PaO_2 \geq 65$ on $FiO_2 < 0.6$	$PaO_2 \leq 65$ on $FiO_2 > 0.6$
pH >7.30	pH ≤ 7.30
PaO_2:$FiO_2 \geq 100$ from baseline	PaO_2:$FiO_2 \leq 100$ from baseline

monitoring, is vital to the success of NPPV therapy. Other factors include location and availability of a wide variety of interfaces to suit the patient's morphological and comfort needs.

NPPV failure should be identified early to avoid unnecessary delays in ETI and IMV. For this reason, several centers offer NPPV therapy in the ICU, high-dependency care units, and respiratory intermediary care units. Staffing ratios and 24-h physician coverage is also important in considering NPPV outside of the ICU. Some of the predictors of NPPV failure include elevated ICU severity of illness scores, presence of ARDS or lobar consolidation, PaO_2/FiO_2 ratio <150 even after 1 h of NPPV, pH– <7.30 on initiation, and failure of pH improvement in 1–2 h.

64.7 Complications of NPPV

Complications of NPPV are predominantly interface related, such as facial discomfort (30–50 %) and skin erythema (20–35 %). Less common (5–10 %) problems include claustrophobia, nasal ulceration, and acneiform rash. Complications related to pressure and flow include nasal congestion (20–50 %), sinus/ear pain (10–30 %), nasal/oral dryness (10–20 %), eye irritation (10–20 %), and gastric distension (5–10 %). Major complications such as aspiration pneumonia, hypotension, and pneumothorax are less than 5 %.

Key Recommendations

- NPPV can be effectively used in the management of ARF.
- NPPV has several benefits, including decreased rates of ETI and IMV, VAP, mortality, and ICU and hospital length of stay.
- Patient selection and early application are crucial.
- A highly committed and motivated team, along with a structured guideline, is important to the success of NPPV.

References

1. Keenan SP, Sinuff T, Cook DJ, Hill NS. Does noninvasive positive pressure ventilation improve outcome in acute hypoxemic respiratory failure? A systematic review. Crit Care Med. 2004;32:2516–23.
2. Brochard L. Noninvasive ventilation for acute respiratory failure. JAMA. 2002;288:932–5.
3. American Thoracic Society/Infectious Diseases Society of America. Guidelines for the management of adults with hospital-acquired, ventilator-associated, and healthcare-associated pneumonia. Am J Respir Crit Care Med. 2005;171:388–416.
4. Carlucci A, Richard JC, Wysocki M, Lepage E, Brochard L. SRLF Collaborative Group on Mechanical Ventilation. Noninvasive versus conventional mechanical ventilation: an epidemiologic survey. Am J Respir Crit Care Med. 2001;163:874–80.

5. Keenan SP, Sinuff T, Cook DJ, Hill NS. Which patients with acute exacerbation of chronic obstructive pulmonary disease benefit from noninvasive positive pressure ventilation? A systematic review of the literature. Ann Intern Med. 2003;138:861–70.
6. Cabrini L, Giovanni L, Oriani A, et al. Noninvasive ventilation and survival in acute care settings: a comprehensive systematic review and metaanalysis of randomized control trials. Crit Care Med. 2015;43:880–8.
7. Nava S, Cuomo AM. Acute respiratory failure in the cancer patient: the role of non- invasive mechanical ventilation. Crit Rev Oncol Hematol. 2004;51:91–103.
8. Azoulay E, Alberti C, Bornstain C, Leleu G, Moreau D, Recher C, Chevret S, et al. Improved survival in cancer patients requiring mechanical ventilatory support: impact of non-invasive ventilatory support. Crit Care Med. 2001;29:519–25.

Noninvasive Versus Invasive Ventilation in Patients with Hematological Malignancies

65

Massimo Antonelli, Giorgio Conti, and Giuseppe R. Gristina

Contents

Abbreviations

AIDS	Acquired immune deficiency syndrome
ALI	Acute lung injury
ARDS	Adult respiratory distress syndrome
ARF	Acute respiratory failure
CPAP	Continuous positive airway pressure
GCS	Glasgow Coma Score
ICU	Intensive care unit
IMV	Invasive mechanical ventilation
NIV	Noninvasive ventilation
PaO_2:FiO_2	O_2 arterial pressure to inspiratory O_2 fraction
PEEP	Positive end-expiratory pressure
PICU	Pediatric intensive care unit
SAPS	Simplified Acute Physiology Score
SOFA	Sequential Organ Failure Assessment Score

M. Antonelli, MD • G. Conti, MD
Institute of Intensive Care and Anesthesiology, Catholic University of the Sacred Heart, Rome, Italy
e-mail: m.antonelli@rm.unicatt.it; g.conti@rm.unicatt.it

G.R. Gristina, MD (✉)
Department of Intensive Care Unit S.Camillo, Forlanini Hospital, Rome, Italy
e-mail: geigris@fastwebnet.it

A.M. Esquinas (ed.), *Noninvasive Mechanical Ventilation: Theory, Equipment, and Clinical Applications*, DOI 10.1007/978-3-319-21653-9_65

65.1 Introduction

In the last two decades, the survival of patients with hematological malignancies has improved because of new chemotherapeutic regimens, bone marrow transplantation, peripheral stem cell rescue, and better supportive measures [1]. At the same time, several investigators have underlined a worsened outcome for granulocytopenic patients requiring supportive therapies in the intensive care unit (ICU), particularly those undergoing tracheal intubation and invasive mechanical ventilation (IMV) for acute respiratory failure (ARF) [2–9], a common complication of hematologic malignancies (and of their treatment), often affected by a poor prognosis. This significantly increased risk of death [3, 5] results from the combination of several different conditions: lung damage induced by opportunistic infections, the direct toxicity of chemotherapy on lung tissue, and complications directly generated by endotracheal intubation. Based on sound evidence on this topic, a consensus exists regarding the use of early noninvasive ventilation (NIV) with the aim of reducing the endotracheal intubation rate and the associated infectious complications [10–12].

65.2 Discussion

Tognet et al. [13] were the first to report interesting clinical results with the intermittent application of NIV in patients with hematologic malignancies; 6 out of 11 patients with ARF were successfully treated with NIV through a face mask, with different levels of pressure support and positive end-expiratory pressure (PEEP). Four years later, Conti and colleagues [14] evaluated the use of NIV delivered via nasal mask in 16 consecutive patients with hematological malignancies and ARF. Fifteen out of 16 patients showed a clear-cut and sustained improvement in gas exchange: PaO_2:FiO_2 after 1 h of treatment increased from 87 ± 22 to 175 ± 64, and continued to improve in the following 24 h ($p<0.01$). Two patients failed to improve, were intubated, and subsequently died from sepsis. Three other patients died from complications unrelated to ARF. Eleven patients were discharged with stable spontaneous breathing after a mean length of ICU stay of 4.3 ± 2.4 days.

In 2001, a prospective, controlled, randomized trial evaluated NIV to avoid intubation and associated complications in immunocompromised patients admitted to the ICU for hypoxemic ARF (PaO_2:FiO_2 < 200), fever, and lung infiltrates [15]. Fifty-two patients (30 patients with hematological malignancies and neutropenia, 18 who received immunosuppressant to prevent rejection after solid organ transplantation, and 4 with acquired immune deficiency syndrome (AIDS)) were randomized to receive conventional treatment (oxygen plus aggressive medical therapy) or NIV plus conventional treatment. NIV was intermittently administered with a face mask. NIV significantly reduced the rate of intubation (46 % vs 77 %, $p=0.003$) and serious complications (50 % vs 81 %, $p=0.02$). Both ICU (38 % vs 69 %, $p=0.03$) and hospital mortality (50 % vs 81 %, $p=0.02$) were also significantly reduced.

These findings show that the early intermittent application of NIV ameliorates the prognosis of immunocompromised patients admitted to the ICU. It is interesting to note that the most impressive results were obtained in the subgroup of patients with hematological malignancies and neutropenia, suggesting a safe, effective, and extensive clinical application of NIV under these conditions.

Ten years later, thanks to advances in equipment technology with performing interfaces and optimal staff training, Squadrone et al. [16] investigated the effectiveness of continuous positive airway pressure (CPAP) delivered through a transparent plastic helmet in the hematological ward, to treat acute lung injury (ALI) and prevent ICU admission and IMV in 40 hematological patients in the early stages of ARF. Patients were randomized to receive oxygen ($N=20$) or oxygen plus CPAP ($N=20$). At randomization, PaO_2:FiO_2 in the control group was 282 ± 41 and in CPAP group was 256 ± 52 mmHg. Fewer patients who received CPAP needed ICU admission for mechanical ventilation compared with controls (4 vs 16 patients; $p=0.0002$). CPAP reduced the relative risk of developing need of ventilatory support to 0.25 (95 % CI; OR 0.10–0.62). Among patients admitted to ICU, the intubation rate was lower in the CPAP group than in the control group (2 vs 14 patients; $p=0.0001$). CPAP reduced the relative risk for intubation to 0.46 (95 % CI: RR 0.27–0.78). These findings suggest that early use of CPAP on the hematological ward in patients with initial derangement of gas exchanges is safe and prevents a worse evolution to ALI requiring IMV in the ICU.

More recently, a large retrospective analysis of prospectively collected data between 2000 and 2006 evaluated 1,302 patients with hematological malignancies admitted with ARF to 158 Italian ICUs [10]. This was the largest report published so far. Only 274 (21 %) of the patients were treated on admission with NIV. Compared with patients receiving IMV since the onset of respiratory failure, those initially treated with NIV were generally younger, with lower Simplified Acute Physiology Score (SAPS) II scores and higher Glasgow Coma Score (GCS). ALI was significantly more frequent in the NIV group, but the prevalence of adult respiratory distress syndrome (ARDS) in the two groups was similar. The IMV and NIV groups also had similar rates of organ failure after ICU admission (434 out of 1028 (42 %) vs 120 out of 274 (44 %); $p=0.64$). Analysis of patients with ALI or ARDS revealed no significant correlation between mortality and type of ventilation (OR 0.77, 95 % CI 0.45–1.30; $p=0.32$), although the IMV subgroup had significantly higher SAPS II scores (means: $58=19$ % vs $49=17$ % in the NIV group, $p<0.0001$). The NIV group exhibited significantly lower ICU and hospital mortality, shorter ventilation periods, and shorter ICU lengths of stay than the IMV group. In a multivariate analysis, after adjustments for group-assignment propensity scores, an initial NIV trial was associated with lower hospital mortality than immediate recourse to IMV (OR 0.73, 95 % CI 0.53–1.00; $p=0.05$). Independent risk factors for mortality included ARDS, septic shock, stroke (on or after ICU admission), and higher SAPS II scores but not neutropenia (OR 1.411; 95 % CI 0.945–1.2106; $p=0.0926$). More than a half (54 %) of the NIV patients never required endotracheal intubation (successful NIV subgroup). In the other 127 (46 %), NIV was replaced with IMV after 3 ± 3 days (unsuccessful NIV subgroup). These two subgroups were similar in terms of age, underlying diseases, organ failure rates at ICU admission, and reasons for ICU admission, but ALI/ARDS was almost twice as common in the unsuccessful NIMV subgroup (42 % vs 24 %; $p=0.002$). Multivariate analysis identified two major risk factors for NIV failure: baseline illness severity reflected by SAPS II scores (OR 2.012, 95 % CI 1.006–4.026; $p=0.048$); and ALI/ARDS at admission (OR 2.266, 95 % CI 1.346–3.816; $p=0.002$). This study indicates that (1) ARF patients with hematological malignancies may represent <1 % of total ICU admissions; (2) NIV is attempted in only around 20 % of these cases; (3) when successful, NIV is generally associated with shorter mechanical ventilation periods and ICU stays, less severe post-admission infections, and lower ICU and hospital mortality; (4) after adjustment for the propensity to receive NIV *ab initio*, the noninvasive approach is significantly associated with lower mortality than immediate IMV; and (5) roughly half of the NIV trials failed, and the patients had to be intubated .

In 2014 and 2015, Azoulay et al. [17, 18] published two studies related to the prognostic impact of ARDS and neutropenia on critically ill patients with malignancies. The data in the first study derived from a cohort of 1,004 patients (86 % with hematological malignancies and 14 % with solid tumors), 44.2 % of whom had neutropenia. According to the Berlin definition [19], 252 (25.1 %) patients had mild, 426 (42.4 %) moderate, and 326 (32.5 %) had severe ARDS due to infectious causes of various origin. Mortality was 59, 63, and 68.5 %, respectively ($p=0.06$). Three hundred and eighty-seven patients (38.6 %) received NIV, 276 (71 %) subsequently required endotracheal ventilation. Hospital mortality was 64 % overall, with a mortality rate higher for severe ARDS. Solid tumors, primary ARDS, and later admission period were associated with lower mortality. Risk factors for higher mortality were allogeneic bone-marrow transplantation, higher Sequential Organ Failure Assessment (SOFA) score, NIV failure, severe ARDS, and invasive fungal infection. This study showed that, in cancer patients, 90 % of ARDS cases were related to documented infection, including one-third due to invasive fungal infections. Mortality decreased over time (from 89 % in 1990–1995 to 52 % in 2006–2011; $p < 0.0001$), but NIV failure was associated with increased mortality. The same group of researchers published a second study aimed at assessing the hospital outcome in 289 critically ill neutropenic cancer patients admitted into the ICU, and at identifying the risk factors for unfavorable outcome. Overall, 131 patients died during their hospital stay (hospital mortality 45.3 %). Four variables were associated with a poor outcome: allogeneic transplantation (OR 3.83; 95 % CI 1.75–8.35), need for IMV (OR 6.57; 95 % CI 3.51–12.32), microbiological documentation (OR 2.33; CI 1.27–4.26), and need for renal replacement therapy (OR 2.77; 95 % CI 1.34–5.74). Ninety-one patients received NIV as first-line intervention for their ARF, but NIV was not a protective factor for mortality.

In the neonatal and pediatric setting, CPAP has been extensively used across the world. Over the last few years there has been a dramatic increase in the utilization of NIV for respiratory support in a variety of pediatric settings. NIV has been recently proposed also in pediatric patients affected by hematological malignancies complicated by hypoxemic ARF of various origins. Piastra et al. [20] successfully treated 23 consecutive immunocompromised children with NIV for early ARDS through a face mask or a helmet. Admission parameters and severity scores between NIV responders and nonresponders were not different, with early and sustained $PaO_2:FiO_2$ improvement in almost 80 % of all cases. Thirteen out of 23 patients (54.5 %) avoided intubation and were discharged from the pediatric intensive care unit (PICU); 10 patients required intubation: 2 of them survived while 8 patients died. NIV responders showed a PICU and hospital mortality significantly lower ($p < 0.001$), and their length of stay in the PICU stay was shorter ($p = 0.03$), with a lower heart and respiratory rate at the end of treatment ($p < 0.001$ and $p = 0.048$, respectively).

These positive results were not confirmed in a later "real-world" study where the authors reported a higher NIV failure (requiring intubation and IMV) and mortality rate in hematological patients with ARF [21]. However, in the same study, a delay from the time of ICU admission and the start of NIV was associated with an increased risk for failure, which was also an independent predictor for worse outcome. These data suggest the need for an early NIV administration but also for a sensitive trigger to identify those patients who do not rapidly respond to NIV and need a prompt endotracheal intubation.

The Society of Critical Care Medicine charged a task force with producing recommendations for the use of NIV as a palliation in patients with terminal diseases and malignancies [22]. The task force suggested use of NIV for patients who choose to forego endotracheal intubation. NIV should be applied after careful discussion of the goals of care, with explicit parameters for success and failure, by experienced personnel, and in appropriate health-care settings.

A similar approach was analyzed by Azoulay et al. [23]. They concluded that, although NIV is increasingly used as a palliative strategy to alleviate the symptoms of respiratory distress in dying patients, more research is needed aimed at identifying benefits from palliative NIV that are not related to patient comfort, a good end-of-life process, or family and caregiver satisfaction.

Conclusion

The survival of patients with hematological malignancies requiring intensive therapy has improved over the years, even though the mortality rate remains close to 50 %. These results were achieved thanks to a better understanding of the mechanisms, improvements to specific therapies, and a more sophisticated approach to organ failures. ARF represents the most frequent complication in these patients. The current management of critically ill hematological patients with ARF admitted to the ICU includes a trial of NIV to avoid endotracheal intubation. However, failure of NIV may lead to an increased mortality.

Knowledge of the specific features and accurate selection of hematological patients to receive NIV are key factors for a good outcome and prognosis. A skilled team and the correct equipment are also two cornerstones for the optimal use of NIV in and out of the ICU. When clinicians chose this strategy, early application and careful evaluation of the potential risks and patient comfort are essential. This is crucial in the pediatric setting. Parameters such as GCS score, aim of NIV, severity of infection, and hemodynamic stability can help in the selection of potential candidates to receive NIV. Patients undergoing allogeneic hematopoietic stem cell transplantation frequently require ICU admission for transplant-related toxicities. In these patients, whose prognosis is often poor, a careful balance between the costs and risks/benefits NIV and IMV is still needed.

Key Major Recommendations

- Patients with hematological malignancies should receive NIV early at the onset of hypoxemia (PaO_2:FiO_2).
- Patients with hematological malignancies receiving NIV should be promptly intubated when there is no improvement in gas exchange after the first hours of NIV.
- Risk factors for higher mortality such as allogeneic bone-marrow transplantation, severely modified SOFA, severe ARDS, and invasive fungal infection should induce on invasive ventilation *ab initio*.
- The option to deliver NIV in pediatric patients with hematological malignancies is safe provided that the risks/benefits ratio is closely respected.
- In patients with hematological malignancies asking to forgo invasive ventilation or at the end of their life, NIV may dignify the last days, allowing a peaceful death and reducing also the psychological stress of the family and caregivers.

References

1. Peigne V, Rusinová K, Karlin L, et al. Continued survival gains in recent years among critically ill myeloma patients. Intensive Care Med. 2009;35:512–8.
2. Lloyd-Thomas AR, Dhaliwal HS, Lister TA, et al. Intensive therapy for life-threatening medical complications of hematologic malignancy. Intensive Care Med. 1986;12:317–24.
3. Denardo SJ, Oye RK, Bellamy PE. Efficacy of intensive care for bone marrow transplant patients with respiratory failure. Crit Care Med. 1989;17:4–6.
4. Crowford W, Schwartz DA, Petersen FB, et al. Mechanical ventilation after bone marrow transplantation. Risk factors and clinical outcome. Am J Respir Crit Care Med. 1988;137:682–7.
5. Blot F, Guignet M, Nitenberg G, et al. Prognostic factors for neutropenic patients in an intensive care unit. Respective roles of underlying malignancies and acute organ failures. Eur J Cancer. 1997;33:1031–7.
6. Ewig S, Torres A, Riquelme R, et al. Pulmonary complications in patients with haematological malignancies treated at a respiratory intensive care unit. Eur Respir J. 1998;12:116–22.
7. Huaringa AJ, Leyva FJ, Giralt SA, et al. Outcome of bone marrow transplantation patients requiring mechanical ventilation. Crit Care Med. 2000;28:1014–7.
8. Benoit DD, Vandewoude KH, Decruyenaere JM, et al. Outcome and early prognostic indicators in patients with a hematologic malignancy admitted to the intensive care unit for a life-threatening complication. Crit Care Med. 2003;31:104–12.
9. Grgić Medić M, Gornik I, Gašparović V. Hematologic malignancies in the medical intensive care unit – Outcomes and prognostic factors. Hematology. 2014. doi:http://dx.doi.org/10.1179/1607845414Y.0000000206.

10. Gristina GR, Antonelli M, Conti G, et al. Noninvasive versus invasive ventilation for acute respiratory failure in patients with hematologic malignancies: a 5-year multicenter observational survey. Crit Care Med. 2011;39:2232–9.
11. Türkoğlu M, Erdem GU, Suyanı E, et al. Acute respiratory distress syndrome in patients with hematological malignancies. Hematology. 2013;18(3):123–30.
12. Argent AC, Biban P. What's new on NIV in the PICU: does everyone in respiratory failure require endotracheal intubation? Intensive Care Med. 2014;40:880–4.
13. Tognet E, Mercatello A, Polo P, et al. Treatment of acute respiratory failure with non-invasive intermittent positive pressure ventilation in hematological patients. Clin Intensive Care. 1994;5:282–8.
14. Conti G, Marino P, Cogliati A, et al. Noninvasive ventilation for the treatment of acute respiratory failure in patients with hematologic malignancies: a pilot study. Intensive Care Med. 1998;24:1283–8.
15. Hilbert J, Grusion D, Vargas F, et al. Noninvasive ventilation in immunosuppressed patients with pulmonary infiltrates, fever and acute respiratory failure. N Engl J Med. 2001;344:481–7.
16. Squadrone V, Massaia M, Bruno B, et al. Early CPAP prevents evolution of acute lung injury in patients with hematologic malignancy. Intensive Care Med. 2010;36:1666–74.
17. Azoulay E, Lemiale V, Mokart D, et al. Acute respiratory distress syndrome in patients with malignancies. Intensive Care Med. 2014;40:1106–14.
18. Mokart D, Darmon M, Resche-Rigon M, et al. Prognosis of neutropenic patients admitted to the intensive care unit. Intensive Care Med. 2015;41:296–303.
19. ARDS Definition Task Force, Ranieri V, Rubenfeld GD, Thompson B, et al. Acute respiratory distress syndrome: the Berlin definition. JAMA. 2012;307(23):2526–33. doi:10.1001/jama.2012.5669.
20. Piastra M, De Luca D, Pietrini D, et al. Noninvasive pressure support ventilation in immunocompromised children with ARDS: a feasibility study. Intensive Care Med. 2009;35(8):1420–7.
21. Adda M, Coquet I, Darmon M, et al. Predictors of noninvasive ventilation failure in patients with hematologic malignancy and acute respiratory failure. Crit Care Med. 2008;36:2766–72.
22. Curtis JR, Cook DJ, Sinuff T, et al. Noninvasive positive pressure ventilation in critical and palliative care settings: understanding the goals of therapy. Crit Care Med. 2007;35:932–9.
23. Azoulay E, Demoule A, Jaber S, et al. Palliative noninvasive ventilation in patients with acute respiratory failure. Intensive Care Med. 2011;37:1250–7.

Noninvasive Mechanical Ventilation in Critically Ill Patients with Hematological Malignancy: Flow Chart, Evidence, and Key Practical Recommendations

66

Pieter Depuydt

Contents

66.1 Introduction

The number of patients with hematological malignancy admitted to the intensive care unit (ICU) is increasing, and there are multiple reasons for this trend. The life expectancy of patients with hematological malignancy is often no longer prohibitive for ICU referral, as therapeutic advances have led to higher cure rates, more extended remission periods, and prolonged survival, even in the presence of active disease. Longer survival also increases the time-at-risk for developing a life-threatening infection or other complication of the disease or its therapy. In addition, new chemotherapeutic or immune-modulating agents and treatment regimes have expanded the spectrum of toxicities and complications. Critical care itself, in general and for

P. Depuydt, MD, PhD
Department of Intensive Care, Ghent University Hospital, De Pintelaan 185, Ghent 9000, Belgium
e-mail: pieter.depuydt@ugent.be

A.M. Esquinas (ed.), *Noninvasive Mechanical Ventilation: Theory, Equipment, and Clinical Applications*, DOI 10.1007/978-3-319-21653-9_66

these patients in particular, has progressed considerably as well, and reluctance to admit these patients to the ICU has largely disappeared. A multicenter prospective study documented an encouraging 39 % hospital survival rate for critically ill patients with hematological malignancy [1].

Acute respiratory failure (ARF) is the main reason for ICU referral of patients with hematological malignancy and is an independent predictor of mortality, especially when mechanical ventilation is required. Noninvasive mechanical ventilation (NIV) has been advocated as the preferable first-line form of ventilatory support in these patients when there is no condition requiring immediate intubation (such as hemodynamic instability, lack of free airway, or imminent respiratory arrest). Over the last decade, the use of NIV in patients with hematological malignancy has increased in everyday practice, mirroring the expanding use of NIV in general ICU patients over a range of types and causes of respiratory failure. In recent years, experience has been gained with the use of NIV in patients with ARF and a do-not-intubate order. This chapter summarizes the recent evidence and controversy regarding the optimal use of NIV in patients with hematological malignancy.

66.2 Analysis and Discussion

66.2.1 Does NIV Improve Outcome in Hematology Patients with ARF?

Enthusiasm for the use of NIV in patients with hematological malignancy is based on the results of a small number of randomized controlled trials (RCTs) and a larger number of observational studies. A pilot RCT in hypoxemic patients with underlying immunosuppression showed lower intubation rates and mortality in patients assigned to the NIV arm compared with the oxygen-only arm. This sparked the initial interest in NIV for patients with hematological malignancy, though it did itself not include patients with malignancy [2]. In a landmark study from 2001, Hilbert et al. [3] made a similar observation of lower intubation rates and mortality in immunocompromised patients assigned to NIV early in the course of ARF, compared with treatment with oxygen only; this study included a significant number of patients with hematological malignancy. In an Italian study of patients with hematological malignancy with incipient ARF in the ward, patients who were randomized to CPAP compared with oxygen required referral to the ICU and intubation less often [4]. In contrast, in a German RCT in allogeneic bone marrow transplant recipients with ARF, NIV did not prevent intubation and had no effect on survival [5].

Apart from these RCTs, a number of observational studies found lower mortality rates in patients with hematological malignancy treated with NIV compared with invasive mechanical ventilation; this finding was not consistent over all studies, however [6–8]. In the interpretation of observational data, one must account for the fact that an association observed in a nonrandomized trial may not reflect causality and that, in a real-life setting, patients eligible for a trial of NIV are different from patients who are immediately intubated. In addition, higher survival rates in patient categories such as "successful NIV" or "NIV only" may overestimate the benefit of NIV as such categorization biases toward a favorable outcome by excluding patients in whom NIV failed. More recent studies have attempted to correct for confounders that obscure the relationship between NIV and outcome. A study that adjusted the association of NIV and mortality for the probability of receiving NIV by a propensity score found a protective effect associated with the use of NIV [6]. The authors of the OUTCOMEREA study group applied a marginal structural model to adjust for the effects of time-dependent covariates in a large dataset of patients treated with first-line NIV as compared with invasive ventilation only, collected over 15 years. An association between lower mortality and NIV was only present in patients with acute-on-chronic respiratory failure (mainly chronic obstructive pulmonary disease (COPD) patients) but not in patients with new-onset ARF, regardless of whether they had underlying immunosuppression [7].

66.2.2 Timing and Place of NIV

In the observational data, the success rate of NIV ranges from 25 to 54 %, but is consistently lower than the NIV success rate in the RCTs (54–90 %). Apart from a more careful patient selection in the RCTs, this difference is likely attributable to a different timing of NIV. In the RCTs, all patients received NIV from the onset of ARF, whereas the time between ARF onset and the initiation of NIV was highly variable (and frequently unknown) in the observational data. Late referral to the ICU, late initiation of NIV, more profound hypoxemia, and additional organ failure have been associated with increased risk for NIV failure. As such, the potential benefit of a trial of NIV is likely optimal when patients are selected in an early stage of ARF. Based upon the available data, NIV should definitely not be used as a last resort to avoid intubation when other therapies have failed. Although in the study by Squadrone et al. [4] a continuous positive airway pressure (CPAP) program was successfully set up in the hematological ward itself, NIV in patients with hematological malignancy preferably should be treated in an ICU setting, given the relatively high risk of NIV failure. Timely and close communication with the attending intensive care physician is therefore essential.

66.2.3 Diagnostic and Therapeutic Approach in NIV-Treated Patients with Hematological Malignancy

Although it has been suggested that NIV offers a certain form of lung protective effect (by preventing alveolar collapse through positive end-expiratory pressure or by limiting the required fraction of inspired oxygen), it is more likely that NIV is a purely supportive therapy that buys time until ARF resolves and that causes less iatrogenic damage than invasive mechanical ventilation. It is important to keep in mind that ARF in patients with hematological malignancy may result from a diverse range of pulmonary insults, both direct and indirect, of which some are more reversible than others. The ultimate prognosis is, to a large extent, defined by the cause of

ARF and, compared with the absence an etiologic diagnosis, being able to identify the cause itself has been associated with better outcome [9]. Initiating NIV should not postpone or obviate the search for the etiology of ARF, and evidently, not the empirical or directed etiologic therapy. NIV may permit and even facilitate bronchoscopy and bronchoalveolar lavage, but imaging with high-resolution computed tomography may be more challenging under NIV.

66.2.4 Avoiding NIV Failure

Failure of NIV is associated with increased mortality. To some extent, this probably relates to failure of the causative therapy directed at the cause of ARF or to a refractory state of ARF. However, unduly prolonging NIV may exert harm by delaying intubation. This is suggested by the observation that late referral to the ICU and an increasing duration of NIV application are independent predictors of mortality [8]. Similarly, in the aforementioned study by Schnell et al. [7], failure of NIV was independently associated with increased mortality after adjustment for time-dependent covariates. Careful selection of patients is therefore essential, not only with regard to the presence of (relative) contraindications for NIV, but also estimating the probability that ARF is likely to be reversed within a short period of time. Efforts should be made to improve tolerance of NIV, but one must bear in mind that persisting discomfort or agitation, especially in hypoxemic ARF, may be an early warning sign of inappropriate use of NIV. Positive pressures should by slowly titrated upward to allow patients to accommodate. Careful adjustment of the ventilator settings while observing patient-ventilator synchrony is important, paying attention to inspiratory and expiratory pressures, trigger sensitivity, and inspiratory and expiratory cycling. Different ventilator modes may be tried under the assumption that no mode has been shown to be superior to another. The patient-ventilator interface should be chosen on an individual basis, preferably trying different types, and a compromise must be achieved between permitting a certain amount of pressure leak and avoiding pressure sores or claustrophobia. Judicious sedation with the use of short-acting agents such as remifentanil and dexmedetomidine may increase the success rate of NIV; however, sedation should not be allowed to mask respiratory deterioration. Attention should be given to try to allow some sleep, to preserve circadian rhythm, and to maintain orientation in time and space. If patients remain dependent on NIV for more than 24–36 h, without signs that ARF is resolving, one should consider cessation of NIV and semi-elective intubation to avoid the adverse effects associated with late NIV failure. Intubation should also be strongly considered at any time if PaO_2/FiO_2 levels fall below 200 or when additional organ failure develops.

66.2.5 NIV in Patients with Hematological Malignancy with a Do-Not-Intubate Order

As NIV permits patients to be awake and to communicate, it is an attractive way to provide mechanical ventilator support while preserving the patient's autonomy and ability to interact with his or her family and loved ones. In addition, it requires only minimal or no sedation, which shortens the time spent in the ICU. Minimal sedation levels are advocated to prevent the occurrence of delirium and perhaps the long-lasting cognitive and functional deficits associated with it. As a trial of NIV may offer a compromise between an increase in the patient's chance to survive an ARF event and a limitation of the risk of embarking on a prolonged ICU stay and its associated complications, it may be of particular value in patients with a do-not-intubate (DNI) order and a potentially reversible ARF event. Although data on this particular use of NIV in patients with hematological malignancy are lacking, a recent prospective observational study in general ICU patients with a DNI order showed that NIV could be successfully applied in more than 60 % of patients [10]. Tolerance of NIV was good to excellent in 34 %, sleep was qualified as good at least one time under NIV in 38 %, and oral intake was possible in 66 %. Importantly, in patients that survived their ICU and hospital stay, functional status afterward was not significantly different compared with the pre-ICU status. Evidently, data on the use of NIV in the specific population of patients with hematological malignancy with a DNI code are eagerly awaited.

66.2.6 NIV in Patients with Hematological Malignancy at the End of Life

A more controversial issue is whether or not NIV should be offered to patients with hematological malignancy with ARF when their disease is refractory or in a terminal phase, and when the aim of therapy is to provide palliation of symptoms rather than to try to extend survival. Although NIV may provide more rapid relief of dyspnea than medication, this may be at the expense of introducing other discomfort such as disruption of sleep, claustrophobia, or pressure sores. The main drawback is that the initiation of NIV subjects the patient to a high-tech procedure in a highly clinical environment at a time when care should move away from aggressive interventions to focus on the creation of comforting surroundings and preparation for a "good death." NIV may offer some precious time to patients and families to say goodbye but may, on the other hand, prolong the dying process and cause additional anxiety and distress. In the absence of good data, offering NIV for this indication should be the exception rather than a rule. If NIV is considered in this setting, it should be for a limited time and in the context of a holistic approach to palliation. At any moment, the benefits, such as permitting time to settle things, say goodbye, or come to terms with death, should be balanced against the discomfort or emotional suffering endured by the patients and their relatives.

Conclusion

NIV is a well-established supportive treatment in patients with ARF and may also be considered as a first-line ventilatory strategy in patients with hematological malignancy, taking into account several caveats. Although NIV can avert intubation and thus improve outcome in a significant number of patients, it may also increase mortality in those patients in whom it fails. The overall impact of

NIV on outcome in patients with hematological malignancy with ARF remains unproven. A subset of patients with hematological malignancy is likely to benefit from NIV, especially those with early-onset ARF, no or limited additional organ failure, and a cause of ARF that is likely to be reversible in a short time. In these patients, a trial of NIV can be offered but should be monitored closely for signs of response or impending failure. NIV should not be allowed to cause delays in intubation when this is appropriate, which is the case when stagnation or progression of organ failure occurs. In addition, NIV may have a role as an upper limit of ventilatory support in selected patients with a DNI order.

Key Major Recommendations

- NIV may be considered in early stages of ARF in patients with hematological malignancy.
- NIV should be avoided in late-stage (>48 h) or severe (PaO_2/FiO_2 <200) ARF in patients with hematological malignancy.
- NIV should be accompanied by a thorough search for the etiology of ARF in patients with hematological malignancy.
- Response to and tolerance of NIV should be carefully assessed, and persisting intolerance or worsening organ failure should prompt intubation.
- Prolonged use of NIV (>48 h) in patients with hematological malignancy should be avoided.

Flow chart:

Decision algorithm regarding choice of type of ventilator support in hematological patient with ARF (and full therapy code)

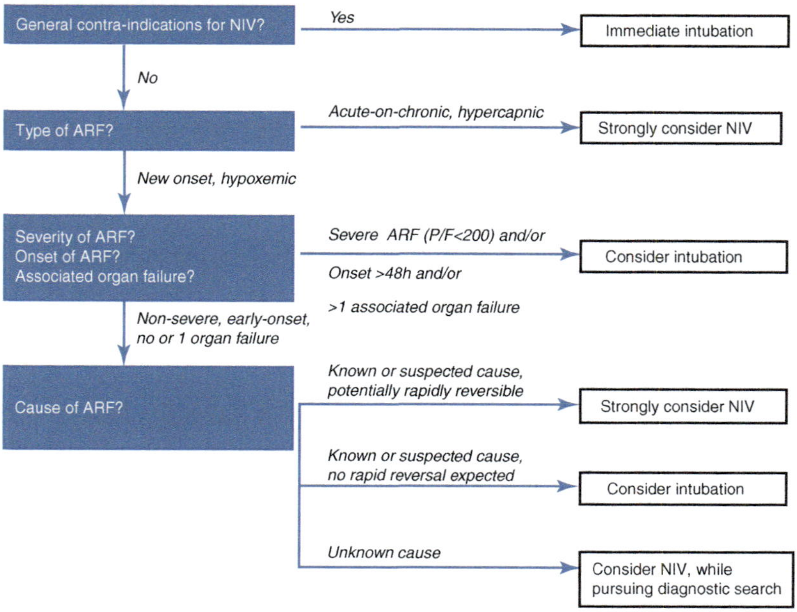

References

1. Azoulay E, Mokart D, Pène F, et al. Outcomes of critically ill patients with hematologic malignancies: prospective multicenter data from France and Belgium. J Clin Oncol. 2013;31:2810–8.
2. Antonelli M, Conti G, Bufi M, et al. Noninvasive ventilation for treatment of acute respiratory failure in patients undergoing solid organ transplantation: a randomized controlled trial. JAMA. 2000;283:235–41.
3. Hilbert G, Gruson D, Vargas D, et al. Noninvasive ventilation in immunosuppressed patients with pulmonary infiltrates, fever, and acute respiratory failure. N Engl J Med. 2001;344:481–7.
4. Squadrone V, Massaia M, Bruno B, et al. Early CPAP prevents evolution of acute lung injury in patients with hematologic malignancy. Intensive Care Med. 2010;36:1666–74.
5. Wermke M, Schiemanck S, Hoffken G, et al. Respiratory failure in patients undergoing allogeneic hematopoietic SCT - a randomized trial on early non-invasive ventilation based on standard care hematology wards. Bone Marrow Transplant. 2012;47:574–80.
6. Gristina G, Antonelli M, Conti G, et al. Noninvasive versus invasive ventilation for acute respiratory failure in patients with hematologic malignancies: a 5-year multicenter observational study. Crit Care Med. 2011;39:2232–9.
7. Schnell D, Timsit JF, Darmon M, et al. Noninvasive mechanical ventilation in acute respiratory failure: trends in use and outcome. Intensive Care Med. 2014;40:582–91.
8. Adda M, Coquet I, Darmon M, et al. Predictors of noninvasive ventilation failure in patients with hematologic malignancy and acute respiratory failure. Crit Care Med. 2008;36:2766–72.
9. Azoulay E, Thiéry G, Chevret S, et al. The prognosis of acute respiratory failure in critically ill cancer patients. Medicine. 2004;83:360–70.
10. Azoulay E, Kouatchet A, Jaber S, et al. Noninvasive mechanical ventilation in patients having declined tracheal intubation. Intensive Care Med. 2013;39:292–301.

Noninvasive Ventilation in Patients with Solid Malignancies

67

Pascal Kingah and Ayman O. Soubani

Contents

P. Kingah, MD
Division of Pulmonary, Critical Care and Sleep Medicine, Wayne State University School of Medicine, Detroit, MI, USA

A.O. Soubani, MD (✉)
Division of Pulmonary, Critical Care and Sleep Medicine, Wayne State University School of Medicine, Detroit, MI, USA

Medical ICU, Harper University Hospital, 3990 John R-3 Hudson, Detroit, MI, 48201, USA

Pulmonary and Critical Care, Karmanos Cancer Center, Detroit, MI, USA
e-mail: asoubani@med.wayne.edu

A.M. Esquinas (ed.), *Noninvasive Mechanical Ventilation: Theory, Equipment, and Clinical Applications*, DOI 10.1007/978-3-319-21653-9_67

67.1 Introduction

Acute respiratory failure (ARF) refers to a rapidly progressive inability of the respiratory system to perform one or both of its gas exchange functions, which includes oxygenation and carbon dioxide elimination. This is usually life threatening especially when it occurs in patients with underlying malignancy. In patients with acute leukemia or lymphoma, the incidence of ARF ranges from 10 to 20 % and increases to 40 % in those with neutropenia or bone marrow transplantation [1, 2]. ARF in patients with solid tumors has a lower incidence of about 1–5 %, with about 44–50 % mortality when these patients were admitted to the intensive care unit (ICU) and required some form of ventilation [3–6]. Recent studies have shown that, in patients with ARF, noninvasive ventilation (NIV) can prevent the need for invasive mechanical ventilation, hence reducing the risks associated with this form of ventilation as well as reducing ICU and hospital stay [7–10]. There have also been reports of lower 30-day mortality with the use of NIV compared with invasive mechanical ventilation [11]. The purpose of this chapter is to provide an overview of the use of NIV in patients with solid malignancies emphasizing on indications and outcome.

67.2 Causes of ARF in Patients with Solid Malignancies

There are a variety of conditions that may cause ARF in patients with solid malignancies (Table 67.1). Infections caused by opportunistic and non-opportunistic organisms are a major consideration. Neutropenia and corticosteroid therapy are risk factors for opportunistic infections in this patient population. Noninfectious etiologies include pulmonary embolism, metastasis, atelectasis from endobronchial lesions causing obstruction, lymphangitic spread, diffuse alveolar hemorrhage, pleural effusions, and hemorrhage from an endobronchial tumor [1, 12, 13]. The treatment of solid malignancies may also contribute to ARF, with drug-induced pulmonary toxicity, radiation-induced pulmonary toxicity, and complications of diagnostic and therapeutic procedures. Post-lung resection ARF reported in the acute setting following lung resection has been related to acute respiratory distress syndrome (ARDS) or atelectasis. Comorbid illnesses including cardiac disease, chronic obstructive pulmonary disease (COPD), asthma, interstitial, and occupational lung diseases could worsen in these patients, predisposing them to develop ARF.

67.3 Outcome of NIV in Patients with Malignancy

Most of the studies that address the use of NIV in cancer patients focus on patients with hematological malignancies (Table 67.2). These studies have shown improved outcome of patients with ARF managed by NIV compared with invasive mechanical ventilation. In one study of 1,302 patients with hematologic malignancies admitted to the ICU with ARF, NIV was attempted in 21 % of these patients and 46 % of

Table 67.1 Causes of acute respiratory failure in patients with solid malignancies

Infectious
Pneumonia
Bacteria
Viral
Post obstructive
Opportunistic infections
Fungal
PCP
Noninfectious
Related to cancer
Airway obstruction
Pulmonary hemorrhage
Lymphangitic pulmonary spread
Pleural effusion
Related to cancer treatment
Drug-induced pulmonary toxicity
Radiation-induced pulmonary toxicity
Complications of diagnostic and therapeutic procedures
Comorbid illnesses
COPD/asthma
Interstitial and occupational lung diseases
Cardiac disease

them later required invasive mechanical ventilation [7]. Favorable outcomes were encountered in NIV patients, with mortality of 46 % compared with 69 % in patients who were initially put on invasive mechanical ventilation and 77 % in patients who failed NIV and later required.

Studies that specifically evaluate the outcome of patients with solid malignancies and ARF treated by NIV are sparse. Two major studies have reported on the use of NIV in patients with solid malignancies. The most recent study by Azoulay et al. [21] in 2014 was a retrospective analysis of data from six previously published retrospective and prospective studies on patients with malignancy admitted to the ICU in 14 university and university-affiliated hospitals in France and Belgium. In this review, there were 147 (14.6 %) patients with solid malignancy, in whom breast and lung cancers were the most commonly encountered. NIV was used in 387 patients, among whom 174 survived and 213 did not survive, with a 64 % overall mortality. Among the 387 patients initiated on NIV, 276 subsequently required mechanical ventilation. NIV failure was strongly associated with the severity of ARDS, with patients failing in the moderate to severe categories by the Berlin definition. Following a multivariate analysis, patients with solid tumors were independently associated with lower mortality, OR 0.51 (0.34–0.77) $p=0.002$. As illustrated in Fig. 67.1, mortality from solid tumors also decreased over time compared with hematologic malignancies.

Table 67.2 Mortality rates, ICU length of stay of patients with malignancy treated with using NIV in studies published in the last two decades (1994–2014)

Author, year	Study design	Type of malignancy	Number of patients on NIPPV	Location	Mean ICU days	NIPPV failure requiring intubation	Hospital mortality rate (%)
Tognet et al. 1994 [14]	Prospective cohort	Hematologic	18	ICU	8.5	12	67
Conti et al. 1998 [8]	Prospective cohort	Hematologic	16	ICU	4.3	1	31.3
Hilbert et al. 2000 [15]	Prospective cohort	Hematologic	64	ICU	7	48	44
Hilbert et al. 2001 [10]	Prospective randomized trial	Hematologic	26	ICU	7	12	50
Azoulay et al. 2001 [16]	Retrospective cohort	Hematologic and Solid organ	48	ICU	7	27	43.7
Principi et al. 2004 [17]	Prospective matched cohort	Hematologic	17	Oncology ward	NR	7	47
Rocco et al. 2004 [18]	Prospective matched cohort	Hematologic Solid organ	19	ICU	9	9	53
Soares et al. 2005 [13]	Prospective cohort	Hematologic and solid organ	19	ICU	NR	NR	37
Adda et al. 2008 [19]	Retrospective	Hematologic	99	ICU	NR	53	61
Depuydt et al. 2010 [21, 24]	Retrospective cohort	Hematologic	166	ICU	6	14	67
Gristina et al. 2011 [7]	Retrospective	Hematologic	274	ICU	9	77	49
Azoulay et al. 2014 [20]	Retrospective	Hematologic and solid organ	387	ICU	NR	276	33
Azevedo et al. 2014 [24]	Prospective cohort	Hematology and solid organ	85	ICU	6	45	55
Lemiale et al. 2014 [1]	Randomized controlled trial	Hematologic and Solid organ	130	ICU	NR	49	0

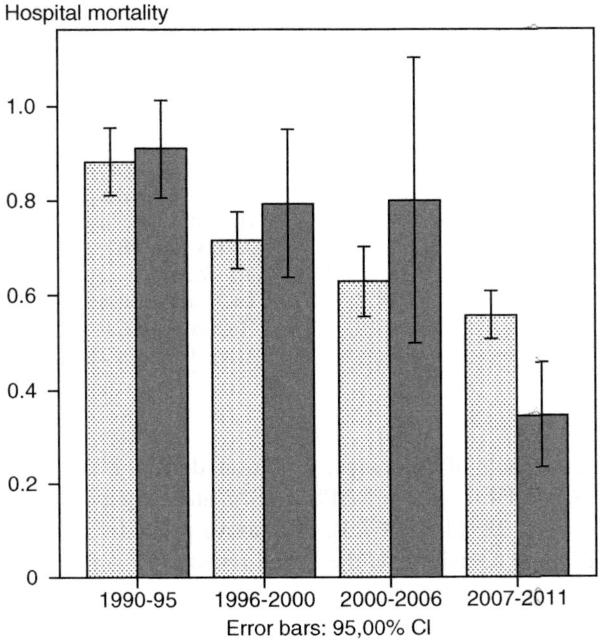

Fig. 67.1 Hospital mortality according to period of admission to the ICU in patients with hematological malignancy (*dotted bars*; $p < 0.0001$) and with solid tumor (*gray bars*; $p < 0.0001$) [21]

The other major study that reported on the use of NIV in solid malignancies was a prospective study by Azevedo et al. [22], which was a multicenter study carried out in 28 ICUs in Brazil. In their patient population, 227 (86 %) patients had solid malignancies and only 36 (14 %) patients had hematologic malignancies. The most frequently encountered malignancies were lung, breast, and lower gastrointestinal cancers. NIV was initially used in 85 patients (32.3 %), and 45 (47.9 %) of these patients required mechanical ventilation. Patients who ended up only using NIV had a mortality of 40 %, whereas those who required mechanical ventilation had a mortality rate of 68.9 %. Reasons for NIV failure were not evaluated in this study. Multivariate analysis to identify independent risk factors for mortality did not reveal that the type of tumor was a risk factor, but significant risk factors for mortality included medical admission, cancer status, tumor as a reason for ventilator support, poor performance status, NIV followed by mechanical ventilation, use of mechanical ventilation only, and higher SOFA (sequential organ failure assessment) scores.

67.4 Predictors of NIV Success and Failure

Major factors found to be associated with NIV failure following multivariate analysis include respiratory rate > 20 breaths per minute, organ failure, particularly renal insufficiency requiring renal replacement therapy, hemodynamic instability requiring vasopressors, ARDS, $PaO_2/FiO_2 < 146$ 1 h after NIV initiation, persistent organ failure over the first few ICU days, pneumonia, pH <7.25, excessive air

Table 67.3 Predictors of success and failure of NIV in patients with malignancy

Major predictors of NIV success	Good performance status especially if ambulatory Absence of airway involvement No recurrence of cancer Age <40
Major predictors of NIV failure	Respiratory rate >20 bpm Renal insufficiency requiring renal replacement therapy Hemodynamic instability requiring pressors ARDS with PaO_2/FiO_2 ratio <146 1 h after NIV pH <7.25 Lack of tolerance to NIV High APACHE II >29 or SAPS II >35 More diffuse pulmonary infiltrates on chest imaging

leak, lack of tolerance, agitation during NIV, high severity of illness scores (APACHE II ≥29 or SAPS II ≥35), and longer duration of NIV dependency [5, 13, 19–21, 23] (Table 67.3). The above predictors should serve as a guideline when making decisions on the initial respiratory support for patients with hematologic malignancy in ARF.

It is also imperative to understand the characteristics of patients with malignancies who have had favorable outcomes with the use of NIV. Following multivariate logistic regression, patient factors that have been associated with favorable outcomes include good performance status, especially if patient is ambulatory, age less than 40, no recurrence of cancer, and absence of airway involvement [13]. Patients with solid tumors were better candidates than those with hematologic malignancy (OR 0.51 (0.34–0.77) $p=0.002$). Patients with ARDS from primary malignancy had better outcomes than those with ARDS from secondary or undermined causes (OR 0.41 (0.2–0.88) $p=0.02$) [21, 22].

67.5 Applications of NIV in Patients with Solid Malignancies

67.5.1 Acute Hypoxic Respiratory Failure

NIV with the use of continuous positive airway pressure (CPAP) has been shown to correct hypoxemia, particularly in patients with pulmonary edema [24]. CPAP offers a high inspired oxygen content, increases mean airway pressure, and improves ventilation to collapsed areas of the lungs by recruitment of under-ventilated lung. This action is similar to positive end-expiratory pressure in mechanically ventilated patients. In patients with malignancies, 90 % of ARDS cases are related to an infection [21]. In patients with moderate to severe ARDS according to the Berlin severity categories, higher NIV failures were noted in recent reports [21, 22]. Approximately 70 % of patients with moderate ARDS failed NIV, and 79.1 % of patients with severe ARDS failed [21]. The use of NIV to treat hypoxia in this group of patients should be avoided.

67.5.2 Acute Hypercapnic Respiratory Failure

NIV unloads inspiratory muscles, hence reducing work of breathing. This, in turn, reduces the respiratory rate and increases alveolar ventilation, which causes a fall in $PaCO_2$. NIV is particularly useful in patients with neuromuscular diseases associated with certain types of solid malignancies leading to hypercapnia [24]. NIV has also been shown to be effective in patients with hypercapnic respiratory failure due to COPD [25].

67.5.3 Treatment of Comorbid Diseases

Patients with COPD are at a much higher risk of developing lung cancer than the average population [26, 27]. Lung cancer remains an important cause of death in patients with COPD [28]. Studies have also shown that patients with hypoxemic acute respiratory failure due to community-acquired pneumonia in COPD respond to the use of NIV [29, 30].

67.5.4 Palliative Treatment in Patients with Do-Not-Intubate Orders

NIV is particularly useful in patients with do-not-intubate (DNI) orders who present with ARF due to causes that could be easily reversible, such as cardiogenic pulmonary edema or COPD exacerbation. The international consensus conference in intensive care medicine approved the use of NIV in patients who have ARF with a reversible cause if the patients are not to be intubated [31]. In 2001, an international consensus that included the American Thoracic Society (ATS), European Society of Intensive Care Medicine (ESICM), Société de Réanimation de Langue Française (SRLF), and the European Respiratory Society (ERS) was the first to address this issue, and considered palliative NIV as appropriate in selected patients in whom endotracheal ventilation is not an option provided the cause of ARF is reversible and NIV improves patient comfort. The Society for Critical Care Medicine (SCCM) task force recommended an approach for deciding when to offer NIV to patients in whom mechanical ventilation could not be performed. This conference, which occurred in 2007, adopted an approach that involved a daily assessment of NIV objectives, which were classified into three categories: NIV as life support for patients with DNI orders, NIV as life support for patients receiving comfort care only, and NIV as life support for patients without any treatment-limitation decisions. Palliative NIV was defined by the first and second categories [32].

In a review on palliative NIV in patients with ARF, Azoulay et al. [33] reported several unanswered questions in the literature available at the time. Their major concerns included the uncertainty whether palliative ventilation increased duration of life or if it extended the dying process, absence of qualitative observational data to determine actual benefits of palliative NIV, and whether palliative NIV should be performed in incapacitated patients to either improve survival or alleviate symptoms of respiratory distress.

A study by Nava et al. [34] evaluated the effectiveness of NIV in reducing dyspnea and the amount of opiates needed in patients with solid malignancy. In this multicenter, multinational randomized controlled trial, 200 patients from seven different countries were randomized to either NIV or oxygen via the Venturi mask. NIV was found to be effective in reducing dyspnea rapidly in the NIV group after the first hour of treatment, and the average change in Borg scale was −0.58, 95 % CI (−0.92 to −0.23). The amount of opiates needed was significantly decreased in the NIV group: 26.9 mg versus 59.4 mg, difference of −32.4 mg, 95 % CI (−47.5 to −17.4). Eleven (11 %) patients in the NIV group discontinued treatment. This was mainly due to mask intolerance and anxiety. Patient selection remains crucial, as NIV should only be attempted on patients who are alert, cooperative, and able to cough [35].

67.5.5 Acute Respiratory Failure Following Surgery

ARF following surgery for underlying solid malignancies is a new and growing indication for NIV. In a study by Yu et al. [36], NIV was used a first-line intervention for patients with ARDS following esophagectomy for esophageal cancer. Intubation was avoided in 30 patients (30/64, 48.4 %). NIV was used as initial treatment in 48 patients and 16 were converted to invasive mechanical ventilation due to active bleeding, hemodynamic instability and neurologic disturbances. Patients treated with NIV had a lower ICU length of stay, 11.5 days compared to 33.1 days in patients on invasive mechanical ventilation. The 28-day hospital mortality rate among patients treated with NIV was much lower as well, 6.25 % compared to 21.9 % in patients who were treated with invasive mechanical ventilation. In this study, the use of NIV appeared to be safe in treating ARDS/ALI following esophagectomy, but conversion to invasive ventilation should be considered early in patients with postoperative complications, including acute kidney injury, cardiac arrest, and patients with severe ARDS [36].

A few earlier studies reported on the use of NIV in patients with ARF following lung resection, but most of the indications for lung resection were for COPD. One of these studies reported that NIV decreased the need for endotracheal intubation and improved outcome [37]. Another study by Auriant et al. [38], in 2001, of patients with ARF following lung resection for lung cancer compared, by randomizing prospectively, standard therapy with and without NIV. In-hospital deaths and subsequent endotracheal intubations were fewer in the NIV group compared with the standard therapy group. In the NIV group, there were 3 deaths out of 24 patients (12.5 %) and in the standard therapy group 9 deaths out of 24 patients (37.5 %), $p=0.045$. Endotracheal intubation with mechanical ventilation was required in 12 out of 24 (50 %) patients with standard care and only 5 out of 24 (20.8 %) in patients randomized to NIV, $p=0.035$. There was no significant difference in ICU length of stay. NIV appears to be safe in reducing the need for mechanical ventilation in patients with lung cancer and respiratory failure following lung resection, although more studies are needed to validate these findings.

67.5.6 NIV and Bronchoscopy

There are limited reports of performing bronchoscopy while the patient is on NIV. The scenarios that would apply to this are either that the patient is already on NIV and needs bronchoscopy for diagnostic or therapeutic purposes or that NIV is started to support the patient's respiratory status during the procedure. In patients with solid malignancies, bronchoscopy may be considered during NIV for bronchoalveolar lavage, removal of secretions, investigation of the source of hemoptysis, obtaining endobronchial biopsies, or performing rigid bronchoscopy for endobronchial treatment of cancer with laser, electrocautery, or cryotherapy. In a study of 40 patients with acute hypoxemic respiratory failure on NIV who underwent bronchoscopy, 53 % of patients were immunosuppressed and 10 % had solid malignancies. The procedure was completed with no major complications in all patients. Mild hypoxemia developed in 5 % of patients. Bronchoalveolar lavage yielded diagnostic information in 68 % of patients [39].

Another study compared NIV and high-frequency nasal cannula (HFNC) during bronchoscopy in critically ill patients with acute hypoxemic respiratory failure [40]. Twenty-five percent of the patients had solid malignancies. Bronchoscopy was well tolerated in all patients except one. Three patients in the NIV group and one patient in the HFNC group were intubated within 24 h after the end of bronchoscopy ($p=0.29$). The conclusion of the study was that NIV was superior to HFNC with regard to oxygenation before, during, and after bronchoscopy in patients with moderate to severe hypoxemia. Performing bronchoscopy while the patient is under NIV requires high skill and expertise by the bronchoscopist and close monitoring of the patient in a critical care environment. Precautions should be in place to intubate the patient immediately if the need arises. Details of bronchoscopy during NIV have been outlined in a review by Esquinas et al. [41].

67.5.7 NIV outside of the ICU

Initiation and monitoring of NIV in patients with ARF is generally recommended to take place in a critical care environment, such as the ICU, respiratory care unit, or intermediate care unit. In these units there is close monitoring of the patient, with a low patient-to-nurse ratio, presence of respiratory care therapists, and involvement by intensivists. There are, however, certain circumstances where NIV can be used outside of the ICU, especially in cancer patients. Instituting NIV early in cancer patients may avoid later intubation and mechanical ventilation, which has traditionally been associated with high mortality. Also, early NIV in patients with cancer and acute hypoxemic respiratory failure has been associated with better outcome. Other factors that may lead to consideration of NIV in cancer patients are lack of ICU beds, patient or family refusal of transfer to the ICU, and the use of this therapy as a palliative tool to relieve dyspnea in patients with advance malignancy. In a questionnaire, 157 respondents from 51 countries (66 %) indicated that they use NIV outside of the ICU, and the common indications were pneumonia in immunocompromised patients (63 %) and palliation (51 %) [42]. There are only few studies in cancer patients that have shown that starting NIV outside of the ICU is clinically feasible with reasonable results [17]. However, the use of NIV outside of the ICU should follow the same precautions as in the ICU, including no hemodynamic or neurologic compromise, no evidence of moderate or severe ARDS (PaO_2/FiO_2 ratio >200), and there should be close monitoring of the patient, and skilled nursing staff present. There should also be detailed hospital policy in place to regulate this application.

67.6 NIV Settings

Similar to invasive mechanical ventilation, administration of NIV has two major modes of ventilation: pressure limited and volume limited. Proportional assist ventilation, which is a relatively new mode that targets patients effort, can also be used [20]. In the pressure-limited mode, the ventilator applies a set pressure both during inspiration and expiration continuously. CPAP of 10 cmH_2O is the recommended level used in several reports, but it could also be titrated from 2.5 to 12.5 cmH_2O using increments of 2–3 cmH_2O [24, 43]. This mode is most useful in correcting hypoxemia and during management of cardiogenic pulmonary edema. Bi-level positive airway pressure (BIPAP) can also be used, which requires setting two different pressure levels, one during inspiration (pressure support) and the other during expiration (CPAP). This mode of NIV is effective in patients with dyspnea and hypercapnic respiratory failure and may be useful in patients with pulmonary infiltrates and hypoxemic respiratory failure. There are no clear recommendations on the pressure settings with this mode of ventilation. The choice of initial pressures depends on factors such as personal experience, clinical setting, arterial blood gases, and patient tolerance. Usually, clinicians start with CPAP of 3–5 cmH_2O and inspiratory pressure of 8–12 cmH_2O above CPAP. If necessary, pressure changes are made gradually, depending on the patient's dyspnea, tolerance, and minute ventilation. Oxygen supplementation should target oxygen saturation above 89 % [44]. Volume-limited Non-invasive Positive Pressure Ventilation (NIPPV) is usually administered via a ventilator that is more expensive, heavier, and has sophisticated alarm systems. It is usually set in assist control mode to allow for spontaneous patient triggering. The backup rate is set slightly below the patient's breathing rate [20].

Conclusion

NIV use in patients with solid malignancies presenting with ARF has been shown to be beneficial in avoiding invasive mechanical ventilation and reducing mortality and hospital length of stay. The main indications for NIV in this patient population are acute hypercapnic respiratory failure, palliative support of respiratory symptoms, treatment of comorbid cardiopulmonary illnesses, and in selected patients with acute hypoxemic respiratory failure, postoperative respiratory failure, and during bronchoscopy. Although NIV offers benefits, patient selection is crucial, as several other studies have revealed that patients with moderate to severe ARDS, high severity of illness, and acute renal failure requiring renal replacement therapy did not benefit from NIV and NIV use resulted in higher mortality once they were intubated. Patient selection remains the primary challenge for clinicians caring for these patients.

References

1. Lemiale V, et al. Identifying cancer subjects with acute respiratory failure at high risk for intubation and mechanical ventilation. Respir Care. 2014;59(10):1517–23.
2. Chaoui D, et al. Incidence and prognostic value of respiratory events in acute leukemia. Leukemia. 2004;18(4):670–5.
3. Muller AM, Gazzana MB, Silva DR. Outcomes for patients with lung cancer admitted to intensive care units. Rev Bras Ter Intensiva. 2013;25(1):12–6.
4. Azoulay E. A new standard of care for critically ill patients with cancer. Chest. 2014;146(2): 241–4.
5. Azoulay E, et al. The prognosis of acute respiratory failure in critically ill cancer patients. Medicine (Baltimore). 2004;83(6):360–70.
6. Azoulay E, Schlemmer B. Diagnostic strategy in cancer patients with acute respiratory failure. Intensive Care Med. 2006;32(6):808–22.
7. Gristina GR, et al. Noninvasive versus invasive ventilation for acute respiratory failure in patients with hematologic malignancies: a 5-year multicenter observational survey. Crit Care Med. 2011;39(10):2232–9.
8. Conti G, et al. Noninvasive ventilation for the treatment of acute respiratory failure in patients with hematologic malignancies: a pilot study. Intensive Care Med. 1998;24(12):1283–8.
9. Rabbat A, et al. Prognosis of patients with acute myeloid leukaemia admitted to intensive care. Br J Haematol. 2005;129(3):350–7.
10. Hilbert G, et al. Noninvasive ventilation in immunosuppressed patients with pulmonary infiltrates, fever, and acute respiratory failure. N Engl J Med. 2001;344(7):481–7.
11. Turkoglu M, et al. Acute respiratory distress syndrome in patients with hematological malignancies. Hematology. 2013;18(3):123–30.
12. Sirithanakul K, et al. Pulmonary complications following hematopoietic stem cell transplantation: diagnostic approaches. Am J Hematol. 2005;80(2):137–46.
13. Soares M, et al. Characteristics and outcomes of cancer patients requiring mechanical ventilatory support for >24 hrs. Crit Care Med. 2005;33(3):520–6.
14. Tognet E, et al. Treatment of acute respiratory failure with non-invasive intermittent positive pressure ventilation in haematological patients. Clin Intensive Care. 1994;5(6):282–8.
15. Hilbert G, et al. Noninvasive continuous positive airway pressure in neutropenic patients with acute respiratory failure requiring intensive care unit admission. Crit Care Med. 2000;28(9): 3185–90.
16. Azoulay E, et al. Improved survival in cancer patients requiring mechanical ventilatory support: impact of noninvasive mechanical ventilatory support. Crit Care Med. 2001;29(3): 519–25.
17. Principi T, et al. Noninvasive continuous positive airway pressure delivered by helmet in hematological malignancy patients with hypoxemic acute respiratory failure. Intensive Care Med. 2004;30(1):147–50.
18. Rocco M, et al. Noninvasive ventilation by helmet or face mask in immunocompromised patients: a case-control study. Chest. 2004;126(5):1508–15.
19. Depuydt PO, et al. The impact of the initial ventilatory strategy on survival in hematological patients with acute hypoxemic respiratory failure. J Crit Care. 2010;25(1):30–6.
20. Mehta S, Hill NS. Noninvasive ventilation. Am J Respir Crit Care Med. 2001;163(2):540–77.
21. Azoulay E, et al. Acute respiratory distress syndrome in patients with malignancies. Intensive Care Med. 2014;40(8):1106–14.

22. Azevedo LC, et al. Outcomes for patients with cancer admitted to the ICU requiring ventilatory support: results from a prospective multicenter study. Chest. 2014;146(2):257–66.
23. Adda M, et al. Predictors of noninvasive ventilation failure in patients with hematologic malignancy and acute respiratory failure. Crit Care Med. 2008;36(10):2766–72.
24. British Thoracic Society Standards of Care Committee. Non-invasive ventilation in acute respiratory failure. Thorax. 2002;57(3):192–211.
25. Hess DR. The evidence for noninvasive positive-pressure ventilation in the care of patients in acute respiratory failure: a systematic review of the literature. Respir Care. 2004;49(7):810–29.
26. Skillrud DM, Offord KP, Miller RD. Higher risk of lung cancer in chronic obstructive pulmonary disease. A prospective, matched, controlled study. Ann Intern Med. 1986;105(4):503–7.
27. Tockman MS, et al. Airways obstruction and the risk for lung cancer. Ann Intern Med. 1987;106(4):512–8.
28. Vestbo J, et al. Evaluation of COPD Longitudinally to Identify Predictive Surrogate Endpoints (ECLIPSE). Eur Respir J. 2008;31(4):869–73.
29. Confalonieri M, et al. Acute respiratory failure in patients with severe community-acquired pneumonia. A prospective randomized evaluation of noninvasive ventilation. Am J Respir Crit Care Med. 1999;160(5 Pt 1):1585–91.
30. Ferrer M, et al. Noninvasive ventilation in severe hypoxemic respiratory failure: a randomized clinical trial. Am J Respir Crit Care Med. 2003;168(12):1438–44.
31. Organized jointly by the American Thoracic Society, the European Respiratory Society, the European Society of Intensive Care Medicine, and the Société de Réanimation de Langue Française, and approved by ATS Board of Directors. International Consensus Conferences in Intensive Care Medicine: noninvasive positive pressure ventilation in acute respiratory failure. Am J Respir Crit Care Med. 2001;163(1):283–91.
32. Curtis JR, et al. Noninvasive positive pressure ventilation in critical and palliative care settings: understanding the goals of therapy. Crit Care Med. 2007;35(3):932–9.
33. Azoulay E, et al. Palliative noninvasive ventilation in patients with acute respiratory failure. Intensive Care Med. 2011;37(8):1250–7.
34. Nava S, Study Authors. Non-invasive ventilation for end-of-life oncology patients–authors' reply. Lancet Oncol. 2013;14(6):e201.
35. Marik PE. Noninvasive positive-pressure ventilation in patients with malignancy. Am J Hosp Palliat Care. 2007;24(5):417–21.
36. Yu KY, et al. Noninvasive positive pressure ventilation for the treatment of acute respiratory distress syndrome following esophagectomy for esophageal cancer: a clinical comparative study. J Thorac Dis. 2013;5(6):777–82.
37. Lefebvre A, et al. Noninvasive ventilation for acute respiratory failure after lung resection: an observational study. Intensive Care Med. 2009;35(4):663–70.
38. Auriant I, et al. Noninvasive ventilation reduces mortality in acute respiratory failure following lung resection. Am J Respir Crit Care Med. 2001;164(7):1231–5.
39. Baumann HJ, Klose H, Simon M, Ghadban T, Braune SA, Hennigs JK, Kluge S. Fiberoptic bronchoscopy in patients with acute hypoxemic respiratory failure requiring noninvasive ventilation–a feasibility study. Crit Care. 2011;15(4):R179.
40. Simon M, Braune S, Frings D, Wiontzek AK, Klose H, Kluge S. High-flow nasal cannula oxygen versus non-invasive ventilation in patients with acute hypoxaemic respiratory failure undergoing flexible bronchoscopy – a prospective randomised trial. Crit Care. 2014;18(6):712.
41. Esquinas A, Zuil M, Scala R, Chiner E. Bronchoscopy during non-invasive mechanical ventilation: a review of techniques and procedures. Arch Bronconeumol. 2013;49(3):105–12.
42. Cabrini L, Esquinas A, Pasin L, Nardelli P, Frati E, Pintaudi M, Matos P, Landoni G, Zangrillo A. An international survey on noninvasive ventilation use for acute respiratory failure in general non-monitored wards. Respir Care. 2015;60(4):586–92.
43. Antonelli M, et al. A multiple-center survey on the use in clinical practice of noninvasive ventilation as a first-line intervention for acute respiratory distress syndrome. Crit Care Med. 2007;35(1):18–25.
44. Bello G, De Pascale G, Antonelli M. Noninvasive ventilation: practical advice. Curr Opin Crit Care. 2013;19(1):1–8.

Part VIII

Hospital Critical Care Applications: Non Invasive Ventilation in Upper Airways, Endoscopy Procedures and Sedation

Noninvasive Ventilation in Difficult Endotracheal Intubation

68

Igor Barjaktarevic, Jeffrey Albores, and David Berlin

Contents

Abbreviations

CPAP Continuous positive airway pressure
ETI Endotracheal intubation
FRC Functional residual capacity
ILM Intubating laryngeal mask

I. Barjaktarevic, MD, MSc • J. Albores, MD
Division of Pulmonary and Critical Care Medicine, David Geffen School of Medicine at UCLA, Los Angeles, CA, USA
e-mail: ibarjaktarevic@mednet.ucla.edu; jalbores@mednet.ucla.edu

D. Berlin, MD (✉)
Division of Pulmonary and Critical Care Medicine, Weill Cornell Medical College, New York, NY, USA
e-mail: berlind@med.cornell.edu

A.M. Esquinas (ed.), *Noninvasive Mechanical Ventilation: Theory, Equipment, and Clinical Applications*, DOI 10.1007/978-3-319-21653-9_68

LMA	Laryngeal mask airway
NIV	Noninvasive positive pressure ventilation
PEEP	Positive end-expiratory pressure

68.1 Introduction

Noninvasive positive pressure ventilation (NIV) is a validated treatment for acute and chronic respiratory failure in selected patients. The need for endotracheal intubation (ETI) and mechanical ventilation is usually considered a failure of NIV. However, the use of NIV immediately before and during ETI may improve the safety of the transition to invasive mechanical ventilation by a number of mechanisms. In this chapter, the use of NIV as an adjuvant to ETI is discussed, with a focus on the use of NIV during a predicted difficult intubation.

68.2 Difficult Intubation

ETI is an essential part of anesthesia care and the support of critically ill patients. Paradoxically, ETI is associated with a number of life-threatening complications. These complications are more likely during "difficult intubation." This is defined as intubation requiring more than three attempts, for longer than 10 min, or the need for use of an alternative intubation device after a failed attempt. Difficult intubation may lead to serious soft tissue damage and is the major cause of death and anoxic brain injury during anesthesia care [1]. The incidence of difficult intubation varies greatly in different series.

Ideally, clinicians should be able to predict whether intubation will be difficult and adjust their airway plan. Although there are a number of useful clinical scales to help predict difficult intubation, they are not highly sensitive or specific. Some of the rules, such as the Mallampati classification, predict the quality of view of the airway using direct laryngoscopy. The Mallampati classification, however, was not designed to predict difficulty with video laryngoscopy nor does it predict difficulty passing the endotracheal tube. The LEMON mnemonic is a more holistic approach to predicting difficult intubation. It includes factors such as mouth opening, cervical mobility, and anatomical obstruction (Table 68.1).

The narrow definition of difficult intubation refers to the placement of the endotracheal tube during laryngoscopy. A broader meaning can include clinical scenarios in which ETI can contribute to clinical deterioration even if laryngoscopy and tube placement are technically easy. Critically ill patients have poor physiologic reserve and have little tolerance of the stressors of ETI. These stressors occur to varying degrees in all patients. While usually insignificant in the healthy population, they can be severe in critically ill patients. For example, patients with respiratory failure and high metabolic rates are intolerant of hypoventilation or apnea during ETI. Similarly, patients with intracranial hypertension or right ventricular failure do not tolerate hypercapnia and hemodynamic consequences of ETI. In these scenarios, we can predict a high risk of deterioration during ETI even if laryngoscopy and tube passage are easy. Of course, the combination of difficult laryngoscopy and tube passage with poor physiologic reserve is the perfect storm of factors that can lead to catastrophic deterioration during ETI. As a

Table 68.1 Mnemonic "LEMON" in evaluation for a potentially difficult airway

Mnemonic	Description
Look externally	Obesity, micrognathia, evidence of previous head and neck surgery or irradiation, presence of facial hair, dental abnormalities (poor dentition, dentures, large teeth), narrow face, high and arched palate, short or thick neck, and facial or neck trauma
Evaluate using the 3:3:2 rule	Normal mouth opening is 3 (of the patient's) fingerbreadths; a normal mandible dimension will likewise allow 3 fingerbreadths between the mentum and the hyoid bone; and the notch of the thyroid cartilage should be 2 fingerbreadths below the hyoid bone
Mallampati classification	In patients with a Mallampati score of 1, the entire posterior pharynx is easily visualized; with a 4, no posterior structures can be seen. Patients with a higher Mallampati grade tend to have poorer visualization during direct laryngoscopy
Obstruction	Evaluation for stridor, foreign bodies, and other forms of sub- and supraglottic obstruction
Neck mobility	Patient with rheumatoid arthritis or suspected traumatic cervical spine injury, and in whom the cervical spine has been immobilized by a cervical collar, have limited neck mobility by definition

result, the rate of complications such as cardiac arrest, hypotension, and critical hypoxemia are much higher in critically ill patients than in anesthesia for elective surgery

68.3 Rationale for NIV in Difficult Intubation

Because NIV can support gas exchange, it is logical to consider its use as a way to improve the safety of difficult intubation. Theoretically, NIV may increase patients' tolerance of prolonged attempts to perform ETI. Therefore, clinicians could consider starting NIV when they predict difficult ETI. Similarly, clinicians could consider placing NIV if the patient will not tolerate even brief periods of apnea. The benefits of NIV as part of a preoxygenation /ventilation strategy have been studied. Alternatively, clinicians could use NIV with a nasal interface to support the patient during oral ETI.

NIV is widely used as an alternative to invasive mechanical ventilation for acute respiratory failure, and although NIV may be effective in preventing the need for ETI, there is a high mortality risk in patients who require ETI despite NIV [2]. Most concerning, there is a high risk of death during emergent ETI after a failed trial of NIV for acute respiratory failure. We speculate that removal of NIV prior to ETI may lead to catastrophic deterioration in gas exchange, partially due to significant lung derecruitment. NIV support during ETI may be an especially attractive idea in the setting of failed NIV and a necessary transition to invasive mechanical ventilation. In this setting, adjusting the settings and mask for NIV may allow the clinician to continue it as partial support of gas exchange during ETI.

68.4 Physiologic Benefits of NIV in ETI

NIV can support the patient during ETI through multiple possible mechanisms (Table 68.2). These mechanisms are reviewed in detail below.

Table 68.2 Physiologic benefits of NIV during ETI

Preoxygenation
Prevention of alveolar de-recruitment
Persistent gas exchange
Splinting upper airways open
Reducing the hemodynamic alterations during ETI
Reduce the level of respiratory distress prior to ETI

68.4.1 Ventilation

Apnea during ETI is usually well tolerated in patients undergoing elective surgical procedures. The rise in PCO_2 during apnea is nonlinear, but approximates 3–4 mmHg · min^{-1}. The rate of PCO_2 rise will be much greater if the patient has an increased metabolic rate. Fever, tissue injury, and systemic inflammation associated with acute illness can greatly increase metabolic rate and CO_2 production. Therefore, clinicians should anticipate complications of ETI in patients with a high metabolic rate and a disease process that makes them intolerant of hypercapnia. In these patients, continuing ventilation during the intubation process may be beneficial.

NIV can improve gas exchange during ETI by cyclically augmenting the transpulmonary pressure gradient to maintain alveolar ventilation. NIV can maintain a satisfactory level of ventilation, even during deep sedation, as demonstrated in a case series of its application in procedural anesthesia [3]. In patients undergoing intubation during spontaneous breathing, NIV can theoretically decrease the work of breathing and improve ventilation by augmenting tidal volumes.

68.4.2 Oxygenation

Traditionally, clinicians perform intubation after induction of anesthesia. After neuromuscular blockade, the lungs recoil to the functional residual capacity (FRC). During apnea, gas exchange continues as mixed venous blood continues to flow to the alveolar capillary bed. Therefore, the FRC is the air reservoir that supplies the circulation with oxygen during apnea. Both the volume of air in the FRC as well as its partial pressure of oxygen determine how quickly arterial desaturation occurs during apnea. The rate of total oxygen consumption in the tissues as well as the magnitude and distribution of pulmonary blood flow also determine the time to desaturation. To lengthen the time before desaturation, clinicians have patients spontaneously breathe high FiO_2 to fill the FRC with pure oxygen. This preoxygenation is effective in patients presenting for anesthesia for elective surgery [4]. However, standard methods of preoxygenation are ineffective due to the deranged physiology of critically ill patients. In critically ill patients, atelectasis commonly reduces FRC and increases the right-to-left shunt fraction. Shock may reduce pulmonary blood flow. Moreover, the high oxygen consumption during acute illness can reduce mixed venous oxygen saturation. All of these factors lead to hypoxia during ETI. Patients with an oxygen saturation less than or equal to 93 % during preoxygenation uniformly desaturate to <90 % during intubation [5].

A number of investigators have shown that NIV may be superior to standard preoxygenation in appropriate scenarios. Through positive pressure, NIV can recruit atelectatic lung in some patients, thereby increasing the size of the FRC and reducing shunt fraction. It can also decrease the work of breathing during spontaneous ventilation. Moreover, by increasing alveolar ventilation, NIV can increase the alveolar oxygen content by CO_2 washout. Finally, NIV can decrease the excessive work of breathing made by critically ill patients. Theoretically, this can raise mixed venous oxygen saturation and improve the effectiveness of preoxygenation. The recruitment and benefit of preoxygenation with NIV can continue even after ETI is completed [6].

Given the success of NIV for preoxygenation, investigators have used NIV during ETI to prevent desaturation. NIV can be a form of apneic oxygenation. If the airway is patent, any high-flow oxygen device can promote the replacement of alveolar gas that flows into the alveolar capillary beds through bulk flow. Therefore, high-flow nasal cannula (HFNC) can be used as an apneic oxygenation method, leading to reduced prevalence of severe hypoxemia during intubation of critically ill patients with mild-to-moderate hypoxemia in a pilot study [7]. However a randomized controlled trial found that HFNC during emergent ETI of patients with severe hypoxemia did not prevent desaturation [8]. It is possible that high-flow devices have limited benefits during ETI because they provide little (if any) lung recruitment and ventilation. NIV during intubation via a nasal interface could theoretically promote lung recruitment through positive end-expiratory pressure (PEEP). The possible benefits of PEEP are especially important because anesthesia and supine positioning cause atelectasis and promote desaturation during ETI.

The ability of NIV to promote alveolar recruitment may be especially important because of denitrogenation. Preoxygenation with high FiO_2 effectively removes inert nitrogen from the alveolar air spaces and blood. Unfortunately, nitrogen normally acts as a pneumatic splint to maintain the patency of unstable lung units. Without nitrogen, the partial pressure of gas is very low in mixed venous blood returning to capillaries. Denitrogenation, therefore, increases the gas pressure gradient from alveoli compared with alveolar capillary blood. After denitrogenation, oxygen will rapidly flow from the alveoli into the capillaries, leading to alveolar instability and atelectasis, a physiological phenomenon also demonstrated on computed tomography imaging [9]. PEEP facilitates alveolar recruitment, which can counteract the adverse effect of denitrogenation on lung recruitment and improve oxygenation. Additionally, nasal NIV during ETI can also aid oxygenation by partially supporting ventilation.

The principle that oxygenation can be supported by nasal NIV throughout the process of intubation has been demonstrated for bronchoscopic [10] and direct laryngoscopic intubation [11].

68.4.3 Splinting the Upper Airways

During deep sedation, airway obstruction commonly occurs at the level of the soft palate. Anesthesia reduces the tone of the pharyngeal muscle dilators, which narrows the anteroposterior diameter of the airway. These effects are most prominent in the supine position. This pattern of airway obstruction in anesthesia is similar to

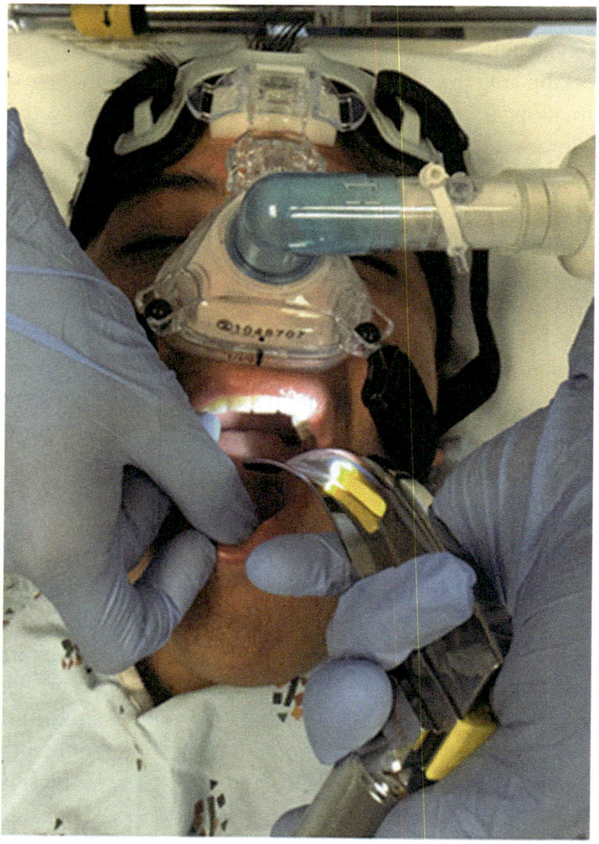

Fig. 68.1 Fiber-optic video images of a patient's hypopharynx demonstrating the pharyngeal splinting action of nasal CPAP (Rothfleisch et al. [12])

obstructive sleep apnea. In both situations, the application of nasal NIV can relieve the airway obstruction. Nasal NIV can displace the soft palate anteriorly, which partially prevents the leakage of air out the oropharynx. Incremental increases in positive airway pressures lead to a linear increase in airway area at a given airway level. Therefore, nasal NIV can serve as a pneumatic splint for the oropharynx during anesthesia. Pilot data demonstrate that this splinting can aide ETI. Figure 68.1 shows fiber-optic video images from a morbidly obese patient's hypopharynx. Nasal NIV (continuous positive airway pressure (CPAP) 20 cm H_2O) relieved upper airway obstruction during fiber-optic-guided nasotracheal intubation [12].

68.4.4 Hemodynamic Effect

Hemodynamic instability commonly complicates ETI in critically ill patients. The hemodynamic effects of NIV during ETI are complex, and it can be difficult to predict their net effect in critically ill patients. NIV can decrease both venous return to the heart and left ventricular afterload. This can effectively treat pulmonary edema from left ventricular failure. Through this mechanism, NIV may be able to improve the safety of ETI. However, positive pressure ventilation frequently decreases cardiac output by decreasing the pressure gradient for venous return to the heart. Additionally, hyperinflation from positive pressure can elevate pulmonary vascular resistance and impede right ventricular output. Therefore, NIV can also worsen hemodynamics before or during ETI. Theoretically, using NIV prior to ETI could make the hemodynamic consequences of positive pressure ventilation manifest prior to ETI, allowing clinicians to treat the hemodynamic instability prior to sedation and ETI.

68.4.5 Patient Comfort and Safety

When respiratory failure is severe, clinicians may be forced to perform urgent ETI before they have had the opportunity to properly assess and prepare the patient for airway management. In select situations, clinicians may use NIV to temporarily stabilize the patient while preparing the patient and equipment for safer ETI. With partial support from NIV, the clinician may be able to use alternative intubation strategies such as bronchoscopic intubation in situations when intubation by direct laryngoscopy will be difficult.

68.5 Procedure

There are several case reports and series published on different procedural techniques using NIV in ETI. Little data exist on the choice of airway interface. For preoxygenation, a full face mask can be used. The full face mask can increase the FiO_2 by limiting the amount of entrained air through the mouth. Moreover, full face masks limit air leak through the mouth and can help maintain PEEP. However, full face masks contribute to upper airway obstruction in anesthetized supine patients by displacing the tongue posteriorly. As discussed above, nasal interfaces can stent the upper airway open and allow oral ETI.

The mode of NIV can influence the effectiveness of ventilation. Patients with noncompliant respiratory systems require higher levels of inspiratory pressure to increase delivered tidal volumes. In this scenario, bi-level positive airway pressure (BIPAP) may be the best mode. Patients with upper airway obstruction may require higher levels of end-expiratory pressure, so CPAP may be appropriate. If the patient is anesthetized, a mode with a set respiratory rate is recommended such as spontaneous/timed (S/T) mode. Regardless of the mode and settings, it is essential to monitor the patient on NIV and determine whether the patient has adequate exhaled tidal volume and minute ventilation. If not, the clinician should evaluate for airway obstruction, excessive leak, dynamic hyperinflation, and inadequate driving pressure.

There are multiple techniques of ETI during NIV (Table 68.3). Aoyama et al. [13] performed fiber-optic-guided intubation during positive pressure ventilation with a laryngeal mask airway (LMA), intubating laryngeal mask (ILM), or endoscopy mask (Patil mask). In this technique, LMA or ILM were initially inserted

Table 68.3 NIV techniques during ETI

Author/report	Procedural technique	Findings
Aoyama et al. Positive pressure ventilation during fiber-optic intubation: comparison of the laryngeal mask airway, intubating laryngeal mask, and endoscopy mask techniques	LMA or ILM inserted followed by insertion of tracheal tube into the tube of the LMA or ILM. Fiber-optic intubation performed with application of 20 cmH_2O PPV through the tracheal tube. In the endoscopy (Patil) mask group, fiber-optic intubation performed while PPV maintained through the Patil mask	Ventilation during intubation with endoscopy mask greater than that with the LMA or ILM, but gastric insufflation was more frequent
Nafeh et al. Fiber-optic tracheal intubation through a Boussignac valve to maintain continuous oxygenation during intubation in severely obese patients: 11 cases	PEEP of 7.5 cmH_2O obtained by a Boussignac valve powered by an oxygen flow of 30 l/min affixed to a face mask. Fiber-optic orotracheal intubation carried out through the Boussignac valve. General anesthesia accomplished when the tracheal tube had advanced to the glottis	None of the severely obese patients experienced decrease in oxygen saturation during this intubation technique
Rothfleisch et al. Facilitation of fiber-optic nasotracheal intubation in a morbidly obese patient by simultaneous use of nasal CPAP	Emergent nasotracheal intubation using a fiber-optic bronchoscope with simultaneous application of CPAP 20 cmH_2O to the contralateral nares using a nasal pillow that helped maintain ventilation and facilitated visualization of anatomic landmarks and translaryngeal passage of the bronchoscope	Fiber-optic video images of this patient's hypopharynx demonstrate the pharyngeal splinting action of nasal CPAP thus applied (Fig. 68.1)
Wong et al. Awake bronchoscopic intubation through an air-Q with the application of BIPAP	BIPAP initially applied for preoxygenation. Single-use air-Q orally inserted in sitting position and BIPAP was applied to the air-Q, followed by the insertion of endotracheal tube via the air-Q to 14 cm. ETT cuff inflated, and BIPAP connected to the ETT through a flexible connector with a bronchoscope port. Bronchoscope advanced through the flexible connector past the well-visualized glottis to the carina. ETT cuff deflated and advanced over the bronchoscope into the trachea. ETT cuff reinflated after confirmation of position	Oxygen saturation 97 % was maintained during the intubation process

Barjaktarevic et al. Bronchoscopic intubation during continuous nasal positive pressure ventilation in the treatment of hypoxemic respiratory failure	BIPAP delivered via nasal interface. Oral airway covered with 5 % lidocaine ointment placed in the oropharynx. After sufficient topical anesthesia, intubating (Williams) airway placed in the oropharynx. ETT inserted into the Williams airway and bronchoscope placed through the ETT and into the distal trachea. ETT inserted into the trachea using the bronchoscope as the stylet. Bronchoscope withdrawn slowly to allow visualization of the tip of the endotracheal tube in good position within the trachea. Nasal NIV then removed (Fig. 68.2)	All 10 patients intubated in the first attempt. Hypotension was the most frequent complication. Mean decrease in oxyhemoglobin saturation during the procedure was $4.7+3.1$
Cataldo et al. The Nasal Oxygenation and Ventilation of the Airway (NOVA) Technique, a new and safer approach to airway management in the critically ill patient	The NOVA technique utilized nasal NIV during direct laryngoscopy and intubation (Fig. 68.3)	Potential elimination of apneic period during intubation

followed by insertion of a tracheal tube into the tube of the LMA or ILM. Fiber-optic intubation was performed during positive pressure ventilation at a pressure of 20 cm H_2O that was continued through the tracheal tube. In the Patil mask group, fiber-optic intubation was performed while positive pressure ventilation was maintained through the Patil mask. The ventilation was better during intubation with the endoscopy mask than that with the LMA or ILM. However, gastric insufflation was also more frequent. This study was performed in patients prior to elective surgery and may not accurately reflect conditions in critically ill patients.

Nafeh et al. [14] performed fiber-optic-guided intubation in 11 severely obese patients while maintaining CPAP with a Boussignac valve (Vygon Medical, Montgomeryville, PA, USA) during the entire intubation procedure. The patients received oral alprazolam or hydroxyzine and nasopharyngeal application of lidocaine 5 %. The patients were placed in a half-sitting position during oxygenation and the anesthesia procedure. PEEP of 7.5 cm H_2O was obtained by a Boussignac valve powered by an oxygen flow of 30 l/min and affixed to a face mask. After initiation of remifentanil, fiber-optic orotracheal intubation was carried out through the Boussignac valve. General anesthesia was accomplished when the tracheal tube had advanced to the glottis. No patient experienced a decrease in oxygen saturation. This study was also performed in elective surgical patients.

Rothfleisch et al. [12] described a case report where they emergently nasotracheally intubated a morbidly obese patient using a fiber-optic bronchoscope with simultaneous application of CPAP 20 cm H_2O to the contralateral nares using a nasal pillow that helped maintain ventilation. The CPAP treatment also facilitated visualization of the anatomic landmarks and translaryngeal passage of the bronchoscope.

Wong et al. [15] described an awake bronchoscopic intubation in an obese patient with a difficult airway and acute respiratory failure. BIPAP was initially applied for preoxygenation given repeated oxygen desaturation. A single-use air-Q was orally inserted in the sitting position and BIPAP was applied to the air-Q, followed by the insertion of endotracheal tube via the air-Q to 14 cm. The endotracheal tube cuff was inflated, and BIPAP was connected to the endotracheal tube through a flexible connector with a bronchoscope port. A bronchoscope was advanced through the flexible connector past the well-visualized glottis to the carina. The endotracheal tube cuff was deflated and advanced over the bronchoscope into the trachea. The endotracheal tube cuff was reinflated after confirmation of position. Oxygen saturation of 97 % was maintained during the intubation procedure.

Barjaktarevic et al. [10] performed bronchoscopic-guided intubation with NIV in 10 patients with acute hypoxemic respiratory failure. These patients were initially treated with NIV, had progressive hypoxemic respiratory failure, subsequently failed NIV, and required rescue ETI. BIPAP was initially delivered via a full face mask that was later changed to a nasal interface in anticipation of rescue orotracheal intubation. Patients were ventilated with nasal NIV and placed in a semi-recumbent position. An oral airway was covered with 5 % lidocaine ointment and placed in the oropharynx. After sufficient topical anesthesia, an intubating (Williams) airway was placed in the oropharynx and systemic sedation was administered (no

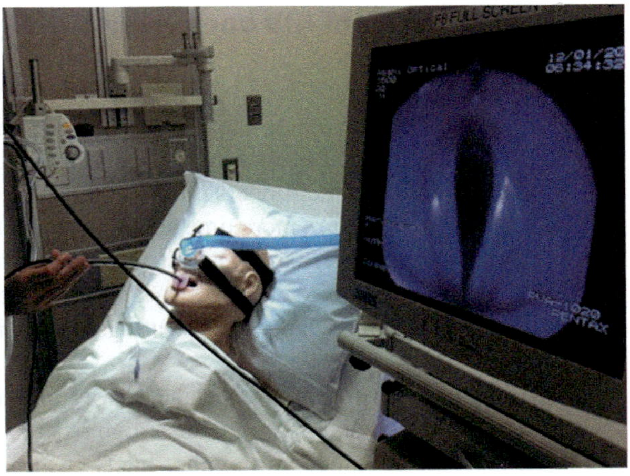

Fig. 68.2 Bronchoscopic intubation during continuous nasal positive pressure ventilation

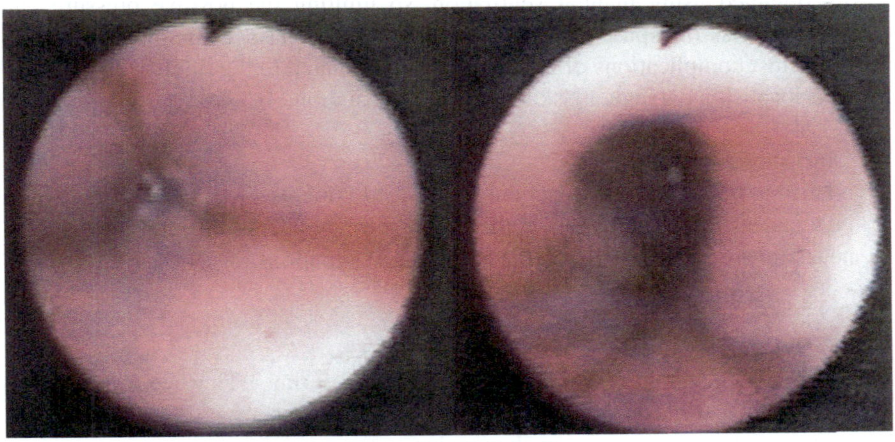

Fig. 68.3 The NOVA technique utilizing nasal NIV during direct laryngoscopy and intubation

neuromuscular blockade was used). The endotracheal tube was inserted into the Williams airway and the bronchoscope was placed through the endotracheal tube and into the distal trachea. The endotracheal tube was then placed into the trachea using the bronchoscope as the stylet. The bronchoscope was withdrawn slowly to allow visualization of the tip of the endotracheal tube in good position within the trachea. The endotracheal tube cuff was inflated, and the tube was attached to the invasive mechanical ventilator circuit. The nasal NIV was then removed (Fig. 68.2).

Cataldo et al. [11] applied the Nasal Oxygenation and Ventilation of the Airway (NOVA) technique with nasal mask NIV during rapid sequence intubation and direct laryngoscopy in critically sick patients requiring ETI (Fig. 68.3). They proposed that partially ventilating a paralyzed patient during rapid sequence intubation may eliminate the apneic period altogether.

68.6 Limitations of NIV during ETI

Application of NIV greatly increases the complexity of ETI. The equipment costs include the use of the ventilator, the disposable airway interface and ventilator tubing, and the personnel to set up the equipment. Adding unfamiliar equipment and procedures can distract practitioners during emergency airway management. Using NIV during ETI may require more time and may not be feasible when there is insufficient time to properly prepare the patient and equipment. Many patients do not tolerate NIV due to patient-ventilator asynchrony. Adequate patient selection and careful titration and adjustment of NIV settings (mode, interface, and pressure titration) are essential.

Blood and excessive secretions in the airway may render NIV ineffective and NIV may need to be avoided in patients at high risk of vomiting and aspirating gastric contents. This complication is more likely if the patient has impaired gastric emptying. The risk exists with an insufflation pressure > 20 cm H_2O, which can be easily obtained using manual ventilation, so limiting the positive pressure can decrease the risk of aspiration [6, 16]. Routine use of a nasogastric tube is not warranted. Most complications of NIV are local and related to the tightly fitting mask, such as local skin damage, mask leak, and eye irritation.

Conclusions

NIV is a well-validated treatment in selected patients with respiratory failure. NIV can also be used to support the patient during ETI. As an emerging concept, new data are needed to define the best clinical situations for its use.

Key Major Recommendations

- Clinicians should consider using nasal NIV during ETI when it will be beneficial to have a pneumatic stent for the upper airway or when it is essential to continue gas exchange during the procedure.

References

1. Henderson JJ, et al. Difficult Airway Society guidelines for management of the unanticipated difficult intubation. Anaesthesia. 2004;59(7):675–94.
2. Antonelli M, et al. Predictors of failure of noninvasive positive pressure ventilation in patients with acute hypoxemic respiratory failure: a multi-center study. Intensive Care Med. 2001; 27(11):1718–28.
3. Strayer RJ, Caputo ND. Noninvasive ventilation during procedural sedation in the ED: a case series. Am J Emerg Med. 2015;33(1):116–20.
4. Weingart SD, Levitan RM. Preoxygenation and prevention of desaturation during emergency airway management. Ann Emerg Med. 2012;59(3):165–75.e1.
5. Davis DP, Hwang JQ, Dunford JV. Rate of decline in oxygen saturation at various pulse oximetry values with prehospital rapid sequence intubation. Prehosp Emerg Care. 2008;12(1):46–51.
6. Baillard C, et al. Noninvasive ventilation improves preoxygenation before intubation of hypoxic patients. Am J Respir Crit Care Med. 2006;174(2):171–7.

7. Miguel-Montanes R, et al. Use of high-flow nasal cannula oxygen therapy to prevent desaturation during tracheal intubation of intensive care patients with mild-to-moderate hypoxemia. Crit Care Med. 2015;43(3):574–83.
8. Vourc'h, M, et al. High-flow nasal cannula oxygen during endotracheal intubation in hypoxemic patients: a randomized controlled clinical trial. Intensive Care Med. 2015;98(1):28–33.
9. Edmark L, et al. Optimal oxygen concentration during induction of general anesthesia. Anesthesiology. 2003;98(1):28–33.
10. Barjaktarevic I, Berlin D. Bronchoscopic intubation during continuous nasal positive pressure ventilation in the treatment of hypoxemic respiratory failure. J Intensive Care Med. 2015; 30(3):161–6.
11. Cataldo S, Pedro M, Lokhandwala B. The Nasal Oxygenation and Ventilation of the Airway (NOVA) technique, a new and safer approach to airway management in the critical ill patient. SOJ Anesthesiol Pain Manag. 2014;1(2):1–4.
12. Rothfleisch R, et al. Facilitation of fiberoptic nasotracheal intubation in a morbidly obese patient by simultaneous use of nasal CPAP. Chest. 1994;106(1):287–8.
13. Aoyama K, et al. Positive pressure ventilation during fibreoptic intubation: comparison of the laryngeal mask airway, intubating laryngeal mask and endoscopy mask techniques. Br J Anaesth. 2002;88(2):246–54.
14. Nafeh S, et al. Fiberoptic tracheal intubation through a Boussignac valve to maintain continuous oxygenation during intubation in severely obese patients: 11 cases. J Clin Anesth. 2011; 23(4):345–6.
15. Wong DT, Wang J, Venkatraghavan L. Awake bronchoscopic intubation through an air-Q(R) with the application of BIPAP. Can J Anaesth. 2012;59(9):915–6.
16. Ho-Tai LM, et al. Gas leak and gastric insufflation during controlled ventilation: face mask versus laryngeal mask airway. Can J Anaesth. 1998;45(3):206–11.

Lung Ultrasound and Noninvasive Ventilation

69

Giovanni Ferrari, Alberto Milan, and Giovanni Volpicelli

Contents

Abbreviations

ACPE	Acute cardiogenic pulmonary edema
ARDS	Acute respiratory distress syndrome
CPAP	Continuous positive airway pressure
DT	Diaphragm thickness
LUS	Lung ultrasound
NIV	Noninvasive ventilation
PEEP	Positive end-expiratory pressure

G. Ferrari (✉)
SC Pneumologia, Ospedale Mauriziano Umberto I, Largo Turati n. 62, Torino, Italy
e-mail: giovanniferrarister@gmail.com

A. Milan
Hypertension Unit, Division of Internal Medicine, Department of Medical Sciences, University Hospital AOU Città della Salute e della Scienza di Torino, University of Torino, Torino, Italy
e-mail: alberto.milan@gmail.com

G. Volpicelli
Department of Emergency Medicine, S.C.D.O, Medicina d'Urgenza, Ospedale Universitario San Luigi Gonzaga, Orbassano, Torino, Italy
e-mail: gio.volpicelli@tin.it

A.M. Esquinas (ed.), *Noninvasive Mechanical Ventilation: Theory, Equipment, and Clinical Applications*, DOI 10.1007/978-3-319-21653-9_69

PS	Pressure support
PTPdi	Transdiaphragmatic pressure-time product
TF	Thickening fraction

69.1 Introduction

Until the end of the last century, the lung was considered an organ poorly accessible to ultrasound, with the exception of the application for the study of pleural effusions. However, notwithstanding its limitations, ultrasound has been increasingly used in the last 15–20 years for examination of the lung in many conditions, such as pneumonia, atelectasis, interstitial syndromes, pneumothorax, and evaluation of diaphragm dysfunction. The advantages of lung ultrasound (LUS) are ease of use at bedside, the repeatability of the examination without exposure to ionizing radiations, and the relatively short learning curve. Many studies have been published demonstrating the diagnostic potential of LUS in several clinical situations, but, to the best of our knowledge, scant literature exists on LUS during noninvasive ventilation (NIV).

This chapter focuses on the importance of LUS in patients undergoing mechanical ventilation. LUS may have an important therapeutic impact in decision-making processes in patients undergoing mechanical ventilation. In the study of Xirouchaki and coworkers [1], LUS changed the clinical behavior in 47 % of patients undergoing mechanical ventilation in the intensive care unit. These changes involved either invasive maneuvers, such as chest tube insertion, bronchoscopy, and continuous veno-venous hemofiltration (CVVH), or noninvasive maneuvers, such as positive end-expiratory pressure (PEEP) titration, recruitment maneuvers, and antibiotic therapy. Moreover, the authors found that one-fifth of the ultrasound examinations revealed findings compatible with diagnoses that were not in the differential diagnosis after the primary evaluation [1].

This chapter examines the potential of LUS in the assessment of alveolar recruitment and the estimation of the work of breathing during NIV, and also the possibility of using LUS as a new index of discontinuation from mechanical ventilation.

69.2 Lung Ultrasound and Alveolar Recruitment during Mechanical Ventilation

In critically ill patients, LUS can be easily performed at bedside. Interstitial syndrome, lung consolidations, and pleural effusion can be easily recognized. According to the first international consensus conference on point-of-care lung ultrasound, the examination targeted to the diagnosis of the interstitial syndrome should be performed in four chest areas per side (an eight-zone examination) [2]. However, the experts validated two other methods: a more rapid anterior two-region scan in critically ill patients and evaluation of 28 rib interspaces in the cardiology setting. LUS showed its potential in the first diagnosis and follow-up of lung consolidations and the differential diagnosis between pulmonary embolism, pneumonia, or compressive and obstructive atelectasis [2]. In lung consolidation, acute respiratory distress syndrome (ARDS), and pulmonary congestion, LUS can be useful to assess semi-quantitatively and monitor changes in lung aeration by observing the progression of four fundamental sonographic patterns: normal aeration, multiple B-lines, coalescent B-lines, and consolidation [2–5].

To the best of our knowledge, there is only one study that has evaluated the use of LUS for the assessment of continuous positive airway pressure (CPAP) treatment in patients with acute cardiogenic pulmonary edema (ACPE) [6]. The authors of this study compared the efficacy of prehospital CPAP plus medical treatment as opposed to oxygen plus medical treatment in patients with ACPE, using LUS to evaluate response to treatment. Although the study suffers from some limitations, the use of LUS to assess the outcome after treatment was of interest. The authors found a significant decrease in the number of B-lines in patients with ACPE treated with CPAP in comparison with standard medical treatment.

Assessment of lung recruitment is important not only in ACPE, but it is also crucial in the management of patients with ARDS. In critically ill patients, LUS has gained an important role in the evaluation of lung consolidations and, according to some studies, LUS can be used as a diagnostic tool for the assessment of lung recruitment induced by PEEP [5, 7].

Assuming that in ARDS the visible ultrasound pattern corresponds to a degree of lung aeration, Bouhemad and coworkers [5] studied prospectively 40 patients with ALI/ARDS undergoing invasive mechanical ventilation. They associated the presence of multiple spaced B-lines with moderate decrease in lung aeration (interstitial syndrome), coalescent B lines with more severe decrease in lung aeration, and lung consolidation containing white points characterized by an inspiratory reinforcement, the so-called dynamic air bronchogram, with complete loss of lung aeration. In the study, the authors used the pressure-volume curve as a gold-standard method to measure lung recruitment and find out that PEEP-induced recruitment could be accurately estimated by LUS. In another study, the authors, using the same re-aeration score, used LUS to assess lung aeration during weaning and concluded that the determination of aeration changes during a spontaneous breathing trial could predict the post-extubation distress more accurately than natriuretic peptides or cardiac filling pressure estimated by echocardiography [8].

There are no original blind studies on lung recruitment during NIV and only one conference abstract, in which the authors evaluated re-aeration score as a predictive tool in patients treated with NIV [9]. In this trial, LUS was performed before starting NIV, after 5 min, and after 60 min of NIV treatment. LUS patterns were defined using the same classification validated in the study of Bouhemad [5]. Out of 16 patients enrolled, 5 failed NIV treatment. A significant difference in re-aeration score between the two groups (patients who failed and patients who were treated successfully with NIV) was found after 1 h of treatment. In this preliminary report, the authors concluded that a re-aeration cut-off value of 0 could predict NIV success, with a sensitivity of 91 % and a specificity of 80 %. No data are provided on gas exchange during treatment and the results must be interpreted cautiously.

However, if confirmed in larger trials, these results might support the use of LUS as an effective tool to evaluate patient response during NIV. This may be extremely useful, because in patients with pneumonia or ARDS, the percentage of failure to NIV treatment is high [10, 11], while, to date, the most reliable variables associated with NIV success are the improvement in gas exchange and a low clinical score as assessed by Simplified Acute Physiology Score (SAPS) II [10, 12]. LUS could be of help in the early recognition of patients who will fail NIV treatment, thus avoiding a possible delay in endotracheal intubation, a condition that is associated with an unfavorable outcome. Further original studies are warranted to establish the reliability of LUS in patients with hypoxemic respiratory failure treated with NIV.

69.3 Diaphragm Ultrasound to Estimate Work of Breathing during NIV

Even if scant literature exists on NIV and LUS, ultrasonography has great diagnostic potential in patients undergoing mechanical ventilation, either invasive or noninvasive. In an elegant study, Vivier et al. [13] hypothesized that measurement of diaphragm thickness (DT) could reflect the magnitude of diaphragmatic work, thereby helping to optimize ventilatory setting. In particular, the relationship between DT and the level of pressure support (PS) was investigated.

Diaphragmatic ultrasound was performed, placing the transducer in the zone of apposition of the diaphragm in the midaxillary line. The thickness of the muscle was recorded in time motion mode [14]. Thickness was measured at end inspiration (Tei) and at end expiration (Tee), and thickening fraction (TF) was assessed with the following formula: Tei – Tee/Tei %. Transdiaphragmatic pressure was recorded by measurement of esophageal and gastric pressure; the transdiaphragmatic pressure-time product (PTPdi) per breath was obtained by measuring the area under the Pdi signal from the onset of its positive deflection to its return to baseline. Out of 14 patients enrolled in the study, the quality of the ultrasound image was good in 12 and not acceptable in only 2. Records of the diaphragm images were obtained initially during spontaneous breathing and subsequently during NIV treatment, at different PS levels (5, 10, and 15 cmH_2O applied randomly). Tidal volume increased with the increase of PS, and the increase in PS was associated with the decrease of PTPdi and of TF. Furthermore, TF correlated significantly with PTPdi [13].

This study is important as it is the first to have evaluated the usefulness of diaphragm ultrasound to assess the work of breathing in patients weaned from MV with noninvasive PS. One of the most important and reliable methods to measure patient muscle effort is PTPdi. However, this method is invasive, requires high expertise, and is only applicable in the setting of research studies. On the other hand, the ease of use and the reproducibility of ultrasound allow frequent bedside reassessment of the patients. In the study of Vivier et al. [13], the authors showed that, during NIV, the thickening of the diaphragm is related to the muscular effort itself and this result, if confirmed by further studies, could be of help in the prediction of weaning from mechanical ventilation.

One of the criticisms that can be made of the measurement of diaphragmatic thickness is its reliability and reproducibility. Cohn and coworkers [15], however, showed that ultrasound measurement of the diaphragm correlated significantly with the measure obtained with a ruler in cadavers. Regarding reproducibility, measurement of diaphragm thickness showed a high intra- and interobserver reproducibility [13, 16], and another study [17] demonstrated that diaphragmatic ultrasound is also highly reproducible in patients under mechanical ventilation.

69.4 Lung Ultrasound and Weaning: Future Applications

The important role of ultrasound in assessing diaphragm function has already been studied, but the attention of the researchers has only more recently focused on the use of LUS in weaning from mechanical ventilation. Before focusing on ultrasound and weaning, the researchers have evaluated diaphragm function in healthy subjects, either assessing diaphragm displacement, either diaphragm thickening during inspiration. One study evaluated diaphragm motion in healthy subjects, identifying normal values of diaphragm excursion [18]. By positioning the probe below the costal margin, between the mid-clavicular and anterior axillary line, the movement of the right hemi-diaphragm could be assessed in most of the patients, while the visualization of the left hemi-diaphragm was more difficult due to the poor acoustic window of the spleen. Mean excursions were measured and reference values for quiet breathing, deep breathing, and voluntary sniffing were assessed.

Diaphragm thickness has been also evaluated in healthy subjects by placing the probe in the zone of the apposition of the diaphragm [15]. Ultrasound measurements were reproducible at different lung volumes, ranging from residual volume to total lung capacity.

The ease of use and the noninvasiveness characteristic of diaphragm ultrasound contrasts with the complicated traditional methods of diaphragm evaluation, some relying also on the use of ionizing radiation. Diaphragm function has been studied, assessing its movement during inspiration [19, 20] and measuring thickening fraction [16]. Both methods are highly reproducible and may detect diaphragm dysfunction and predict weaning failure. If compared with traditional methods used to assess diaphragm function (measurement of trans-diaphragmatic pressure, phrenic nerve stimulation, fluoroscopy, and electromyography), ultrasound is simple, rapid, and noninvasive. Ultrasound can be repeated several times without any risk to the patient, providing important information on his or her respiratory function.

Alhough there is the need for confirmation by further studies, available literature data suggest that ultrasound of the diaphragm has an important potential in predicting patients who may fail a weaning attempt. However, as no data exist in literature on the use of LUS in weaning from NIV, future research should be particularly addressed to the investigation of the role of diaphragm ultrasound in patients undergoing NIV.

Conclusions

LUS has widespread application in clinical practice in assessing and monitoring many pulmonary conditions. However, scant literature exists on the application of ultrasound during NIV. Future studies on LUS may provide physicians with important data regarding how to titrate extrinsic PEEP in patients undergoing

NIV or assess patient-ventilator asynchrony [21]. One of the future applications will be the application of diaphragm evaluation for the assessment of the patient with acute respiratory failure undergoing NIV.

References

1. Xirouchaki N, Kondili E, Prinianakis G, et al. Impact of lung ultrasound on clinical decision making in critically ill patients. Intensive Care Med. 2014;40(1):57–65.
2. Volpicelli G, Elbarbary M, Blaivas M, et al. International evidence-based recommendations for point-of-care lung ultrasound. Intensive Care Med. 2012;38(4):577–91.
3. Agricola E, Bove T, Oppizzi M, et al. "Ultrasound comet-tail images": a marker of pulmonary edema: a comparative study with wedge pressure and extravascular lung water. Chest. 2005; 127(5):1690–5.
4. Bouhemad B, Liu ZH, Arbelot C, et al. Ultrasound assessment of antibiotic-induced pulmonary reaeration in ventilator-associated pneumonia. Crit Care Med. 2010;38(1):84–92.
5. Bouhemad B, Brisson H, Le-Guen M, et al. Bedside ultrasound assessment of positive end-expiratory pressure-induced lung recruitment. Am J Respir Crit Care Med. 2011;183(3): 341–7.
6. Strnad M, Prosen G, Borovnik Lesjak V. Bedside lung ultrasound for monitoring the effectiveness of prehospital treatment with continuous positive airway pressure in acute decompensated heart failure. Eur J Emerg Med. 2014. doi:10.1097/MEJ.0000000000000205.
7. Arbelot C, Ferrari F, Bouhemad B, et al. Lung ultrasound in acute respiratory distress syndrome and acute lung injury. Curr Opin Crit Care. 2008;14(1):70–4.
8. Soummer A, Perbet S, Brisson H, et al. Ultrasound assessment of lung aeration loss during a successful weaning trial predicts postextubation distress*. Crit Care Med. 2012;40(7): 2064–72.
9. Nobile L, Beccaria P, Zambon M et al. Lung ultrasound reaeration score: a useful tool to predict non-invasive ventilation effectiveness. 34th international symposium on intensive care and emergency medicine. Crit Care. 2014;18(Suppl 1):P1–502.
10. Antonelli M, Conti G, Esquinas A, et al. A multiple-center survey on the use in clinical practice of noninvasive ventilation as a first-line intervention for acute respiratory distress syndrome. Crit Care Med. 2007;35(1):18–25.
11. Rana S, Jenad H, Gay PC, et al. Failure of non-invasive ventilation in patients with acute lung injury: observational cohort study. Crit Care. 2006;10(3):R79.
12. Antonelli M, Conti G, Moro ML, et al. Predictors of failure of noninvasive positive pressure ventilation in patients with acute hypoxemic respiratory failure: a multi-center study. Intensive Care Med. 2001;27(11):1718–28.
13. Vivier E, Mekontso Dessap A, Dimassi S, et al. Diaphragm ultrasonography to estimate the work of breathing during non-invasive ventilation. Intensive Care Med. 2012;38(5): 796–803.
14. Wait JL, Nahormek PA, Yost WT, et al. Diaphragmatic thickness-lung volume relationship in vivo. J Appl Physiol (1985). 1989;67(4):1560–8.
15. Cohn D, Benditt JO, Eveloff S, et al. Diaphragm thickening during inspiration. J Appl Physiol (1985). 1997;83(1):291–6.
16. Ferrari G, De Filippi G, Elia F, et al. Diaphragm ultrasound as a new index of discontinuation from mechanical ventilation. Crit Ultrasound J. 2014;6(1):8.
17. Goligher EC, Laghi F, Detsky ME, et al. Measuring diaphragm thickness with ultrasound in mechanically ventilated patients: feasibility, reproducibility and validity. Intensive Care Med. 2015;41(4):642–9.

18. Boussuges A, Gole Y, Blanc P. Diaphragmatic motion studied by m-mode ultrasonography: methods, reproducibility, and normal values. Chest. 2009;135(2):391–400.
19. Lerolle N, Guérot E, Dimassi S, et al. Ultrasonographic diagnostic criterion for severe diaphragmatic dysfunction after cardiac surgery. Chest. 2009;135(2):401–7.
20. Kim WY, Suh HJ, Hong SB, et al. Diaphragm dysfunction assessed by ultrasonography: influence on weaning from mechanical ventilation. Crit Care Med. 2011;39(12):2627–30.
21. Matamis D, Soilemezi E, Tsagourias M, et al. Sonographic evaluation of the diaphragm in critically ill patients. Technique and clinical applications. Intensive Care Med. 2013;39(5): 801–10.

Noninvasive Ventilation in Cardiac Procedures: Key Technical and Practical Implications

70

Francesco Sbrana, Bruno Formichi, and Antonio Pisano

Contents

Abbreviations

AMI	Acute myocardial infarction
AS	Aortic stenosis
CPAP	Continuous positive airway pressure
EPAP	Expiratory positive airway pressure
FiO_2	Inspiratory oxygen fraction
ICU	Intensive care unit
IPAP	Inspiratory positive airway pressure

F. Sbrana, MD
Lipid Apheresis Unit, Fondazione Toscana Gabriele Monasterio, Via Moruzzi, 1, Pisa 5614, Italy
e-mail: francesco.sbrana@ftgm.it

B. Formichi, MD
Division of Anesthesia and Intensive Care, National Research Council – Institute of Clinical Physiology and Fondazione Toscana Gabriele Monasterio, Via Moruzzi, 1, Pisa 5614, Italy
e-mail: formichi@ifc.cnr.it

A. Pisano, MD (✉)
Cardiac Anesthesia and Intensive Care Unit, A.O.R.N. "Dei Colli" – Monaldi Hospital, via L. Bianchi 80131, Naples, Italy
e-mail: antoniopisanoMD@libero.it

A.M. Esquinas (ed.), *Noninvasive Mechanical Ventilation: Theory, Equipment, and Clinical Applications*, DOI 10.1007/978-3-319-21653-9_70

MR	Mitral regurgitation
NIV	Noninvasive ventilation
$PaCO_2$	Arterial partial pressure of CO_2
PCI	Percutaneous coronary intervention
PEEP	Positive end-expiratory pressure
PSV	Pressure support ventilation
SaO_2	Arterial oxygen saturation
TAVI	Transcatheter aortic valve implantation
TEE	Transesophageal echocardiography

70.1 Introduction

Noninvasive ventilation (NIV) is broadly used in patients with both chronic and acute respiratory failure, both inside and outside the intensive care unit (ICU). Moreover, NIV may be applied to allow safe sedation in several clinical contexts and increasingly is used to treat or even prevent postoperative pulmonary complications after major surgery. Today, NIV is also increasingly used during nonsurgical cardiac procedures in which there is an actual risk of respiratory distress or failure, such as percutaneous coronary interventions (PCI) performed in patients with pulmonary edema secondary to acute myocardial infarction (AMI), as well as percutaneous valve procedures, which mostly involve high-risk patients who often need sedation. Finally, the use of NIV to aid less-invasive diagnostic cardiac procedures such as transesophageal echocardiography (TEE) has been reported.

Although some concerns regarding the use of NIV in these procedures may exist, a team well trained in managing NIV often may carry them out safely, even in highly compromised patients. The following sections describe the use of NIV in the cardiac catheterization laboratory, during percutaneous cardiac valve procedures, to aid TEE examination, and during electrophysiological procedures, focusing on both technical and clinical aspects.

70.2 Cardiac Catheterization Laboratory

Procedures performed in the cardiac catheterization laboratory include coronary angiography, PCI, percutaneous closure of septal defects, and transcatheter cardiac valve stents [1]. Coronary angiography and PCI are usually performed without sedation and/or ventilatory support. Accordingly, these procedures do not need anesthesia care, except when respiratory distress or hemodynamic instability coexist, due to AMI, pulmonary edema, or heart failure.

Yamamoto and colleagues [2] successfully used NIV in 261 patients with pulmonary edema (secondary or not to AMI) undergoing coronary angiography and PCI. In this retrospective, single-center study, patients received continuous positive airways pressure (CPAP) via a full or total face mask using a BiPAP Vision machine

(Respironics, Murrysville, PA, USA) as first-line treatment. The initial positive end-expiratory pressure (PEEP) was 4–10 cmH_2O and was subsequently adjusted to improve patient comfort. Inspiratory oxygen fraction (FiO_2) was set to achieve an arterial oxygen saturation (SaO_2) > 95 %. If the patient complained of dyspnea at 30 min after initiation of CPAP treatment, NIV with a bi-level positive airway pressure (BiPAP) modality was started. NIV effectively improved oxygenation and lowered the tracheal intubation rate in patients with cardiogenic pulmonary edema of all etiologies, including AMI.

Whereas percutaneous closure of septal defects is usually performed under general anesthesia with tracheal intubation, transcatheter cardiac valve procedures can be also performed in awake patients with sedation and the aid of NIV [3, 4], as discussed in the following section.

70.3 Percutaneous Cardiac Valve Procedures

Surgery is the standard of care for valve diseases such as aortic stenosis (AS) or mitral regurgitation (MR). However, percutaneous procedures represent an alternative in patients for whom the risk of surgery is considered too high, due to older age, poor general health status, or severe comorbidities. In particular, about 30 % of patients with AS belongs to this "inoperable"/high-risk subset [3]. In these patients, transcatheter aortic valve implantation (TAVI) allows minimization of surgical stress (by avoiding sternotomy and cardiopulmonary bypass, and decreasing the duration of intervention). Moreover, TAVI can usually be performed under local anesthesia, thus avoiding the potential risks of general anesthesia, tracheal intubation, and mechanical ventilation [4]. However, the supine position, which is necessary during the procedure (usually lasting at least 1.5 h), is often poorly tolerated by orthopneic patients, especially when respiratory diseases coexist. Accordingly, sedation is generally required, with possible further worsening of respiratory function and gas exchanges.

Guarracino and colleagues reported the use of NIV during TAVI in five patients with orthopnea and severe chronic pulmonary disease (pulmonary fibrosis in four patients and silicosis in one patient) [4], as well as in patients undergoing transfemoral [5] or transaxillary [3] TAVI who needed intraprocedural TEE, which may contribute to respiratory impairment. The five patients with severe pulmonary comorbidities underwent CoreValve (Medtronic, CV Luxembourg) implantation and received pressure support ventilation (PSV) by a Vision NIV ventilator (Respironics Inc., Murrysville, PA, USA) connected to an adult oronasal mask (VIP 75™ 7500 Series V masks™, Hans Rudolph, Inc., Kansas City, MO, USA). PSV was initially set at 8–12 cmH_2O, with a PEEP of 4–6 cmH_2O and a FiO_2 of 0.35–0.5, and was subsequently adjusted to maintain a SaO_2 >92 % and an arterial partial pressure of CO_2 ($PaCO_2$) <50 mmHg. All patients were adequately sedated to be comfortable during the entire procedure. No complications occurred.

Theoretically, even percutaneous mitral repair (mitral clip) could be performed in awake patients with the aid of NIV [6], which may also allow safe intraprocedural TEE (see below). However, to the authors' knowledge, there are no literature reports in this regard.

70.4 TEE

TEE has been used for many years both as a diagnostic tool, mostly in patients with severe cardiac diseases (e.g., atrial fibrillation, prosthetic valve dysfunction, and infective endocarditis), and as a monitoring adjunct for percutaneous cardiac procedures, including TAVI and, more recently, mitral clip, which are usually performed in high-risk patients [3–5, 7]. Because TEE often causes temporary arterial blood gas worsen during and after examination, respiratory failure and/or severe cardiac arrhythmias may occur in frail patients undergoing diagnostic or intraprocedural TEE [5]. For example, orthopneic patients may develop respiratory failure due to the supine position, in addition to the presence of the probe [6]. Moreover, because TEE is a relatively invasive procedure, possibly causing pain, dangerous reflexes, and emotional distress, sedation is often required to perform the exam. However, sedation itself, besides the examination-related stress, may cause cardiorespiratory failure, while general anesthesia may result in significant complications, primarily respiratory, and is generally poorly tolerated by high-risk cardiac patients [5, 6, 8].

The use of NIV to aid TEE examination in severely ill, high risk patients has been suggested in recent years [3, 5, 8]. Indeed, under these circumstances, NIV could both improve patient tolerance to the examination and allow safe sedation.

Guarracino et al. [3, 5] reported the use of NIV via a modified face mask to support TEE examination in severe, orthopneic cardiac patients undergoing transcatheter aortic valve implantation or valvuloplasty. The TEE probe was passed through a vertical hole obtained on the anterior part of an adult oronasal NIV mask (VIP 75 7500 Series V masks) by a surgical cutter. No air leakage was observed. PSV, with an inspiratory positive airway pressure (IPAP) of 8–12 cmH_2O, a PEEP of 4–6 cmH_2O, and a FiO_2 of 0.35–0.5 was used. NIV was administered for the entire procedure and for the following 2 hours, and appeared to be effective in allowing orthopneic patients to lie in the supine position and in preventing respiratory failure due to sedation.

More recently, Pisano et al. [8] performed TEE during NIV through a helmet in a poorly cooperative ICU patient, with multiple severe comorbidities, who developed cardiorespiratory failure following high-risk replacement of a malfunctioning mitral mechanical prosthesis. No change of ventilator settings or modality (PSV) was necessary. Tidal volumes, respiratory rate, arterial blood gases, and hemodynamic parameters remained unchanged during and after the procedure. Moreover, NIV allowed adequate sedation, thus avoiding general anesthesia and tracheal intubation.

However, a technical issue limits the possibility of performing TEE through a helmet. In fact, the airtight ports for catheters or probes available on helmets are not large enough to allow insertion and movements of the TEE probe. Pisano and colleagues used the larger airtight port that is located on the Castar R Next helmet

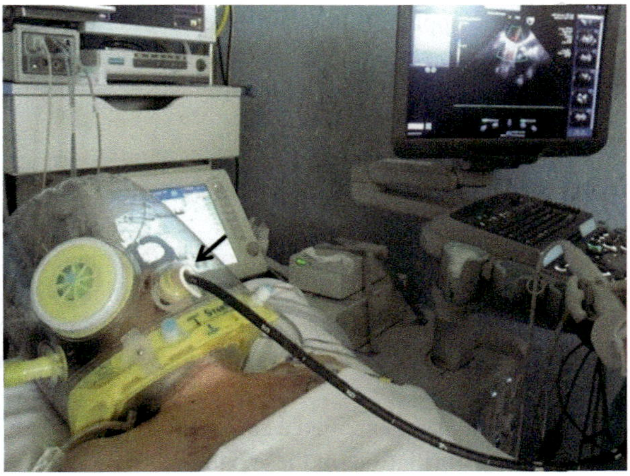

Fig. 70.1 TEE examination through a non-invasive ventilation helmet in a sedated patient. Part of a tracheostomy foam dressing is used as an airtight sleeve (*arrow*). Reproduced from Pisano et al. [8]

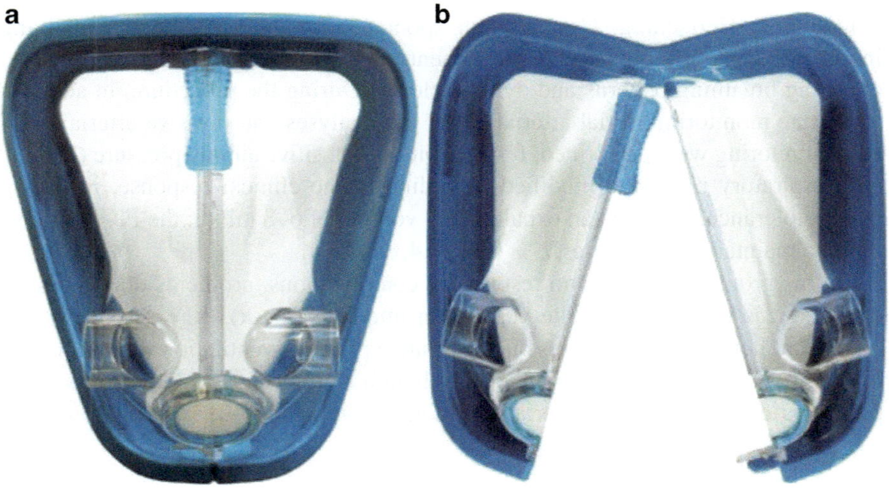

Fig. 70.2 The Janus full face mask. (**a**). Closed. (**b**). Opened. Courtesy of Biomedical (Florence, Italy)

(StarMed, Mirandola, Italy), after removing the inner airtight sleeve. The resulting gross air leakage was avoided by using part of a tracheostomy foam dressing (Pharmaplast, Alexandria, Egypt), rolled up around the portion of the probe that crossed the helmet, as an airtight sleeve (Fig. 70.1). The availability on NIV helmets of a multipurpose airtight port, allowing insertion and adequate movements of the TEE probe, may be desirable if further research will confirm safety and effectiveness of this, as well as other endoscopic procedures, through NIV helmets.

Conversely, oronasal masks provided with an airtight port for endoscopy, which also allows TEE examination, are already available on the market. In particular, an openable full face mask exists (Janus, Biomedical, Florence, Italy) (Fig. 70.2), which can be applied to the patient even after the TEE probe has been positioned, allowing NIV to start, if necessary (unexpected respiratory distress or need of sedation) without stopping the exam [6].

70.5 Electrophysiological Procedures

Patients undergoing electrophysiological mapping, which is a catheter-based procedure for ventricular arrhythmias, or catheter ablation for atrial fibrillation are required to lie motionless on the table for several hours, and repeated stimuli from ablation are sometimes painful. For these reasons, patients usually need deep sedation or general anesthesia.

Sbrana et al. [9] described a case series of patients who underwent catheter ablation for atrial fibrillation. In these patients, NIV and deep sedation were started after trans-septal puncture. NIV was performed through a latex-free total face mask (Respironic®, Murrysville, PA, USA) (Fig. 70.3) connected to a Garbin ventilator (Linde Inc., Herrsching, Germany) in spontaneous/temporized mode, applying incorporated algorithms to improve patient-ventilator synchrony by adjusting to changing breathing patterns and dynamic leaks. During the procedure, in addition to routine monitoring, serial arterial blood gas analyses and invasive arterial pressure monitoring were performed. IPAP, expiratory positive airway pressure (EPAP), and respiratory rate were modified according to the clinical response, including patient tolerance, to obtain an exhaled tidal volume of 6–8 ml/kg; the FiO_2 requirement to maintain SaO_2 above 92 % was ≤ 0.4.

In this group of patients, no respiratory complications, problems due to gastric distention, issues related to the ventilation interface (mask), NIV discomfort, or significant hemodynamic effects due to positive pressure ventilation were reported. Furthermore, these patients maintained (although with respiratory parameters in the physiological range) better arterial blood gases and acid–base balance compared

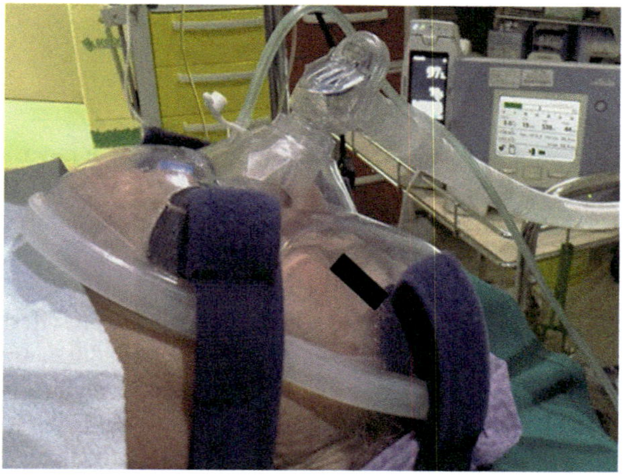

Fig. 70.3 A patient ventilated through the Respironic® latex-free total face mask during catheter ablation for atrial fibrillation

with a deep sedation group without NIV [10]. Finally, a continuous monitoring of tidal volume, air leak, and actual minute ventilation during the entire procedure contributed to patient safety.

Key Major Recommendations

- NIV should be considered in patients with pulmonary edema (including patients with acute myocardial infarction) undergoing coronary angiography and PCI.
- NIV may have an additional role in the anesthetic management of percutaneous cardiac valve procedures (TAVI and mitral clip) and electrophysiological procedures.
- The use of NIV to aid TEE examination in severely ill, high-risk patients could both improve patient tolerance to the examination and allow safe sedation.
- Skilled personnel, adequate monitoring, and appropriate ventilatory interfaces allow the safe use of NIV during most cardiac procedures, minimizing complications in frail or high-risk patients.

References

1. Hamid A. Anesthesia for cardiac catheterization procedures. Heart Lung Vessel. 2014; 6(4):225–31.
2. Yamamoto T, Takeda S, Sato N, et al. Noninvasive ventilation in pulmonary edema complicating acute myocardial infarction. Circ J. 2012;76(11):2586–91.
3. Guarracino F, Covello RD, Landoni G, et al. Anesthetic management of transcatheter aortic valve implantation with transaxillary approach. J Cardiothorac Vasc Anesth. 2011;25: 437–43.
4. Guarracino F, Cabrini L, Baldassarri R, et al. Noninvasive ventilation for awake percutaneous aortic valve implantation in high-risk respiratory patients: a case series. J Cardiothorac Vasc Anesth. 2011;25(6):1109–12.
5. Guarracino F, Cabrini L, Baldassarri R, et al. Non-invasive ventilation-aided transoesophageal echocardiography in high-risk patients: a pilot study. Eur J Echocardiogr. 2010;11:554–6.
6. Cabrini L, Zangrillo A, Landoni G. Preventive and therapeutic noninvasive ventilation in cardiovascular surgery. Curr Opin Anaesthesiol. 2015;28(1):67–72.
7. Peterson GE, Brickner ME, Reimold SC. Transesophageal echocardiography: clinical indications and applications. Circulation. 2003;107(19):2398–402.
8. Pisano A, Angelone M, Iovino T, et al. Transesophageal echocardiography through a noninvasive ventilation helmet. J Cardiothorac Vasc Anesth. 2013;27(6):e78–81.
9. Sbrana F, Ripoli A, Formichi B. Safety and utility of noninvasive ventilation during deep sedation for catheter ablation of atrial fibrillation. J Cardiothorac Vasc Anesth. 2014;28(1):e6–8.
10. Sbrana F, Ripoli A, Formichi B. Anesthetic management in atrial fibrillation ablation procedure: adding non-invasive ventilation to deep sedation. Indian Pacing Electrophysiol J. 2015 (in press). doi:10.1016/j.ipej.2015.07.003

Noninvasive Mechanical Ventilation During Bronchoscopy: Key Technical and Clinical Evidence

71

Raffaele Scala

Contents

71.1 Introduction

Among the procedures that are routinely used in both general intensive care units (ICUs) and respiratory intensive care units (RICUs), bronchoscopy and noninvasive mechanical ventilation (NIMV) constitute "musts" for clinicians who face challenging scenarios in critically ill patients. Flexible bronchoscopy (FBO) represents a well-defined step in the diagnostic flowchart of severe community-acquired and hospital-acquired pneumonia, as well as acute interstitial lung diseases [1]. This is due to its wide range of ancillary diagnostic procedures, including bronchoalveolar lavage (BAL), protected specimen brush (PSB), transbronchial need aspiration, transbronchial lung biopsy (TBLB) and endobronchial ultrasound [1]. Although it

R. Scala, MD, FCCP
Respiratory Ward and Pulmonary Intensive Care Unit, S. Donato Hospital,
Via Nenni, 8 -52100, Arezzo, Italy
e-mail: raffaele_scala@hotmail.com

A.M. Esquinas (ed.), *Noninvasive Mechanical Ventilation: Theory, Equipment, and Clinical Applications*, DOI 10.1007/978-3-319-21653-9_71

has less major application, rigid bronchoscopy (RB) plays a crucial role in performing interventional procedures (laser, argon plasma, and stent position) in critical patients with tracheal or main bronchial stenosis, massive hemoptysis, and inhaled foreign body, especially in pediatric patients [2].

NIMV includes negative and positive pressure ventilatory techniques that have been shown to achieve the "goals of mechanical ventilation" (i.e., unload respiratory muscles, improve pulmonary gas exchange, and increase alveolar ventilation) without the risk of conventional mechanical ventilation (CMV)-correlated complications. Because of the tremendous technological improvements in ventilators and interfaces, positive-pressure NIMV (ppNIMV) has become the first-line ventilatory treatment in different patterns of acute respiratory failure (ARF), including acidotic chronic obstructive pulmonary disease (COPD) exacerbations, cardiogenic pulmonary edema, and immunosuppressed conditions. Compared with standard medical therapy, ppNIMV reduces the rate of endotracheal intubation (ETI) and its complications, as well as mortality and length of stay in hospital [3]. Conversely, negative-pressure NIMV (npNIMV), mainly delivered by an "iron lung," is now performed only in a few expert centers to manage selected patients (e.g., COPD exacerbations nonresponsive to ppNIMV, respiratory distress syndrome, and weaning difficulty, especially in pediatric patients) [4].

In this chapter, the rationale, clinical indications, scientific evidence, practical issues, and risks for the synergistic use of bronchoscopy during NIMV are reported.

71.2 Pitfalls of Bronchoscopy and NIMV

Even with its widespread application in the ICU/RICU, bronchoscopy can be challenging and risky in nonintubated patients with ARF. This is the case with diagnostic FBO in subjects admitted to the ICU/RICU for severe hypoxemia caused by lung infiltrates of unknown origin. Performing bronchoscopy in critically ill patients presents potential complications that can be related to the procedure itself, patient-related factors, and the bronchoscopist's experience. The cardiopulmonary pathophysiological effects of FBO have been well investigated [1, 2].

The bronchoscope occupies 10–15 % of the normal tracheal lumen, causing an increase in resistance of the airway and a drop in tidal volume with the augmentation of work of breathing. Consequently, the patient develops a rapid shallow breathing pattern with a risk of impending respiratory muscle fatigue, worsening of gas exchange, and the need for mechanical ventilation. Because of the incomplete expiratory lung emptying, FBO can facilitate "air trapping" with a generation of intrinsic positive end-expiratory pressure (PEEP), which is particularly deleterious in COPD [1, 2].

Hypoxemia occurs with insertion of the bronchoscope into the trachea and becomes worse when BAL is performed, as a consequence of ventilation-perfusion (V/Q) mismatch. The application of suction through the bronchoscope channel lowers airway pressure at the end of expiration, facilitating early alveolar closure and hypoxemia. As a matter of a fact, FOB induces arterial oxygen pressure (PaO_2) to decrease between 10 and 20 mmHg [1, 2]. The use of analgo-sedation during FBO to reduce patient discomfort may worsen gas exchange further through drug-induced hypoventilation. These pulmonary changes persist after the procedure is completed, and the time that the gas exchange takes to normalize ranges from 15 min in normal subjects to several hours in patients with lung disease. All this justifies the use of supplemental O_2 in patients undergoing FBO at risk of oxygen desaturation [1].

FBO-induced sympathetic stimulation and hypoxemia can lead to an increase in heart rate and cardiac output with the heart's augmented oxygen consumption. Decreased intrathoracic pressure caused by the augmented respiratory muscle efforts (i.e., deeper negative transdiaphragmatic swings during inspiration) produces an increase in both right ventricular preload and left ventricular afterload. Consequently, FBO may trigger cardiac arrhythmias in 11–40 % of the cases and, less frequently, cardiogenic pulmonary edema and acute coronary syndrome, especially in patients with preexisting heart disease [1].

Thoracic societies recommend avoiding FBO and BAL in patients with hypoxemia that cannot be corrected to at least a PaO_2 of 75 mmHg or to an oxygen saturation (SpO_2) of ≥90 % with supplemental oxygen [1]. In these higher-risk patients, when noninvasive diagnostic tests are not conclusive, avoiding FBO means being compelled to use empirical treatment. As a consequence, when bronchoscopy is mandatory, only CMV can assure adequate ventilation during the maneuver. Unfortunately, CMV is not free of complications.

Cardiopulmonary pathophysiological changes observed during FBO are more exaggerated during intervention procedures performed with RB, especially because of airway obstruction by the bronchoscope, prolonged suctioning, low inspiratory fraction of O_2 (FiO_2) (to prevent laser combustion), and respiratory depression resulting from analgo-sedation [2].

Despite its increasing clinical application in critical respiratory patients, the failure rate of ppNIMV varies between 5 and 60 %, depending on numerous factors, including the cause of ARF, excessive secretions, hypercapnic encephalopathy (HE), agitation, patient-ventilator asynchrony, and sleep disturbances [5]. Unsuccessful ppNIMV was found to be independently associated with death, especially in patients with "de novo" hypoxemic ARF [3]. Among all causes, inefficacy in spontaneously clearing airways of an excessive burden of secretions plays an important role in determining ppNIMV failure in 33–61 % of cases [3, 5]. This is a result of the noninvasive interfaces that do not allow direct access into the airways (Table 71.1).

71.3 Rationale for the Combined Use of NIMV and FBO

There is a strong pathophysiological rationale for combining bronchoscopy and NIMV for the management of respiratory critical patients because the limitations of one technique may be counterbalanced by the properties of the other. In other words, NIMV may be of help in performing safe bronchoscopy in ARF patients, and FBO may increase the chance of success in patients at risk of NIMV failure.

Table 71.1 Advantages and disadvantages of bronchoscopy and noninvasive ventilation

Bronchoscopy	Noninvasive ventilation
Advantages	
Diagnosis in suspected pneumonia	Improving gas exchange
Diagnosis in diffuse lung diseases	Reduced work of breathing
Clearing of mucous from airway	Reduced heart work-load
Treatment of airways obstruction	Avoidance of ETI and CMV
Disadvantages	
Increased airway's resistance	Failure in case of burden of secretion
Increased work of breathing	
Worsening of gas exchange	
Increased heart workload	

ppNIMV is able to prevent and correct the cardiopulmonary alterations induced by bronchoscopy through three mechanisms: (1) compensation of the bronchoscope-correlated extra-resistive work of breathing by means of the unloading of respiratory muscles leading to a more favorable breathing pattern and diaphragmatic load-force relationship; (2) improvement of pulmonary gas exchange due to a better V/Q ratio and the correction of hypoventilation; and (3) counterbalancing of the increased heart workload by means of a marked relief of respiratory muscle effort with a reduced negative inspiratory intrathoracic pressure. Keeping the patient on ppNIMV after bronchoscopy may prevent the derangement of lung function that can last several hours after the procedure [6].

As a result of the clearing the airways in the early phases of ppNIMV, FBO may improve ventilation and, therefore, reduce the need for ETI in patients with an unfavorable balance between excessive burden of secretions and inefficient spontaneous clearance after the failure of chest physiotherapeutic techniques [6].

Three different acute scenarios of synergistic interaction between FBO and ppNIMV may be encountered in the ICU/RICU environment: (1) patients on O_2 therapy who undergo diagnostic FBO under ppNIMV assistance (for prevention of mandatory noninvasive or invasive ventilatory support in O_2-supported patients); (2) patients already on ppNIMV who undergo diagnostic FBO under ventilation (for prevention of CMV in ppNIMV-supported patients); and (3) patients requiring ETI for an excessive burden of bronchial secretions who undergo early therapeutic and diagnostic FBO during ppNIMV (as an alternative to mandatory CMV in ppNIMV plus FBO-supported patients) (Fig. 71.1).

71.4 Clinical Evidence of NIMV-Bronchoscopy Synergy

The majority of the published studies have used ppNIMV to prevent respiratory deterioration in spontaneously breathing hypoxemic patients undergoing FBO who do not still require ppNIMV for ARF [6] (Table 71.2). Antonelli et al. [7] were the first to report on ppNIMV-assisted FBO; they performed BAL in eight immunocompromised

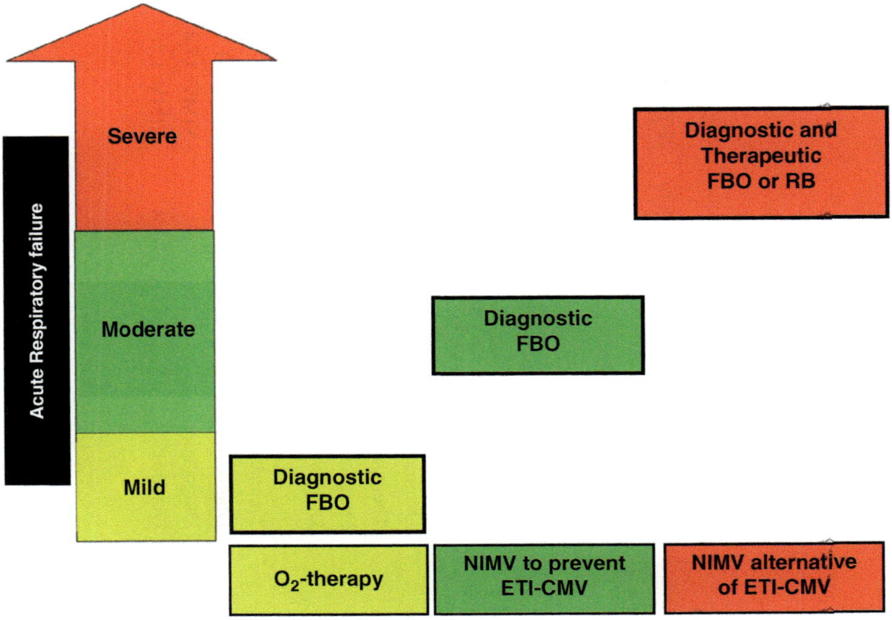

Fig. 71.1 Potential scenarios for synergistic application of bronchoscopy and noninvasive ventilation according to the severity of acute respiratory failure, the baseline support of the patients, and the purposes of bronchoscopy. *FBO* flexible bronchoscopy, *NIMV* noninvasive mechanical ventilation, *ETI-CMV* endotracheal intubation conventional mechanical ventilation, *RB* rigid bronchoscopy

patients with severe hypoxemia ($PaO_2/FiO_2 \leq 100$ mmHg) due to suspected pneumonia. The use of ppNIMV was associated with significant improvements in PaO_2/FiO_2 and SpO_2 during bronchoscopy. FBO with NPPV was well tolerated, and no patient required ETI. Two patients died 5–7 days after FBO from unrelated complications of the underlying illness. A causative pathogen was identified by BAL in all patients, and six of them responded to treatment and survived hospital admission.

In a subsequent study, Da Conceicao et al. [8] investigated the feasibility of ppNIMV-assisted FBO in a 10 COPD patients admitted to ICU for pneumonia with hypoxemic-hypercapnic ARF ($PaO_2=53\pm13$ mmHg; $PaCO_2=67\pm11$ mmHg). During FBO with ppNIMV, SpO_2 increased from 91 ± 4.7 % at baseline to 97 ± 1.7 %.9. There were no changes in $PaCO_2$ and PaO_2 during the hour following the end of procedure. FBO under NIPPV was performed without complications and was well tolerated in 8 patients. No patient required ETI within 24 h, and all patients survived.

In the first randomized controlled trial (RCT), conducted on 30 patients with $PaO_2 \leq 125$ mmHg despite high-flow oxygen mask (i.e., 10 l/min) requiring diagnostic FBO, Maitre et al. [9] showed significantly higher SpO_2 values during FBO and 30 min thereafter with CPAP, compared with oxygen-therapy, using a new device open to the atmosphere (CPAP Boussignac). Not only did the patients in the oxygen group develop hypoxemia during FBO, but 5 patients in the oxygen group (compared with none in the CPAP group) also required ventilatory assistance (1

Table 71.2 Studies on the combined use of FBO and ppNIMV in acute respiratory failure

Author, year	Study	No. patients	ARF pattern	Support pre-FBO	Indication FBO	FBO procedure	ETI (%)
Antonelli, 1996	Prospective	NIMV: 8	Hypoxemic	Oxygen	Diagnostic	BAL	NIMV: 0
Da Conceicao, 2000	Prospective	NIMV: 10	Hypoxemic-hypercapnic	Oxygen	Diagnostic	BAL	NIMV: 0
Maitre, 2000	RCT	CPAP: 15	Hypoxemic	Oxygen	Diagnostic	BAL, br. biopsy	CPAP: 6.7
		O_2: 15					O_2: 46.7
Antonelli, 2002	RCT	NIMV: 13	Hypoxemic	Oxygen	Diagnostic	BAL	NIMV: 7.7
		O_2: 13					O_2: 15.4
Chiner, 2010	Prospective	NIMV: 35	Hypoxemic	Oxygen	Diagnostic	BW, PSB,BAL,	0
					Therapeutic	br. biopsy	
Heunks, 2010	Prospective	NIMV: 12	Hypoxemic	Oxygen	Diagnostic	BAL	NIMV: 8.3
Scala, 2010	Case control	NIMV: 15	Hypoxemic-hypercapnic	NIMV	Diagnostic	BAL	NIMV: 20
		CMV: 15			Therapeutic		
Baumann, 2011	Prospective	NIMV: 40	Hypoxemic	NIMV	Diagnostic	BAL	NIMV 10
Clouzeau, 2011	Prospective	NIMV: 23	Hypoxemic	NIMV	Diagnostic	BAL	NIMV: 17.4
Agarwall, 2012	Prospective	NIMV: 6	Hypoxemic	Oxygen	Diagnostic	BAL, TBLB	NIMV: 1.7

ppNIMV and 4 CMV) within 6 h following the procedure ($p=0.003$). A causative infectious agent was identified in 14 cases, with two diagnoses of carcinomatous lymphangitis (one by BAL and one by bronchial biopsy); fat embolism and drug-induced hypersensitivity pneumonia were diagnosed in 2 patients.

Subsequently, in another RCT involving 26 patients with nosocomial pneumonia and $PaO_2/FiO_2 \leq 200$ mmHg, Antonelli et al. [10] evaluated the effectiveness and safety of ppNIMV versus conventional oxygen supplementation before, during, and after diagnostic FBO. Application of ppNIMV was associated with increase in PaO_2/FiO_2 by 82 %, in contrast to a decline in PaO_2/FiO_2 of 10 % in the oxygen group during FBO. Furthermore, in the ppNIMV group, PaO_2/FiO_2 remained higher, heart rate was lower, and there was no reduction in mean arterial pressure in comparison with a 15 % decrease from the baseline in the control group 60 min after FBO. Eighteen patients had significant growth of a pathogen found in BAL fluid. One patient in the ppNIMV group and 2 patients in the control group required non emergency ETI. Four patients in the ppNIMV group and 7 patients in the oxygen group died from complications of their underlying disease 5–7 days after study entry. The same group also found the helmet for delivering NIMV to be safe in avoiding gas exchange deterioration in 4 hypoxemic patients [11].

Chiner et al. [12] evaluated nasal mask for delivering ppNIMV while the FBO was performed orally using a bite block sealed with an elastic glove finger in 35 patients with a mean PaO_2/FiO_2 of 168. A total of 35 bronchoaspirates, 21 PSB, 11 BAL, and 8 bronchial biopsies were performed. In contrast to other studies, patients developed hypoxemia during the procedure, with SpO_2 decreasing to 86 % during FBO, probably as a result of excessive mouth-air leaks during nasal NIMV. The clinical course was favorable in 66 %; there was a relatively high rate of need of CMV (11 % of the cases occurring 5 ± 4 days after FBO) and in-hospital mortality (33 % of the cases occurring 3 ± 2 days after FBO), mainly correlated with the underlying disease.

Heunks et al. [13] reported the use of a novel total face mask for delivering NIMV during diagnostic FBO in 12 hypoxemic patients (mean $PaO_2/FiO_2=192\pm23$). The procedure was successful in all patients; in only 1 patient SpO_2 decreased to 86 % during FBO. A microbiological diagnosis was established in 8 of 12 patients.

All the reported studies have shown that ppNIMV is able to ensure adequate gas exchange during FBO in spontaneously breathing hypoxemic patients, thus avoiding ET. There is only one study that reported the use of FBO in patients with hypoxemic ARF requiring ppNIMV before the procedure. Baumann et al. [14] evaluated 40 hypoxemic patients requiring ppNIMV ($PaO_2/FiO_2=176\pm54$) who underwent FOB for suspected pneumonia. FBO was successfully performed without complications. BAL yielded diagnostic information in 68 % of the patients. The mean PaO_2/FiO_2 ratio improved at the end of FBO after 120 min. Four patients (10 %) required ETI during the first 8 hours after the procedure.

Agarwal et al. [15] published a pilot experience of ppNIMV-assisted FBO for performing BAL and TBLB in six severely hypoxemic patients ($PaO_2/FiO_2 < 200$) with diffuse interstitial lung diseases. There was significant improvement in respiratory rate and PaO_2/FiO_2, and significant decline in heart rate after application of ppNIMV. FBO was well tolerated and all subjects maintained $SpO_2 > 92\ \%$ during the procedure. One subject required ETI due to hemoptysis. There was no evidence of pneumothorax in any subject. A definite diagnosis was obtained in five (two malignancies, one lymphoma, one sarcoidosis, and one pneumocystis pneumonia) of the six patients only with TBLB, which enabled their successful management. Although the authors concluded that ppNIMV-assisted TBLB is feasible in patients with ARF and diffuse pulmonary infiltrates, this approach should be performed only in centers showing wide experience with both ppNIMV and FBO, as well as with the management of TBLB complications (i.e., pulmonary hemorrhage and pneumothorax). More studies are required to adequately define the utility and safety of NIMV-assisted TBLB.

The last scenario of a synergistic interaction between the two techniques deals with the usefulness of FBO as therapeutic tool to avoid ppNIMV failure in ARF patients with an excessive burden of secretions [6]. In the context of decompensated COPD patients requiring ETI because of impaired mucous clearance, Scala et al. [16] postulated that the early suction of secretions with FBO performed during ppNIMV is feasible and effective. In a matched case-control study, the authors compared 15 acutely decompensated COPD patients with copious secretion retention and HE resulting from community-acquired pneumonia undergoing early FBO plus BAL during ppNIMV in an expert RICU with 15 controls receiving CMV in the ICU. Two hours of ppNIMV plus FBO significantly improved gas exchange, sensorium, and cough efficiency without major complications (e.g., cardiovascular events, emergent ETI, or pneumothorax). Improvement in $PaCO_2$ and pH, hospital mortality, and durations of hospitalization and ventilation were similar in both groups. ppNIMV significantly reduced serious infectious complications compared with CMV, as well as the need for tracheostomy. Even though this ppNIMV strategy may be a successful alternative to CMV in selected COPD patients within expert units, larger RCTs are necessary to confirm this result and, therefore, to test the efficacy of the FBO-ppNIMV protocol applied to an earlier time course of COPD decompensations when ETI is not mandatory by comparing ppNIMV alone versus ppNIMV with early FBO [16].

71.5 Special Situations

71.5.1 Difficult Intubation

The combined use of FBO and ppNIMV to perform ETI may be useful in peculiar clinical contexts. In a RCT performed on 32 patients with an anticipated difficult intubation in ear-nose-throat surgery, Bourgain et al. [17] demonstrated that, during FBO performed under propofol, ppNIMV improves ventilation efficiency compared with spontaneous breathing. ETI is particularly risky and difficult in patients with severe hypoxemic ARF who deteriorate despite a trial of ppNIMV. The lack of clear benefit of ppNIMV in these patients is at least in part due to an increased mortality risk during rescue ETI. Maintaining ppNIMV during ETI may prevent alveolar de-recruitment and derangement of gas exchange. This concept was demonstrated by Bailard et al. [18] in a RCT study conducted on 53 hypoxemic patients requiring ETI in ICU. The authors showed that SpO_2 values were significantly greater if pre-oxygenation before ETI was performed with ppNIMV rather than with a conventional non-rebreather bag-valve mask.

In the first pilot French study, Da Conceiçao et al. [19] assessed the feasibility and safety of a new technique of FBO-assisted naso-tracheal-intubation with ppNIMV delivered via an adapted endoscopic facial mask under conscious sedation in 16 patients with hypoxemic-hypercapnic ARF ($PaCO_2 = 64 \pm 26$ mmhg, $PaO_2/FiO_2 = 142 \pm 70$) who required CMV due to late ppNIMV failure. The FBO intubation was performed without any failure or complication. SpO_2 significantly improved during ETI with values kept over 90 % during the procedure. In another US pilot study, Barjaktarevic et al. [20] reported a series of 10 nonconsecutive hypoxemic patients who developed failure of ppNIMV via full face mask, showing a PaO_2/FiO_2 ratio < 100. The subjects were orally intubated under the guide of FBO, keeping ppNIMV delivered via the nasal route. Adopting this new technique, ETI was successfully performed without major complications; one-third of the patients developed arterial hypotension, mainly correlated with the use of analogo-sedation. Only a mild drop in SpO_2 (4.7 ± 3.1 %) was reported during the procedure. These preliminary experiences require confirmation by large RCTs comparing conventional versus FBO-guided ETI under ppNIMV in patients with impending ppNIMV failure. It may be speculated that this new procedure for rescue ETI in case of ppNIMV failure is likely to be more advantageous in patients with predicted or proven difficult direct laryngoscopy.

71.5.2 Obstructive Sleep Apnea Syndrome

Patients with obstructive sleep apnea syndrome (OSAS) are at high risk of developing severe hypoxemia under and after sedation during surgical or endoscopic procedures [21]. This is particularly true in the case of FBO performed with the use of sedatives, which may precipitate the collapse of airways in OSAS patients and augment the degree of FOB-induced hypoxemia. ppNIMV counteracts negative inspiratory pressures and the hypotonicity of the upper airway muscles in OSAS patients. The positive pressure generated by ppNIMV allows for the laryngeal structures to be identified as the device passes the hypopharynx and is introduced through the vocal chords. This aspect is fundamental in OSAS patients with predicted difficult intubation [21].

71.5.3 Interventional Procedures During RB

The application of intermittent positive pressure and jet-ventilation are the two standard ventilatory modes that guarantee effective ventilation during RB. Patients can also be managed with assisted spontaneous breathing. Unfortunately, these ventilatory strategies have important limitations during RB, such as requirement of higher FiO_2, ineffective control of ventilatory output with risk of acidosis, need for higher doses of opioids, and prolonged recovery time [2, 22].

In two RCTs, Vitacca et al. [23, 24] demonstrated that, compared with both assisted spontaneous breathing and external high-frequency oscillation, npNIMV delivered by a poncho-wrap to support interventional RB procedures under general anesthesia, was associated with less incidence and severity of respiratory acidosis, less requirement of increased O_2 supply, lower use of opioids, shorter recovery time, and less need for assisted-manual ventilation.

71.6 Practical Issues

It is recommended that FBO NIMV procedures should be performed in an ICU or RICU setting, or a standard bronchoscopy room capable of dealing with any cardiopulmonary complications and the management of airways [6]. ppNIMV should be initiated at least 15–20 min before bronchoscopy. There are no published papers comparing the different ventilatory modes. The easiest mode of assisting FBO in hypoxemic patients consists of delivering CPAP by means of a Boussignac system with a face mask [6, 9]. This system accelerates the air molecules in the form of microjets that generate a "virtual valve" through a turbulence effect. The gas velocity transforms into pressure, depending on the flow of gas provided. Usually, CPAP is set at 10 cmH_2O with FiO_2 of 1.0 and then the pressure is eventually increased, based on SpO_2 values. As this CPAP device remains open to the atmosphere, it has the advantage of allowing easy maintenance of a positive pressure and CPAP delivery while FBO is being performed [9].

Pressure-support ventilation has been the most commonly used mode of ppNIMV [3, 5, 6]. An initial pressure support of 10 cmH_2O is recommended during the procedure, with low PEEP levels (e.g., 5 cmH_2O) [6]. With advanced ventilators provided with a double-tube circuit and accurate ventilatory monitoring, pressure support is titrated to achieve an expiratory tidal volume of 8–10 ml/kg and respiratory rate below 25 min^{-1}. FiO_2 is initially set at 0.5 and then changed to achieve SpO_2 values above 90 %; accordingly, an ICU ventilator capable of delivering FiO_2 from high-pressure sources is recommended [16].

NIMV setting adjustments can be made during the procedure [6]:

(a) If there is hypoxemia despite FiO_2 1.0, PEEP may be increased by steps of 2 cmH_2O until SpO_2 ≥90 % is reached; patients who remain hypoxemic despite high FiO_2 and PEEP levels are not good candidates for NIMV-assisted FBO.
(b) Hypercapnia and respiratory acidosis have to be corrected by raising pressure support levels to improve effective alveolar ventilation before FBO.

Regarding the interfaces, almost all types of masks have been used. The most widely used are orofacial masks [6]. Currently, endoscopic face masks usually

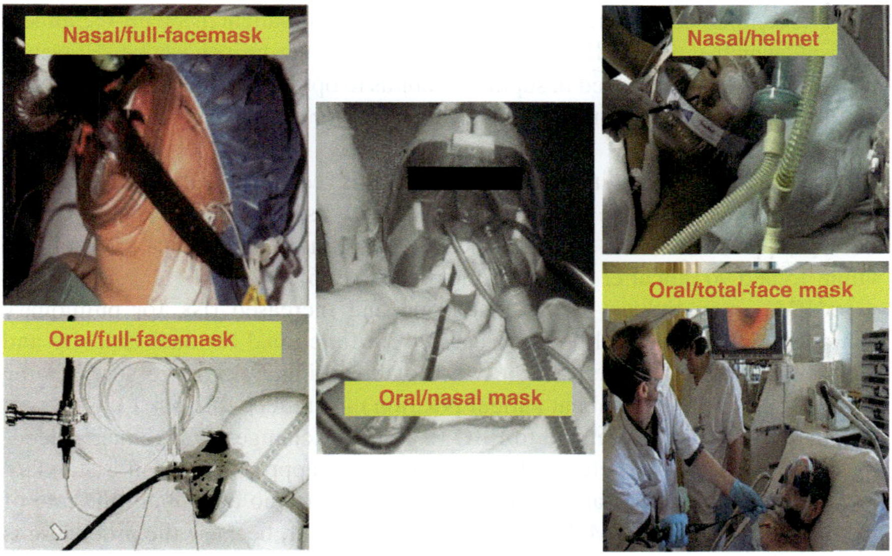

Fig. 71.2 Different combinations of access of the bronchoscope into the airways (nasal or oral route) and interfaces used for delivering noninvasive ventilation

have two orifices: one for the administration of gas and a second that is sealed and distensible as it allows for an endoscope to be introduced. FBO with ppNIMV can be performed with a helmet [11] or a total face mask [13]. Chiner et al. [12] used a handmade system of a membrane made out of a latex glove coupled with a bite block with a small incision; this maintains the pressure administered by the ventilator through a nasal mask, and bronchoscopy is carried out orally with good results.

The bronchoscope can be introduced through both the nasal and oral routes, depending on the mask used and operator experience [6] (Fig. 71.2). With face masks, the nasal or oral pathways can be used. The introduction of the bronchoscope into the nares through the face mask can be a difficult step, as the bronchoscope has to be considerably manipulated, which not only prolongs the procedure but can also cause trauma to the nasal mucosa. To facilitate easy passage, the bronchoscope is initially passed through the face mask, and the tip of bronchoscope is gently passed through the nose until the vocal cords are visible. With the helmet, either nasal or oral entry can be used, with the patient sitting or in supine decubitus [11]. Likewise, the use of Boussignac CPAP, because it is an open system, allows for oral or nasal entry [6, 9].

Delivery of ppNIMV does not necessarily imply greater sedation. For topical anesthesia, lidocaine is used as with standard FBO. Some authors propose the use of analgesic (opioids) and/or sedative drugs (benzodiazepines, propofol) for FBO under ppNIMV to reduce patient discomfort, but it is essential to have experience in drug management [6].

It is recommended to carry out the procedure with the patient in a semi-recumbent position, which is implied by the anterior entry of the bronchoscope. However, ppNIMV itself has been used in supine decubitus to optimize respiratory parameters in other explorations such interventional cardiology or in suspected dynamic airway collapse [6].

As in all interventions in high-risk patients, it is recommended to keep the time as shorter as possibile. The mean duration of NIMV-assisted FBO is approximately 8 min [6]. ppNIMV should be maintained with a setting similar to that prior to FBO within 15 and 90 min after the end of the procedure [6].

ppNIMV may induce gastric distension and increased risk for pulmonary aspiration. The abdominal pressure can reduce functional residual capacity and add a restrictive component to the work of breathing. Lower pressures of the ventilator and semi-recumbent patient position may reduce this risk [3, 6]. There are other complications related to FBO (e.g., gas exchange derangement, bleeding, poor collaboration, etc.), whose resolution is approached as in a standard FBO with prompt ETI availability [1, 2, 6]. There are no data about the rate of pneumothorax during NIMV-assisted TBLB. However, because the procedure is performed under positive pressure, the risk should not to be underestimated as pneumothorax was reported as a complication during both acute and chronic ppNIMV. Accordingly, facilities for inserting chest drainage should be promptly available. Less frequently, there may be major cardiovascular complications (malignant arrhythmias, acute coronary syndrome, cardiac arrest), which can be minimized through proper patient selection and monitoring during bronchoscopy. Nasal or facial injuries appear only after prolonged NIMV use [6].

Contraindications of this procedure are those of ppNIMV itself, such as cardiac arrest, severe encephalopathy, gastrointestinal bleeding, severe hemodynamic instability, history of facial surgery or trauma, recent esophageal-gastric interventions, and inability to protect the airway [3, 5, 6]. There are other absolute contraindications of bronchoscopy itself, such as recent acute coronary syndrome, severe arrhythmias, and severe coagulopathies if biopsy is planned [1, 2, 6].

Conclusions

An increasing amount of data suggest the use of bronchoscopy during NIMV in ARF to avoid or reduce the need of ETI. Despite a strong rationale for the combined use of the two techniques, there is not still enough evidence for a large-scale application of this strategy in all clinical scenarios. The majority of the available data are in favor of the "help" given by NIMV to diagnostic bronchoscopy in high-risk hypoxemic patients. Preliminary findings report the successful help given by early bronchoscopy to NIMV in patients with hypoxemic-hypercapnic ARF who are likely to fail because of hypersecretion. This combined approach should be performed only in centers with wide experience with both NIMV and bronchoscopy, where close monitoring and ETI facilities are promptly available.

Key Major Recommendations

- Some scenarios represent contraindications for NIMV and bronchoscopy, such as severe hypoxemia for the latter and accumulated tracheobronchial secretions for the former.
- There is a strong pathophysiological rationale for combining bronchoscopy and NIMV for the management of respiratory critical patients because the limitations of one technique may be counterbalanced by the properties of the other.
- ppNIMV is helpful to support diagnostic FBO in high-risk hypoxemic patients, and FBO may increase the chance of ppNIMV success by removing the burden of secretion
- npNIMV is the more effective ventilatory mode to support patients during the interventional procedure performed with RB in general anesthesia.
- The bronchoscopy-NIMV combined procedure must be performed only in the ICU or RICU setting, or whenever there is a suitable monitoring of the patient and a team with good expertise in both techniques and in the management of airways (i.e., ETI) and cardiopulmonary complications.

References

1. Du Rand IA, Blaikley J, Booton R, et al. British Thoracic Society Bronchoscopy Guideline Group. British thoracic society guideline for diagnostic flexible bronchoscopy in adults: accredited by NICE. Thorax. 2013;68(Suppl 1):i1–i44
2. Wahidi MM, Herth FJ, Ernst A. State of the art: interventional pulmonology. Chest. 2007;131:261–74.
3. Nava S, Hill N. Non-invasive ventilation in acute respiratory failure. Lancet. 2009;374:250–9.
4. Corrado A, Gorini M. Negative-pressure ventilation: is there still a role? Eur Respir J. 2002;20:187–97.
5. Ozyilmaz E, Ugurlu AO, Nava S. Timing of noninvasive ventilation failure: causes, risk factors, and potential remedies. BMC Pulm Med. 2014;14:19.
6. Esquinas A, Zuil M, Scala R, et al. Bronchoscopy during non-invasive mechanical ventilation: a review of techniques and procedures. Arch Bronconeumol. 2013;49:105–12.
7. Antonelli M, Conti G, Riccioni L, et al. Noninvasive positive-pressure ventilation via face mask during bronchoscopy with BAL in high-risk hypoxemic patients. Chest. 1996;110:724–8.
8. Da Conceiçao M, Genco G, Favier JC, et al. Fiberoptic bronchoscopy during noninvasive positive-pressure ventilation in patients with chronic obstructive lung disease with hypoxemia and hypercapnia. Ann Fr Anesth Reanim. 2000;19:231–6.
9. Maitre B, Jaber S, Maggiore SM, et al. Continuous positive airway pressure during fiberoptic bronchoscopy in hypoxemic patients. A randomized double-blind study using a new device. Am J Respir Crit Care Med. 2000;162:1063–7.
10. Antonelli M, Conti G, Rocco M, et al. Noninvasive positive-pressure ventilation vs conventional oxygen supplementation in hypoxemic patients undergoing diagnostic bronchoscopy. Chest. 2002;121:1149–54.

11. Antonelli M, Pennisi MA, Conti G, et al. Fiberoptic bronchoscopy during noninvasive positive pressure ventilation delivered by helmet. Intensive Care Med. 2003;29:126–9.
12. Chiner E, Sancho-Chust JN, Llombart M, et al. Fiberoptic bronchoscopy during nasal non-invasive ventilation in acute respiratory failure. Respiration. 2010;80:321–6.
13. Heunks LM, de Bruin CJ, van der Hoeven JG, et al. Noninvasive mechanical ventilation for diagnostic bronchoscopy using a new face mask: an observational feasibility study. Intensive Care Med. 2010;36:143–7.
14. Baumann HJ, Klose H, Simon M, et al. Fiberoptic bronchoscopy in patients with acute hypoxemic respiratory failure requiring noninvasive ventilation–a feasibility study. Crit Care. 2011;15:R179.
15. Agarwal R, Khan A, Aggarwal AN, et al. Bronchoscopic lung biopsy using noninvasive ventilatory support: case series and review of literature of NIV-assisted bronchoscopy. Respir Care. 2012;57:1927–36.
16. Scala R, Naldi M, Maccari U. Early fiberoptic bronchoscopy during noninvasive ventilation in patients with decompensated chronic obstructive pulmonary disease due to community acquired pneumonia. Crit Care. 2010;14:R80.
17. Bourgain JL, Billard V, Cros AM. Pressure support ventilation during fibreoptic intubation under propofol anaesthesia. Br J Anaesth. 2007;98:136–40.
18. Baillard C, Fosse JP, Sebbane M, et al. Noninvasive ventilation improves preoxygenation before intubation of hypoxic patients. Am J Respir Crit Care Med. 2006;174:171–7.
19. Da Conceiçao M, Favier JC, Bidallier I, et al. Fiber-optic intubation with non-invasive ventilation with an endoscopic facial mask. Ann Fr Anesth Reanim. 2002;21:256–62.
20. Barjaktarevic I, Berlin D. Bronchoscopic intubation during continuous nasal positive pressure ventilation in the treatment of hypoxemic respiratory failure. J Intensive Care Med. 2015;30:161–6.
21. Corso RM, Gregoretti C, Braghiroli A, et al. Practice guidelines for the perioperative management of patients with obstructive sleep apnea: navigating through uncertainty. Anesthesiology. 2014;121:664–5.
22. Cavaliere S, Venuta F, Foccoli P, et al. Endoscopic treatment of malignant airway obstructions in 2008 patients. Chest. 1996;11:1536–42.
23. Natalini G, Cavaliere S, Vitacca M, et al. Negative pressure ventilation vs. spontaneous assisted ventilation during rigid bronchoscopy. A controlled randomised trial. Acta Anaesthesiol Scand. 1998;42:1063–9.
24. Natalini G, Cavaliere S, Seramondi V, et al. Negative pressure ventilation vs external high frequency oscillation during rigid bronchoscopy. A controlled randomized trial. Chest. 2000;118:18–23.

Sedation and Analgesia for Noninvasive Ventilation in Intensive Care

72

Yalim Dikmen

Contents

Abbreviations

ARF	Acute respiratory failure
COPD	Chronic obstructive pulmonary disease
ETI	Endotracheal intubation
ICU	Intensive care unit
NPPV	Noninvasive positive pressure ventilation
PaO_2/FiO_2	Ratio of arterial oxygen tension to fractional inspired oxygen concentration

72.1 Introduction

The use of noninvasive positive pressure ventilation (NPPV) in patients with acute respiratory failure is increasing dramatically. It is now considered the first-line treatment in certain types of acute respiratory failure such as acute exacerbations of

Y. Dikmen
Department of Anesthesiology and Reanimation, Cerrahpasa Medical School, Istanbul University, Istanbul, Turkey
e-mail: ydikmen@istanbul.edu.tr

A.M. Esquinas (ed.), *Noninvasive Mechanical Ventilation: Theory, Equipment, and Clinical Applications*, DOI 10.1007/978-3-319-21653-9_72

chronic obstructive pulmonary disease (COPD), acute cardiogenic edema, asthma, and in patients with immunosuppression. The main aim of NPPV in these settings is to avoid endotracheal intubation (ETI) by correcting gas exchange, relieving symptoms of dyspnea, and decreasing work of breathing. It is now known that avoiding intubation prevents complications associated with invasive mechanical ventilation, decreases rates of nosocomial infections, and shortens length of intensive care unit (ICU) and hospital stay.

These positive effects of NPPV are dependent on patient tolerance during ventilation, and it may be difficult in the presence of claustrophobic sensation, excessive air leaks around the interface, and patient-ventilator dys-synchronies. These may necessitate the presence of health-care staff at the bedside during the initial hours of application. If the patient learns to breathe through the ventilator, and if the support may overcome the respiratory distress (i.e., correct gas exchange and unload respiratory muscles without causing too much dyssynchrony) then the need for help and reassurance decreases. As a result of skin lesions caused by the mask, abdominal distension, dryness of upper airways, and neuropsychological distress, patient discomfort may worsen, leading to poor acceptance of NPPV. In these instances, application of a sedative may increase patient tolerance and help to avoid endotracheal intubation.

72.2 Discussion

Although sedation and analgesia are well established in patients with invasive ventilation, the use of sedatives and analgesics during NPPV is a controversial issue. An updated guideline for management of pain, agitation, and delirium in the ICU has been published [1]. This guideline suggests the use of opioid analgesics and lighter levels of sedation, with scales to assess depth of sedation; however, it does not address the use of analgesics and sedation in patients on noninvasive ventilation.

In general, the use of sedatives and narcotic analgesics may be seen as relatively contraindicated because they can depress the level of consciousness, interfere with upper airway reflexes, and may lead to endotracheal intubation. On the other hand, use of sedatives and/or opioids may be helpful in alleviating agitation and dyspnea in patients with respiratory distress and may increase patients' tolerance to NPPV. The success of noninvasive ventilation may depend on patient acceptance and tolerance of the mask interface. In an epidemiologic survey conducted by Carlucci et al. [2], tolerance to the mask was significantly lower in patients who failed noninvasive ventilation. In this study, 52 of 108 patients required early termination of noninvasive ventilation, and in 22 % of these cases the reason for failure was the patient's refusal to continue NPPV. Another survey showed that the physicians perceived mask tolerance as one of the most important problems in NPPV application [3]. In this web-based survey on the use of noninvasive ventilation in general wards, 67.5 % of the respondents reported patient refusal or mask intolerance as problems associated with NPPV.

In the setting of mask intolerance or patient agitation, sedation or analgesics can be considered. On the other hand, as sedative and opioid analgesic drugs also have anxiolytic effects and depress respiratory drive and central perception, they may be helpful in patients with respiratory distress by alleviating symptoms associated with dyspnea [4]. These drugs along with other non-pharmacologic interventions have the potential to increase patient tolerance and acceptance, and NPPV success in patients with ARF.

There is currently no established protocol or consensus on the use of sedatives and analgesics during noninvasive ventilation, and the effects of sedation and analgesia during NPPV remain controversial due to a lack of knowledge and experience. One survey study published in 2007 investigated the sedation practices during noninvasive ventilation [5]. In this study, 790 physicians from Europe and North America responded to the survey, indicating varying rates of sedative use and differing choices of sedatives and hand restraints. In general, the use of sedatives and analgesics was low; the percentages of North American and European physicians who used sedatives and analgesics more than 25 % of the time were 45 % and 26 %, respectively. North Americans used sedatives and analgesics more frequently than their European counterparts, and intensive care physicians were more likely to use them than other physicians. The drugs chosen for sedation and analgesia were mainly benzodiazepines (33 % of the respondents) and opioids (22 % of the respondents); regimens containing propofol or dexmedetomidine were quite infrequent (7 % and 5 %, respectively). Drug choice was dependent on clinical experience and lack of effect on respiratory drive. Only 14 % of the respondents reported the use of a specified protocol for sedation during NPPV, and assessment was done by clinical observation rather than sedation scales (63 % vs 32 %).

The practices observed in this study may be considered outdated today in the light of the new guidelines [1] and findings of the studies showing the association of benzodiazepines with delirium [6]. These literature show a need for avoidance of benzodiazepine use in intensive care patients and applying analgosedation where opioids play a major role, in addition to use of scales and protocols to keep the sedation levels as light as possible.

In general, sedation may not be needed routinely during noninvasive ventilation, but there may be some situations, mainly poor acceptance, in which sedatives may be indicated. Before initiating any sedative, the physician should keep in mind that the chosen interface and ventilator mode can be a contributing factor to patient discomfort. Face masks with tight fittings or large leaks from around the mask, continuous high flow provided by the ventilator, or patient ventilator dyssynchrony may be the factors associated with patient agitation and refusal of the mask [7]. The physician should be ready to choose different interfaces to improve patient comfort and change ventilator settings according to patient comfort.

72.2.1 Sedative and Analgesic Drugs

The ideal sedative should be effective in controlling anxiety and discomfort without causing respiratory depression or depression of upper airway reflexes. The level of sedation should easily be titrated to keep the patient awake or easily arousable [8].

Table 72.1 Doses of sedative drugs used in NPPV [8]

Drug	Bolus dose	Infusion dose
Dexmedetomidine	1 μ/kg	0.2–0.7 μg/kg/h
Midazolam	0.05 mg/kg	0.05–0.1 mg/kg/h
Remifentanil	–	0.025 μg/kg/min
Propofol	–	0.4 μg/ml (down to 0.2 ml – target plasma concentration)

For this purpose, propofol and benzodiazepines are used as the drugs of choice. However, reports claiming unwanted effects of benzodiazepines, and the introduction of the α-adrenergic agonist dexmedetomidine, have shifted the choice away from benzodiazepines. The advent of short-acting synthetic morphine derivatives has made analgosedation using drug combinations more feasible. The doses of sedative drugs used during NPPV are listed in Table 72.1.

In a study conducted by Conti et al. [9], the effects of sufentanil on respiratory drive, respiratory pattern, and gas exchange were investigated in intubated patients during pressure support ventilation. In this study, no changes in hemodynamic or respiratory parameters were observed with the use of 0.2–0.3 μg/kg/h sufentanil infusion for 24 h. Newer drugs have a better safety profile than sufentanil and are used in ICUs for sedation and analgesia in intubated patients.

There are several recent studies, where remifentanil and dexmedetomidine is used to facilitate NPPV in patients whom refuse this treatment due to intolerance. Both drugs have shorter half-life and lower risk of unwanted effects.

Rocco et al. [10] reported 61 % of 36 patients with acute hypoxemic failure, who refused NPPV, were able to receive the treatment after sedation with remifentanil (0.025 μg/kg/min). The mortality rate in the successfully ventilated patient group was 14 %, whereas it was 50 % in the patients who required ETI despite remifentanil infusion. In a pilot study conducted on 12 patients who refused NPPV, only 4 needed ETI with the infusion of remifentanil [11]. The authors concluded that the use of remifentanil sedation was safe and effective in patients who refused noninvasive ventilation.

Huang et al. [12] compared dexmedetomidine and midazolam in NPPV failure due to patient refusal in a randomized study. Of the 62 treated patients with cardiogenic pulmonary edema, 20 had failed NPPV despite sedative infusions. The failure rate was 44.8 % in the midazolam group and 21.2 % in the dexmedetomidine group. The reasons for NPPV failure were inability to increase PaO_2/FiO_2 ratio, worsening hemodynamic status, and inability to cope with secretions. In patients with successful NPPV, dexmedetomidine resulted in shorter ICU stay and lower rates of respiratory infections, although the success rate and mortality were similar in both groups.

In a randomized, double-blind, controlled trial, dexmedetomidine was compared with placebo in patients receiving NPPV for ARF [13]. The patients were randomized to study groups within 8 h of NPPV, and received infusions for 72 h or until intubation or weaning. The study failed to show any advantage of initiating dexmedetomidine with noninvasive ventilation on tolerance, the patients were not selected from the ones who had intolerance to interface or agitation.

Propofol is widely used for conscious sedation during diagnostic interventions. It provides an easily controllable level of sedation with fast recovery after cessation of drug application. Clouzeau et al. [14] used propofol during fiber-optic bronchoscopy in patients with acute hypoxemic respiratory failure with noninvasive pressure support. The authors reported that an infusion regimen targeting plasma propofol concentrations was safe and effective in relieving patient discomfort without any adverse effects.

All of the above publications were reports of the results of preliminary or pilot studies with limited numbers of patients, generally with intolerance to NPPV. Although not conclusive, there are signs of a beneficial effect of analgosedation to relieve discomfort and improve patient acceptance of noninvasive ventilation. An important aspect of these studies is that all of them were conducted in ICUs, where all means of monitoring are available. The issue of whether sedation can be used in settings other than ICUs is controversial, and it may be dangerous because patients cannot be monitored as closely as in the ICU environment. It would be reasonable to admit the patients who refuse NPPV to the ICU to provide sedation before initiating invasive ventilation (i.e., endotracheal intubation).

Key Major Recommendations

- Use of sedation by titrating to a predetermined level may be beneficial in patients who refuse NPPV due to intolerance to interface, air leaks, or respiratory distress by increasing the success of noninvasive ventilation.
- The choice of drugs for sedation must be made considering their ease of dose titration and unwanted respiratory and cardiovascular effects.
- If necessary, sedation should be applied with the patient under close monitoring, preferably in the ICU.

References

1. Barr J, Fraser GL, Puntillo K, et al. American College of Critical Care Medicine. Clinical practice guidelines for the management of pain, agitation, and delirium in adult patients in the intensive care unit. Crit Care Med. 2013;41:263–306. doi:10.1097/CCM.0b013e3182783b72.
2. Carlucci A, Richard JC, Wysocki M, et al. Noninvasive versus conventional mechanical ventilation. An epidemiologic survey. Am J Respir Crit Care Med. 2001;163:874–80.
3. Cabrini L, Esquinas A, Pasin L, et al. An international survey on noninvasive ventilation use for acute respiratory failure in general non-monitored wards. Respir Care. 2015;60:586–92. doi:10.4187/respcare.03593.
4. Mahler DA. Opioids for refractory dyspnea. Expert Rev Respir Med. 2013;7:123–34. doi:10.1586/ers.13.5; quiz 135.
5. Devlin JW, Nava S, Fong JJ, et al. Survey of sedation practices during noninvasive positive-pressure ventilation to treat acute respiratory failure. Crit Care Med. 2007;35:2298–302.
6. Mehta S, Cook D, Devlin JW, et al. Prevalence, risk factors, and outcomes of delirium in mechanically ventilated adults. Crit Care Med. 2015;43:557–66. doi:10.1097/CCM.0000000000000727.
7. Longrois D, Conti G, Mantz J, et al. Sedation in non-invasive ventilation: do we know what to do (and why)? Multidiscip Respir Med. 2014;4(9(1)):56. doi:10.1186/2049-6958-9-56.

8. Scala A. Sedation during non-invasive ventilation to treat acute respiratory failure. Shortness of Breath. 2013;2:35–43.
9. Conti G, Arcangeli A, Antonelli M, et al. Sedation with sufentanil in patients receiving pressure support ventilation has no effects on respiration: a pilot study. Can J Anaesth. 2004;51:494–9.
10. Rocco M, Conti G, Alessandri E, et al. Rescue treatment for noninvasive ventilation failure due to interface intolerance with remifentanil analgosedation: a pilot study. Intensive Care Med. 2010;36:2060–5. doi:10.1007/s00134-010-2026-y.
11. Constantin JM, Schneider E, Cayot-Constantin S, et al. Remifentanil-based sedation to treat noninvasive ventilation failure: a preliminary study. Intensive Care Med. 2007;33:82–7.
12. Huang Z, Chen YS, Yang ZL, et al. Dexmedetomidine versus midazolam for the sedation of patients with non-invasive ventilation failure. Intern Med. 2012;51:2299–305.
13. Devlin JW, Al-Qadheeb NS, Chi A, et al. Efficacy and safety of early dexmedetomidine during noninvasive ventilation for patients with acute respiratory failure: a randomized, double-blind, placebo-controlled pilot study. Chest. 2014;145:1204–12.
14. Clouzeau B, Bui HN, Guilhon E, et al. Fiberoptic bronchoscopy under noninvasive ventilation and propofol target-controlled infusion in hypoxemic patients. Intensive Care Med. 2011; 37(12):1969–75. doi:10.1007/s00134-011-2375-1.

Use of Noninvasive Ventilation in the Course of Extracorporeal Membrane Oxygenation

73

Adriano Peris, Maria Cristina Cozzolino, and Morena Ferraro

Contents

Abbreviations

ARDS	Acute respiratory distress syndrome
COPD	Chronic obstructive pulmonary disease
$ECCO_2R$	Extracorporeal CO_2 Removal
ECMO	Extracorporeal membrane oxygenation
IMV	Invasive mechanical ventilation
NIV	Noninvasive ventilation

73.1 Introduction

Over the years, the therapeutic approach to respiratory failure in its various forms was based on a mechanistic approach. The most important innovation was the replacement of natural ventilation controlled by the negative pressure of the pleura

A. Peris (✉) • M.C. Cozzolino • M. Ferraro
Emergency and TRauma ICU-Regional ECMO Referral Center,
Careggi Teaching Hospital-Florence (ITA), Florence, Italy
e-mail: perisa@aou-careggi.toscana.it

A.M. Esquinas (ed.), *Noninvasive Mechanical Ventilation: Theory, Equipment, and Clinical Applications*, DOI 10.1007/978-3-319-21653-9_73

with a positive pressure induced by an external device that is still based on the biomechanical principles of more than 50 years ago. Invasive mechanical ventilation (IMV), which is technologically more advanced in its expression, requires the transfer of a flow of gas at positive pressure at the level of the carina. This type of ventilation is optimized in the presence of a complete adaptation of the patient and a nonoffensive ventilation mode, meeting the needs of the lung-chest wall system, using triggers and automatic detection of compliance.

Noninvasive mask ventilation is still included in the initial stages of anesthesia and is considered to be preparatory ventilation in conditions of respiratory failure awaiting definitive clinical decisions, such as tracheal intubation, or optimization of extrapulmonary physiological parameters that might prevent intubation. Clinical studies have established that it is possible to continue without intubation, maintaining positive ventilation even for prolonged periods of time, by exploiting the recruitability of lung areas to low ventilation-perfusion ratio and contextually maintaining a gas flow for the CO_2 wash-out. In this new setting, there is little new knowledge about the physiology of positive pressure ventilation. The skills of the operators have had to gradually be oriented to the appropriate choice of sedation techniques, optimization of cardiocirculatory function, and physiotherapy. Widespread use of noninvasive ventilation (NIV) has stimulated clinicians to improve the capability to anticipate the conditions of low compliance with NIV treatment, thus preventing hypoxia and acidosis, both of which synergistically lead to emergency intubation and hinder the subsequent recovery of the lung.

The limit of a system of this type, with, on the one hand, a perfectly working device (a ventilator) and, on the other, a patient who is tolerant and perfectly adapted to the ventilation, is that it is unstable system. In acute conditions, NIV requires the reversibility of the pathophysiological process underlying the respiratory failure, and therefore its stability is time correlated.

The extension of the therapeutic window is especially useful to avoid tracheal intubation, which is an important morbidity factor. Especially in patients at high infectious risk, prevention of bacterial colonization and multidrug resistance are decisive factors for the prevention of mortality and can even contribute to the completion of therapeutic programs such as lung transplantation. In some centers where extracorporeal membrane oxygenation (ECMO) is routinely applied in patients who are candidates for lung transplant or in the presence of acute respiratory distress syndrome (ARDS) refractory to treatment, protocols have been developed that apply NIV associated with ECMO. The attractive hypothesis of this association is essentially based on the possibility of ensuring ventilation without intubation even for long periods, and consequently avoiding prolonged use of sedative drugs and opioids. With this approach, it is possible to maintain the patient's ability to participate in the ventilation and physiotherapy with beneficial effects on the recovery phase. Maintaining NIV is also facilitated, in theory, by the use of ECMO, thanks to the stability of oxygenation, carbon dioxide blood content, and blood pH, preventing phases of distress that can lead to NIV failure and subsequent invasive ventilation.

73.2 Discussion and Analysis

ECMO is an important therapeutic strategy that was developed and first used over 40 years ago to support an adult patient with refractory respiratory failure. Recent evidence suggests that ECMO may positively impact survival in adult patients with refractory respiratory failure [1]. Over the past decades, the use of extracorporeal respiratory support has increased and different modalities have been described. Veno-venous ECMO may be initiated as a treatment strategy for patients with severe acute respiratory failure, including ARDS. Additionally, partial extracorporeal support systems have been suggested for less severe respiratory failure. These devices prevalently remove carbon dioxide from blood, providing limited oxygenation. For a long time, the approach of replacing the failing native lung with an artificial organ was used as a salvage therapy for patients with profound gas-exchange abnormalities despite IMV. The advantages of the technique are well established, but there are also well-known disadvantages, such as an increased risk for nosocomial pneumonia, neurological disorders associated with prolonged analog-sedation, and activation of inflammation, leading to ventilator-induced lung injury [2].

In the last decade, some groups have began to consider ECMO as an alternative to IMV in selected groups of patients; this approach is frequently called "awake ECMO." In theory, several activities could play a positive role during awake ECMO, such as spontaneous feeding, physiotherapy, and interaction with relatives and medical staff. An important factor is the preservation of diaphragm function; furthermore, the well-known detrimental effects of IMV (barotrauma, pneumothorax, decrease in cardiac output, ventilation-associated pneumonia, and ventilator-associated lung injury) can be avoided [3].

During awake ECMO, different devices for supplementary oxygen delivery can be used, ranging from oxygen facial mask to NIV. The use of ventilatory support such as continuous positive airway pressure/NIV could be necessary to exploit residual oxygenation function of the native lung or to prevent progressive lung derecruitment.

73.2.1 Application Fields

The most important indication for awake ECMO is as a bridge to lung transplantation, to avoid muscle deconditioning, neuromuscular complications, and hospital-acquired infections caused by intubation and sedation. Numerous centers have reported the strategy of employing ECMO as a bridge to lung transplantation without invasive ventilation. Fuehner et al. [4] evaluated the outcomes of patients treated with the awake ECMO strategy as a bridge to transplantation. Patients in the awake ECMO group required shorter postoperative IMV and showed a trend toward a shorter postoperative hospital stay. Crotti et al. [5] found that patients who maintain spontaneous breathing on NIV during ECMO bridging have a lower morbidity before and after lung transplantation.

Another application field for NIV and "awake extracorporeal support" is for the treatment of patients with severe chronic obstructive pulmonary disease (COPD).

For patients experiencing acute respiratory failure due to a severe exacerbation of COPD, NIV has been shown to significantly reduce mortality and hospital length of stay compared with respiratory support with IMV. Lower mortality has been reported in patients successfully treated with NIV compared with IMV, and NIV has thus become a standard of care in severe exacerbation of COPD [6]. Despite continued improvements in NIV administration, refractory hypercapnia and hypercapnic acidosis necessitate IMV. On the other hand, particularly in this group of patients, the use of IMV frequently leads to lung damage and concomitant complications, such as pneumothorax and pneumomediastinum. This suggests that any technique that increases the avoidance of IMV in severe COPD exacerbation is likely to be of clinical benefit.

The use of extracorporeal CO_2 removal ($ECCO_2R$) has been reported in acute exacerbations of COPD. This is a strategy that could reduce the requirement of IMV. In the study of Kluge et al. [7], 21 patients treated with partial $ECCO_2R$, at the point of failing support with NIV were compared retrospectively with patients who had been treated conventionally with IMV after failing NIV. The results of this study showed that 90 % of the patients treated with $ECCO_2R$ did not require intubation and invasive respiratory support. Moreover, this group showed a trend toward reduced length of hospital stay.

A novel concept is the use of awake ECMO in patients with ARDS to avoid the complications of invasive ventilation. Wiesner et al. [8] reported a single case of awake ECMO in a 26-year-old woman with ARDS following septic shock who failed NIV and refused invasive ventilation. The patient fully recovered and was discharged from the hospital 8 days after decannulation. Hoeper et al. [9] described six cases of ARDS treated with ECMO instead IMV; the patients suffered from isolated lung failure and most were immunocompromised, potentially obtaining particular benefit from avoiding endotracheal intubation. Of course this strategy will not replace IMV as the standard ARDS treatment, but it may become a feasible alternative in carefully selected patients in which one might consider the use of ECMO during NIV treatment.

Conclusions

NIV is now a widespread therapeutic approach in patients with several causes of respiratory failure. Referral centers for respiratory failure and ARDS treatment should develop procedures that can be applied in patients needing respiratory support with the purpose of preventing intubation. Currently, the most intuitive ECMO application in cooperative patient is the preemptive treatment of patients affected by end-stage lung disease, particularly cystic fibrosis, awaiting lung transplant. In the last 5 years, respiratory failure associated with flu outbreaks, especially the influenza A (H1N1) pandemic flu, has increased the use of ECMO, leading to better knowledge of this therapeutic approach in ARDS patients. Some centers have extended the use of extracorporeal support in patients with ARDS initially treated with NIV. Although the use of awake ECMO in acute hypoxic respiratory failure is still under investigation and the subject of debate, considering the safety of NIV treatment during ECMO, this approach should be implemented through specific clinical procedures as a feasible therapeutic strategy in selected patients with ARDS.

The main limiting factor to this approach is represented by the late involvement of ECMO referral centers in the treatment of patients with ARDS, usually after the failure of conventional treatment. A future approach, based on early involvement of experienced centers during the earliest stages of respiratory failure, can provide the opportunity to increase the number of patients treated with the awake ECMO strategy. Of course, the use of NIV treatment in patients undergoing extracorporeal support, even with the low blood-flow technique ($ECCO_2R$), should be restricted to selected centers highly experience in extracorporeal treatment.

Key Major Recommendations

- Use the awake ECMO strategy in patients awaiting lung transplant.
- Implement specific clinical procedures of NIV treatment during ECMO support in patients with ARDS.
- Involve referral ECMO centers early in the treatment of patients with ARDS, using awake ECMO as the main target and indicator of efficacy.
- ECMO should be restricted to selected centers that are highly experienced in extracorporeal treatment.

References

1. Patroniti N, Zangrillo A, Pappalardo F, et al. The Italian ECMO network experience during the 2009 influenza A(H1N1) pandemic: preparation for severe respiratory emergency outbreaks. Intensive Care Med. 2011;37(9):1447–57.
2. Schmidt M, Pellegrino V, Combes A, et al. Mechanical ventilation during extracorporeal membrane oxygenation. Crit Care. 2014;18(1):203.
3. Nosotti M, Rosso L, Tosi D, et al. Extracorporeal membrane oxygenation with spontaneous breathing as a bridge to lung transplantation. Interact Cardiovasc Thorac Surg. 2013;16(1):55–9.
4. Fuehner T, Kuehn C, Hadem J, et al. Extracorporeal membrane oxygenation in awake patients as bridge to lung transplantation. Am J Respir Crit Care Med. 2012;185(7):763–8.
5. Crotti S, Iotti GA, Lissoni A, et al. Organ allocation waiting time during extracorporeal bridge to lung transplant affects outcomes. Chest. 2013;144(3):1018–25.
6. Chandra D, Stamm JA, Taylor B. Outcomes of noninvasive ventilation for acute exacerbations of chronic obstructive pulmonary disease in the United States, 1998–2008. Am J Respir Crit Care Med. 2012;185(2):152–9.
7. Kluge S, Braune SA, Engel M, et al. Avoiding invasive mechanical ventilation by extracorporeal carbon dioxide removal in patients failing noninvasive ventilation. Intensive Care Med. 2012;38(10):1632–9.
8. Wiesner O, Hadem J, Sommer W, et al. Extracorporeal membrane oxygenation in a nonintubated patient with acute respiratory distress syndrome. Eur Respir J. 2012;40(5):1296–8.
9. Hoeper MM, Wiesner O, Hadem J, et al. Extracorporeal membrane oxygenation instead of invasive mechanical ventilation in patients with acute respiratory distress syndrome. Intensive Care Med. 2013;39(11):2056–7.

Noninvasive Ventilation Outside the ICU

74

Laura Pasin, Pasquale Nardelli, and Alessandro Belletti

Contents

Abbreviations

AHRF	Acute hypoxemic respiratory failure
ALI	Acute lung injury
ARDS	Acute respiratory distress syndrome
ARF	Acute respiratory failure
COPD	Chronic obstructive pulmonary disease
ICU	Intensive care unit
NIV	Noninvasive ventilation

L. Pasin, MD (✉) • P. Nardelli, MD • A. Belletti, MD
Department of Anesthesia and Intensive Care, IRCCS San Raffaele Hospital, Via Olgettina 60, Milan 20132, Italy
e-mail: pasin.laura@hsr.it; nardelli.pasquale@gmail.com; belletti.ale@gmail.com

A.M. Esquinas (ed.), *Noninvasive Mechanical Ventilation: Theory, Equipment, and Clinical Applications*, DOI 10.1007/978-3-319-21653-9_74

74.1 Introduction

The use of noninvasive ventilation (NIV) for the treatment of patients with acute respiratory failure (ARF) has markedly increased in the last decades. Currently, NIV can be considered the first-choice therapy in the treatment cardiogenic pulmonary edema, chronic obstructive pulmonary disease (COPD) exacerbations, and acute hypoxemic respiratory failure (AHRF), especially in immunocompromised patients. In addition to these well-established indications, NIV is also commonly used in conditions in which response to NIV is less clear, including asthma, chronic neuromuscular and neurologic diseases, and pneumonia in non-immunocompromised patients. The increasing knowledge of NIV efficacy and physicians' familiarity with managing this technique have been accompanied by a progressive reduction of the number of available intensive care unit (ICU) beds worldwide. Therefore, as confirmed by a recent international web-based survey, the use of NIV in general wards is common and growing [1, 2]. In fact the percentage of hospitals using NIV in general wards was reported to have increased from 10 % in 2005 [3] to 66 % in 2014 [1].

74.2 Discussion and Analysis

74.2.1 Evidence of NIV Success

According to published evidence, NIV treatment is supported by a large number of randomized clinical trials showing a statistically significant mortality reduction in patients affected by ARF in different contexts, such as weaning from invasive mechanical ventilation, respiratory acidosis, acute exacerbation of COPD, and AHRF [4].

Strong evidence from meta-analyses of randomized clinical trials has proved that the addition of NIV to standard medical care improves the outcome of patients with acute cardiogenic pulmonary edema or COPD exacerbation [5, 6]. Nonetheless, NIV can be used to support patients with ARF from other etiologies. In fact, an international web-based survey [1] showed that, worldwide, other frequent causes of ARF commonly treated by NIV outside the ICU are neuromuscular diseases, postoperative ARF, and pneumonia in immunocompromised patients. Moreover, NIV is often prescribed in non-immunocompromised patients with pneumonia, in asthma and thoracic trauma, or as a palliative treatment.

However, while the effectiveness of NIV in avoiding the need for endotracheal intubation and reducing related mortality in patients with AHRF has been widely supported in recent decades, the efficacy of NIV in AHRF that is not related to COPD or acute pulmonary edema is debated. Currently, controversies still exist regarding NIV application in community-acquired pneumonia, acute asthma, post-extubation respiratory failure, chest trauma, rapidly progressive neurological diseases, acute lung injury (ALI), and acute respiratory distress syndrome (ARDS).

Table 74.1 Contraindications to NIV application

Absolute:
Inability to protect airways
Significantly altered mental status
Inability to cooperate with wearing and fitting mask
Apnea
Respiratory arrest
Shock
Pneumothorax
Recent facial fractures
Recent esophageal, laryngeal, or gastric surgery
Rapid clinical deterioration
Inadequate staff to closely monitor the patients in case of deterioration
Relative:
Significant chest trauma
Nausea and vomiting
Agitation
Cardiac arrhythmias
Cardiac ischemia or acute myocardial infarction

Patients with community-acquired pneumonia treated with NIV were often associated with poor outcome in the literature. However, more recent studies reported better outcomes in patients treated with NIV in this context [8]. Therefore, large, randomized clinical trials are needed to confirm these recent, positive findings. On the contrary, recent reviews on the use of NIV in acute asthma concluded that there is not enough evidence to support the use of NIV in this setting and that medical treatment alone may usually be effective [7].

Regarding post-extubation respiratory failure, no trials have proved the benefit of NIV treatment in ARF during the first 48–72 h after extubation. Furthermore, one multicenter randomized clinical trial even found an increased mortality rate in the group of patients treated with NIV, probably due to delayed reintubation. As a result, current guidelines suggest that NIV should not be routinely used in patients who develop post-extubation respiratory failure [9].

Current evidence does not support the routine use of NIV in patients with ALI/ARDS and chest trauma because of lack of well-designed randomized clinical trials [8, 10].

74.2.2 Optimal Use of Noninvasive Ventilation

Regardless the underlying cause of ARF and the above-discussed limitations of NIV application, patients with exclusion criteria for NIV should be carefully identified. Absolute and relative contraindications to NIV are presented in Table 74.1.

The identification of the right patients likely to benefit from NIV therapy can be considered the key to NIV success outside ICU, along with the recognition of NIV failure and avoiding delayed intubation when indicated. However, it is not always easy to identify which patients will initially benefit from treatment. Usually, subjects likely to fail NIV are older, with a lower level of consciousness, more severe hypoxia, tachypnea, and respiratory acidosis. Moreover, clinical signs that can be unclear on presentation generally become more definitively predictive of NIV failure if they persist after 2 h of starting NIV [11, 12].

No current guidelines suggest the use of one specific interface among the others, nor one mode of noninvasive positive-pressure ventilation, a model of ventilator, or an optimal triggering for NIV application [9]. Nonetheless available evidence on patients with ARF suggests that the first choice of interface should be the oronasal mask or full face mask. Different interfaces should be available in case of patient intolerance to the oronasal mask or full face mask, or if complications such as facial cutaneous lesions occur.

Conclusions

The use of NIV in general wards is common and growing worldwide. Strong published evidence has proved that the addition of NIV to standard care improves outcomes of patients with COPD exacerbation or acute cardiogenic pulmonary edema. Controversies still exist regarding NIV application in conditions in which response to NIV is less clear, such as community-acquired pneumonia, acute asthma, post-extubation respiratory failure, chest trauma, rapidly progressive neurological diseases, ALI, and ARDS. Therefore large, well-designed, randomized clinical trials are needed in these settings. Moreover, definitive and specific guidelines and protocols for the management of NIV in the general ward are warranted.

Key Major Recommendations

- The use of NIV outside ICU should be encouraged, expecially in patients with COPD exacerbation or acute cardiogenic pulmonary edema.
- Patients with exclusion criteria for NIV should be carefully identified.
- Early recognition of NIV failure, avoiding delayed intubation when indicated is one of the keypoint of NIV success outside ICU.
- The first choice interface should be the oronasal mask or the full face mask but different interfaces should be always available in case of patients' intolerance.
- Improvement in staff training and introduction of standardized protocols could help making NIV safer and more common when applied in general non-monitored wards.

References

1. Cabrini L, Esquinas A, Pasin L, Nardelli P, Frati E, Pintaudi M, Matos P, Landoni G, Zangrillo A. An international survey on noninvasive ventilation use for acute respiratory failure in general non-monitored wards. Respir Care. 2015;60(4):586–92. doi: 10.4187/respcare.03593.
2. Cabrini L, Antonelli M, Savoia G, Landriscina M. Non-invasive ventilation outside of the intensive care unit: an Italian survey. Minerva Anestesiol. 2011;77(3):313–22.
3. Burns KE, Sinuff T, Adhikari NK, Meade MO, Heels-Ansdell D, Martin CM, Cook DJ. Bilevel positive pressure ventilation for acute respiratory failure: survey of Ontario practice. Crit Care Med. 2005;33(7):1477–83.
4. Landoni G, Comis M, Conte M, Finco G, Mucchetti M, Paternoster G, Pisano A, Ruggeri L, Alvaro G, Angelone M, Bergonzi PC, Bocchino S, Borghi G, Bove T, Buscaglia G, Cabrini L, Callegher L, Caramelli F, Colombo S, Corno L, Del Sarto P, Feltracco P, Forti A, Ganzaroli M, Greco M, Guarracino F, Lembo R, Lobreglio R, Meroni R, Monaco F, Musu M, Pala G, Pasin L, Pieri M, Pisarra S, Ponticelli G, Roasio A, Santini F, Silvetti S, Székely A, Zambon M, Zucchetti MC, Zangrillo A, Bellomo R. Mortality in Multicenter Critical Care Trials: An Analysis of Interventions With a Significant Effect. Crit Care Med. 2015;43(8):1559–68. doi: 10.1097/CCM.0000000000000974.
5. Lightowler JV, Wedzicha JA, Elliott MW, Ram FS. Noninvasive positive pressure ventilation to treat respiratory failure resulting from exacerbations of chronic obstructive pulmonary disease: Cochrane systematic review and meta-analysis. BMJ. 2003;326:185–9. [PMC free article] [PubMed]
6. Masip J, Roque M, Sánchez B, Fernández R, Subirana M, Expósito J. Noninvasive ventilation in acute cardiogenic pulmonary edema. Systematic review and meta-analysis. JAMA. 2005; 294:3124–30.
7. Lim WJ, Mohammed Akram R, Carson KV, Mysore S, Labiszewski NA, Wedzicha JA, Rowe BH, Smith BJ. Non-invasive positive pressure ventilation for treatment of respiratory failure due to severe acute exacerbations of asthma. Cochrane Database Syst Rev. 2012;12:CD004360. doi: 10.1002/14651858.CD004360.pub4.
8. Ferrer M, Torres A. Noninvasive ventilation for acute respiratory failure. Curr Opin Crit Care. 2015;21(1):1–6. doi:10.1097/MCC.0000000000000173.
9. Keenan SP, Sinuff T, Burns K, Canadian Critical Care Trials Group/Canadian Critical Care Society Noninvasive Ventilation Guidelines Group, et al. Clinical practice guidelines for the use of noninvasive positive-pressure ventilation and noninvasive continuous positive airway pressure in the acute care setting. CMAJ. 2011;183(3):E195–214.
10. Karcz MK, Papadakos PJ. Noninvasive ventilation in trauma. World J Crit Care Med. 2015;4(1):47–54. doi:10.5492/wjccm.v4.i1.47. eCollection 2015.
11. Hill NS. Where should noninvasive ventilation be delivered? Respir Care. 2009;54(1):62–70.
12. Confalonieri M, Garuti G, Cattaruzza MS, Osborn JF, Antonelli M, Conti G, et al. A chart of failure risk for noninvasive ventilation in patients with COPD exacerbation. Eur Respir J. 2005;25(2):348–55.

Part IX

Non Invasive Ventilation in Sleep Medicine

Anatomical, Physical, and Psychological Factors of NIV Interfaces

75

Zoltan Tomori, Viliam Donic, Pavol Torok, and Josef Firment

Contents

Abbreviations

AHI	Apnea hypopnea index
ARDS	Adult respiratory distress syndrome
AspR	Aspiration reflex
CPAP	Continuous positive airway pressure
e-sigh	Extended sigh

Z. Tomori (✉) • V. Donic
Department of Human Physiology, Faculty of Medicine, Safarik University, Kosice, Slovak Republic
e-mail: zoltan.tomori@upjs.sk

P. Torok
Faculty of Medicine, Clinic of Anesthesiology and Intensive Medicine, East-Slovakian Institute of Heart and Vascular Diseases, Safarik University, Kosice, Slovak Republic

J. Firment
Faculty of Medicine, Clinic of Anesthesiology and Intensive Medicine, University PJ Safarik, Kosice, Slovakia

A.M. Esquinas (ed.), *Noninvasive Mechanical Ventilation: Theory, Equipment, and Clinical Applications*, DOI 10.1007/978-3-319-21653-9_75

CR	Cough reflex
EEG	Electroencephalogram
EMG	Electromyogram
ExpR	Expiration reflex
NIPPV	Noninvasive positive pressure ventilation
NIV	Noninvasive ventilation
Pcrit	Critical pressure
PEEP	Positive end-expiratory pressure
SAHS	Sleep apnea hypopnea syndrome
SDB	Sleep-disordered breathing
TI	Inspiratory time
UA	Upper airways
UANP	Upper airway negative pressure

75.1 Introduction

75.1.1 Anatomical and Physical Factors of NIV Interfaces

The upper airways (UA), as the crossroads of the respiratory and gastrointestinal systems, have a valvular function, *serving respiration* in addition to providing swallowing and other gastrointestinal functions, as well as speech, psychological, and other activities. The function and mechanisms of the UA are complex, largely depending on the balance of two main factors: *anatomically imposed mechanical loads* (one-third of cases) and *neuromuscular factors* (two-thirds of cases). *Structural anatomical changes* include hypertrophy of tonsils, adenoid vegetations in children, retrognathia, and various craniofacial variations, as well as increased fatty tissue deposition around the pharynx and submucosal edema, narrowing the pharyngeal lumen. *The neuromuscular factors* are realized by different sphincter mechanisms and various airway reflexes. The upper, medial, and lower pharyngeal constrictors represent the sphincters. Pharyngeal dilation results from phasic activation of M. genioglossus (GG), supported by tonic contraction of the tensor palatini.

75.1.2 Analysis of the NIV Effects and Their Comparison to Airway Reflexes

The effect of *breathing through a tracheal tube* and/or *the UA* on the respiratory drive was analyzed in dogs [2]. A tracheal tube containing a fenestration allowed communication also with the UA, and could differentiate the reflex effect of *the negative or positive pressure, acting either from the lower or upper airways. After tracheal occlusion with closed fenestration*, the inspiratory time (TI) of both the increasing diaphragmal electromyogram (EMG) activity and the decreasing tracheal pressure was prolonged during wakefulness and sleep, weakening *the inhibitory effect of lung inflation, caused by the Hering-Breuer inflation reflex. After tracheal and nasal occlusion*, the opening of fenestration *allowed transmission of negative intrathoracic pressure but not the flow to the UA*. Therefore, TI was further prolonged, but the change was smaller, indicating an additional but weaker inhibitory effect from the UA receptors. In addition, the *UA negative pressure reflexively activated the dilatory GG muscle* during both wakefulness and sleep (rapid eye movement and non-rapid eye movement). Therefore, there was *no collapse of the UA* and the tracheal and mouth pressure practically did not differ [2]. In anesthetized rats, a negative pressure (> −20 cmH_2O) in the UA *increased the activity of UA muscle* and changed the thoracic respiratory outflow. This stabilized the UA and minimized the collapsing stress to which it is subjected during inspiration. In the response to UA transmural pressure changes, the *tongue retractor and pharyngeal constrictor muscles* also play a role in keeping the UA patent. After a tracheal closure during expiration, the next inspiration was postponed, imitating central sleep apnea [3].

Noninvasive intermittent positive pressure ventilation (NIPPV) with 4 cmH_2O in a nonsedated neonatal lamb through a tracheostomy evoked active glottal narrowing, resulting from a decrease in the crico-thyroidal (CT) dilator and increase in the thyro-arytenoideus (TA) constrictor EMG in response to stimulation of tracheo-broncho-pulmonary receptors but not from the upper airways. However, similar positive pressure applied to the totally isolated UA did not evoke laryngoconstriction, but during the inspiratory phase in the lamb, breathing though a tracheotomy, there was an increase of airway pressure in the mask and an increased activation of CT-dilator muscle [6]. Vocal cord adduction was induced in cats by application of negative pressure to lower airways and even more strongly from the subglottal area [7]. These seemingly contradictory results can be explained partly by use of different conditions: various animal species compared with humans, premedication, anesthesia, possible damage of laryngeal nerve supply during vagotomy, and sleep or wakefulness. However, they are in agreement with the effect of two distinct airway reflexes: *the sniff- and gasp-like aspiration reflex* (AspR), characterized by *deep inspiration and laryngo-dilation*, elicited from the *naso- and oro- pharynx,* and the so-called *expiration reflex* (ExpR), manifesting with *laryngo-constriction and prompt expiration*, evoked from the larynx and lower airways by mechanical contact and by negative or positive pressure stimulation [4].

UA negative pressure (UANP) influences the diaphragmal inspiratory activity not only in animals *but also in infants.* Compared with separate occlusion of lower airways, brief occlusion of upper and lower airways reduced the maximum airway pressure and the slope of airflow rate with a threshold of suction pressure −4 cmH_2O and latency around 0.12 s, suggesting that *UA suction reflexively inhibits the thoracic inspiratory muscles* [5].

75.2 Assessment of UA Resistance: UA Patency/Collapsibility

The UANP reflex, with afferents in the trigeminal, glossopharyngeal, and superior laryngeal nerves, can modify the lumen of UA by activation of dilatory muscles (GG and tensor palatini), as well as the upper, medial, and lower constrictors [6, 7].

The valvular function of the UA influences both the *airway patency* (measured by pharyngeal resistance) and the *anatomical airway narrowing/collapsibility* (reflected by necessary positive end-expiratory pressure) observed in patients with *severe sleep apnea hypopnea syndrome* (SAHS), with apnea hypopnea index 75/h. The UANP, in addition to primary activation, also induces *a secondary inhibition of GG muscle activity* to prevent aspiration by allowing UA collapsibility together with modification of diaphragmal activity.

75.3 Discussion

Full face masks are used more frequently in NIV in acute cases to avoid analgo-sedation and prevent laryngeal swelling caused by intubation [8, 9]. NIV can be *applied in clinical wards 24 h a day*, with a possibility of gradual weaning. *In chronic conditions, use of a nasal mask is preferred*, for less static dead space and fewer skin irritations and claustrophobic effects, and because it allows better comfort for eating, drinking, expectoration, and communication [10, 11]. Nasal pillows or plugs and mouthpieces are used less often [1].

75.3.1 Valvular Function of UA during Sleep

The valvular function of UA changes significantly during sleep, particularly in patients with *sleep-disordered breathing* (SDB) manifested by snoring. In adult patients with SAHS, there is a *collapse of the UA,* which occurs at low negative and even positive inspiratory airway pressures. The critical pressure (*Pcrit*) separating SAHS patients from healthy subjects is *–5 cmH2O*. The occlusion of the UA is caused *by passive mechanical loads in one-third* of cases and by active neuromuscular compensation in *two-thirds*. However, closing of the UA also develops at less negative Pcrit in children with mild SDB, compared with controls, indicating a higher pharyngeal collapsibility. The lowest positive nasal pressure allowing effective flow at maintained airway patency was tested. The mean value of this so-called *flow-dependent positive airway pressure* in SAHS patients was 6.6 ± 1.2 cmH_2O. The *closing Pcrit* in SAHS patients is less negative than the opening pressure, and both change dynamically throughout the respiratory cycle and in various stages of sleep, as well as in different body positions during sleep.

A change of valvular system activity allows stimulation of various regions of the airways during NIV, resulting in different effects. Animal experiments indicated that mechanical and other methods of stimulation of the upper and lower airways evokes three different airway reflexes. *Stimulation of the oro- and nasopharynx* evokes *strong inspiratory effort* (gasp or sniff-like aspiration reflex, or AspR), caused by reflex activation of the brainstem inspiratory generator. A similar reaction can also be evoked *by a voluntary sniff.* On the contrary, *stimulation of the larynx evokes strong expiratory effort* (expiration reflex, or ExpR), as a result of reflex activation of the brainstem expiratory generator. Stimulation of the lower airways

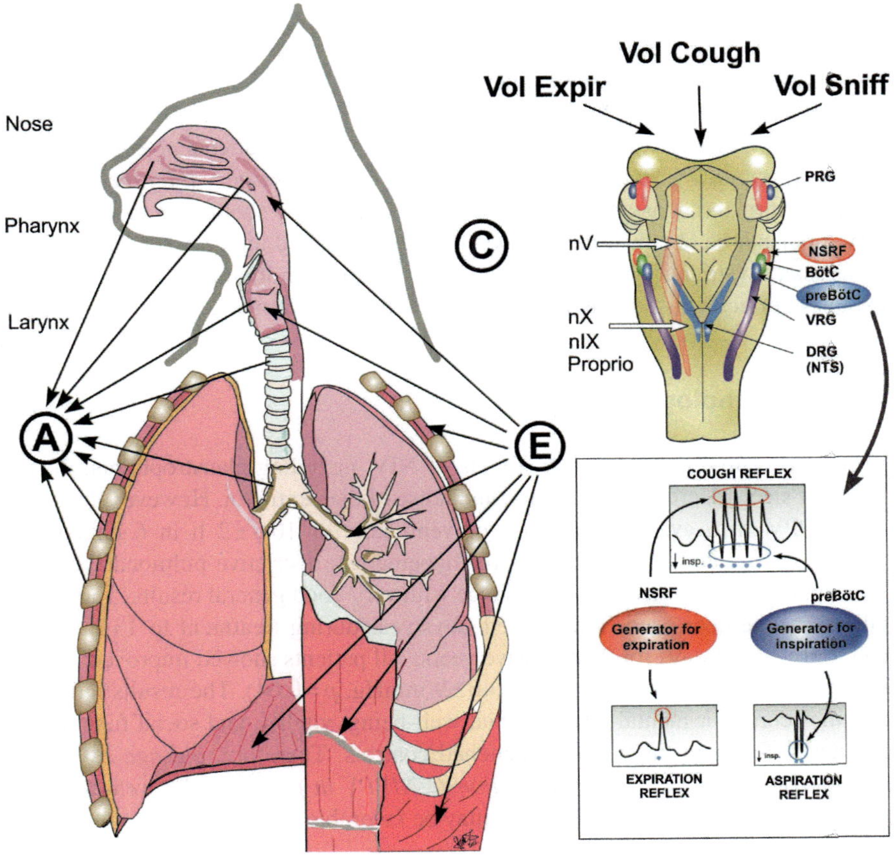

Fig. 75.1 Reflex arch indicating the afferent (*A*), central (*C*), and efferent (*E*) components of the AspR, ExpR, and cough reflex and their voluntary counterparts (From Tomori et al. [4])

evokes the *cough reflex, characterized by deep inspiration, followed by rapid and strong expiratory effort, caused by reflex activation of the inspiratory and followed subsequently by the expiratory generator*. [4, 12–15] The afferent (A), central (C), and efferent (E) parts of these three airway reflexes are indicated in Fig. 75.1.

Obesity and craniofacial abnormalities significantly influence the collapsibility of upper airways in patients with SDB. On the other hand, *GG muscle contraction evoked by electrical stimulation increased the cross-sectional area of both the velopharynx and nasopharynx* and decreased the critical pressure from 1.2 ± 3.3 to −0.7 ± 3.8 cmH_2O without affecting pharyngeal stiffness in patients with SDB. *Sitting posture* and *sniffing position decreases the collapsibility of passive pharynx in patients*. UA anatomic loads in combination with mechanical trauma, caused by snoring and apneic episodes, can initiate an inflammatory process. This can lead to a series of *ultrastructural changes*, aggravating neuromechanical defects manifesting in SAHS. In *adult respiratory distress syndrome* (ARDS), there is a decrease of alveolar volume (alveolar derecruitment), where continuous positive airway pressure (CPAP) improves oxygenation. A recruitment maneuver with *extended sigh* (e-sigh), using CPAP with high values (>40 cmH_2O) for 40 min, can be adapted to the patient according to flow volume curves and positive end-expiratory pressure (PEEP) >15 cmH_2O. Such treatment also evokes in most patients *alveolar recruitment and increase in tidal volume* and *better cardiorespiratory tolerance.* Similar high pressure and constantly increased PEEP, induced by shortening of the expiratory time, can be obtained using *a patented device* called the *ParaVent* from Kalas (Povazska Bystrica, Slovakia), providing alveolar recruitment in addition to an expulsive effect adjustable in patients with pulmonary edema [13].

75.3.2 Psychological Factors

There are many unpleasant side effects of NIV, including claustrophobia, disturbance of sleep, decrease of mobility, and noise of the ventilator. However, domiciliary NIPPV with average daily use of ventilator for 10.5 ± 2 h in 6 patients of 79 ± 3 years treated 31 ± 17 months for hypercapnic restrictive-pulmonary disease indicated good tolerance and compliance with very good general results. The hospitalization rate decreased from 40 ± 31 days/year during treatment to 13 ± 14 days and to 0.8+−0.4 days for 2 successive years. All patients showed improved arterial blood gases (from $PaCO_2$ 66 ± 10 to 46 ± 9 mmHg, $p = 0.04$). The results indicated that the scores for mental health, social well-being, vitality, and social functioning did not differ from those of age-matched controls. Therefore, *old age cannot be considered per se as a contraindication to NIPPV in patients with well-accepted indications*, and the cost/benefit ratio may be favorable.

Conclusion

Anatomical, physical, and psychological factors provide many advantages for successful application of NIV, indicated and performed according to guidelines, and including NIPPV in the older population. Modification of NIV using larger volume has therapeutic use, or when applied preferentially to upper or lower airways through provocation of valvular function, it also has a reflex effect, typical of the region involved.

Key Major Recommendations

Benefits of the chapter are proposals for non-invasive ventilation using a mask for management of respiratory failure in patients:

- Minimalizing leakage around the mask with a tight fit, preventing interface that does not cause side effect.
- Using a comfortable interface that does not cause side effects.
- Providing a compensation for leakage with increased volume or pressure.

The aim of successful NIV is to maximize ventilation and improve patient-ventilator synchrony[1].

References

1. Elliott MW. The interface: crucial for successful noninvasive ventilation. Eur Respir J. 2004;23:7–8.
2. Eastwood PR, Curran AK, Smith CA, et al. Effect of upper airway negative pressure on inspiratory drive during sleep. J Appl Physiol. 1998;84:1063–75.
3. Ryan S, Mc Nicholas WT, Regan RG, et al. Reflex respiratory response to changes in upper airway pressure in the anaesthetized rat. J Physiol. 2001;537:251–65.
4. Tomori Z, Donic V, Benacka R, et al. Reversal of functional disorders by aspiration, expiration, and cough reflexes and their voluntary counterparts. Front Respir Physiol. 2012; article 00467: 1–14. doi: 10.3389/fphys.2012.
5. Thach BT, Shaft GL, Pickens DL, et al. Influence of upper airway negative pressure reflex on response to airway occlusion in sleeping infants. J Appl Physiol. 1989;67:749–55.
6. Horner RL, Innes JA, Holden HB, et al. Afferent pathway(s) for pharyngeal dilatory reflex to negative pressure in man: a study of upper airway anaesthesia. J Physiol. 1991;436:31–44.
7. Patil SP, Schneider H, Marx JJ, et al. Neuro mechanical control of upper airway patency during sleep. Appl Physiol. 2007;102:547–56.
8. Eckert DJ, McEvoy RD, George KE, et al. Genioglossus reflex inhibition to upper-airway negative pressure stimuli during wakefulness and sleep in healthy males. J Physiol. 2007;582: 1193–205.
9. Horner RL. Contribution of passive mechanical loads and active neuromuscular compensation to upper airway collapsibility during sleep. J Appl Physiol. 2007;102:510–2.
10. Schwartz AR, Patil SP, Schneider H, et al. Modeling pathogenic mechanisms of upper airway function in the molecular age. Eur Respir J. 2008;32:255–8.
11. Constantin JM, Jaber S, Futier E, et al. Respiratory effects of different recruitment maneuvers in acute respiratory distress syndrome. Crit Care. 2008;12(2):R50. doi:10.1186/cc6869.
12. Tomori Z, Donic V. Influence of down regulation and up-regulation of cough using airway reflexes and breathing maneuvers: chapter 1. In: Esquinas AM, editor. Noninvasive ventilation in high-risk infections and mass casualty events. Wien: Springer; 2014. p. 3–6.
13. Donic V, Torok P, Tomori Z. Preventing the spread of aerosol infection during application of high-frequency jet ventilation by mask. In: Esquinas AM, editor. Noninvasive ventilation in high-risk infections and mass casualty events. Wien: Springer; 2014. p. 45–7.
14. Korpas J, Tomori Z. Cough and other respiratory reflexes. Karger Basel. 1979. p. 379.
15. Tomori Z, Donic V, Benacka R, Jakus J, Gresova S. Resuscitation and auto resuscitation by airway reflexes in animals. Cough. 2013;9(1):21. doi:10.1186/1745-9974-9-21.

Identification of Therapeutic CPAP for the Treatment of Obstructive Sleep Apnea: Key Major Topics and Clinical Implications

76

Oreste Marrone, Adriana Salvaggio, Anna Lo Bue, and Giuseppe Insalaco

Contents

Abbreviations

AASM	American Academy of Sleep Medicine
AHI	Apnea/hypopnea index
CPAP	Continuous positive airway pressure
OSA	Obstructive sleep apnea
REM	Rapid eye movement

O. Marrone, MD (✉) • A. Salvaggio, MD • A. Lo Bue, MD • G. Insalaco, MD
Italian National Research Council – Institute of Biomedicine and Molecular Immunology, Palermo, Italy
e-mail: marrone@ibim.cnr.it; salvaggio@ibim.cnr.it; annalobue@yahoo.it; insalaco@ibim.cnr.it

A.M. Esquinas (ed.), *Noninvasive Mechanical Ventilation: Theory, Equipment, and Clinical Applications*, DOI 10.1007/978-3-319-21653-9_76

76.1 Introduction

Continuous positive airway pressure (CPAP) counterbalances forces leading to upper airway narrowing or collapse during sleep and is the most widely used treatment for obstructive sleep apnea (OSA). In patients with OSA, progressively higher CPAP levels applied during sleep turn obstructive apneas into hypopneas, hypopneas into continuous inspiratory flow limitation, with or without snoring, and flow limitation into unobstructed breathing (Fig. 76.1). When breathing becomes unobstructed, "respiratory arousals," that is, arousals that may follow increased inspiratory efforts associated with obstructed breathing, are eliminated, while sleep becomes more stable and sleep cycles more regular, contributing to improvements in subjective sleep quality, daytime sleepiness, and quality of life usually observed after already few nights of CPAP application [1]. In addition, relief of upper airway obstruction is associated with resolution of intermittent hypoxemia and hemodynamic swings that accompany obstructive events, with a consequent reduction in long-term morbidity and mortality [2].

The objectives of OSA treatment are elimination of symptoms and of health risks related to upper airway obstruction during sleep. If treatment by CPAP is planned, patients must be previously instructed and adapted. These aspects are beyond the scope here. In this chapter, we will review procedures for choosing modalities to define therapeutic CPAP levels and will discuss their effectiveness. In fact, several methods may be adopted to identify which pressure must be prescribed to each patient, sometimes leading to different results. Today, however, according to European experts, the best procedures to establish the effective CPAP level remain unknown [3].

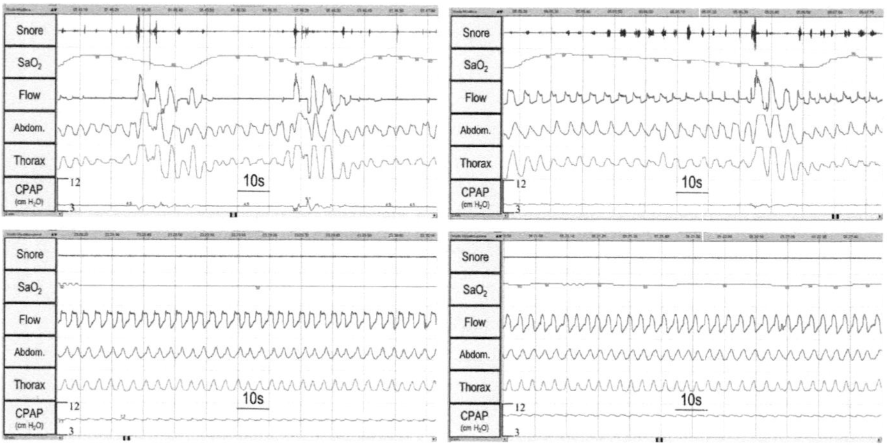

Fig. 76.1 Example of effects of increasing CPAP levels on sleep breathing pattern in a patient with obstructive sleep apnea. Upper left panel: obstructive apneas; *upper right panel*: obstructive hypopnea; *lower left panel*: inspiratory flow limitation, no hypopnea; *lower right panel*: unobstructed breathing

76.2 Analysis and Discussion

Monitoring during sleep can allow observation of the effects of CPAP on breathing, and help to identify the pressure to prescribe. CPAP titration consists of the application of various CPAP levels during sleep to find the pressure that may best correct respiratory disorders.

Manual CPAP titration in the sleep laboratory is the oldest titration method. It is performed during a full night polysomnographic recording, while a technician manually modifies pressure administered by a CPAP device. All signals generally recorded during polysomnography have an important role: electroencephalogram, electrooculogram, and chin electromyogram for recognition of sleep stages and arousals; body position to control CPAP effects in each posture; pressure at the mask to monitor the CPAP level that is administered; and signals for detection of snoring, airflow, respiratory movements, and oxyhemoglobin saturation to observe modifications in breathing characteristics as CPAP level is changed. In particular, as regards airflow, monitoring by a pneumotachograph is recommended, as a flattened shape in the inspiratory portion of the flow signal recorded by this method is indicative of flow limitation. The titration polysomnographic study should include the recording of some rapid-eye-movement (REM) sleep and of some sleep time in the supine posture, inasmuch as REM sleep, and, even moreso, supine posture, may require the application of higher CPAP levels [4]. The American Academy of Sleep Medicine (AASM) allows split-night polysomnographies (first part of the night for diagnosis, last part for CPAP titration), provided that the diagnostic part of the polysomnogram lasts a minimum of 2 hours and documents an apnea/hypopnea index (AHI: number of apneas + hypopneas per hour of sleep) of at least 40, while the CPAP titration part is carried out for more than 3 hours, including REM sleep with the patient in the supine position [5].

More recently, automatic CPAP titration by means of "auto-CPAP" machines has been introduced ("autotitration"). Auto-CPAP devices are designed to automatically deliver a variable CPAP level that should correspond to the lowest required pressure in each moment. Today, most auto-CPAP devices are designed to eliminate all obstructive events and inspiratory flow limitation, and to distinguish central apneas with open airway, not requiring pressure augmentations, from apneas with a closed airway. They are able to record several types of information during their application, including pressures delivered, air leaks, and respiratory events detected, and can usually calculate AHI. Principles of operation of auto-CPAP devices can be different. Likewise, their efficacy may differ among patients, although several modern devices are effective in the correction of upper airway obstruction and reliable in the vast majority of patients.

Autotitration can be performed with the application of an auto-CPAP device during a standard polysomnographic study. A technician may assist autotitration, with the task to control the polysomnographic recording and the patient. Analysis of the polysomnographic study allows us to verify the relationship between pressures that have been delivered and breathing characteristics, sleep architecture, and body postures. In this way, it is possible to select the CPAP level that proves most appropriate for correction of upper airway obstruction. This method is recognized as a valid alternative to traditional manual titration [6], but differences in costs and time required for the two procedures are limited.

As an alternative to the search for optimal CPAP with polysomnography, unassisted autotitration without any monitoring, except that provided by the auto-CPAP machine itself, has been introduced. With this method, an auto-CPAP is given to the patient for nocturnal self-application. Data collected and elaborated by the machine are downloaded, and periods with excessive air leaks are discarded from analysis. The 90th or 95th percentile pressure (i.e., the pressure that is not exceeded for 90 or 95 % of the time of the auto-CPAP application) is usually considered equivalent to the manually titrated pressure. Lack of external monitoring during auto-CPAP application can lead to errors in the recognition of optimal CPAP level. Both administration of excessively high pressures and under-correction of obstruction are possible. Erroneous pressure administration may go undetected if no monitoring in addition to the one performed with the auto-CPAP itself is done. AHI calculated by the auto-CPAP machines may help to identify some unsatisfactory autotitrations. Recent studies have validated the values of AHI calculated by some auto-CPAP devices. However, reliability of these calculations depends on the software of each device and may vary between machines [7].

The pressure to prescribe to each patient has been indicated as "optimal" pressure. It should correspond to the lowest CPAP that eliminates upper airway obstruction in all sleep stages and body postures. However, the real need to fully correct all degrees of upper airway obstruction is uncertain [8], and the application of very high CPAP levels for the purpose of preventing any obstructive episode may be counterproductive, because it may result in the appearance of central apneas or in discomfort that may discourage patients from treatment. In fact, the AASM considers optimal titrations those resulting in AHI <5, but still adequate those where the AHI is reduced by 75 % even though it remains >10 [4]. However, an AHI >10 is representative of a significant alteration of the breathing pattern, and even the AASM recommends repeating CPAP titration if the number of residual events during CPAP is high.

The strongest argument against nocturnal monitoring for very precise determinations of a CPAP level to prescribe is that the pressure needed to fully open the upper airway can vary not only within nights, mainly in association with sleep stage or posture changes, but also between nights. Today, the existence of a precise optimal pressure is questioned [9], and the role of single-night, either manual or automatic, titrations, not to speak of split-night procedures, is discussed.

As polysomnographic monitoring for multiple nights is not easily feasible and has high costs, it has been proposed that unassisted autotitration without external monitoring be performed for several nights. The average of the 90th or 95th percentile pressures on all nights of auto-CPAP application could represent an appropriate pressure for treatment. Progressive adaptation of the patient during consecutive nights to sleep with CPAP could prevent errors associated with poor sleep quality or lack of REM sleep, minimize errors due to the absence of an external monitoring, and enhance successive compliance to treatment. Some cases of poor performance of the auto-CPAP machine may remain undetected if no nocturnal instrumental monitoring is performed. However, even simple cardiorespiratory monitoring performed after autotitration while wearing CPAP at the fixed level previously determined may be helpful in identifying uncommon but possible cases of unsatisfactory autotitrations. In our experience, a disadvantage of unassisted autotitration is that, despite previous training, not all patients are able to start sleeping with CPAP if they do not initially have a support from a caregiver.

The number of nights for the unassisted autotitration method is not standardized. A small number of nights could make it an economical procedure because of the lack of complex monitoring and analysis, and of technical assistance. Multiple-night unassisted autotitration has been recognized as a possible valid alternative to polysomnographic titration, but with recommendations to rely on auto-CPAP devices that have been better validated and to strictly keep in touch patients after initiation of CPAP treatment [6]. However, it has been shown that, in a subset of patients, inter-night variability of the effects of each pressure level is so high that no single effective pressure for prescription can be identified. In such patients the usefulness of any CPAP titration would be limited, and the most appropriate CPAP treatment will be by means of variable pressure levels, such as those delivered by auto-CPAP devices [10].

To further simplify CPAP prescription procedures, it has been proposed, rather than titrating CPAP, to prescribe a pressure calculated by means of predictive equations. Different predictive equations for therapeutic CPAP have been elaborated. Calculated pressure values differ to some extent according to the equation. Generally, agreement between calculated and titrated values decreases when extreme (very low or very high) pressure levels are required by the patient for treatment [11]. Today, predictive equations are not considered reliable substitutes for titration [8].

In the last years, it has been emphasized that CPAP prescription and long-term treatment should carefully take into consideration a patient's symptoms, life quality, tolerance and adherence to treatment, and, possibly, benefits on blood pressure control. These effects may, to some extent, guide clinicians to modify the pressure previously prescribed on the basis of the results of nocturnal monitoring [12]. However, it must be kept in mind that, in some cases, clinical criteria may lead to erroneous interpretations of the effectiveness of CPAP on respiratory disorders. In fact, improvement in sleepiness may occur despite incomplete resolution of upper airway obstruction, due to a placebo effect or, on the contrary, sleepiness may persist despite normal breathing; compliance to treatment may be good even with subtherapeutic pressure; and OSA treatment does not always result in effects on blood pressure.

It has been investigated whether untreated asymptomatic OSA may have prognostic implications. In this regard, contrasting results have been reported. However, the results of most studies suggest that, in asymptomatic subjects, OSA may be less dangerous, but it is not harmless [13], especially in patients with severe disorders. Therefore, incomplete correction of respiratory disorders may expose patients to persistence of increased cardiovascular risk, and an instrumental monitoring is advisable, at least before CPAP prescription or after treatment initiation, even in patients highly compliant to the treatment and with a good correction of symptoms.

Conclusions

CPAP prescription can be a challenging task. It should simultaneously ensure the correction of upper airway obstruction during sleep, the reversal of the symptoms related to OSA, and good adherence to the treatment. These aims are promptly obtained in many, but not all patients. In fact, an optimal pressure for the correction of obstructive events may be difficult to recognize in some patients, or may fluctuate between nights. Furthermore, evaluation of therapeutic pressure based on objective nocturnal recordings, patient's symptoms, or compliance to treatment may show some differences. A careful instrumental and clinical evaluation should lead to the prescription of a CPAP treatment that may be the most appropriate for each patient.

Key Major Recommendations

- Before prescribing CPAP, choose an instrumental monitoring that may be reliable for the identification of the best pressure. For most patients, different options are available, provided that an expert physician evaluates their outcomes.
- Prescribe to each patient the CPAP level that may best eliminate obstructive respiratory events.
- Evaluate subjective and clinical findings after initiation of CPAP treatment, whatever the procedure that has been adopted for CPAP prescription.
- Take into consideration subjective indications given by each patient to slightly modify the therapeutic pressure or to reconsider CPAP titration.

References

1. Giles TL, Lasserson TJ, Smith BH, White J, Wright J, Cates CJ. Continuous positive airways pressure for obstructive sleep apnoea in adults. Cochrane Database Syst Rev. 2006;(3):CD001106.
2. Kendzerska T, Mollayeva T, Gershon AS, Leung RS, Hawker G, Tomlinson G. Untreated obstructive sleep apnea and the risk for serious long-term adverse outcomes: a systematic review. Sleep Med Rev. 2014;18:49–59.
3. Fischer J, Dogas Z, Bassetti C, Berg S, Grote L, Jennum P, Levy P, et al. Standard procedures for adults in accredited sleep medicine centres in Europe. J Sleep Res. 2012;21:357–68.
4. Kushida C, Chediak A, Berry R, Brown LK, Gozal D, Iber C, et al. Clinical guidelines for the manual titration of positive airway pressure in patients with obstructive sleep apnea. J Clin Sleep Med. 2008;4:157–71.
5. Kushida CA, Littner MR, Morgenthaler T, Alessi CA, Bailey D, Jack Coleman J, et al. Practice parameters for the indications for polysomnography and related procedures: an update for 2005. Sleep. 2005;28:499–521.
6. Morgenthaler TI, Aurora RN, Brown T, Zak R, Alessi C, Boehlecke B, et al. Practice parameters for the use of autotitrating continuous positive airway pressure devices for titrating pressures and treating adult patients with obstructive sleep apnea syndrome: an update for 2007. An American Academy of Sleep Medicine report. Sleep. 2008;31:141–7.

7. Schwab RJ, Badr SM, Epstein LJ, Gay PC, Gozal D, Kohler M, et al. An official American Thoracic Society Statement: continuous positive airway pressure adherence tracking systems. The optimal monitoring strategies and outcome measures in adults. Am J Respir Crit Care Med. 2013;188:613–20.
8. Sanders MH, Montserrat JM, Farré R, Givelber RJ. Positive pressure therapy. A perspective on evidence-based outcomes and methods of application. Proc Am Thorac Soc. 2008;5:161–72.
9. Farré R, Navajas D, Montserrat JM. Is there an optimal nasal pressure for treating obstructive sleep apnea–and if so, what is it? Sleep. 2013;36:463–4.
10. Callahan CY, Norman RG, Taxin Z, Mooney AM, Rapoport DM, Ayappa I. Multinight recording and analysis of continuous positive airway pressure airflow in the home for titration and management of sleep disordered breathing. Sleep. 2013;36:535–45.
11. Marrone O, Salvaggio A, Romano S, Insalaco G. Automatic titration and calculation by predictive equations for the determination of therapeutic continuous positive airway pressure for obstructive sleep apnea. Chest. 2008;133:670–6.
12. Fitzpatrick MF, Alloway CED, Wakeford TM, MacLean AW, Munt PW, Day AG. Can patients with obstructive sleep apnea titrate their own continuous positive airway pressure? Am J Respir Crit Care Med. 2003;167:716–22.
13. Mirrakhimov AE. Non drowsy obstructive sleep apnea as a potential cause of resistant hypertension: a case report. BMC Pulm Med. 2012;12:16.

Dual-Mode Noninvasive Mechanical Ventilation: Key Technical and Practical Applications

77

Grazia Crescimanno, Andrea Vianello, and Oreste Marrone

Contents

Abbreviations

AVAPS	Average volume-assured pressure support
COPD	Chronic obstructive pulmonary disease
CRF	Chronic respiratory failure
HI-PS	High-intensity pressure support
HRQL	Health-related quality of life
IBW	Ideal body weight

G. Crescimanno, MD (✉)
Italian National Research Council, Institute of Biomedicine and Molecular Immunology, Palermo, Italy

Department of Pneumology, Villa Sofia – Cervello Hospital, Palermo, Italy
Via Ugo La Malfa, 153, Palermo 90146, Italy
e-mail: grazia.crescimanno@ibim.cnr.it

A. Vianello, MD
Respiratory Pathophysiology Division, University-City Hospital of Padova, Padua, Italy
e-mail: avianello@qubisoft.it

O. Marrone, MD
Italian National Research Council, Institute of Biomedicine and Molecular Immunology, Palermo, Italy
e-mail: marrone@ibim.cnr.it

A.M. Esquinas (ed.), *Noninvasive Mechanical Ventilation: Theory, Equipment, and Clinical Applications*, DOI 10.1007/978-3-319-21653-9_77

iVAPS	Intelligent volume-assured pressure support
NMD	Neuromuscular disease
OHS	Obesity hypoventilation syndrome
PEEP	Positive end-expiratory pressure
PS	Pressure support
PSV-VS	Pressure support ventilation volume security
PSV-VTG	Pressure support ventilation with guaranteed volume
$PtCO_2$	Transcutaneous carbon dioxide pressure
VAPS	Volume-assured pressure support

77.1 Introduction

The primary goal of mechanical ventilation is the maintenance of adequate gas exchanges, which can be achieved either by volume or pressure ventilation. During pressure ventilation, the airway pressure is fixed and the tidal volume is variable. An increase in pulmonary resistance can lead to a drop in tidal volume and to alveolar hypoventilation. During volume ventilation, tidal volume is fixed, whereas the airway pressure is variable and depends on the respiratory system mechanics and patient effort. An increase in respiratory drive, for example, due to fever, can result in insufficient alveolar ventilation and asynchrony. In the past, volume ventilation has been extensively used to guarantee a constant volume in acute patients with altered chest wall compliance and airway resistance, as well as in patients with different kinds of respiratory failure who require continuous ventilator support during sleep. However, since recent studies have shown that pressure ventilation is more comfortable than volume ventilation [1] and can compensate better if there are leaks [2], new ventilatory modes have been designed and developed to offer volume stability and avoid disadvantages related to volume ventilation. These news modes, called "dual-control modes" or "volume target pressure ventilation," are hybrid modes aimed at administering pressure ventilation and, at the same time, ensuring that the target tidal volume is reached despite changes in airway resistance or pulmonary elastance conditions [3]. In simple terms, they combine the advantages of volume ventilation (constant tidal volume and preservation of minute ventilation) and pressure ventilation (adaptability of flow to patient's requirements, i.e., variable flow). Dual-mode ventilators were initially developed for invasive mechanical ventilation in the intensive care environment, but their use has progressively extended to noninvasive ventilation (NIV), both for hospital and home utilization.

77.2 Principles of Operation and Setting of Dual-Control Modes of Ventilation

Although dual-control modes can work in different ways, they all assure stable arterial CO_2 levels by maintaining adequate minute ventilation when impedance of the respiratory system increases. Dual-control "within a breath" refers to a technique whereby the ventilator, after the setting of a minimal inspiratory pressure, switches to volume control in the middle of a breath if the target volume cannot be reached by the pressure ventilation mode. In this option, the flow changes from decelerated to fixed, so as to warrant the desired tidal volume, while the inspiratory pressure passively increases. An acronym generally used to indicate ventilators working with this modality is PSV-VTG (pressure support ventilation with guaranteed volume).

Dual-control "breath to breath" ventilators work in a way that, if the tidal volume decreases, the pressure progressively varies from breath to breath within a preset pressure range until the desired target volume is reached. Acronyms generally used for ventilators working with this modality are PSV-VS or PSV-VG (pressure support ventilation-volume security or -volume guaranteed), and AVAPS (average volume-assured pressure support) (Fig. 77.1).

The iVAPS (intelligent volume-assured pressure support) is a dual-control mode in which the target is not tidal volume (like PSV-VT and AVAPS) but alveolar ventilation. It is an autotitrating mode of ventilation that has appeared on the market in recent years. While taking into account a predicted anatomical dead space, it varies respiratory rate and pressure support within preset limits to maintain a target alveolar ventilation. If ventilation falls below the target, the ventilator responds to the change quicker than the previous dual-control ventilators, increasing pressure support at a higher rate.

In dual-control ventilators, the target tidal volume must always be set. In addition, depending on the ventilator algorithm, minimal and maximal pressure, inspiratory flow rate, or inspiratory time may be required to set. There are no official recommendations about which target tidal volume should be set, and in most centers, indications provided by manufacturers are adopted. According to these indications, in most studies, dealing with patients with different diseases, the minimal tidal volume was set at about 8 ml/kg of ideal weight, with a range between 7 and 12. However, no comparative studies between settings have been performed. Both in the within-a-breath and in the breath-to-breath modes, if the preset minimal target volume is too low, it may lead to an increase in respiratory rate, which may cause an increase in the work of breathing. Instead, if the set tidal volume is too high, the ventilator may raise the pressure support and possibly cause barotrauma or hemodynamic compromise, or lead to the appearance of intrinsic positive end-expiratory pressure (PEEP).

In the breath-to-breath mode, the pressure range is manually or automatically set. If the maximum set pressure limit is too high it could not only cause barotrauma but also an undesired increase in the delivered volume. On the other hand, if the minimal preset inspiratory pressure is too low, the drop in pressure that follows leaks may cause hypoventilation.

In the within-a-breath mode, inspiratory flow rate or time is set. If the minimal inspiratory flow rate is set too low, lung inflation may be slow, with a late switch from pressure to volume control and an undesired prolongation of inspiratory time. An inspiratory time that is too long can cause expiratory asynchrony.

77.2.1 Consequences of Leaks on Efficacy of Ventilation

An important issue to address is the behavior of volume target mode in the presence of unintentional leaks. Contal et al. [4] tested seven home ventilators on a bench model adapted to simulate leaks. They found that tidal volume provided by the

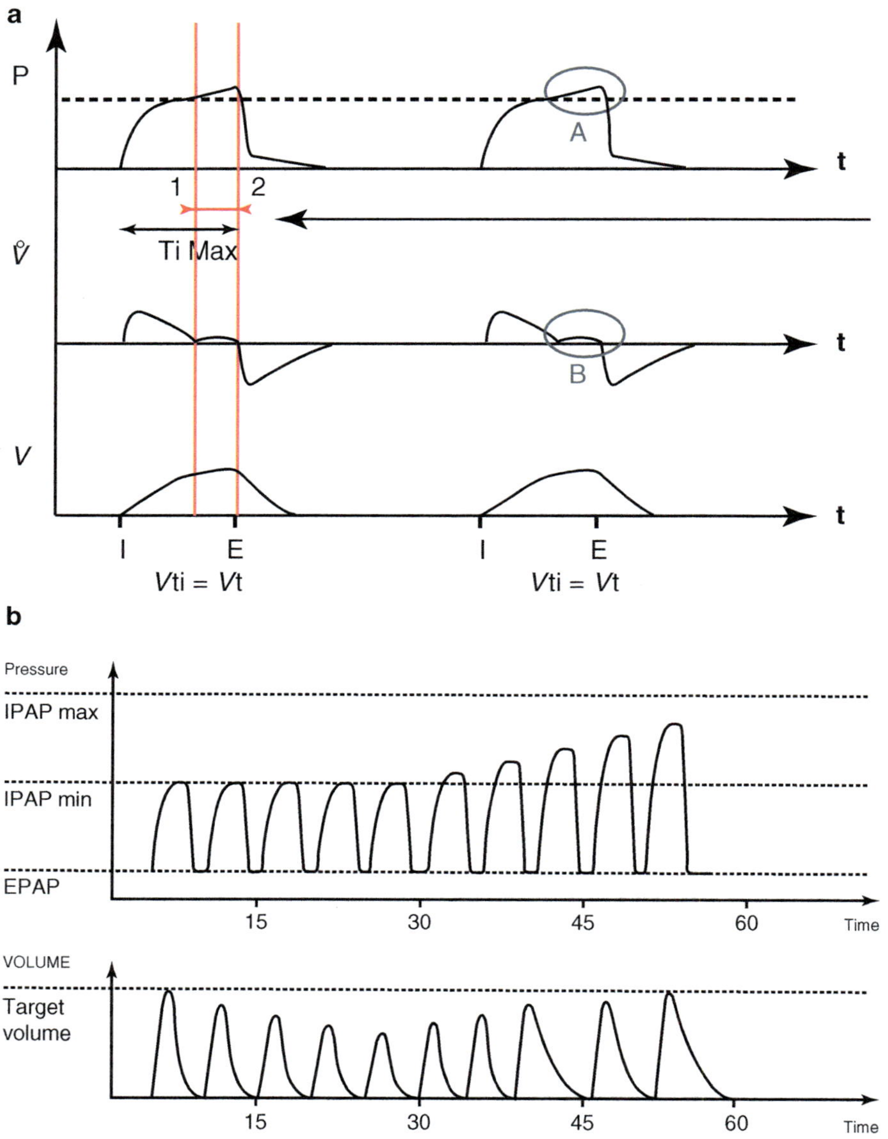

Fig. 77.1 *Upper panel A*: dual-control "within-a-breath" mode. The figure shows that, if the target volume cannot be reached by the pressure ventilation mode, the ventilator switches from pressure to volume control. The flow changes from decelerated to fixed (**b**) and inspiratory pressure passively increases (**a**). Target volume (*Vt*) is adjusted according to the measured inspiratory volume (*Vti*). Ti max = preset maximum inspiratory time. (Reproduced with permission from ResMed). *Lower panel B*: Dual-control "breath-to-breath" mode. The figure shows that if the tidal volume is not reached, the pressure progressively increases from breath to breath within a preset pressure range until the desired target volume is obtained (Reproduced with permission from Philips Respironics)

software in the presence of leaks was underestimated by all devices, and that, for most devices, bias increased with higher insufflation pressures. Similarly, Lujàn et al. [5] evaluated the reliability of the tidal volume provided by five ventilators in a bench test with simulated leaks. They found that all the tested ventilators underestimated tidal volume, and that the higher the leak, the higher the difference between the estimated and the actual tidal volume. By contrast, Sogo et al. [6], who evaluated the same ventilators in similar conditions, found that inspiratory leaks were followed by overestimates of tidal volume by most of ventilators. They also found that, in the presence of expiratory leaks, the behaviors of each of the tested ventilators were different; three ventilators underestimated and one ventilator overestimated the tidal volume. Independently from these contrasting results, which may be the result of different study designs and protocols, it is important to emphasize that, when large leaks occur, data provided by the ventilator software may not always be reliable. In clinical practice, where the behavior of leaks is often erratic, this may translate into a difficult assessment of patients' ventilation. Inclusion of algorithms that calculate the pressure loss as a function of the flow exiting the ventilator may increase the reliability of tidal volume estimation.

Tidal volume estimation by dual-control ventilators during air leaks may vary with circuit configuration. Khirani et al. [7] studied the ability of seven home dual-mode ventilators to maintain the preset minimal target volume during leaks with different circuit configurations. They reported that all studied ventilators with a single-limb circuit were able to maintain the minimal preset tidal volume during leaks; only one ventilator overcompensated during prominent leaks. By contrast, with the exception of one ventilator model, all the studied ventilators with a single circuit and an expiratory valve, or with a double circuit, failed to maintain the minimal tidal volume during leaks, because they misinterpreted leaks as an increase in tidal volume and therefore decreased their inspiratory pressure to the minimal preset level. Similar results were reported by Carlucci et al. [8]. However, Lujan et al. [9] have shown that the introduction of a random leak also influences the performance of commercial ventilators with a single-limb circuit, and that inspiratory leaks decrease the delivered tidal volume, with an important clinical impact in terms of hypoventilation. Thus, an effective estimation of ventilation during leaks may depend on the circuit and the configuration of the ventilator and may vary with the ventilator model. The loss of accuracy in estimated tidal volume may also cause patient-ventilator asynchrony, although this point has not been specifically addressed in most of the previously cited studies.

77.2.2 Clinical Trials on Dual-Mode Ventilators (Table 77.1)

77.2.2.1 Clinical Trials on the PSV-VTG Ventilation Mode

A precursor of modern dual-mode ventilators was described by Amato et al. [10] in 1992. These authors published the results of a clinical trial, performed in intubated patients with acute respiratory failure, which compared a dual mode of ventilation,

Table 77.1 Major trials on Dual-mode NIV available in the literature

Authors	Ventilator	Setting	Patients	Duration	Outcomes with target mode
Storre et al. (2006)	Synchrony Cross-over	Fixed PS vs AVAPS 7–10 ml/kg IBW Pressure max 30 cmH_2O	10 stable OHS	6 weeks	Improved nocturnal gas exchange; no variation in sleep quality and HRQL
Janssen et al. (2009)	Synchrony Cross-over	Fixed PS vs AVAPS 8–10 ml/kg AB Pressure max 30 cmH_2O	12 stable OHS	2 nights	Improved nocturnal gas exchange; decreased comfort, subjective and objective sleep quality
Crisafulli et al. (2009)	Synchrony Cross-over	Fixed PS vs AVAPS 8 ml/kg IBW Pressure max 30 cmH_2O	9 stable COPD	2 weeks	No variation in diurnal gas exchange and comfort Better subjective sleep efficiency
Jaye et al. (2009)	AutoVPAP Cross-over	Fixed PS vs iVAPS Autotitrating Pressure max 21 cmH_2O	20 stable NMD	2 months	No differences in nocturnal gas exchange and sleep quality
Ambrogio et al. (2009)	Synchrony Cross-over	Fixed PS versus AVAPS 8 ml/kg IBW or 110 % of baseline VT Pressure max 30 cmH_2O	28 stable CRF	2 nights	No differences in nocturnal gas exchange and sleep quality; greater minute ventilation
Crescimanno et al. (2011)	Idea Ultra Cross-over	Fixed PS versus PSV-VG 8–10 ml/kg IBW Pressure max 20 cmH_2O	28 stable NMD	2 nights	No differences in nocturnal gas exchange, comfort and subjective sleep quality; more asynchrony
Murphy et al. (2012)	Synchrony Parallel group	Fixed PS versus AVAPS 8–10 ml/kg IBW Pressure max 22 cmH_2O	46 stable Super OHS	3 months	No differences in daytime gas exchanges
Briones Claudett et al. (2013)	Synchrony Parallel group	Fixed PS vs AVAPS 8–12 ml/kg IBW and after stability 6–8 ml/kg Pressure max 26 cmH_2O	22 acute COPD	1–2–3–12–24 h	More rapid improvement of diurnal gas exchange and recovery of consciousness (GCS)

Ekkernkamp et al. (2014)	STELLAR Cross-over	Fixed HI-PS vs iVAPS Autotitrating Pressure max 25 cmH_2O	14 COPD	2 nights 6 weeks	No differences in nocturnal gas exchanges and sleep quality in short term, greater decrease in $PtCO_2$ and better subjective sleep quality long term with iVAPS
Kelly et al. (2014)	STELLAR Cross-over	Fixed PS vs iVAPS Autotitrating Pressure max 18 cmH_2O	18 mixed CRF	1 month	No differences in nocturnal gas exchanges and sleep quality. Better compliance in naïve patients
Oscroft et al. (2014)	STELLAR Parallel group	Fixed PS vs iVAPS Autotitrating Pressure max 25 cmH_2O	34 stable COPD	3 months	No differences in daytime and nocturnal gas exchanges or compliance
Storre et al. (2014)	VIVO 40–50 Cross-over	Fixed HI-PS vs PS-VT 8 ml/kg IBW/110 % Vt pressure max 35 cmH_2O	10 COPD	3 months	No differences in nocturnal gas exchange, tolerance, sleep quality

PS pressure support, *AVAPS* average volume-assured pressure support, *OHS* obesity hypoventilation syndrome, *HRQL* health-related quality of life, *COPD* chronic obstructive pulmonary disease, *iVAPS* intelligent volume pressure support, *NMD* neuromuscular disease, *IBW* ideal body weight, *HI-PS* high intensity pressure support, *PtCO2* transcutaneous carbon dioxide pressure, *CRF* chronic respiratory failure called volume-assured pressure support (VAPS), and operating with within-a-breath, volume ventilation. The authors concluded that this new mode of ventilation was beneficial in terms of improvement in blood gases, workload, and synchrony.

Only one study compared PSV-VTG ventilation with conventional noninvasive pressure support ventilation (PSV), which is the most widely used ventilation modality [11]. In this study, the possible role of PSV-VTG in patients affected by neuromuscular disease was evaluated in a cross-over, short-term, randomized study. The results showed that PSV-VTG did not offer any advantage in comparison with pressure support, and that it could predispose to patient-ventilator asynchronies.

77.2.2.2 Clinical Trials on AVAPS

AVAPS has been more extensively studied than the within-a-breath mode, both in acute and stable patients. Several clinical trials have been published that compared AVAPS with PSV. Most studies were done on patients ventilated during sleep.

In 2006, Storre et al. [12] performed a long-term study (6 weeks) on clinically stable patients affected by obesity-hypoventilation syndrome (OHS). They found a significantly lower nocturnal transcutaneous CO_2 during AVAPS than during PSV without differences in sleep quality and comfort. In 2008, Janssen et al. [13] performed a similar study on 12 patients affected by OHS using the AVAPS mode, and similarly concluded that it controlled nocturnal hypoventilation better than PSV, but at the expense of a slight worsening in objective and subjective sleep quality and in comfort of ventilation. In the following year, Crisafulli et al. [14] reported similar effects on arterial blood gases and no difference in comfort with NIV between AVAPS and PSV in 9 patients with chronic obstructive pulmonary disease (COPD). Ambrogio et al. [15] explored the role of AVAPS in patients affected by obstructive or restrictive chronic respiratory failure and, unlike Janssen, did not observe any improvement in sleep quality with AVAPS with respect to fixed PSV. However, they found that minute ventilation was higher during AVAPS than during PSV. Another study on OHS was performed in super-obese patients by Murphy et al. in 2012 [16]. In that study, no difference between effects of AVAPS and fixed-level PSV on daytime gas exchanges was found after three months of follow-up. Briones Claudett et al. [17] have carried out a prospective interventional controlled study in 22 patients with COPD exacerbation and hypercapnic encephalopathy. Interestingly, they observed a more rapid recovery of patients treated with AVAPS than with PSV, although they were not able to demonstrate differences in terms of length of hospital stay or days on NIV. Finally, Storre et al. [18] compared AVAPS with high-intensity PSV in 10 COPD patients. They did not find differences in tolerance, sleep quality, health-related quality of life, exercise capacity, and lung function.

77.2.2.3 Clinical Trials on IVAPS

Four studies have been published about clinical effects of iVAPS. The first clinical trial was performed by Jaye et al. [19] in 2009 in 20 patients with neuromuscular diseases. The authors reported that iVAPS and standard bi-level ventilation produced comparable control of nocturnal blood gases in these patients. These results were confirmed by a second study performed in 2014 by the same group in patients naïve to NIV [20]. Ekkernkamp et al. [21] compared the impact of iVAPS and of PSV in patients with COPD at different times after their initiation. They found no differences in the short term, but some advantages in gas exchange and subjective sleep quality after 6 weeks. By contrast, Oscroft et al. [22], in a long-term study in patients with COPD found similar physiological outcomes under iVAPS or bi-level ventilation.

Conclusions

In recent years, hybrid modes have been developed to overcome some drawbacks of volume and pressure ventilation. The advantages of dual-mode ventilators have not yet been definitely established. Some studies have examined only technical aspects of dual ventilation and not clinical observations on patients. Among clinical studies, overall, 4 of 12 reported a more rapid improvement in gas exchange using dual-mode ventilators than traditional pressure ventilators. However, results reported so far are inconsistent, possibly due to the different algorithms and circuit configurations of the ventilators used for comparisons with dual-control ventilators. Additionally, in most trials, the recruited patients were already accustomed to some mode of NIV before using a dual-volume targeting mode. Little information is available on the effects of dual-mode ventilators on sleep quality and patient ventilator-interaction.

In the future, it will be necessary to standardize the nomenclature for dual modes of NIV. Besides, further clinical studies are needed. In fact, while ventilator manufacturers need to demonstrate engineering success in a lung model to obtain marketing approval both in the United States and in Europe, individual patients' responses to alternative modes of ventilation may greatly differ in clinical practice. This should be born in mind when new modes of ventilation are tested.

Key Major Recommendations

- Take into consideration how the ventilator algorithm works to assure target volume.
- Prefer a single-limb circuit configuration.
- Consider dual modes if you need to use high pressures either in the acute or long-term setting.
- Consider dual modes if long-term patient adherence to treatment is expected to be inadequate.
- Monitor the patient's unintentional leaks and do not use dual modes if they cannot be governed.

References

1. Betensley AD, Khalid I, Crawford J, et al. Patient comfort during pressure support and volume controlled-continuous mandatory ventilation. Respir Care. 2008;53:897–902.

2. Mehta S, McCool FD, Hill NS. Leak compensation in positive pressure ventilators: a lung model study. Eur Respir J. 2001;17:259–67.
3. Branson RD, Davis Jr K. Dual control modes: combining volume and pressure breaths. Respir Care Clin N Am. 2001;7:397–408.
4. Contal O, Vignaux L, Combescure C, et al. Monitoring of noninvasive ventilation by built-in software of home bilevel ventilators: a bench study. Chest. 2012;141:469–76.
5. Luján M, Sogo A, Pomares X, et al. Effect of leak and breathing pattern on the accuracy of tidal volume estimation by commercial home ventilators: a bench study. Respir Care. 2013; 58:770–7.
6. Sogo A, Montanyà J, Monsó E, et al. Effect of dynamic random leaks on the monitoring accuracy of home mechanical ventilators: a bench study. BMC Pulm Med. 2013;13:75.
7. Khirani S, Louis B, Leroux K, et al. Harms of unintentional leaks during volume targeted pressure support ventilation. Respir Med. 2013;107:1021–9.
8. Carlucci A, Schreiber A, Mattei A, et al. The configuration of bi-level ventilator circuits may affect compensation for non-intentional leaks during volume-targeted ventilation. Intensive Care Med. 2013;39:59–65.
9. Luján M, Sogo A, Grimau C, et al. Influence of dynamic leaks in volume-targeted pressure support non invasive ventilation: a bench study. Respir Care. 2015;60:191–200.
10. Amato MB, Barbas CS, Bonassa J, et al. Volume-assured pressure support ventilation (VAPSV). A new approach for reducing muscle workload during acute respiratory failure. Chest. 1992;102:1225–34.
11. Crescimanno G, Marrone O, Vianello A. Efficacy and comfort of volume-guaranteed pressure support in patients with chronic ventilatory failure of neuromuscular origin. Respirology. 2011;16:672–9.
12. Storre JH, Seuthe B, Fiechter R, et al. Average volume-assured pressure support in obesity hypoventilation: a randomized crossover trial. Chest. 2006;130:815–21.
13. Janssens JP, Metzger M, Sforza E. Impact of volume targeting on efficacy of bi-level non-invasive ventilation and sleep in obesity-hypoventilation. Respir Med. 2009;103:165–72.
14. Crisafulli E, Manni G, Kidonias M, et al. Subjective sleep quality during average volume assured pressure support (AVAPS) ventilation in patients with hyperapnic COPD: a physical pilot study. Lung. 2009;187:299–305.
15. Ambrogio C, Lowman X, Kuo M, et al. Sleep and non-invasive ventilation in patients with chronic respiratory insufficiency. Intensive Care Med. 2009;35:306–13.
16. Murphy PB, Davidson C, Hind MD, et al. Volume targeted versus pressure support non-invasive ventilation in patients with super obesity and chronic respiratory failure: a randomised controlled trial. Thorax. 2012;67:727–34.
17. Briones Claudett KH, Briones Claudett M, Sang Wong MC, et al. Noninvasive mechanical ventilation with average volume assured pressure support (AVAPS) in patients with chronic obstructive pulmonary disease and hypercapnic encephalopathy. BMC Pulm Med. 2013;13:12.
18. Storre JH, Matrosovich E, Ekkernkamp E, et al. Home mechanical ventilation for COPD: high-intensity versus target volume noninvasive ventilation. Respir Care. 2014;59:1389–97.
19. Jaye J, Chatwin M, Dayer M, et al. Autotitrating versus standard noninvasive ventilation: a randomised crossover trial. Eur Respir J. 2009;33:566–71.
20. Kelly JL, Jaye J, Pickersgill RE, et al. Randomized trial of 'intelligent' autotitrating ventilation versus standard pressure support non-invasive ventilation: impact on adherence and physiological outcomes. Respirology. 2014;19:596–603.
21. Ekkernkamp E, Storre JH, Windisch W, et al. Impact of intelligent volume-assured pressure support on sleep quality in stable hypercapnic chronic obstructive pulmonary disease patients: a randomized, crossover study. Respiration. 2014;88:270–6.
22. Oscroft NS, Chadwick R, Davies MG, Quinnell TG, Smith IE. Volume assured versus pressure preset non-invasive ventilation for compensated ventilatory failure in COPD. Respir Med. 2014;108:1508–15.

Results of Servo-ventilation and Other Ventilatory Modes in Sleep Apnea Syndrome: Key Topics and Practical Implications

78

Dominic Dellweg, Markus Wenzel, and Jens Kerl

Contents

78.1 Introduction

Sleep apnea is comprised of different breathing abnormalities that occur during sleep. These syndromes can mainly be divided into disorders with airflow obstruction and into disorders with altered respiratory drive, as well as the combination of both [1]. For patients with obstructive sleep apnea, continuous positive airway pressure (CPAP), which was first introduced in 1981, is the usual form of treatment [2]. CPAP can be applied in form of a fix pressure or in an automatic mode in which the CPAP machine titrates treatment pressure to measured indices of airflow obstruction [3]. Pressure therapies applying different pressure levels during inspiration and expiration might be used in case of pressure intolerance and allow for lower pressures during expiration without compromising airway patency [4].

Breathing disorders with altered respiratory drive in adults have to be separated according to their etiology:

1. Primary central sleep apnea
2. Central apnea with Cheyne-Stokes respiration
3. Central sleep apnea of high altitude

D. Dellweg, PhD (✉) • M. Wenzel, MD • J. Kerl, MSc
Department for Respiratory Medicine, Critical Care and Sleep Medicine, Kloster Grafschaft, Annostr. 1, Schmallenberg 57392, Germany
e-mail: d.dellweg@fkkg.de; m.wenzel@fkkg.de; j.kerl@fkkg.de

A.M. Esquinas (ed.), *Noninvasive Mechanical Ventilation: Theory, Equipment, and Clinical Applications*, DOI 10.1007/978-3-319-21653-9_78

4. Central sleep apnea related to other (e.g., neurologic) diseases
5. Central sleep apnea syndrome provoked by medication, drugs, and substances
6. Pressure therapy-induced central apnea (complex sleep apnea)

These entities are the domain of more sophisticated ventilation modes, which will be reviewed in this chapter.

78.2 Ventilator Modes for Sleep Syndromes with Altered Respiratory Drive

During centrally mediated apneas, there is no isometric contraction of the respiratory muscles, resulting in cessation of respiratory flow. CPAP given in this instance will not generate a breath in the absence of an inspiratory effort. CPAP might improve central apneas in heart failure patients by other mechanisms, such as preload reduction, but it does not have an impact on mortality in these patients [5]. For this reason, central apnea syndromes have become the domain of ventilator modes with different pressures during inspiration and expiration, usually known as bi-level or BIPAP (bi-level positive airway pressure) therapy, or more sophisticated modes that change pressure levels in view of the patient's breathing effort. In general, cessation of respiratory drive occurs when carbon dioxide is lowered below the apneic threshold [6], measured in the carotid body chemoreceptors [7]. Chronic hyperventilation with a reduction of the CO_2 baseline appears to play an important role here because baseline CO_2 will be closer to the apneic threshold [8–10]. For this reason, elevation of CO_2 by means of increased inspiratory CO_2 fraction of the addition of dead space to ventilation can ameliorate central apneas [11].

During an apnea, CO_2 rises until breathing stimulus reappears. The stability of this feedback system of breathing control depends on the magnitude of the loop gain. Loop gain is the mathematical ratio of breathing response to the magnitude of the perturbation [12]. If the response is too high, reflected by a ration greater than 1, a steady correction will not be achieved [12]. In this instance, it is of importance that any type of pressure therapy should be targeted to lower the loop gain ratio. Figures 78.1, 78.2, and 78.3 illustrate modes of functioning of bi-level-S, bi-level-ST, and servo-ventilation in patients with central apneas. It is obvious that S-mode ventilation will augment the emergence of central apneas because ventilation supports spontaneous breath but fails to give support during central apneas. S-mode ventilation will therefore increase the loop gain ratio (Fig. 78.1). ST-mode ventilation does not really impact loop gain ratio because ventilator support is given during the patient's efforts as well as during times of apneas (Fig. 78.2). Servo-ventilation, in contrast, decreases the loop gain ratio because ventilator support compensates for the patient's respiratory pattern because pressure support is given in disproportion to spontaneous breaths (Fig. 78.3).

On the basis of this pathophysiological background, it is not surprising that the usual bi-level noninvasive positive-pressure ventilation (NPPV) might even worsen breathing patterns dominated by central apneas [13]. Proportional-assist ventilation, on the other hand, which applies pressure in proportion to the patient's effort,

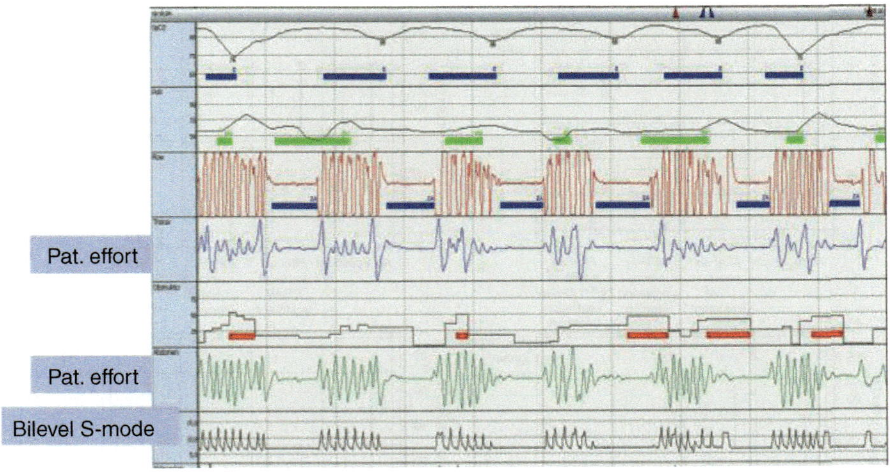

Fig. 78.1 Functioning of a bi-level ventilator in the spontaneous mode (S-mode). Notice that patient ventilation is augmented while no support is given during phases of apnea

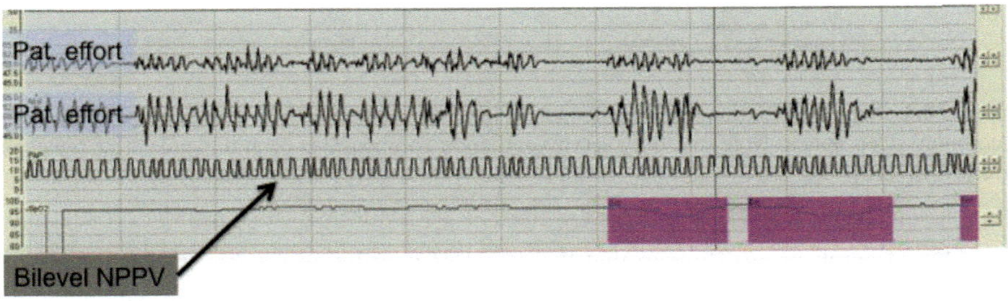

Fig. 78.2 Functioning of a bi-level ventilator in the spontaneous-timed mode (ST-mode). Notice that ventilator support is given during breathing efforts as well as during apneas

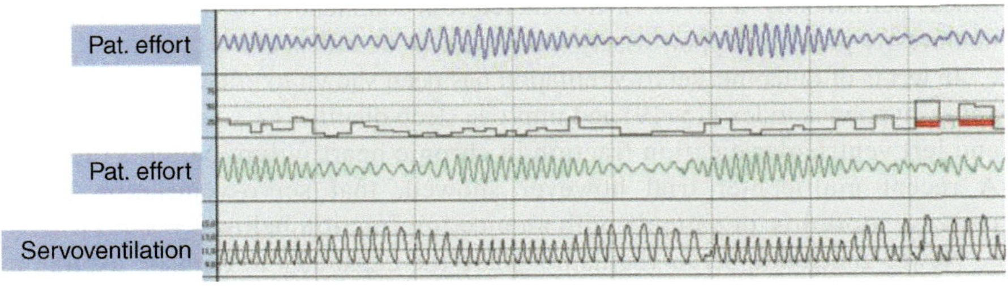

Fig. 78.3 Functioning of a servo-ventilator. Notice that ventilator support is given disproportionately to breathing efforts

promotes periodic breathing [14]. If ventilation is given in disproportion to patient effort, it is likely to improve central apneic breathing patterns. Servo-ventilation has such a disproportional approach, and several studies have shown the superiority of different servo-ventilators in this instance [15–17].

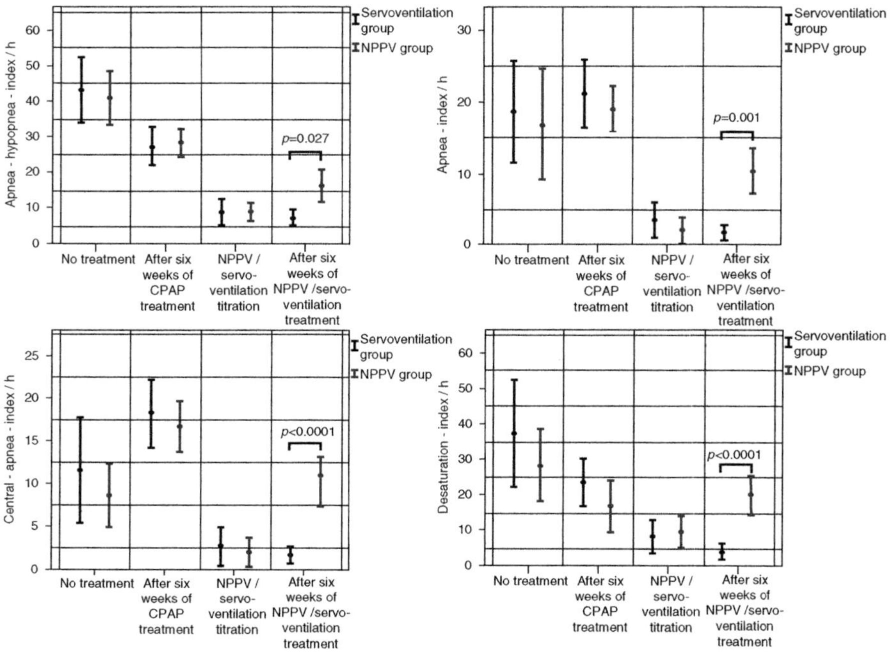

Fig. 78.4 Servo-ventilation compared with bi-level ventilation (IPPV group) in patients with complex sleep apnea. Note that only servo-ventilation compensates central events after 6 weeks follow-up [18]

Our research group showed that the effect of ventilation on the human breathing pattern can change over time [18]. In this randomized controlled trial in patients with persistent CPAP-induced central apneas, known as complex sleep apnea, bi-level ventilation improved central breathing pattern in the short term, but resulted in reemergence of central apneas after 6 weeks. Servo-ventilation, on the other hand, compensated apneas permanently (Fig. 78.4). It is therefore recommended to choose the type of noninvasive pressure support wisely and reevaluate treatment effect over time.

In terms of outcome, servo-ventilation has been shown to effectively reduce the apnea-hypopnea index [15–19] and improve sleep quality [17], quality of life [20], and left ventricular ejection fraction in chronic heart failure patients [20, 21]. A recent multicenter trial however showed, that servo-ventilation might increase mortality in patients with an ejection fraction below 45 % [22].

Newer-generation servo-ventilators share the capability to regulate expiratory pressure according to the grade of upper airway obstruction using techniques that are also used in automatic CPAP devices (APAP).

It is important to know that function differs between servo-ventilators. Due to patent law, different companies have developed different algorithms. The main goal of servo-ventilators is to keep ventilation constant. Whereas some devices measure the actual flow and are programmed to keep flow constant, others detect relative minute ventilation in shifting timeframes. Algorithms providing automatic back-up rates as well as autotitration of expiratory pressure are also different between servo-ventilators. For this reason, these devices are not arbitrarily interchangeable but must be titrated individually to each patient [23, 24].

More sophisticated feedback control systems have been introduced for the treatment of central and mixed sleep apnea, but they appear to have a low tolerance [25]. Studies comparing this approach to conventional servo-ventilation are missing to date.

Conclusion

For obstructive sleep apnea, conventional CPAP therapy remains the gold standard. Central apneas, however, require a more targeted approach. Central apneas are usually caused by variations in CO_2 regulation. To achieve CO_2 homeostasis, ventilation must compensate for apneas without augmentation of uncompromised breathing efforts. Servo-ventilators deliver pressure disproportional to the patient's own breathing effort and stabilize the human CO_2 feedback-control system.

References

1. Guilleminault C, Tilkian A, Dement WC. The sleep apnea syndromes. Annu Rev Med. 1976;27:465–84.
2. Sullivan CE, Issa FG, Berthon-Jones M, et al. Reversal of obstructive sleep apnoea by continuous positive airway pressure applied through the nares. Lancet. 1981;1:862–5.
3. Randerath W, Parys K, Lehmann D, et al. Self-adjusting continuous positive airway pressure therapy based on the measurement of impedance. A comparison of free pressure variation and individually fixed higher minimum pressure. Respiration. 2000;67:272–9.
4. Wenzel M, Kerl J, Dellweg D. Expiratory pressure reduction (C-Flex Method) versus fix CPAP in the therapy for obstructive sleep apnoea. Pneumologie. 2007;61:692–5.
5. Bradley TD, Logan AG, Kimoff RJ, et al. Continuous positive airway pressure for central sleep apnea and heart failure. N Engl J Med. 2005;353:2025–33.
6. Dempsey JA. Crossing the apnoeic threshold: causes and consequences. Exp Physiol. 2005;90:13–24.
7. Nakayama H, Smith CA, Rodman JR, et al. Carotid body denervation eliminates apnea in response to transient hypocapnia. J Appl Physiol. 2003;94:155–64.
8. Xie A, Rutherford R, Rankin F, et al. Hypocapnia and increased ventilatory responsiveness in patients with idiopathic central sleep apnea. Am J Respir Crit Care Med. 1995;152:1950–5.
9. Xie A, Skatrud JB, Puleo DS, et al. Apnea-hypopnea threshold for CO_2 in patients with congestive heart failure. Am J Respir Crit Care Med. 2002;165:1245–50.
10. Hanly P, Zuberi N, Gray R. Pathogenesis of Cheyne-Stokes respiration in patients with congestive heart failure. Relationship to arterial PCO_2. Chest. 1993;104:1079–84.
11. Thomas RJ. Alternative approaches to treatment of central sleep apnea. Sleep Med Clin. 2014;9:87–104.
12. White DP. Pathogenesis of obstructive and central sleep apnea. Am J Respir Crit Care Med. 2005;172:1363–70.
13. Johnson KG, Johnson DC. Bilevel positive airway pressure worsens central apneas during sleep. Chest. 2005;128:2141–50.
14. Younes M, Ostrowski M, Thompson W, et al. Chemical control stability in patients with obstructive sleep apnea. Am J Respir Crit Care Med. 2001;163:1181–90.
15. Allam JS, Olson EJ, Gay PC, et al. Efficacy of adaptive servoventilation in treatment of complex and central sleep apnea syndromes. Chest. 2007;132:1839–46.

16. Arzt M, Wensel R, Montalvan S, et al. Effects of dynamic bilevel positive airway pressure support on central sleep apnea in men with heart failure. Chest. 2008;134:61–6.
17. Teschler H, Dohring J, Wang YM, et al. Adaptive pressure support servo-ventilation: a novel treatment for Cheyne-Stokes respiration in heart failure. Am J Respir Crit Care Med. 2001; 164:614–9.
18. Dellweg D, Kerl J, Hoehn E, et al. Randomized controlled trial of noninvasive positive pressure ventilation (NPPV) versus servoventilation in patients with CPAP-induced central sleep apnea (complex sleep apnea). Sleep. 2013;36:1163–71.
19. Morgenthaler TI, Gay PC, Gordon N, et al. Adaptive servoventilation versus noninvasive positive pressure ventilation for central, mixed, and complex sleep apnea syndromes. Sleep. 2007;30:468–75.
20. Philippe C, Stoica-Herman M, Drouot X, et al. Compliance with and effectiveness of adaptive servoventilation versus continuous positive airway pressure in the treatment of Cheyne-Stokes respiration in heart failure over a six month period. Heart. 2006;92:337–42.
21. Oldenburg O, Schmidt A, Lamp B, et al. Adaptive servoventilation improves cardiac function in patients with chronic heart failure and Cheyne-Stokes respiration. Eur J Heart Fail. 2008; 10:581–6.
22. Cowie MR, Woehrle H, Wegscheider K, et al. Rationale and design of the SERVE-HF study: treatment of sleep-disordered breathing with predominant central sleep apnoea with adaptive servo-ventilation in patients with chronic heart failure. Eur J Heart Fail. 2013;15:937–43.
23. Javaheri S, Brown LK, Randerath WJ. Clinical applications of adaptive servoventilation devices: part 2. Chest. 2014;146:858–68.
24. Javaheri S, Brown LK, Randerath WJ. Positive airway pressure therapy with adaptive servoventilation: part 1: operational algorithms. Chest. 2014;146:514–23.
25. Oldenburg O, Bitter T, Wellmann B, et al. Trilevel adaptive servoventilation for the treatment of central and mixed sleep apnea in chronic heart failure patients. Sleep Med. 2013;14: 422–7.

Contribution of Back-Up Respiratory Rate Setting in Noninvasive Ventilation

79

Jean-Paul Janssens, Dan Adler, Patrick Pasquina, and Olivier Contal

Contents

Abbreviations

ABG	Arterial blood gases
ACV	Assist-control ventilation
BURR	Back-up respiratory rate
CHRF	Chronic hypercapnic respiratory failure
COPD	Chronic obstructive pulmonary disease
CPAP	Continuous positive airway pressure

J.-P. Janssens, MD (✉) • D. Adler, MD • P. Pasquina
Division of Pulmonary Diseases, Geneva University Hospitals,
4-6 rue Gabrielle-Perret-Gentil, Geneva 14 1211, Switzerland
e-mail: jean-paul.janssens@hcuge.ch; dan.adler@hcuge.ch; patrick.pasquina@hcuge.ch

O. Contal, PhD
University of Health Sciences, Lausanne, Switzerland
e-mail: olivier.contal@hesav.ch

A.M. Esquinas (ed.), *Noninvasive Mechanical Ventilation: Theory, Equipment, and Clinical Applications*, DOI 10.1007/978-3-319-21653-9_79

EPAP	Expiratory positive airway pressure
HMV	Home mechanical ventilation
LTOT	Long-term oxygen therapy
NIV	Noninvasive ventilation
NPPV	Noninvasive positive pressure ventilation
$PaCO_2$	Arterial partial pressure of carbon dioxide
P_{CRIT}	Pharyngeal critical pressure
PEEPi	Intrinsic positive end-expiratory pressure
PS	Pressure support
PSG	Polysomnography
$PtcCO_2$	Transcutaneous partial pressure of carbon dioxide
PTPes	Pressure time product based on esophageal pressure
RR	Respiratory rate
S	Spontaneous mode
S/T	Spontaneous/timed mode

79.1 Introduction

Although crucial in clinical practice, few publications report details of ventilator settings for long-term home mechanical ventilation (HMV), and clinical practices may vary considerably from one center to another. Recommendations for ventilator settings for HMV have been summarized by a task force of the American Association for Sleep Medicine (AASM) [1]. However, these guidelines suggest a polysomnography (PSG)-based titration of NIV (which is difficult to implement in many countries) and reflect the experience of sleep laboratories dealing mostly electively with sleep-disordered breathing and obesity hypoventilation. This chapter comments on the use of a back-up respiratory rate (BURR) mostly in pressure-cycled home ventilation, based on the available published studies.

Noninvasive (or invasive) ventilation for HMV can be provided using volume- or pressure-cycled ventilators. Volume-cycled devices are usually used either in *controlled* (respiratory rate is determined by the ventilator irrespective of the patient's efforts) or *assist-control modes* (respiratory rate is determined by the ventilator but the patient may receive either controlled or assisted breaths). Usually, BURR is set either just below the spontaneous respiratory rate (RR) or slightly higher than spontaneous RR [2, 3]. Indeed, BURR frequencies used with volume-cycled devices are on average slightly higher than those set on pressure-cycled bi-level devices [2, 3]. A controlled mode, or a high BURR in an assist-control mode, is frequently used in patients with neuromuscular disorders whose inspiratory muscles are too weak to trigger the ventilator: a high BURR allows the patient to be passively and comfortably ventilated. High BURR may also allow the ventilator to "capture" the patients' respiratory mode and correct abnormal respiratory patterns (i.e., high respiratory rate/low tidal volume or episodes of nocturnal tachypnea).

79.2 Bi-Level Pressure Cycled Ventilation: S (Spontaneous) or S/T (Spontaneous/Timed) Mode?

Use of a BURR in certain groups of patients is a subject of controversy. It is generally accepted that, in patients at risk to develop nocturnal alveolar hypoventilation and/or central apnea, the use of a BURR is recommended, or even mandatory [1]. Such is the case for most neuromuscular disorders. For the same reason, several centers prefer volume-cycled to pressure-cycled devices in these indications, irrespective of whether ventilation is invasive (tracheotomy) or not: volume-cycled devices guarantee a tidal volume and minute ventilation set by the clinician (although leaks may compromise their efficacy); furthermore, until recently, these devices had alarms that were not present on many pressure-cycled home ventilators. These devices do not usually provide an "S" (spontaneous) mode option.

When central hypoventilation and/or central apnea can be reasonably excluded, AASM guidelines recommend the "S" mode as a default setting for HMV [1]. There is very little support for this option in published data. In an early study, Restrick et al. [4] found no difference in terms of nocturnal SpO_2 and daytime arterial blood gas (ABG) levels between pressure support ventilation and assist-control ventilation with a BURR in a heterogeneous group of 12 patients under noninvasive ventilation (NIV) for chronic hypercapnic respiratory failure (CHRF). No sleep studies were performed, however, and the results of ACV on correction of $PaCO_2$ were suboptimal. Casanova et al. [5] performed a 1-year randomized controlled trial comparing long-term oxygen therapy (LTOT) with LTOT plus NIV in 52 patients with chronic obstructive pulmonary disease (COPD). NIV was provided using a bi-level pressure support (PS) ventilator set in a *spontaneous* ("S") mode. No sleep studies were performed. Five patients interrupted the study in the NIV group because of intolerance to NIV (the reason reported by the authors was "too high pressures," although average inspiratory positive airway pressure was 12 ± 2 cmH_2O). After 1 year, none of the physiological or clinical outcomes had improved significantly in the NIV plus LTOT group versus the control subjects. In a 3-month randomized controlled trial of 36 patients with obesity hypoventilation, Piper et al. [6] compared CPAP with bi-level PS in an "S" mode, after exclusion of patients with severe nocturnal CO_2 retention or residual hypoxemia after CPAP titration. There was no report of sleep-disordered breathing induced by bi-level ventilation, and tolerance and clinical impact of both modes were similar. Total sleep time, sleep efficiency, respiratory disturbance index during rapid-eye-movement (REM) and non-REM sleep, and Epworth Sleepiness Scale did not differ significantly between CPAP and bi-level ventilation.

In post hoc analysis from a randomized controlled study of volume-targeted PS versus fixed PS for obesity hypoventilation ($n = 46$ patients completed the trail), Murphy et al. [7] found that patients who had a higher proportion of pressure-controlled breaths delivered by the ventilator (>50 %) had significantly higher improvements in nocturnal oximetry and capnometry measures. A study by Contal et al. [8] aimed to compare the impact of no BURR ("S" mode) versus either low BURR or high BURR in 10 stable patients with obesity hypoventilation syndrome (OHS), on long term HMV, and all using the same device. All subjects underwent

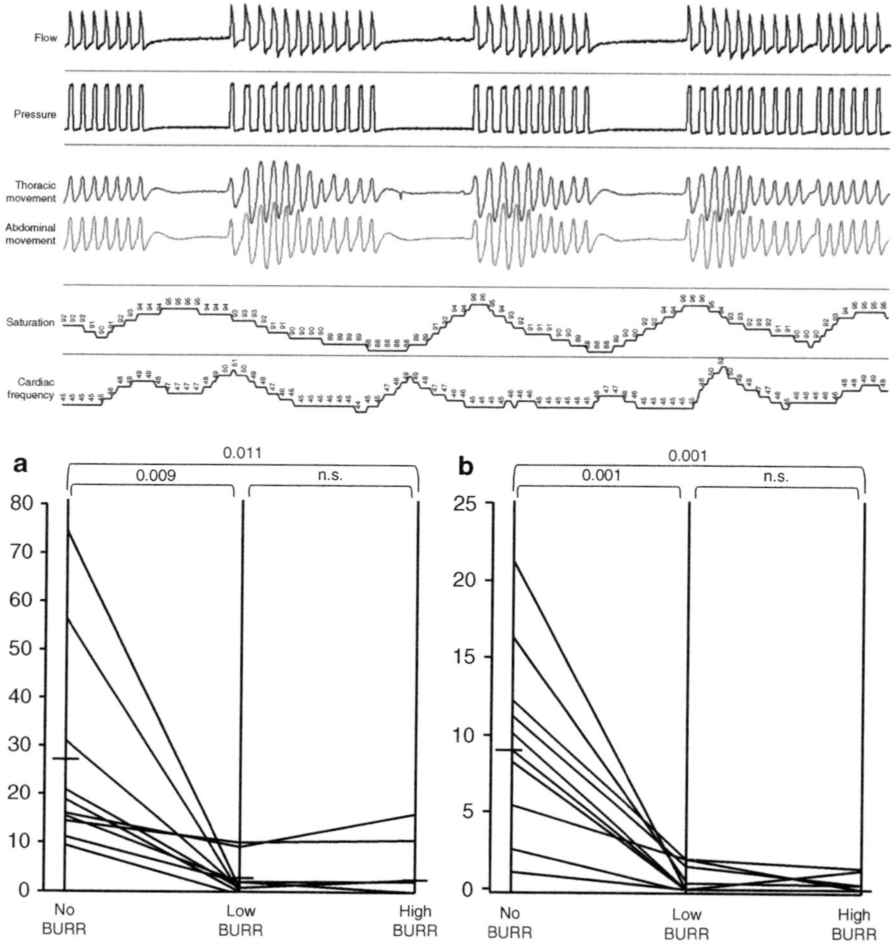

Fig. 79.1 (**a**) Occurrence of central apnea in patients under NIV for stable OHS: impact of absence of BURR. From *top* to *bottom*: flow, pressure, thoracic, and abdominal movements; SpO_2 and pulse rate. (**b**) Changes in central apnea-hypopnea index and mixed apnea-hypopnea index according to absence of BURR, low BURR, or high BURR in patients under NIV for stable OHS (Adapted from Ref. [8])

three consecutive sleep studies with either no BURR, low BURR, or high BURR, in random order, and without any other change in ventilator settings. Absence of BURR was associated with a marked increase in both central and obstructive events, suggesting that at least a low BURR was necessary to prevent central events induced by positive pressure ventilation (Fig. 79.1). Increase in obstructive events without any BURR may have been related to too low expiratory positive airway pressure (EPAP) values. However, interestingly, both low and high BURR stabilized the upper airways and decreased simultaneously central, mixed, and obstructive events.

Correction of obstructive events with high BURR might be related to airway pressure being always above P_{CRIT} (pharyngeal critical pressure, which reflects upper airway collapsibility). Quality of sleep was subjectively lower with a high BURR, although excellent tolerance to a high BURR has been reported.

In normal subjects, Parreira et al. [9] compared the quality of sleep under bi-level NPPV, using either an "S" mode or a BURR of 17 or 25/min; under NPPV with an "S" mode, periodic breathing and central apneas were common, sometimes with large drops in SpO_2.

79.3 High or Low BURR in COPD

Fauroux et al. [10] performed a physiological study in 10 patients with cystic fibrosis (age 15.0 ± 4.4 years), comparing work of breathing (WOB) with volume- and pressure-cycled ventilators at different frequencies of BURR. The authors showed that increasing BURR decreased WOB estimated by pressure time product based on esophageal pressure (PTPes)/min, and that PTPes/min was lowest at the highest BURR tolerated.

Adjusting BURR may also be critical in COPD. In acute respiratory failure, the respiratory drive of patients with COPD is high, and use of a BURR is probably unnecessary (Nicholas Hart, personal communication). However, in CHRF related to COPD, Dreher et al. [11] have suggested that "high intensity" ventilation (combining high pressure support and high BURR) may be more efficient for correction of ABG, improving dyspnea, and daytime Pulmonary Function Tests (PFT) than "low-intensity" ventilation (lower pressure support and BURR). This concept has been challenged by Murphy et al. [12] in a randomized 12-week cross-over trial, comparing "high-intensity" ventilation (i.e., high pressure and high BURR, set at 16 ± 2/min) with "high pressure" with a low BURR (set at 6/min). The authors found no difference in any of the physiological endpoints tested (mean nocturnal usage, ABG, objective and subjective sleep quality, and health-related quality of life (HRQL), albeit for the respiratory domain of the Severe Respiratory Insufficiency (SRI) Questionnaire). Noteworthy is the high rate of drop-outs in this study because of intolerance to NIV.

Thus, although "high-intensity" ventilation appears to have a favorable impact on major physiological and subjective endpoints, the contribution of the "high BURR" component may be of minor importance. BURR settings may, in fact, have different impacts according to patient phenotype, Intrinsic positive end-expiratory pressure (PEEPi), and importance of airway obstruction. Adler et al. [13] studied a specific phenotype of severe COPD with hyperinflation and "deventilation dyspnea" (i.e., sustained and invalidating dyspnea after cessation of NIV). The author's hypothesis was that too high pressure support led to progressive dynamic hyperinflation during nocturnal ventilation, leading to increased PEEPi, patient-ventilator asynchrony (PVA), and discomfort when interrupting NIV. Decreasing pressure support, slightly increasing BURR, and time to peak pressure improved PVA and morning discomfort without increasing $PtcCO_2$.

79.4 Respiratory Rate and Data Provided by Ventilator Software

Most home ventilators now provide built-in software that summarizes compliance, pattern of use, average tidal volume and minute ventilation, leaks, apnea and hypopnea, and respiratory rate. Some devices estimate the actual RR of the patient, and the percentage of respiratory cycles triggered (or cycled) by the patient (or the ventilator). This information theoretically allows determination of the extent to which the patient triggers the ventilator, or is "captured" and passively ventilated by the device. In a cross-sectional description of ventilator data provided by built-in software in 150 patients, the percentage of respiratory cycles triggered by the ventilator was highest in patients with neuromuscular disorders (23 %) versus the other indications combined (on average 50–65 %), reflecting a common practice, which is to "capture" the RR of these patients [14].

The reliability of this information is influenced by leaks: a low percentage of inspiratory cycles triggered by the patient may either result from ineffective inspiratory efforts, or may reflect a patient "controlled" by the ventilator, and resting on the BURR. The analysis of this information is further subject to the reliability of monitoring of leaks, which changes markedly from one device to another, and according to the level of pressure support [15].

79.5 Items to Be Explored

The use of a BURR seems to impact on respiratory centers and have a stabilizing effect on obstructive, mixed, and central events, although this should be confirmed in settings other than OHS. Use of a high BURR in COPD remains controversial. Although it may favor a more appropriate ventilator mode in severe COPD, it does not seem to be a necessary component of the "high-intensity" ventilation proposed by certain German groups. New automated devices with auto-adjusting pressure support, EPAP, and BURR are potentially an important breakthrough to facilitate implementation of home NIV. However, they must be tested and – until they are clearly independently validated – require monitoring by respiratory polygraphy or polysomnography.

Conclusion

There is little evidence to support the use of a spontaneous mode in HMV. If this option is chosen, the clinician must be aware that the absence of a BURR may be associated with an increase in central apnea, or hypopnea, as clearly described in normal subjects and patients with OHS. It may also further destabilize the upper airway. Conversely, a BURR may paradoxically stabilize upper airways. Use of a high BURR may improve PVA, may decrease work of breathing in certain groups of patients, and is frequently used in neuromuscular disorders. Although there are few publications describing ventilator settings by diagnostic group, the most frequent option, in bi-level pressure support, is the use of a BURR just below spontaneous respiratory rate.

Take Home Messages

- Spontaneous mode (absence of BURR) is associated with an increase in central apnea and hypopnea in normal subjects and subjects with OHS and may destabilize upper airway.
- There is little evidence to support the use of a spontaneous mode in home mechanical ventilation. If this option is chosen, the impact must be monitored by nocturnal polygraphy or polysomnography.
- "High-intensity ventilation" combining high pressure support and high BURR may increase the benefit of NIV on arterial blood gases, symptoms, and PFT in stable hypercapnic COPD. The contribution of high BURR in this setting has, however, been challenged.
- High BURRs are commonly used in neuromuscular disorders to reduce the risk of central apnea, hypopnea, and hypoventilation and allow the patient to be passively ventilated.
- The interaction between BURR and respiratory centers in central apnea-hypopnea syndromes requires further study.

References

1. Berry RB, Chediak A, Brown LK, et al. Best clinical practices for the sleep center adjustment of noninvasive positive pressure ventilation (NPPV) in stable chronic alveolar hypoventilation syndromes. J Clin Sleep Med. 2010;6:491–509.
2. Janssens JP, Derivaz S, Breitenstein E, et al. Changing patterns in long-term noninvasive ventilation: a 7-year prospective study in the Geneva Lake area. Chest. 2003;123: 67–79.
3. Leger P, Bedicam JM, Cornette A, et al. Nasal intermittent positive pressure ventilation. Long-term follow-up in patients with severe chronic respiratory insufficiency. Chest. 1994;105:100–5.
4. Restrick LJ, Fox NC, Braid G, et al. Comparison of nasal pressure support ventilation with nasal intermittent positive pressure ventilation in patients with nocturnal hypoventilation. Eur Respir J. 1993;6:364–70.
5. Casanova C, Celli BR, Tost L, et al. Long-term controlled trial of nocturnal nasal positive pressure ventilation in patients with severe COPD. Chest. 2000;118:1582–90.
6. Piper AJ, Wang D, Yee BJ, et al. Randomised trial of CPAP vs bilevel support in the treatment of obesity hypoventilation syndrome without severe nocturnal desaturation. Thorax. 2008;63:395–401.
7. Murphy PB, Davidson C, Hind MD, et al. Volume targeted versus pressure support non-invasive ventilation in patients with super obesity and chronic respiratory failure: a randomised controlled trial. Thorax. 2012;67:727–34.
8. Contal O, Adler D, Borel JC, et al. Impact of different backup respiratory rates on the efficacy of noninvasive positive pressure ventilation in obesity hypoventilation syndrome: a randomized trial. Chest. 2013;143:37–46.
9. Parreira VF, Delguste P, Jounieaux V, et al. Effectiveness of controlled and spontaneous modes in nasal two-level positive pressure ventilation in awake and asleep normal subjects. Chest. 1997;112:1267–77.
10. Fauroux B, Louis B, Hart N, et al. The effect of back-up rate during non-invasive ventilation in young patients with cystic fibrosis. Intensive Care Med. 2004;30:673–81.

11. Dreher M, Storre JH, Schmoor C, et al. High-intensity versus low-intensity non-invasive ventilation in patients with stable hypercapnic COPD: a randomised crossover trial. Thorax. 2010;65:303–8.
12. Murphy PB, Brignall K, Moxham J, et al. High pressure versus high intensity noninvasive ventilation in stable hypercapnic chronic obstructive pulmonary disease: a randomized crossover trial. Int J Chron Obstruct Pulmon Dis. 2012;7:811–8.
13. Adler D, Perrig S, Takahashi H, et al. Polysomnography in stable COPD under non-invasive ventilation to reduce patient-ventilator asynchrony and morning breathlessness. Sleep Breath. 2012;16:1081–90.
14. Pasquina P, Adler D, Farr P, et al. What does built-in software of home ventilators tell us? An observational study of 150 patients on home ventilation. Respiration. 2012;83:293–9.
15. Contal O, Vignaux L, Combescure C, et al. Monitoring of noninvasive ventilation by built-in software of home bilevel ventilators: a bench study. Chest. 2012;141:469–76.

Nasal High Flow: Novel Approach for Ventilatory Assist During Sleep

80

Hartmut Schneider and Jason P. Kirkness

Contents

Abbreviations

BiPAP	Bi-level positive airway pressure
COPD	Chronic obstructive pulmonary disease
CPAP	Continuous positive airway pressure
ICU	Intensive care unit
LTOT	Long-term oxygen therapy
NIV	Noninvasive mechanical ventilation
OSA	Obstructive sleep apnea

H. Schneider, MD PhD (✉) • J.P. Kirkness, PhD
Division of Pulmonary, Critical Care and Sleep Medicine, Johns Hopkins University, Baltimore, MD, USA
e-mail: hschnei3@jhmi.edu

A.M. Esquinas (ed.), *Noninvasive Mechanical Ventilation: Theory, Equipment, and Clinical Applications*, DOI 10.1007/978-3-319-21653-9_80

80.1 Introduction

Respiratory failure is the most common complication of pulmonary and chest wall disorders. An open nasal cannula system for delivering warm and humidified air or oxygen at higher flow rates (2–50 l/min) has been shown to assist ventilation in the acute setting in adults and children as well as in the subacute setting to ease respiratory symptoms in patients with severe, end-stage respiratory failure. The concept of delivering high flow through an open nasal cannula (NHF) has been extended to assist ventilation during sleep. This chapter reviews the medical and technical requirements needed to use NHF during sleep and their effects on ventilation. The reason for this review is the promise of NHF becoming an alternative to conventional ventilatory assist such as nocturnal oxygen, positive pressure support, and nocturnal ventilation.

80.2 Sleep-Disordered Breathing

It is well established that sleep plays a vital restorative role in maintaining health across the life span and particularly in patients with underlying cardiopulmonary disease. It is increasingly recognized, however, that sleep is a vulnerable state that can augment cardiopulmonary stress and induce disturbances in breathing pattern and blood gas exchange that are subsumed as sleep-disordered breathing.

Sleep-disordered breathing has generally been attributed to pathogenic alterations in either the upper airway or ventilatory control leading to reductions in tidal volumes, tachypnea, and increased work of breathing. Continuous and bi-level positive airway pressure (CPAP and BiPAP) and noninvasive ventilation (NIV) via a nasal/facial mask are the mainstream treatment for sleep-disordered breathing, but adherence rates are even lower than those for long-term oxygen treatment (LTOT) [1]. Thus, a majority of patients with severe chronic obstructive pulmonary disease (COPD) and obstructive sleep apnea (OSA) are insufficiently treated because they cannot tolerate a nasal mask or oxygen cannula. For these patients, NHF of warm and humidified air may represent an alternative means to improve sleep-disordered breathing.

80.3 Medical and Technical Requirements for Using NHF during Sleep

NHF of oxygen or room air through an open nasal cannula was first introduced to improve oxygenation in infants and children with hypoxic respiratory failure. It was then extended to adult pulmonary care to improve outcomes for patients in various intensive care unit (ICU) settings. An extensive review of the use of NHF in the acute and subacute settings are provided elsewhere [2, 3] in several reviews. There are, however, several technical and medical necessities uniquely required for using NHF to treating sleep-disordered breathing:

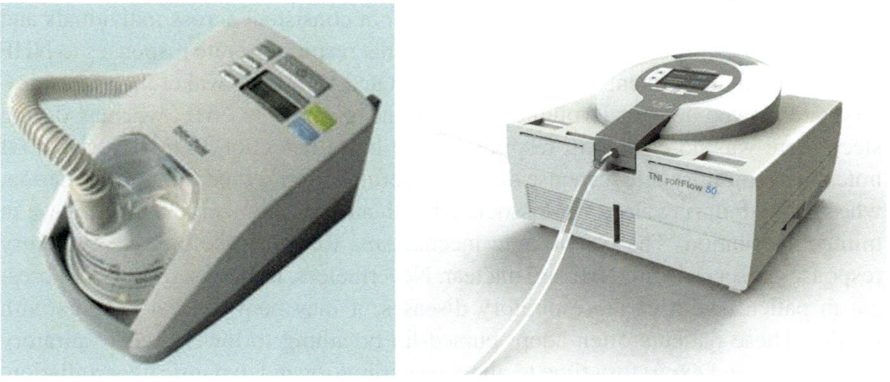

Fig. 80.1 NHF devices for use during sleep in the home. *Left*: myAIRVO™, *Right*: TNI® softFlow

1. Minimal noise due to turbulent nasal expiratory airflow. Flow rates are lower than commonly used in the ICU (i.e., 10–35 l/min, most use 20–25 l/min).
2. Optimal comfort through individual temperature (30–35 °C) and humidification (80–95 % RH) preference.
3. Appropriate portability and independence from wall or tank pressured airflow.
4. Adequacy for home requires negligible or no side effects due to cannula size or position in the nares. Cannula to nares cross-sectional area ratio is ideally <80 % and does not disperse water droplets.
5. Improved sleep quality (immediate efficacy) on the first night.
6. Approved medical device reimbursable for home use.

Although several NHF medical devices (e.g., TNI® softFlow, TNI® medical AG, Würzburg, Germany; Precision Flow, Vapotherm, Exeter, NH, USA; myAIRVO™, Fisher & Paykel, East Tamaki, Auckland, NZ) and cannula systems (AcuCare HFNC, ResMed, Bella Vista, Australia; Optiflow, Fisher & Paykel, East Tamaki, Auckland, NZ; Salter-Style® 1600HF, Salter Labs, Arvin, CA, USA) exist for use in various hospital settings using pressurized air outlets, the most commonly use devices that are suited for use during sleep at home, illustrated in Fig. 80.1, meet all of the aforementioned technical requirements.

80.4 Effect of Sleep on Ventilatory Responses to NHF

Whereas most studies demonstrate a marked improvement in oxygenation with increasing air-flow rates, inconsistencies exist with regard to the respiratory pattern response to NHF. The majority of studies tested responses to NHF during wakefulness. Although some patients may have stayed awake throughout the protocols, others may have dozed off, given the comfort and relief of respiratory stress with NHF. In particular, several studies indicate that patients reduce their respiratory rates when using NHF, but this response was not consistent across individuals and between studies [4]. One study demonstrated that respiratory rate responses to NHF were markedly dependent on the sleep/wake state [4]. During wakefulness, respiratory rate slowed and tidal volume increased in response to NHF, whereas during sleep there was no change in respiratory rate but a reduction in tidal volume. Of note, the respiratory rate response during wakefulness preserved minute ventilation, whereas NHF during sleep was associated with an approximately 20 % decrease in minute ventilation. The physiologic mechanisms for the wakefulness ventilatory responses observed with NHF are unclear. Nevertheless, if these responses are present in patients with cardiorespiratory diseases, it may help to treat patients with COPD. These patients often adopt pursed-lip breathing to lower their respiratory rate and prolong expiratory time to alleviate expiratory and dynamic hyperinflation. Pursed-lip breathing is, however, associated with an increased work of breathing and patients cannot maintain this pattern over a longer time period. NHF responses, in fact, resemble the breathing pattern of pursed-lip breathing. Thus, NHF may provide a therapeutic benefit for patients who cannot or will not adopt a slow and deep breathing pattern. NHF may also be beneficial for subjects who have high dead space ventilation due to tachypnea or a rapid, shallow breathing pattern, particularly during sleep. NHF may help to prevent development of respiratory failure in patients who suffer from increased ventilatory loads during sleep.

80.5 Mechanisms of Action

Although nasal high flow increases pharyngeal pressure (see Fig. 80.2), it differs from CPAP during the expiratory phase [5]. The contribution of the cannula size/nasal valve area and nasal cannula flow rate determine expiratory pressure. There are two main explanations for the difference in expiratory resistance responses between NHF and CPAP. NHF exerts a jet-flow effect that creates a pressure gradient across the flow-restricted nose segment, whereas CPAP increases the pressure at the nares without creating a further pressure gradient across the valve area. Furthermore, CPAP only minimally increases pressure during expiration, indicating that air-flow resistance during expiration remained relatively constant with CPAP. Stiffening of the nasal passage may also contribute to a greater expiratory resistance with increasing expiratory air flow. Regardless of the mechanism, NHF is not like minimal CPAP; rather, it serves as a means to increase resistance to expiratory air. When NHF is present, the pressure at onset of inspiration remains above atmosphere for most of the inspiratory phase, raising the driving pressure for inspiration. Despite similar patient acceptance [6], improvements in inspiratory air-flow dynamics and increases in expiratory resistance make NHF a distinctly different form of ventilatory assistance compared with CPAP.

Several studies have examined the effect of NIV or CPAP on ventilation and gas exchanges in patients with COPD. Increasing levels of CPAP increases minute ventilation without a change in arterial blood gases, indicating that patients' ventilatory responses to CPAP would differ from responses to NHF. Likewise, NHF would also differ from responses to NIV. During NIV, nasal or facial masks impose added

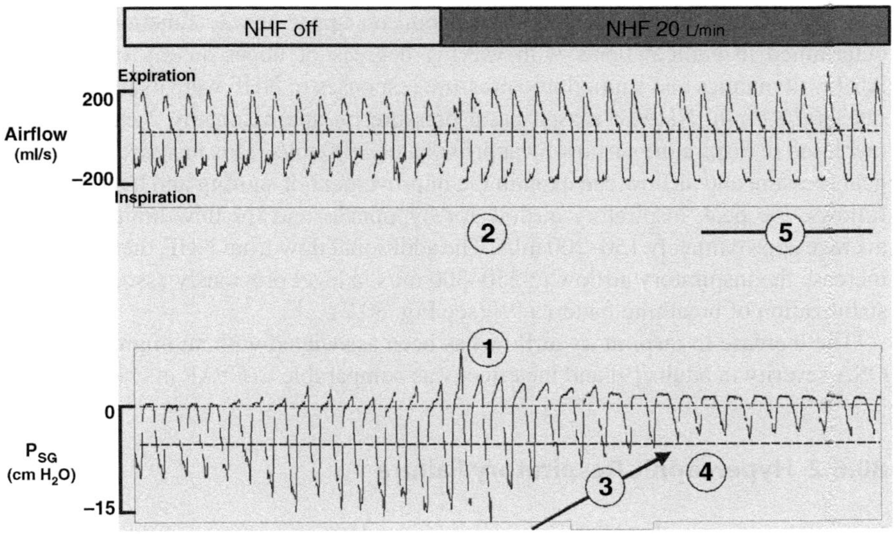

Fig. 80.2 Effects of NHF at 20 l/min on upper airway obstruction. Mechanisms by which NHF alleviates inspiratory airflow limitation (for details, see Schneider et al. [9])

dead-space volume. Improvements in alveolar ventilation must first overcome this added dead-space volume, which often requires the application of either high tidal volumes or high transpulmonary pressures, both of which are rarely well tolerated. In vitro imaging methods utilizing flow-dependent tracer-gas clearance models demonstrated increasing dead-space washout with increasing NHF rates. An anatomically based model established complete tracer-gas removal from the nasal cavities within 1.0 s. The level of clearance in the nasal cavities increased by 1.8 m /s for every 1.0/min increase in the rate of NHF, which is capable of reducing dead-space re-breathing [7].

A reduction in dead-space volume to assist breathing has been used in patients with tracheotomies by insufflating fresh air into the tracheal tube. In these studies, reductions in dead-space volumes as low as 40 ml have been shown either to decrease arterial CO_2 from 46 to 40 mmHg, if tidal volume remained unchanged, or to reduce minute ventilation and work of breathing with no or only minimal reductions in arterial CO_2 [8]. The ventilatory responses to nasal NHF, therefore, resemble more those of tracheal gas insufflation. Thus, the principles of tracheal gas insufflation appear more suitable to explaining physiologic and clinical responses of nasal NHF than CPAP and NIV.

80.6 Clinical Implications of NHF During Sleep

80.6.1 High Flow Alleviates Upper Airway Obstruction

Several studies in patient populations demonstrate that NHF increases the end-expiratory pressure. These increases are sufficient to alleviate inspiratory flow limitation in adults and children. Several studies to date have been published to confirm this hypothesis. NHF's mechanism of action on upper airway function was first determined in adult patients with varying degrees of upper airway obstruction. Airflow dynamics and supraglottic pressure responses to NHF were examined. At a rate of 20 l/min, NHF increased nasal pressure by approximately 2 cmH_2O, and increased in inspiratory airflow by approximately 100 ml/s. This increase in pharyngeal pressure and airflow can explain the improvement of snoring and hypopneas as follows: the peak inspiratory airflow for hypopneas and for flow-limited breaths average approximately 150–200 ml/s. The additional flow from NHF, therefore, will increase the inspiratory airflow to 250–300 ml/s, a level previously associated with stabilization of breathing patterns [9] (see Fig. 80.2).

The increase in inspiratory airflow has been associated with an improvement in OSA severity in adults [9] and the effect was comparable to CPAP in children [10].

80.6.2 Hypercapnic Respiratory Failure

New evidence exists that NHF may improve ventilation even in the absence of upper airway obstruction. In patients with a mild degree of COPD (Global Initiative on Obstructive Lung Disease (GOLD) I–II), the use of NHF during sleep has been associated with a reduction in arterial CO_2 compared with room air. In another study, NHF was used during wakefulness in addition to supplemental oxygen since patients had severe COPD (Gold IV) requiring oxygen treatment [11]. In these patients, NHF and supplemental oxygen also reduced respiratory rate, and lowered arterial CO_2 by more than 10 % in some individuals, indicating that alveolar ventilation had improved and ventilation had become more effective with NHF. Moreover, there are an increasing number of case reports and even randomized clinical trials showing that the application of NHF daily or nightly improves overall health outcomes. However, whether nocturnal use of NHF can prevent nocturnal hypercapnia and improve daytime outcomes similar to NIV remains to be established.

80.6.3 Obesity Hypoventilation

Additional data regarding ventilator support independent of inspiratory flow limitation is available from studies of children. McGinley et al. [10] demonstrated that, in patients with rapid shallow breathing, NHF markedly reduced the respiratory rate and inspiratory duty cycle, even if inspiratory flow limitation was not fully restored (see Fig. 80.3). The precise mechanism for improving gas exchange and efficacy of ventilation is not fully understood. It is possible that NHF may have reduced CO_2 production by lowering work of breathing, or it reduced the dead-space ventilation by washing out anatomic dead space of the nasal cavity. Alternatively, NHF may have reduced intrapulmonary dead space by opening up atelectasis through slight increase in positive end-expiratory pressure. Regardless of the mechanism, the data from patients with COPD indicate that nasal insufflations reduced the load of breathing, particularly in patients with rapid shallow breathing pattern. Nevertheless,

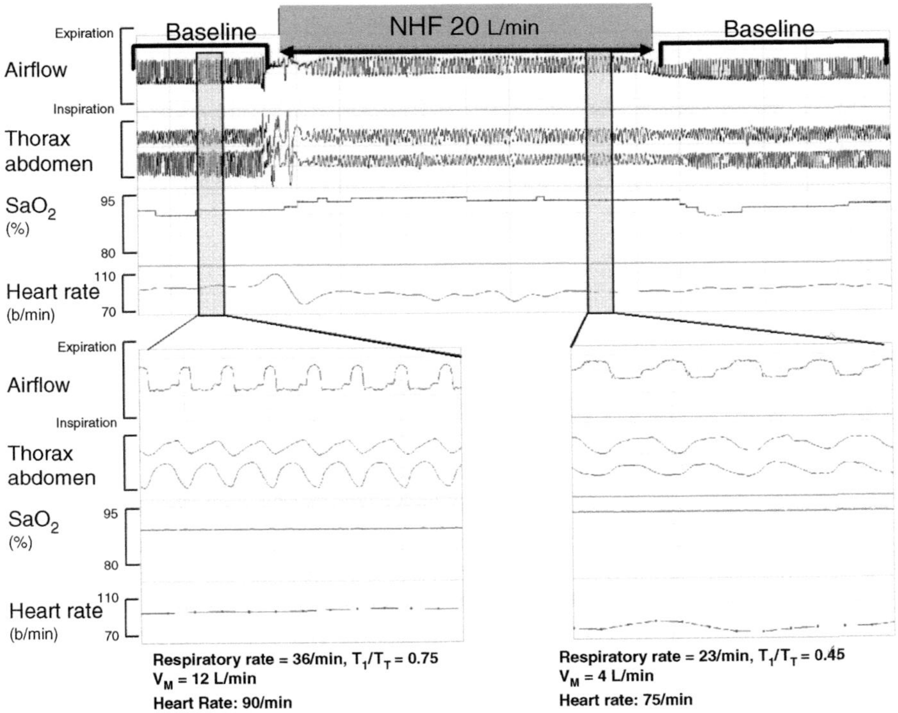

Fig. 80.3 Changes in respiratory pattern in obesity hypoventilation. The effect of NHF on a rapid shallow breathing pattern in an obese child (10 years old) demonstrates that both the respiratory rate and the minute ventilation decrease substantially. Note also that the oxygenation improves and heart rate is lowered, indicating improved gas exchange and reduction in sympathetic activity

additional clinical studies are warranted to determine NHF's effectiveness in these patients.

80.6.4 Overlap (COPD/OSA) Syndrome

Investigators have demonstrated that the prevalence of nocturnal hypoxemia increases with the severity of COPD in a large, multi-center, community-based cohort study, and that the presence of nocturnal hypoxemia cannot be predicted from daytime PaO_2 levels. Although the pathogenesis of nocturnal hypoxemia in COPD is unclear, it is likely due to decreases in neuroventilatory drive that normally occur during sleep and particularly during rapid-eye-movement sleep. A loss of drive to upper airway dilator muscles during sleep leads universally to the development of partial or complete upper airway obstruction, also known as inspiratory airflow limitation or OSA. The combination of OSA and COPD is a well-recognized risk factor for worse outcomes and, thus, justifies the separate term of an overlap syndrome. In contrast, less evidence exists for inspiratory airflow limitation without

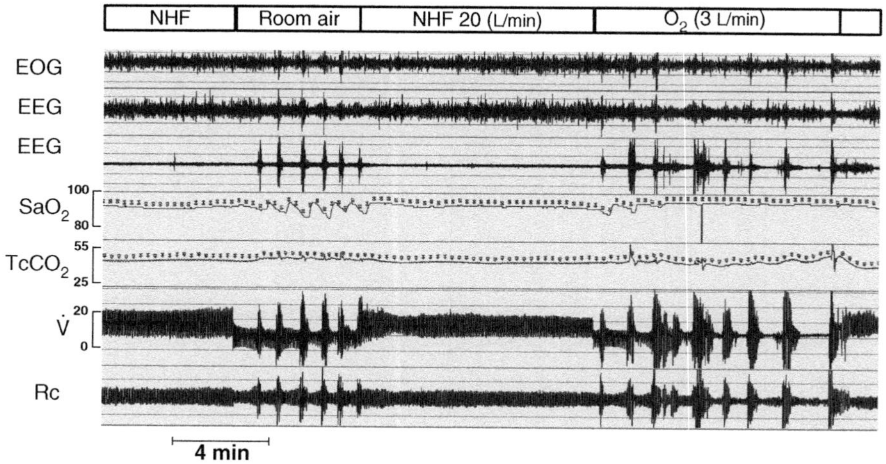

Fig. 80.4 Overlap syndrome. Effects of NHF and oxygen in a 75-year-old patient with COPD with hypopnea during sleep. For details, see the text

sleep apnea. Although inspiratory airflow limitation is well tolerated in normal subjects during sleep, in COPD, however, even subtle degrees of inspiratory airflow limitation can compromise ventilation, nocturnal oxygenation, and sleep quality. In an effort to stabilize ventilation in COPD subjects during sleep, investigators have administered oxygen and heliox. These treatments have been largely ineffective, presumably because these interventions did not mitigate airflow limitation during either inspiration or expiration. An alternative therapy is suggested by investigators who have demonstrated low levels of CPAP to be effective in relieving inspiratory and expiratory flow limitation. Fig. 80.4 shows a recording example of a sleep and breathing pattern of a 74-year-old patient who had inspiratory flow limitation leading to repetitive hypopneas with intermittent hypoxia and sleep fragmentation. NHF stabilized breathing pattern while on room air (left and middle NHF period). On oxygen at 3 l/min (right period), the patient developed severe sleep apnea of longer duration compared with the hypopneas on room air and stronger arousal responses as noted by larger tidal volumes in the inter-apneic periods. Note that the oximeter signal on oxygen remained constant at 98 %. This example shows that NHF can stabilize breathing pattern in patients with overlap syndrome who have mild upper airway obstruction (hypopneas rather than apneas) and that the use of oxygen can worsen the breathing pattern. This recording example also amplifies that oximetry alone is not sufficient to detect worsening in breathing pattern.

80.7 Summary: Clinical Implications of NHF During Sleep

An open nasal cannula system delivering warm and humidified air at a flow rate of 20 l/min (NHF) can effectively lower ventilatory requirements to provide ventilatory assistance for disordered breathing during sleep in those with COPD. A reduction in dead-space ventilation, alterations in inspiratory air-flow dynamics, and increases in expiratory resistance make NHF a distinctly different form of ventilatory assistance compared with CPAP. NHF may also play a role in protecting patients with respiratory failure, as it can reduce arterial CO_2 and alleviate rapid shallow breathing, thereby increasing efficacy of breathing. Although there is evidence that daily or nightly use improves overall health outcomes, it remains to be established whether nocturnal use of NHF can prevent nocturnal hypercapnia and improves daytime outcomes similar to NIV.

References

1. McEvoy RD, Pierce RJ, Hillman D, Esterman A, Ellis EE, Catcheside PG, O'Donoghue FJ, Barnes DJ, Grunstein RR. Nocturnal non-invasive nasal ventilation in stable hypercapnic COPD: a randomised controlled trial. Thorax. 2009;64:561–6.
2. Lee JH, Rehder KJ, Williford L, Cheifetz IM, Turner DA. Use of high flow nasal cannula in critically ill infants, children, and adults: a critical review of the literature. Intensive Care Med. 2013;39:247–57.
3. Sotello D, Rivas M, Mulkey Z, Nugent K. High-flow nasal cannula oxygen in adult patients: a narrative review. Am J Med Sci. 2015;349:179–85.
4. Mundel T, Feng S, Tatkov S, Schneider H. Mechanisms of nasal high flow on ventilation during wakefulness and sleep. J Appl Physiol. 2013;114:1058–65.
5. Parke R, McGuinness S, Eccleston M. Nasal high-flow therapy delivers low level positive airway pressure. Br J Anaesth. 2009;103:886–90.
6. Sowho MO, Woods MJ, Biselli P, McGinley BM, Buenaver LF, Kirkness JP. Nasal insufflation treatment adherence in obstructive sleep apnea. Sleep Breath. 2014;19(1):351–7.
7. Moller WG, Celik S, Feng P, Bartenstein G, Meyer O, Eickelberg O, Schmid O, Tatkov S. Nasal high flow clears anatomical dead space in upper airway models. J Appl Physiol. 2015. DOI: 10.1152/japplphysiol.00934.2014
8. Tagaito Y, Schneider H, O'Donnell CP, Smith PL, Schwartz AR. Ventilating with tracheal gas insufflation and periodic tracheal occlusion during sleep and wakefulness. Chest. 2002;122:1742–50.
9. Schneider H, O'hearn DJ, Leblanc K, Smith PL, O'Donnell CP, Eisele DW, Peter JH, Schwartz AR. High-flow transtracheal insufflation treats obstructive sleep apnea. A pilot study. Am J Respir Crit Care Med. 2000;161:1869–76.
10. McGinley B, Halbower A, Schwartz AR, Smith PL, Patil SP, Schneider H. Effect of a high-flow open nasal cannula system on obstructive sleep apnea in children. Pediatrics. 2009;124:179–88.
11. Nilius G, Franke KJ, Domanski U, Ruhle KH, Kirkness JP, Schneider H. Effects of nasal insufflation on arterial gas exchange and breathing pattern in patients with chronic obstructive pulmonary disease and hypercapnic respiratory failure. Adv Exp Med Biol. 2013;755:27–34.

NIV Adaptation Process: Implications of Team: Key Practical Recommendations and Evidence

81

Pawel J. Kuca and Witold Z. Tomkowski

Contents

Abbreviations

COPD	Chronic obstructive pulmonary disease
CPAP	Continuous positive airway pressure
EPAP	Expiratory positive airway pressure
IPAP	Inspiratory positive airway pressure
NIV	Noninvasive mechanical ventilation
OSA	Obstructive sleep apnea
pCO_2	Partial pressure of carbon dioxide
PEEP	Positive end-expiratory pressure
RF	Respiratory failure
RFT	Respiratory function tests
UL	Unintentional leak

P.J. Kuca, MD, PhD (✉) • W.Z. Tomkowski, MD, PhD
Cardio-Respiratory Intensive Care, National Tuberculosis and Lung Diseases Research Institute, Plocka 26, Warsaw 01-138, Poland
e-mail: pawel.jan.kuca@gmail.com; w.tomkowski@igichp.edu.pl

A.M. Esquinas (ed.), *Noninvasive Mechanical Ventilation: Theory, Equipment, and Clinical Applications*, DOI 10.1007/978-3-319-21653-9_81

81.1 Introduction

Over the past two decades, noninvasive ventilation (NIV) has assumed a central role in the treatment of patients with hypoxemic and hypercapnic respiratory failure (RF) in the acute or chronic setting. The main advantage of NIV in acute RF is avoiding endotracheal intubation and its related complications, preventing severe sedation and tracheostomy, improving patient comfort, and preserving defense mechanisms [1]. The most convincing evidence supporting NIV use in the acute setting has been shown for patients with exacerbation of chronic obstructive pulmonary disease (COPD) or acute cardiogenic pulmonary edema. The clinical indications for NIV have increased in recent years and are now well defined for the treatment of chronic RF secondary to restrictive thoracic diseases and for COPD as high-intensity NIV. Results indicate that, for patients with chronic restrictive RV who use it, NIV improves quality of life, prolongs survival, enhances gas exchange, and provides better sleep quality.

Once the decision to start NIV has been made, it is essential to choose a proper ventilator, ventilation mode, and interface, and to construct a detailed plan for adequate location for and precise monitoring of the use of NIV [1]. Adaptation process plays an important role in the efficacy and safety of NIV treatment. Unfortunately, this problem is poorly addressed in the literature. Moreover, current international guidelines are usually disease-specific and concentrate on technical aspects of NIV in acute RF. Therefore, a deeper understanding of adherence and nonadherence for specific forms of NIV – continuous positive airway pressure (CPAP) in the treatment of patients with obstructive sleep apnea (OSA) – may be helpful for detecting critical factors for NIV adaptation success in other conditions. Educational, supportive, and behavioral interventions to improve adaptation for CPAP in adult populations with OSA are reviewed.

Implementation protocols for NIV in acute RF, significant for adaptation, have been precisely described by British Thoracic Society Standards of Care Committee and Canadian Critical Care Society NIV Guidelines Group. Two adaptation strategies for chronic setting have been described: one for patients with COPD, based on high-intensity NIV and started in the hospital, and another for patients with restrictive, neuromuscular, and obesity problems with ventilation, with hospital or home implementation.

At the end common problems with adaptation process, depended on staff members or organizing structure, and troubles with equipment malfunctions, important for adaptation, were discussed.

81.2 Lessons from CPAP Adherence and Nonadherence for OSA

CPAP is the standard treatment for OSA, first described by Sulivan et al. in 1981. CPAP has been demonstrated to improve daytime performance, reduce daytime sleepiness, reduce automobile accidents, normalize sleep architecture, decrease blood pressure, and reduce other cardiovascular events. To reach these beneficial effects, CPAP should be used regularly. CPAP adherence in patients with OSA has been intensively studied. The main endpoint of most studies was CPAP usage time per night. Despite the efficacy of CPAP in reversing sleep apnea, of those studies using the cut point of at least 4 h per night to define adherence, 29–83 % of patients were nonadherent [2].

One important way to improve adherence is to understand that the pattern of adherence that is established early, within the first week of treatment, predicts long-term use. It is also important to know that there are many patients who refuse to consider treatment for OSA because of the nature of CPAP as a mechanical mask- and machine-based therapy. This nonacceptance of therapy is therefore the crucial cause of nonadherence. It has been observed that improvements in symptoms, daytime sleepiness, neurological behavior, blood pressure, and quality of life occur with greater use. Some studies suggest that even low levels of application provide some benefits. Other studies have demonstrated a dose-response relationship [2]. In fact, any use is better than no use, but greater gains in clinical outcomes may be obtained with longer nightly durations of CPAP therapy.

Various factors associated with good adherence can be identified, including patient characteristics (female gender, increasing age), parameters of disease severity, aspects of the technological interface, factors related to the initial exposure to CPAP, and psychological and social variables. Patient education is recommended in all patients receiving CPAP therapy for OSA before, during, and shortly after the initiation of treatment. There is stronger support for the symptomatic severity of OSA to influence adherence. Increased nasal resistance affects CPAP use and initial acceptance of this treatment. Initial presentation of CPAP in a supportive, controlled environment may influence adherence outcomes. There is a strong suggestion that having someone available to reinforce the important benefits of the treatment, to immediately troubleshoot any interface-related problems, and to provide education may enhance CPAP adherence. There have been reports that the sensation of claustrophobia may interfere with use. The initial perception of CPAP as a desirable and effective treatment may be a critical factor in patient acceptance of CPAP. Patient perception of the risk of the illness, benefit of treatment, and volition to use the therapy, formed during the first week, also affect adherence. Social support, partner interaction, and partner sleep quality were important for the adherence to treatment [2].

There are three interventions that improve CPAP adherence in patients with OSA: humidification of the airway, patient selection for different modalities of CPAP, and behavioral interventions [3]. It was concluded in a Cochrane review that, in CPAP-naive patients with severe OSA, low-quality evidence indicates that supportive interventions that encourage people to continue to use their CPAP machines increase usage compared with usual care. Moderate-quality evidence shows that a short-term educational intervention results in a modest increase in CPAP usage. Low-quality evidence indicates that behavioral therapy leads to a large increase in CPAP machine usage [4].

Our current understanding of CPAP adherence suggests that adherence is a multifactorial, complex, clinical problem that requires similarly designed approaches to effectively address poor CPAP adherence in the OSA population. It recognizes the significance of adaptation to NIV in the acute and chronic settings.

81.3 Adaptation to NIV in the Acute Setting

The use of NIV to treat patients with acute RF has been expanded in the last two decades. NIV is particularly indicated in COPD with respiratory acidosis, acute hypercapnic RF secondary to chest wall deformity or neuromuscular diseases, cardiogenic pulmonary edema, and weaning from tracheal intubation [5].

NIV is not suitable for all patients with RF. If used indiscriminately, patients who would be managed more appropriately by tracheal intubation will receive suboptimal treatment. Use of NIV in patients in whom it is unlikely to be beneficial is also undesirable. It is essential that NIV be applied in an appropriate clinical area by trained staff using the optimal ventilator mode, settings, and interface for the patient with adequate monitoring [6].

Sequential steps for delivering NIV in patients with acute RF are presented in Fig. 81.1. Figure 81.2 provides a practical explanation of all steps for NIV starting in acute RF [5].

Adaptation of NIV in a unit requires education, a program of development, and an opportunity to provide feedback to the team [7]. The main reasons for low use of NIV are lack of physician knowledge, inappropriate NIV equipment, poor previous experience, and inadequately trained staff. Experience in NIV is the most important precondition for success in adaptation of NIV in acute patients. The location for starting NIV should have facilities for monitoring, rapid access to endotracheal

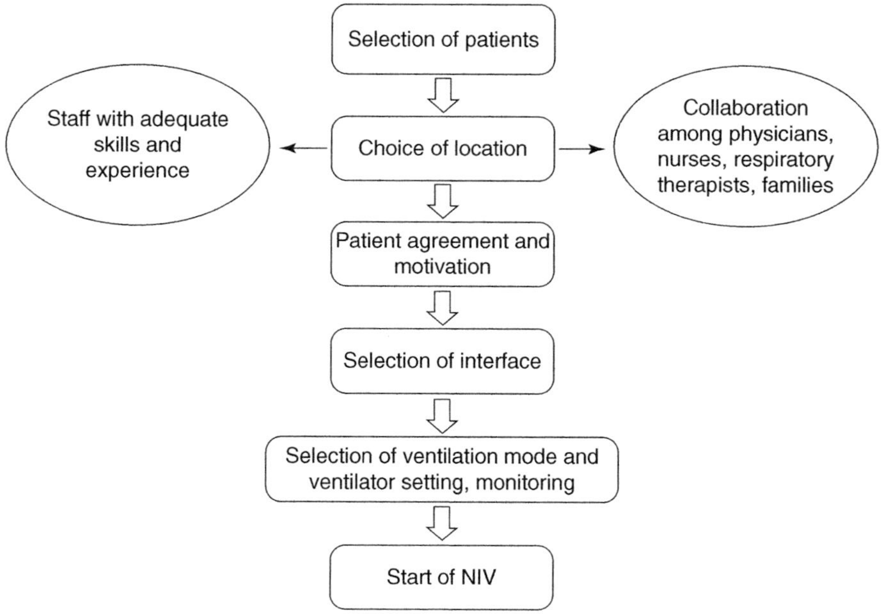

Fig. 81.1 Sequential steps for delivering NIV in patients with acute RF [1]

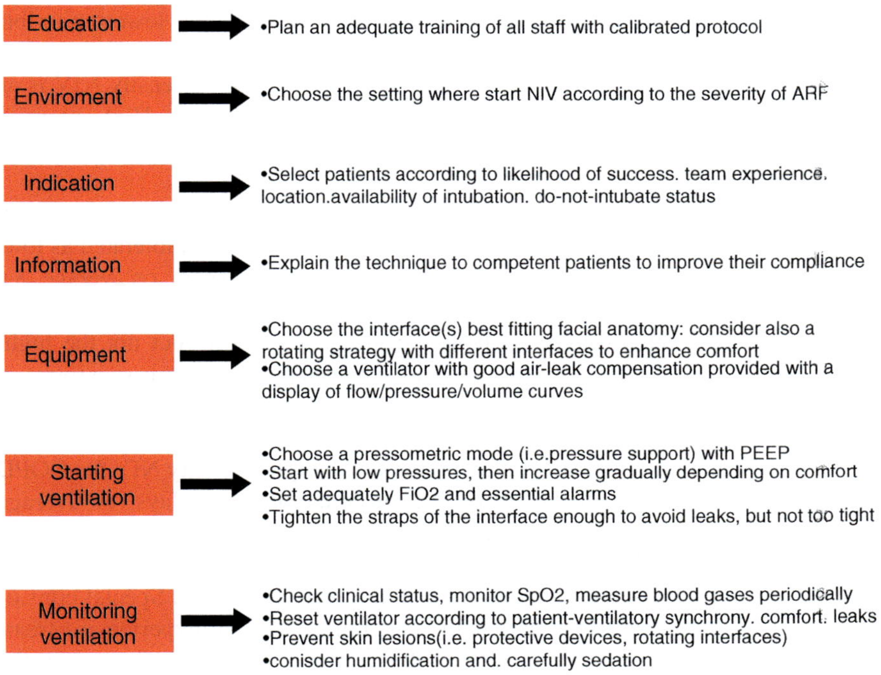

Fig. 81.2 Practical explanation for all steps for NIV starting in acute RF [5]

intubation and invasive ventilation, and an adequate number of experienced staff. The model of hospital care varies from country to country. The most important factors in determining where NIV should be started are need for monitoring, monitoring capabilities of the unit, experience of the staff, and time response to NIV. NIV should be started early, immediately after the patient's consent, because a delay may permit further deterioration and increase the likelihood of failure. The physician has an obligation to identify the disease to be treated with NIV and to exclude from NIV patients with contraindications. Continuous monitoring is needed to verify the clinical efficacy. Adherence to NIV may be improved by providing suitable humidification, and patient comfort may be improved by a soft sedation. Patient motivation is a critical issue for adaptation during NIV to enhance favorable outcomes [7].

81.4 Adaptation to NIV in the Chronic Setting

There are two important and distinct strategies for the use of NIV in the chronic setting: one COPD and another in restrictive thoracic diseases, obesity hypoventilation syndrome, and neuromuscular disorders with chronic RF.

The rationale for long-term NIV for COPD patients is still disputed. Fortunately, a promising NIV technique has been described and introduced into clinical practice [8]. High-intensity NIV is defined as long-term (chronic) NIV aimed at maximally improving gas exchange. This means that the patient should achieve normocapnia or, if hypercapnia cannot be totally avoided, the lowest possible level of pCO_2 in arterial blood using high ventilatory settings, as maximally tolerated or necessary. From the physiological point of view, high-intensity NIV is an effective procedure and improves several variables and parameters. High-intensity NIV now is the first-choice method for home mechanical ventilation in patients with COPD.

This approach clearly contrasts with the conventional, low-intensity approach. It might be speculated that high-intensity NIV would not be as well tolerated as low-intensity NIV in COPD. In fact, the opposite is true: patients spent, on average, 3.6 more hours per day on NIV when using high-intensity NIV compared with the low-intensity strategy. Interestingly, dropouts occurred in the low- but not the high-intensity group. More effective ventilation, as achieved by more aggressive forms of NIV, results in better patient adherence, which is attributable to improved quality of life and more effectively ameliorated symptoms [8].

An important part of the adaptation process with high-intensity NIV for COPD patients consume is the time spent on the introduction. More days (on average 2.5) were spent in the hospital to acclimatize patients to high-intensity NIV compared with low-intensity NIV. Other important factors include greater amounts of leakage during night ventilation and induction in cardiac output. Special consideration should be given to patients with heart failure and antihypertensive treatment. High-intensity NIV is typically established in a step-wise approach in the hospital [8]. The typical order of single steps for initiation and optimal adaptation, as well as pitfalls and problem-solving advice for individual tracks of the adaptation process, have been precisely described by Windisch [8] and are presented in Table 81.1.

Great progress has been made in NIV modalities for the treatment of restrictive chronic RF. NIV improves quality of life, prolongs survival, enhances gas exchange, and provides better sleep quality. Currently, indications are well defined for patients with neuromuscular and chest wall diseases, complications of tuberculosis, obesity hypoventilation syndrome, and other syndromes involving alveolar hypoventilation [9].

Most patients committed to chronic NIV undergo the traditional adaptation and follow-up in hospital. The period of adaptation to NIV for patients who are initiating treatment usually takes place on a scheduled in-patient basis, although it has been reported to have been undertaken successfully in day hospitals, outpatient clinics, and even in the patient's home. Good infrastructure, adequate equipment, and home-care staff have allowed home treatment to be as efficient as conventional hospitalization [9]. Possibly more important than where the adaptation process takes place is the motivation, experience, and dedication of the caregivers assigned to carry it out. In fact, adaptation and follow-up in the patient's home is as efficient as that conducted within the hospital framework, but with the added benefit of utilizing the patient's family environment. Table 81.2 lists steps for adaptation and the follow-up protocol for chronic NIV in stable patients with chronic restrictive RF.

Table 81.1 Practical approach for high-intensity NIV adaptation and problem solving in patients with COPD [8]

Adaptation approach for high-intensity NIV
Use NIV in the daytime first, with the primary aim of establishing tolerance, but also with control of blood gases and vital parameters including blood pressure
Start with assisted NIV first For this purpose, the lowest back-up respiratory rate and most sensitive trigger threshold are typically used in addition to low inspiratory positive airway pressure (IPAP) levels, normally ranging between 12 and 16 cmH_2O Expiratory positive airway pressure (EPAP) levels are low at this time
Once assisted NIV is tolerated, carefully increase IPAP in a step-wise approach until maximal tolerance is reached, usually up to 30 (range 20–40) cmH_2O The tolerated maximum may differ greatly between individuals
Increase the respiratory rate just beyond the spontaneous rate (not more) to establish controlled ventilation, but avoid excessively high respiratory rate settings that cause dynamic hyperinflation
Set EPAP to avoid dynamic hyperinflation according to subjective comfort (usually 3 and 6 cmH_2O), and, similarly, set the inspiratory:expiratory ratio to 1:2 or lower EPAP settings may be higher when upper airway obstruction is simultaneously treated (COPD + obstructive sleep apnea syndrome)
Once daytime tolerance is acceptable, apply nocturnal NIV Do not apply nocturnal NIV too early when the patient is not comfortable with daytime NIV
Adjust ventilator settings according to subjective tolerance and nocturnal monitoring of blood gases. Sometimes settings can be modified considerably at the first control visit in the hospital after the patient has been acclimatized to NIV at home for some weeks
Problem solving in adaptation to high-intensity NIV
Tolerance of higher IPAP levels can last from minutes to several days or even weeks: individual adjustment is inevitable Sometimes significant modification of settings is feasible at the first control in-hospital visit after having discharged patients for acclimatization in the home environment
In cases of coexisting upper airway obstruction, higher EPAP levels are required On the other hand, higher EPAP reduces the effective IPAP (which is IPAP minus EPAP); thus, avoid high EPAP levels if not required
For controlled NIV (final aim), respiratory rates are typically set to 1 $breath \cdot min^{-1}$ higher than during spontaneous breathing; thus, avoid excessively high respiratory rates, even though controlled ventilation is the aim
Try out several masks For nocturnal NIV, use oronasal masks because of potentially substantial leakage; for daytime NIV, a nasal mask is often better tolerated
Several days in hospital are usually necessary to establish high-intensity NIV
Use humidification in cases of dry mucous membrane
Leakage is unavoidable, but should be kept as low as possible
Gastrointestinal side-effects can be managed by medication, positioning, and adjustment (reduction) of ventilator settings; here, pressure-limited NIV is superior to volume-limited NIV
Care must be taken in patients with preexisting cardiac disease because high-intensity NPPV may induce a reduction in cardiac output

Table 81.2 Adaptation and follow-up protocol for chronic NIV in stable patients with chronic restrictive RF

(a) Adaptation to chronic NIV (hospital and home)

	Day 1	Day 2	Day 3/4	Day 4/5	Day 5/6
Pneumonologist	Initial visit Adaptation Parameters	Clinical visit Tolerance Synchrony	Clinical visit Tolerance Synchrony Modification parameters	Clinical visit Tolerance Synchrony	Discharge visit
Nurse	Clinical visit Tolerance Training	Clinical visit Tolerance Problems	Clinical visit Tolerance Problems	Clinical visit Arterial gases Pulse oximetry	Clinical visit
Physiotherapist		Training Visit Respiratory exercises	Training Visit Respiratory exercises		
Comments	Quality of life questionnaire (SF-36), Borg dyspnea score and degree of dependency (Barthel index) are measured. We decide the type of mask the patient will use and we adapt it. We initiate ventilation, 2 h/morning and 2 h/afternoon, with no nocturnal ventilation.	Continue with daily ventilation, 2 h/morning and 2 h/afternoon.	We initiate nocturnal ventilation (for at least 6 h).	Only nocturnal ventilation. We assess ventilation efficacy with: arterial blood gases at baseline (3 h after ending nocturnal ventilation); Nocturnal pulse oximetry with ventilation. If hypoxemia is not corrected, oxygen can be added.	If the results are acceptable (disappearance or decrease of hypercapnia to at least 10 mmHg, with normal pH), the patient is discharged.

(b) Chronic NIV follow-up (home or pulmonary outpatient consultation)

	Pneumonologist	Nurse	Physiotherapist
1st month	Clinical visit	Arterial gases	
3rd month	Clinical visit RFT	SF-36 questionnaire and Borg scale Arterial gases Nocturnal pulse oximetry	Clinical visit
6th month	Clinical visit RFT	SF-36 questionnaire and Borg scale Arterial gases Nocturnal pulse oximetry	Clinical visit

Modified from Domenech-Clar et al. [9]. *RFT* respiratory function tests

81.5 Common Problems in the Adaptation Process

81.5.1 Malfunction of Equipment

The most frequent problems during adaptation are related to low compliance, patient discomfort, high unintentional leaks (ULs), and insufficient correction of arterial blood gases. Many equipment malfunctions are easy to diagnose during a detailed medical history with a systematic checklist of ventilator-associated symptoms. ULs are the most common problem in NIV, both in the acute and the chronic setting. Poor compliance may also be precisely assessed by ventilation software. Psychiatric or cognitive disorders may interfere with compliance. Phobias related to masks and claustrophobia may be improved through hypnosis or behavioral therapy [10].

Good communication and a structured discharge plan adapted to the individual are required. The patients, families, and caregivers should complete competency training on how to operate the equipment, identify simple problems, and when and how to seek advice [10]. In all families, reassessment and retraining as well as provision of problem-solving plans are necessary. Written information and educational materials should be available during and after adaptation.

81.5.2 Physiotherapist's Role in Adaptation

In many countries, the assessment, education, and care of patients with pulmonary disorders in acute and chronic settings are managed by pulmonologists and nurses. During the first 1–2 h of NIV, clinicians' time with the patients is intensive and leads to adaptation success. In a few specialized hospitals, some physiotherapists are trained and involved in patients' adaptation to NIV, but the role of physiotherapists is still undefined. They should be involved as an important part of the care team in monitoring physiological responses to therapies, supervising exercise training, and performing airways clearance techniques in cases requiring more intensive treatment.

Conclusions and Key Major Recommendations

- The process of adaptation to NIV is complex and many sequential steps for successful NIV delivery in patients with acute and chronic RF are needed.
- The successful adaptation to NIV in acute settings is determined by proper selection of patients, interface, ventilation mode, and monitoring. The patient's status is usually severe, therefore, patient agreement and motivation are important but not determinative for adaptation success. Close monitoring in an appropriate location are of primary importance for NIV adaptation.
- Adaptation to NIV in patients with chronic RF needs support not only in the patient-machine interaction. Many psychological, social, and behav-

ioral factors influence adaptation to chronic NIV. Some information comes from the adherence to CPAP in the OSA population. Step-by-step adaptation procedures are proposed for high-intensity NIV in COPD and for restrictive chronic RF diseases.

- In all steps, effective patient–health-care provider communication should be an integral part of practice before and during adaptation of NIV. It may enhance favorable NIV outcome.

References

1. Bello G, Depascale G, Antonelli M. Noninvasive ventilation: practical advice. Curr Opin Crit Care. 2013;19:1–8.
2. Weaver TE, Grunstein RR. Adherence to continuous positive airway pressure therapy. The challenge to effective treatment. Proc Am Thorac Soc. 2008;5:173–8.
3. Esquinas Rodriguez AM, Scala R, Soroksky A, et al. Clinical review: humidifiers during noninvasive ventilation – key topics and practical implications. Crit Care. 2012;16:203.
4. Wozniak DR, Lasserson TJ, Smith I. Educational, supportive and behavioural interventions to improve usage of continuous positive airway pressure machines in adults with obstructive sleep apnea. Cochrane Database Syst Rev. 2014;(1):CD007736.
5. Scala R, Latham M. How to start a patient on NIV. In: Elliott MW, Nava S, Schonhofer B, editors. Principles and practice of non-invasive ventilation and weaning. London): Horder Arnold; 2010. p. 70–83.
6. British Thoracic Society Standards of Care Committee. Non-invasive ventilation in acute respiratory failure. Thorax. 2002;57:192–211.
7. Diaz-Lobato S, Mayorales-Alises S. Setting up and organizing a noninvasive ventilation unit for hospital and home therapy. Arch Bronconeumol. 2005;41:579–83.
8. Windisch W. Noninvasive positive pressure ventilation in COPD. Breathe. 2011;8:114–23.
9. Domenech-Clar R, Nauffal-Mansur D, Compte-Torreo L, et al. Adaptation and follow-up to noninvasive home mechanical ventilation: ambulatory versus hospital. Respir Med. 2008;102:1521–7.
10. Simonds AK. Risk management of the home ventilator dependent patient. Thorax. 2006;61:369–71.

Adherence to and Complications of CPAP in Obstructive Sleep Apnea: Key Determinants

82

Ahmed S. BaHammam, Aisha Hussain, and Mohammad Al-Asmri

Contents

A.S. BaHammam, MD, FRCP (✉)
Department of Medicine, The University Sleep Disorders Center, College of Medicine, King Saud University, Strategic Technologies Program of the National Plan for Sciences and Technology and Innovation, Box 225503, Riyadh 11324, Saudi Arabia
e-mail: ashammam2@gmail.com

A. Hussain, MD • M. Al-Asmri, MD
Department of Medicine, The University Sleep Disorders Center, College of Medicine, King Saud University, Riyadh, Saudi Arabia
e-mail: aishssain@gmail.com; drmdasmri2006@gmail.com

A.M. Esquinas (ed.), *Noninvasive Mechanical Ventilation: Theory, Equipment, and Clinical Applications*, DOI 10.1007/978-3-319-21653-9_82

Abbreviations

AHI	Apnea hypopnea index
ATS	American Thoracic Society
CPAP	Continuous positive airway pressure
ESS	Epworth sleepiness scale
MSLT	Multiple sleep latency test
OSA	Obstructive sleep apnea
PAP	Positive airway pressure

82.1 Introduction

Obstructive sleep apnea (OSA) is a disorder that is characterized by obstructive apneas and hypopneas resulting from repetitive collapse of the upper airway during sleep, which is attributed to several causes that can be classified into anatomical factors such as maxillofacial structure changes or redundant soft tissues of the upper airway and physiological factors such as defects in upper airway muscles and function. OSA is a serious medical illness. If left untreated, OSA increases both morbidity and mortality [1, 2]. OSA has been shown to increase the risk of hypertension, stroke, and cardiovascular complications [1, 2]. Moreover, OSA increases the risk of motor vehicle accidents.

Continuous positive airway pressure (CPAP) is the treatment of choice for OSA. It is an effective therapy that reduces morbidity and mortality; however, CPAP adherence remains a major obstacle [3]. CPAP compliance has been reported to range from 20 to 84 %, depending on the design of the study, the definition of compliance, and the population examined [4].

This chapter discusses CPAP compliance, factors that influence compliance, how to monitor CPAP compliance, interventions to improve CPAP compliance, and common side effects of CPAP therapy.

82.2 Definition of Good CPAP Compliance

The question of how much CPAP use equates to good adherence is not clearly known because there is a dose-response relationship between the duration of CPAP use and clinical improvement in several outcome parameters [3, 5]. An accepted definition of good CPAP adherence is CPAP usage for at least 4 h/night on more than 70 % of nights during the duration of assessment [6]. However, there is no good evidence to support this definition. Data suggest that usage of CPAP for as little as 2 h results in improvement in certain outcomes such as daytime sleepiness, as reflected by the Epworth sleepiness scale (ESS) and the multiple sleep latency test (MSLT) [7, 8]. Furthermore, a number of studies including randomized controlled trials have demonstrated improvements in functional outcomes, cognitive function, and blood pressure in patients treated with CPAP for less than 4 h/night, 70 % of the nights [6, 9–11]. Therefore, it is not correct to label patients who use CPAP for less than 4 h as noncompliant. An official American Thoracic Society (ATS) statement on CPAP use defined CPAP users as adherent to therapy if they use CPAP regularly for more than 4 h/night or if they use CPAP more than 2 h/night and have clinical improvement in OSA-related symptoms such as daytime sleepiness or quality of life or improvement in OSA-associated health impairments such as hypertension and diabetes [5]. This definition is more comprehensive because it takes into account the clinical improvements with CPAP use even if patients do not meet the strict criteria of 4 h/night and 70 % of the time. Nevertheless, therapists should always aim for full-time CPAP use during sleep.

82.3 Factors That May Affect CPAP Adherence

Several studies have been conducted to define factors that influence or predict CPAP use and adherence. These factors can be categorized into (1) factors related to patients' characteristics and disease features; (2) psychological and social factors; (3) factors related to the CPAP device and its side effects; and (4) factors related to CPAP titration protocol.

82.3.1 Factors Related to Patients' Characteristics and Disease Features

An association has been reported between CPAP adherence and the severity of OSA as expressed by the apnea hypopnea index (AHI), oxygen desaturation (time spent with oxygen saturation <90 % during sleep), and daytime sleepiness [12–16]. However, this association was found to be weak when other factors were included in the analysis [3]. Several studies reported that race might influence CPAP adherence. The available data suggest lower CPAP adherence in African Americans than Caucasians [17–19]. Moreover, lower socioeconomic status has been reported to be associated with worse adherence to CPAP in subjects with good standardized access to health care and treatment [17].

82.3.2 Factors Related to the CPAP Device and Its Side Effects

The technology of CPAP therapy has developed significantly since its first description in 1981 [20]. In spite of this, around 60 % of patients experience side effects that may influence their adherence [21, 22].

Heated humidification has been developed to adjust inhaled air humidity and temperature to improve acceptance and hence adherence. Although heated humidification reduces inhaled air dryness [23], studies that examined the use of heated humidity with CPAP delivery reported inconsistent findings [24, 25]. The effect of heated humidification during CPAP therapy is influenced by several factors, including air leak, interface, room temperature, temperature of inhaled gas, humidity of the environment, airflow, and pressure used [26]. Future studies are needed assess the role of humidification during CPAP titration in patients with mouth breathing and patients requiring high positive airway pressure.

A new advancement in CPAP technology is the development of auto-titrating CPAP and pressure relief (Flex-technology). In general, studies have shown no clinically significant improvement in adherence by using the new technology. Two meta-analyses have assessed the differences between auto-titrating CPAP and conventional CPAP in the treatment of OSA. Ayas et al. [27] reported that auto-titrating CPAP and conventional CPAP were similar in adherence rates, elimination of respiratory events, and improvement of subjective sleepiness. In a recent meta-analysis that included 24 randomized controlled trials, Stanley et al. [28] reported improved CPAP compliance by 11 min per night and reduced sleepiness as measured by the ESS by 0.5 points in the auto-titrating CPAP group. However, the reported improvements in ESS and compliance are not of clinical significance [28]. Nevertheless, auto-titrating CPAP may enhance adherence in subgroups of patients who have persistent side effects, those needing higher CPAP pressure, and young patients [29, 30].

Pressure relief CPAP (C-Flex™, Phillips Respironics, Murrysville, PA, USA) was developed to solve pressure-intolerance reported by some patients. Studies that assessed the effect of pressure relief CPAP have reported conflicting results [31–35]. A randomized, controlled trial that included four sites in the United States and Germany reported no difference in CPAP adherence among patients who used pressure relief CPAP compared with conventional CPAP at 30, 90, and 180 days [33]. Another 3-month, double-blinded, parallel-arm randomized controlled trial compared compliance with C-Flex versus conventional CPAP, and analyzed objective and subjective sleepiness and vigilance among patients with severe OSA [32]. There were no significant differences between groups in terms of CPAP compliance, subjective sleepiness, sleep quality, health-related quality of life, or treatment comfort. Moreover, there was no significant difference between the two groups in the sleep latency values measured by the modified maintenance of wakefulness test [32]. Nevertheless, pressure release or flex mode may be helpful for patients who complain of discomfort during breathing on CPAP, especially when exhaling.

82.3.3 Psychological and Social Factors

Several studies have demonstrated that depression is common among OSA patients [36]. Theoretically, the presence of depression may influence the adherence to CPAP therapy in OSA patients. Previous studies have reported conflicting results. In a questionnaire-based study that assessed self-reported adherence to CPAP therapy in 178 established CPAP users, depression was associated with lower CPAP use [37]. On the other hand, a study that objectively assessed the adherence of 122 OSA patients to CPAP therapy 1 month after beginning CPAP treatment reported no effect of depression on CPAP adherence [38]. Two other small studies found no association between CPAP use and depression [39, 40]. A study that used 1 week of home-based auto-CPAP titration and monitored adherence objectively in 240 CPAP-naive OSA patients reported depression as an independent predictor of fewer hours of auto-CPAP use [41]. However, most of the previous studies did not control for confounders that may influence adherence, such as OSA symptoms (e.g., daytime sleepiness) or comorbid conditions of OSA and depression (e.g., insomnia). Future studies should examine the effect of treatment of depression on CPAP acceptance and adherence, and should control for possible confounders that may interact with depression and influence CPAP adherence.

Social factors have also been shown to affect CPAP adherence in OSA patients. CPAP users who are married or in a live-in relationship show higher compliance compared with those who live alone [39, 42]. A spouse or partner may provide feedback about the effect of CPAP therapy such as elimination of symptoms and improvement in quality of life, which could contribute to higher CPAP compliance [43].

82.3.4 Factors Related to CPAP Titration Protocol

The first exposure of patients to CPAP is a critical factor that may influence subsequent adherence. CPAP titration can be done during a full-night, in-laboratory therapeutic sleep study (following a full-night diagnostic sleep study) or using a split-night protocol (both diagnostic study and CPAP titration are combined in one study). Moreover, titration can be done using unattended auto-titrating CPAP. Studies that compared the full-night, in-laboratory therapeutic sleep study with the split-night sleep study have shown that the protocol used does not influence CPAP adherence [44]. Studies that compared CPAP adherence between unattended auto-titrating CPAP and in-laboratory titration reported conflicting results regarding adherence rates [45]. An earlier retrospective study that examined the effect of in-laboratory sleep study and CPAP titration against unattended auto-titrating CPAP at home on subsequent CPAP adherence reported no difference in the number of nights of CPAP use between the two groups; however, patients who underwent in-laboratory titration used CPAP for more hours per night compared with patients who underwent unattended auto-titrating CPAP (4.1 vs 2.9 h; $p<0.05$) [46]. More recent studies, however, showed no clinically significant differences in adherence rates between the two titrating protocols [47, 48]. In a multicenter, randomized clinical trial comparing home-based unattended portable monitoring for diagnosis and auto-titrating CPAP with in-laboratory sleep study and CPAP titration [47], CPAP adherence (defined as percentage of night used ≥4 h) was 12.6 % higher among the auto-titrating CPAP group [47]. Therefore, unattended CPAP titration is an acceptable option in patients with a high likelihood of moderate to severe OSA.

82.4 How to Track CPAP Adherence

Earlier studies that reported CPAP adherence relied on self-reports. Self-reports overestimate CPAP use by approximately 1 h/night when compared with objectively measured CPAP use [49–51]. To overcome this inaccuracy, the manufacturers of CPAP machines developed tracking systems to monitor CPAP adherence and efficacy. Hour meter recording systems, which measure machine-on time, were developed initially and, subsequently, mask-on recording systems were developed. Data are stored in the CPAP machine and can be downloaded to a computer through a card containing a microprocessor chip, a modem, or a web-based server, which allows objective measurement of CPAP therapy adherence [22]. New tracking systems provide information about residual sleep-disordered breathing, hours of CPAP use, and mask leak, and some systems provide a number of different flow signals [5]. CPAP adherence can be reliably determined from CPAP tracking systems, which provide important information to the treating team. As a result, third-party players such as Medicare mandate the use of CPAP adherence tracking systems to continue reimbursement for CPAP beyond the first 3 months of treatment [5]. However, the residual respiratory events and leak data from CPAP tracking systems are not as easy to interpret and the definitions of these parameters are inconsistent between manufacturers and not well validated [5]. Tracking systems can be used on all positive airway pressure devices used to treat OSA patients, including conventional CPAP, auto-titrating CPAP, and bi-level PAP devices. An official statement from the ATS recommends standardization of nomenclature on the CPAP tracking reports [5]. Despite the above-mentioned limitations, tracking systems are helpful in daily clinical practice to solve problems related to the device such as air leaks, treat residual respiratory events, and enhance CPAP adherence. Nevertheless, studies are needed to document the usefulness of the CPAP tracking systems and to assess their effects on OSA outcomes.

82.5 Interventions to Improve CPAP Adherence

A multidisciplinary approach is needed to improve adherence to CPAP therapy through proper orientation, psychological and social support, and education provided to the patient about the disease, its complications, and benefits of CPAP therapy [21, 39]. Based on studies that examined different interventional strategies to enhance CPAP adherence, interventions can be categorized as supportive, educational, and behavioral. Supportive interventions focus on support, "reinforcement," and enhanced access to health-care services. Educational interventions emphasize enhancing patient knowledge about the diagnosis and treatment of OSA. Behavioral intervention strategies use cognitive behavioral therapy by expert interventionists to enhance adherence. A recent Cochrane meta-analysis that included 30 randomized parallel controlled trials assessed the effectiveness of educational, supportive, and behavioral strategies in encouraging CPAP adherence in CPAP-naive patients with severe OSA [52]. Compared with usual care, supportive ongoing interventions increased machine usage by about 50 min per night (low-quality evidence), and increased the number of participants who used their machines for longer than 4 h/night from 59 to 75 % (low-quality evidence) [52]. Educational interventions increased machine usage by about 35 min per night (moderate-quality evidence), and increased the number of participants who used their machines for longer than 4 h/night from 57 to 70 % (low-quality evidence). Behavioral therapy led to substantial improvement in average machine usage of 1.44 h per night (low-quality evidence) and increased the number of participants who used their machines for longer than 4 h/night from 28 to 47 % (low-quality evidence) [52].

82.6 Common CPAP Complications

More than 65 % of patients who use a CPAP machine complain of some side effects during usage [21]. Nevertheless, most of these side effects can be resolved. The most commonly encountered problems are mask leaks, nasal congestion, and removal of mask during sleep [53, 54]. It is estimated that up to two-thirds of patients do not adhere to CPAP because of side effects [21]. Table 82.1 presents common problems encountered during CPAP use and the proposed solutions.

Table 82.1 Common problems during CPAP use and proposed solutions

Problem	Causes	Possible interventions
Claustrophobia	Anxiety Face mask	Use CPAP machine gradually; try to increase an hour at a time every night. Use CPAP and apply the mask while watching TV or listening to music. Do not overtighten the straps on the mask.
Difficulty tolerating blowing air	High pressure	Use "ramp" feature on the machine. Use auto-CPAP or pressure relief (Flex technology) Relaxation and desensitization techniques. ENT evaluation to check for possible nasal obstruction.
Leaky mask/air leak	Poorly fitting mask Improperly adjusted straps Incorrect mask size High pressure	Try adjusting the mask and interface straps to get a better fit. Refit the mask, making sure it does not sit too high on the nasal bridge. Apply the mask while air is blowing through the circuit to help seal the mask on contact. Try nasal pillows or a different style of mask.
Skin irritation or pressure sores	Wrong mask size Dirty mask Headgear not adjusted properly	Try different masks or nasal pillows until a comfortable mask is found. Good hygiene of the mask. Make sure not to overtighten the mask.
Unintentionally removing the CPAP device during sleep	Nose is congested Mask discomfort	Check for proper mask fit or size. Using a chin strap may help keep the device on the patient's face. Advise patient to use a heated humidifier. Review desensitization techniques with the patient. Activate the disconnect alarm if available. Treat nasal congestion if existing.

(continued)

Table 82.1 (continued)

Problem	Causes	Possible interventions
Dry mouth/ mouth breather	Wrong mask size Air leak Patient sleeps with his/her mouth open Headgear not adjusted properly	Refit for a different mask or try a full face mask. A chin strap may help in keeping the mouth closed. Advise patient to use a heated humidifier.
Annoyed by the noise/noisy machine	Dirty air filter Faulty machine	Make sure the air filter is clean Check the device with the medical supplier to ensure it is working properly. Wear earplugs.
Air in the stomach/ aerophagia	High pressure Air swallowing	Start with a low CPAP pressure and increase the pressure gradually. Try not to use high pillows that can block the airways. Eat dinner 3–4 h before sleep. Usually disappears with continuous use
Dry, stuffy nose	Nasal congestion	Use heated humidifier. Prescribe a nasal steroid spray or normal saline.
Eye discomfort or irritation	Wrong mask size Mask not fit properly	Try a different type of mask or nasal pillows. Adjust the mask, do not overtighten.
Air hunger	Mask leak	Check mask or interface leak. Check CPAP setting if needed to adjust the ramp. Use chin strap if the patient sleeps with his/ her mouth open.

82.6.1 Mask Intolerance and Claustrophobia

One of the most common side effects of CPAP use is mask intolerance due to the wrong choice of style or size of mask or claustrophobia. Proper mask selection is an important step in management. Mask selection should take into consideration patient preferences, air leak, and adequate fit. Patients may develop anxiety and complain of feelings of suffocation. Claustrophobia occurs in approximately 15 % of CPAP users and has been associated with lower CPAP adherence [55]. To solve this problem, patients may be asked to hold the mask up to the face without fixing the straps. Once they feel comfortable, they can fix the straps. Additional techniques such as biofeedback and progressive muscle relaxation before applying CPAP may help [56]. Using alternative masks with smaller size such as nasal pillows may help reducing claustrophobia and anxiety [57, 58]. Another common side effect related to masks is mask leakage, which may cause eye dryness and irritation and dry mouth and throat. Moreover, mask leak may increase the risk of developing central apneas, which may decrease CPAP compliance [59].

82.6.2 Nasal Congestion or Dryness

Nasal problems such as nasal congestion, dryness, and rhinorrhea are frequently encountered among CPAP users. Air leak may increase the risk of developing nasal dryness, congestion, and rhinorrhea. Therefore, air leak should be ruled out in patients with nasal symptoms. Topical inhaled steroids are frequently prescribed to treat nasal symptoms among CPAP users. A randomized, double-blinded, placebo-controlled study that evaluated the effect of inhaled nasal steroids on nasal symptoms and CPAP use reported no significant difference in CPAP compliance or nasal symptoms between the two groups [60]. Heated humidifiers have been used to ameliorate nasal symptoms. When nasal steroids were compared with heated humidifiers, the group using heated humidifiers had fewer nasal symptoms with CPAP use [61]. Patients who have low compliance because of nasal obstruction due to nasal pathology such as nasal septal deviation or inferior turbinate hypertrophy may benefit from surgical intervention [62].

82.6.3 Nasal Bridge Redness or Ulceration

Nasal bridge redness or ulceration result from the wrong choice of the mask or excessive tightening of mask straps. Patients may tighten the straps to reduce air leak around the mask. It is essential to choose the mask with the best fit and to train patients on the correct way of applying masks.

82.6.4 Gastric Distension

Some patients complain of gastric distension when using CPAP. These symptoms are usually transient and disappear with regular use.

Conclusion

OSA is a common medical problem with serious medical complications. CPAP is an effective treatment that reduces the risk of several complications if used regularly during sleep. However, patient adherence to CPAP therapy is a major challenge for the treating team. New technology allows the treating team to assess CPAP compliance and the presence of residual respiratory events or air leak with more accuracy. Several factors have been associated with poor compliance, including side effects of the CPAP machine. Therefore, support, education, and behavioral therapy are needed to improve CPAP adherence among patients. Additionally, close follow-up of patients on CPAP therapy, particularly in the first few week of CPAP use, is essential to enhance CPAP compliance.

Recommendations

- OSA is a common disorder with serious comorbidities. Therefore, every effort should be made to diagnose and treat OSA patients.
- CPAP is an effective therapy for OSA; however, adherence to therapy is a major obstacle. Therefore, CPAP adherence should be monitored regularly over time.
- CPAP compliance should be assessed using the new tracking systems.
- Intensive educational and support programs with frequent follow-up of patients on CPAP are recommended to enhance adherence.
- Most of the problems arising during CPAP therapy can be resolved during follow up.

Acknowledgment This work was supported by a grant the Strategic Technologies Program of the National Plan for Sciences and Technology and Innovation in the Kingdom of Saudi Arabia.

Conflicts of Interest The authors have no conflicts of interest to declare.

References

1. Foster GD, Sanders MH, Millman R, et al. Obstructive sleep apnea among obese patients with type 2 diabetes. Diabetes Care. 2009;32(6):1017–9.
2. Martinez-Garcia MA, Campos-Rodriguez F, Catalan-Serra P, et al. Cardiovascular mortality in obstructive sleep apnea in the elderly: role of long-term continuous positive airway pressure treatment: a prospective observational study. Am J Respir Crit Care Med. 2012;186(9):909–16.
3. Sawyer AM, Gooneratne NS, Marcus CL, et al. A systematic review of CPAP adherence across age groups: clinical and empiric insights for developing CPAP adherence interventions. Sleep Med Rev. 2011;15(6):343–56.
4. Alotair HA, Bahammam AS. Continuous positive airway pressure compliance in Saudi men and women with sleep apnea. Saudi Med J. 2008;29(7):1064–5.
5. Schwab RJ, Badr SM, Epstein LJ, et al. An official American Thoracic Society statement: continuous positive airway pressure adherence tracking systems. The optimal monitoring strategies and outcome measures in adults. Am J Respir Crit Care Med. 2013;188(5):613–20.
6. Weaver TE, Maislin G, Dinges DF, et al. Relationship between hours of CPAP use and achieving normal levels of sleepiness and daily functioning. Sleep. 2007;30(6):711–9.
7. Antic NA, Catcheside P, Buchan C, et al. The effect of CPAP in normalizing daytime sleepiness, quality of life, and neurocognitive function in patients with moderate to severe OSA. Sleep. 2011;34(1):111–9.
8. Weaver TE, Chasens ER. Continuous positive airway pressure treatment for sleep apnea in older adults. Sleep Med Rev. 2007;11(2):99–111.
9. Aloia MS, Knoepke CE, Lee-Chiong T. The new local coverage determination criteria for adherence to positive airway pressure treatment: testing the limits? Chest. 2010;138(4):875–9.

10. Engleman HM, Martin SE, Deary IJ, et al. Effect of CPAP therapy on daytime function in patients with mild sleep apnoea/hypopnoea syndrome. Thorax. 1997;52(2):114–9.
11. Faccenda JF, Mackay TW, Boon NA, et al. Randomized placebo-controlled trial of continuous positive airway pressure on blood pressure in the sleep apnea-hypopnea syndrome. Am J Respir Crit Care Med. 2001;163(2):344–8.
12. Engleman HM, Martin SE, Deary IJ, et al. Effect of continuous positive airway pressure treatment on daytime function in sleep apnoea/hypopnoea syndrome. Lancet. 1994;343(8897):572–5.
13. Kribbs NB, Pack AI, Kline LR, et al. Effects of one night without nasal CPAP treatment on sleep and sleepiness in patients with obstructive sleep apnea. Am Rev Respir Dis. 1993;147(5):1162–8.
14. Krieger J. Long-term compliance with nasal continuous positive airway pressure (CPAP) in obstructive sleep apnea patients and nonapneic snorers. Sleep. 1992;15(6 Suppl):S42–6.
15. Reeves-Hoche MK, Meck R, Zwillich CW. Nasal CPAP: an objective evaluation of patient compliance. Am J Respir Crit Care Med. 1994;149(1):149–54.
16. Sin DD, Mayers I, Man GC, et al. Long-term compliance rates to continuous positive airway pressure in obstructive sleep apnea: a population-based study. Chest. 2002;121(2): 430–5.
17. Billings ME, Auckley D, Benca R, et al. Race and residential socioeconomics as predictors of CPAP adherence. Sleep. 2011;34(12):1653–8.
18. Billings ME, Rosen CL, Wang R, et al. Is the relationship between race and continuous positive airway pressure adherence mediated by sleep duration? Sleep. 2013;36(2):221–7.
19. Wallace DM, Wohlgemuth WK. Does race-ethnicity moderate the relationship between CPAP adherence and functional outcomes of sleep in US veterans with obstructive sleep apnea syndrome? J Clin Sleep Med: JCSM: Off Publ Am Acad Sleep Med. 2014;10(10): 1083–91.
20. Sullivan CE, Issa FG, Berthon-Jones M, et al. Reversal of obstructive sleep apnoea by continuous positive airway pressure applied through the nares. Lancet. 1981;1(8225):862–5.
21. Engleman HM, Wild MR. Improving CPAP use by patients with the sleep apnoea/hypopnoea syndrome (SAHS). Sleep Med Rev. 2003;7(1):81–99.
22. Weaver TE, Sawyer AM. Adherence to continuous positive airway pressure treatment for obstructive sleep apnoea: implications for future interventions. Indian J Med Res. 2010;131:245–58.
23. Martins De Araujo MT, Vieira SB, Vasquez EC, et al. Heated humidification or face mask to prevent upper airway dryness during continuous positive airway pressure therapy. Chest. 2000;117(1):142–7.
24. Esquinas AM, Bahammam AS. Humidification during CPAP titration: an unresolved issue. Sleep Breathing. 2013;17(2):439–40.
25. Yu CC, Luo CM, Liu YC, et al. The effects of heated humidifier in continuous positive airway pressure titration. Sleep Breath. 2013;17(1):133–8.
26. Esquinas Rodriguez AM, Scala R, Soroksky A, et al. Clinical review: humidifiers during noninvasive ventilation – key topics and practical implications. Crit Care. 2012;16(1):203.
27. Ayas NT, Patel SR, Malhotra A, et al. Auto-titrating versus standard continuous positive airway pressure for the treatment of obstructive sleep apnea: results of a meta-analysis. Sleep. 2004;27(2):249–53.
28. Ip S, D'Ambrosio C, Patel K, et al. Auto-titrating versus fixed continuous positive airway pressure for the treatment of obstructive sleep apnea: a systematic review with meta-analyses. Syst Rev. 2012;1:20.
29. Hukins C. Comparative study of autotitrating and fixed-pressure CPAP in the home: a randomized, single-blind crossover trial. Sleep. 2004;27(8):1512–7.
30. Massie CA, McArdle N, Hart RW, et al. Comparison between automatic and fixed positive airway pressure therapy in the home. Am J Respir Crit Care Med. 2003;167(1):20–3.
31. Aloia MS, Stanchina M, Arnedt JT, et al. Treatment adherence and outcomes in flexible vs standard continuous positive airway pressure therapy. Chest. 2005;127(6):2085–93.

32. Bakker J, Campbell A, Neill A. Randomized controlled trial comparing flexible and continuous positive airway pressure delivery: effects on compliance, objective and subjective sleepiness and vigilance. Sleep. 2010;33(4):523–9.
33. Dolan DC, Okonkwo R, Gfullner F, et al. Longitudinal comparison study of pressure relief (C-Flex) vs. CPAP in OSA patients. Sleep Breath. 2009;13(1):73–7.
34. Marshall NS, Neill AM, Campbell AJ. Randomised trial of compliance with flexible (C-Flex) and standard continuous positive airway pressure for severe obstructive sleep apnea. Sleep Breath. 2008;12(4):393–6.
35. Nilius G, Happel A, Domanski U, et al. Pressure-relief continuous positive airway pressure vs constant continuous positive airway pressure: a comparison of efficacy and compliance. Chest. 2006;130(4):1018–24.
36. Ejaz SM, Khawaja IS, Bhatia S, et al. Obstructive sleep apnea and depression: a review. Innov Clin Neurosci. 2011;8(8):17–25.
37. Kjelsberg FN, Ruud EA, Stavem K. Predictors of symptoms of anxiety and depression in obstructive sleep apnea. Sleep Med. 2005;6(4):341–6.
38. Poulet C, Veale D, Arnol N, et al. Psychological variables as predictors of adherence to treatment by continuous positive airway pressure. Sleep Med. 2009;10(9):993–9.
39. Lewis KE, Seale L, Bartle IE, et al. Early predictors of CPAP use for the treatment of obstructive sleep apnea. Sleep. 2004;27(1):134–8.
40. Stepnowsky Jr CJ, Bardwell WA, Moore PJ, et al. Psychologic correlates of compliance with continuous positive airway pressure. Sleep. 2002;25(7):758–62.
41. Law M, Naughton M, Ho S, et al. Depression may reduce adherence during CPAP titration trial. J Clin Sleep Med: JCSM: Off Publ Am Acad Sleep Med. 2014;10(2):163–9.
42. Gagnadoux F, Le Vaillant M, Goupil F, et al. Influence of marital status and employment status on long-term adherence with continuous positive airway pressure in sleep apnea patients. PLoS One. 2011;6(8):e22503.
43. Cartwright R. Sleeping together: a pilot study of the effects of shared sleeping on adherence to CPAP treatment in obstructive sleep apnea. J Clin Sleep Med: JCSM: Off Publ Am Acad Sleep Med. 2008;4(2):123–7.
44. Gay P, Weaver T, Loube D, et al. Evaluation of positive airway pressure treatment for sleep related breathing disorders in adults. Sleep. 2006;29(3):381–401.
45. Xu T, Li T, Wei D, et al. Effect of automatic versus fixed continuous positive airway pressure for the treatment of obstructive sleep apnea: an up-to-date meta-analysis. Sleep Breath. 2012;16(4):1017–26.
46. Means MK, Edinger JD, Husain AM. CPAP compliance in sleep apnea patients with and without laboratory CPAP titration. Sleep Breath. 2004;8(1):7–14.
47. Rosen CL, Auckley D, Benca R, et al. A multisite randomized trial of portable sleep studies and positive airway pressure autotitration versus laboratory-based polysomnography for the diagnosis and treatment of obstructive sleep apnea: the HomePAP study. Sleep. 2012;35(6): 757–67.
48. Skomro RP, Gjevre J, Reid J, et al. Outcomes of home-based diagnosis and treatment of obstructive sleep apnea. Chest. 2010;138(2):257–63.
49. Kribbs NB, Pack AI, Kline LR, et al. Objective measurement of patterns of nasal CPAP use by patients with obstructive sleep apnea. Am Rev Respir Dis. 1993;147(4):887–95.
50. Engleman HM, Asgari-Jirhandeh N, McLeod AL, et al. Self-reported use of CPAP and benefits of CPAP therapy: a patient survey. Chest. 1996;109(6):1470–6.
51. Rauscher H, Formanek D, Popp W, et al. Self-reported vs measured compliance with nasal CPAP for obstructive sleep apnea. Chest. 1993;103(6):1675–80.
52. Wozniak DR, Lasserson TJ, Smith I. Educational, supportive and behavioural interventions to improve usage of continuous positive airway pressure machines in adults with obstructive sleep apnoea. Cochrane Database Syst Rev. 2014;(1):CD007736.
53. Olsen S, Smith S, Oei T, et al. Health belief model predicts adherence to CPAP before experience with CPAP. Eur Respir J. 2008;32(3):710–7.

54. Pepin JL, Leger P, Veale D, et al. Side effects of nasal continuous positive airway pressure in sleep apnea syndrome. Study of 193 patients in two French sleep centers. Chest. 1995;107(2):375–81.
55. Chasens ER, Pack AI, Maislin G, et al. Claustrophobia and adherence to CPAP treatment. West J Nurs Res. 2005;27(3):307–21.
56. Edinger JD, Radtke RA. Use of in vivo desensitization to treat a patient's claustrophobic response to nasal CPAP. Sleep. 1993;16(7):678–80.
57. Ryan S, Garvey JF, Swan V, et al. Nasal pillows as an alternative interface in patients with obstructive sleep apnoea syndrome initiating continuous positive airway pressure therapy. J Sleep Res. 2011;20(2):367–73.
58. Zhu X, Wimms AJ, Benjafield AV. Assessment of the performance of nasal pillows at high CPAP pressures. J Clin Sleep Med: JCSM: Off Publ Am Acad Sleep Med. 2013;9(9):873–7.
59. Montesi SB, Bakker JP, Macdonald M, et al. Air leak during CPAP titration as a risk factor for central apnea. J Clin Sleep Med: JCSM: Off Publ Am Acad Sleep Med. 2013;9(11):1187–91.
60. Strobel W, Schlageter M, Andersson M, et al. Topical nasal steroid treatment does not improve CPAP compliance in unselected patients with OSAS. Respir Med. 2011;105(2):310–5.
61. Massie CA, Hart RW, Peralez K, et al. Effects of humidification on nasal symptoms and compliance in sleep apnea patients using continuous positive airway pressure. Chest. 1999;116(2):403–8.
62. Poirier J, George C, Rotenberg B. The effect of nasal surgery on nasal continuous positive airway pressure compliance. Laryngoscope. 2014;124(1):317–9.

"Deventilation Syndrome" in CPAP Users with Obstructive Sleep Apnea: Clinical Impact and Solutions

83

Çiğdem Akyol Beyoğlu, Aylin Özdilek, and Emre Erbabacan

Contents

Abbreviations

AHI	Apnea hypopnea index
Auto-PEEP	Auto-positive end-expiratory pressure
COPD	Chronic obstructive pulmonary disease
CPAP	Continue positive airway pressure
NIV	Noninvasive ventilation
OSA	Obstructive sleep apnea
OSAS	Obstructive sleep apnea syndrome
PAP	Positive airway pressure

Ç. A. Beyoğlu, MD (✉) • A. Özdilek, MD • E. Erbabacan, MD
Department of Anesthesiology and Reanimation, Cerrahpasa School of Medicine, Istanbul University, Istanbul, Turkey
e-mail: cigdem-akyoll@hotmail.com; draylinnizamoglu@yahoo.com; emreerbabacan@hotmail.com

A.M. Esquinas (ed.), *Noninvasive Mechanical Ventilation: Theory, Equipment, and Clinical Applications*, DOI 10.1007/978-3-319-21653-9_83

PSG	Polysomnography
PVA	Patient-ventilator asynchrony
RERAs	Respiratory effort-related arousals

83.1 Introduction

Obstructive sleep apnea (OSA) is a common respiratory sleep disorder that is characterized by repetitive partial or complete collapse of the upper airway. Repeated episodes of pharyngeal collapse lead to cessation of airflow for 10 or more seconds, identified as apneas, and decrease in airflow by 30 %, called hypopneas [1]. Diagnosis is based on the sum of apneas and hypopneas per hour of sleep. The hallmark symptom is excessive daytime sleepiness and impaired functioning in daily activities. Fortunately, there are several kinds of treatment for OSA patients, including weight loss, pharmacological treatment, surgery and continuous positive airway pressure (CPAP). The most effective treatment is CPAP, which uses a mask to deliver a calibrated level of pressure to keep the airway open, thus significantly attenuating the occurrence of apneas and hypopneas [2]. However, nocturnal noninvasive mechanical ventilation (NIV) in OSA patients may result in severe morning deventilation dyspnea, commonly named "deventilation syndrome," just after interruption of the NIV therapy [3, 4]. This aspect of OSA CPAP use is a newer topic in the literature, and the mechanisms and treatment are controversial. In this chapter, we review a detailed description of deventilation syndrome, the pathways that cause it, its clinical impact, and solutions.

83.2 Discussion and Analysis

OSA is a sleep-related disorder characterized by intermittent partial or complete collapse of upper airway during sleep, despite ongoing breathing efforts. It affects 2–4 % of the middle-aged population [5]. When airway obstruction occurs, the inspiratory airflow can be either reduced or completely absent [1]. These respiratory events may lead to intermittent hypoxemia and hypercapnia, cortical arousals, and surges of sympathetic activity [5]. Respiratory effort-related arousals (RERAs) are defined as arousals from sleep that do not technically meet the definitions of apneas or hypopneas but do disrupt sleep [6]. The brain responds to the lack of oxygen by alerting the body and cessation of inspiration, and restores the breath as a reflex mechanism.

It seems that gender, age, and weight are risk factors for OSA, but the basic pathology is not defined clearly. The underlying causes are thought to be the upper airway anatomy, response capability of the upper airway dilator muscles to respiratory challenge during sleep, the propensity to wake from increased respiratory drive during sleep, the stability of the respiratory control system, and the potential for state-related changes in lung volume to influence these factors [7]. Mechanistically, in addition to central respiratory drive, the genioglossus is modulated by local reflex mechanisms that respond to negative pharyngeal pressure [7]. Rapid changes in negative intrapharyngeal pressure activate the muscle. Reduction in oropharyngeal muscle tone provokes the upper airway obstruction. According to Poiseuille's law, if a tube's diameter decreases, there must be an increase in pressure to maintain a flow rate, whether for a gas or a liquid. In the upper airway, this can be supplied by creating a more negative intrathoracic pressure. This results in further narrowing of the upper airway and obstruction and worsens the clinical impact.

OSA symptoms include snoring, gasping for air, non-restorative sleep, daytime sleepiness, poor memory and attention, cognitive dysfunction, depression, and anxiety. Symptoms are related to short-term and transient sleep breath disorder events and impairment of sleep quality. The disorder is defined as obstructive sleep apnea syndrome (OSAS) when at least five apnea or hypopnea episodes occur in 1 h with clinical symptoms such as daytime sleepiness.

Apnea hypopnea index (AHI) is used as a classification of the severity of the disease. AHI is calculated by dividing the number of apnea and hypopnea events by the number of hours of sleep. Using the AHI, OSA can be classified as mild (AHI 5–14), moderate (AHI 15–29), and severe (AHI $\geq$ 30). Clinical symptoms are as follows:

Mild OSA: Involuntary sleepiness during activities that require little attention, such as watching TV or reading

Moderate OSA: Involuntary sleepiness during activities that require some attention, such as meetings and presentations

Severe OSA: Involuntary sleepiness during activities that require more active attention, such as talking or driving

Overnight polysomnography (PSG) is the gold standard for the diagnosis of OSA. Overnight PSG is performed by a technician in a sleep laboratory. Multiple physiologic signals are monitored during sleep that fall into three branches: cardiac, respiration, and sleep deepness. A trained polysomnogram technologist and a sleep physician analyze the collected data. The data gives a strong opinion about the patient's airflow, how it affects the physiologic status, and an accurate course of the disease. It is a preferable way to decide CPAP device parameters under PSG, so that incorrect pressure settings can be recognized easily.

Positive airway pressure (PAP) therapy is the gold standard and the most effective noninvasive treatment modality for OSA patients. Applying positive pressure to the upper airway continuously prevents the pharyngeal muscles from collapsing and keeps the airway open. However, in some cases, patients suffer from severe dyspnea just after interruption of NIV after an entire night of treatment with NIV. Patients cannot get out of the bed or perform daily activities at least 30 min after cessation of NIV [3]. This is called "deventilation syndrome," and possible pathways and treatment are controversial. To highlight the mechanisms underlying deventilation dyspnea, it is important to understand the role of CPAP in patients with OSA.

83.2.1 CPAP

CPAP supplies a continuous, constant supra-atmospheric pressure to the airway in both inspiration and expiration by pressure of the ventilator circuit. It is the most common and effective respiratory therapy for OSA patients [1]. The CPAP device is a high-flow generator that pumps compressed room air via a bellows system. The generator provides a continuous positive pressure to the upper airway via a low-resistance breathing circuit and a mask connected at the end. Every mask has its own exhalation valve, which directly influences the leak level. Air leaks may also result from gaps between the mask and skin or mouth, leaks during nasal ventilation, or nasal leaks during mouthpiece ventilation. Pressure requirements differ according to the leak level. Mask leaks can be avoided by using compatible masks fitted to the mouth, nose, or face. Patients must be educated about not mouth breathing while sleeping if using a nasal mask or not using the nostrils to breathe if using a mouth mask.

Interfaces used for CPAP therapy have a direct impact on CPAP compliance and treatment success. Leaks are usually well tolerated, but a large level of leaks may affect ventilator cycling adversely and result in arousals. Therefore, devices that can compensate for leak are desirable. Leakage compensation capability differs by NIV device. The important issue is to achieve a harmony between the patient, interface, and device. The internal dead space of NIV masks varies by mask style and may influence the hypercapnia and leak levels, so it must therefore be kept in mind.

The CPAP device increases the flow when the pressure is low in inspiration and decreases the flow when the pressure is high in expiration, so it supplies the continuous positive pressure. The lowest pressure level to eliminate the upper airway obstruction during sleep is the "optimal" CPAP. An appropriate CPAP therapy eliminates the clinical symptoms such as snoring and cortical arousals, provides a satisfactory sleep pattern, and improves quality of life.

Conventionally, CPAP parameters are set up in sleep laboratory under PSG by a sleep technician [5]. It is performed in a limited time in one night and the parameters are not changed after the appropriate adjustments. More recently, auto-CPAP devices have been introduced to deliver variable pressure levels related to the requirements of the patient during sleep to optimize the pressure. An auto-CPAP automatically titrates the minimum pressure level required for the patient. The device does not deliver a constant pressure, rather, it measures the resistance in the patient's breathing and provides the minimum pressure at a set time. The efficacy of auto-CPAP machines is variable, and they collect data to guide the clinician to examine the efficacy of the therapy.

The best method is to set the CPAP device parameters during PSG to ensure the efficacy of the treatment. The optimum pressure level is the lowest one applied to the patient to keep the airway open. The aim of this treatment is to eliminate the following respiratory events: apneas, hypopneas, RERAs, and snoring [6]. Patient-ventilator asynchrony (PVA) and discomfort may occur when the clinician fails to optimize the ventilator parameters. Technical properties of the machine, such as trigger efficiency, pressurization speed, and air leak compensation, are important in optimizing the ventilator settings. PVA is frequent in patients who are thought to be treated efficiently [8].

83.3 Mechanisms Underlying Deventilation Syndrome

83.3.1 PVA

PVA is suggested to be the main problem leading to deventilation syndrome [3]. The PVA index is the number of asynchrony events divided by the total respiratory rate as the sum of number of ventilator cycles (triggered or not) and unrewarded efforts × 100. It is used to determine the severity of asynchrony.

83.3.1.1 Auto-Positive End-Expiratory Pressure

Auto-positive end-expiratory pressure (auto-PEEP) is also referred to as occult PEEP, intrinsic PEEP, or dynamic hyperinflation. Auto-PEEP is one of the most important reasons for PVA [8]. In patients with obstructive airways disease, increased resistance leads to ineffective inspiration and expiration. Auto-PEEP occurs when expiration is ineffective and the air is trapped in the alveoli. The patient feeling air hunger increases the velocity of inspiration to get air into the lungs. When air gets into the lungs it cannot get out because of the obstruction. Incomplete emptying of the lungs leads to an excessive amount of air at the end of the expiratory phase. This leads to stretching of the lungs (hyperinflation) and impairment of the diaphragmatic contractility.

Residual pressure formed at the end of expiration exceeds the atmospheric pressure. Air flow cannot be reestablished until there is a pressure gradient from the mouth to the alveoli. The patient needs to increase the effort to initiate inspiratory airflow. Spontaneously breathing patients with air-trapping must generate a negative pressure equal to the level of auto-PEEP to initiate inspiratory flow. Hyperinflation and high end-expiratory pressure, at the end, lead to the increased work of breathing and development of rapid-shallow breathing. This promotes dynamic hyperinflation and increases auto-PEEP.

The airway obstruction should be improved to break this vicious cycle. Applying CPAP is the most effective way to treat air trapping and auto-PEEP. The key to administration of CPAP is to set the CPAP level higher than the auto-PEEP because air trapping worsens if CPAP pressure remains under the auto-PEEP level.

Reflex mechanisms from both chemoreceptors and mechanoreceptors that control the activity of pharyngeal dilator muscles are reduced during sleep [9]. Impaired activity of the pharyngeal dilator muscle during sleep plays a critical role in determining airway collapse in OSA patients. It has been observed that, during wakefulness, the activity of the pharyngeal dilator muscles in OSA patients is increased to overcome compromised pharyngeal anatomy. Once awake, the patient's improved pharyngeal dilator muscle tone overcomes the adverse forces causing obstruction and hyperinflation in the lungs. This is the recovery period from deventilation dyspnea.

83.3.1.2 Trigger Asynchrony

Ineffective triggering, auto-triggering, and double-triggering can be monitored during CPAP treatment in patients with. In patients with OSA, ineffective triggering and double-triggering are the most commonly seen patterns of PVA. [10]. Ineffective triggering is a lack of ventilatory response to patient's effort. High pressure support levels and high tidal volumes result in auto-PEEP, which leads to hyperinflation, especially in patients with chronic obstructive pulmonary disease (COPD) overlapping. Patients cannot override the existing PEEP and the effort cannot initiate the ventilator cycle. Adjusting the ventilator settings can significantly reduce PVA frequency. Reducing the pressure support level is the most effective method of eliminating PVA related to ineffective triggering [8, 10]. Auto-triggering is a cycle delivered by the ventilator without patient triggering. Reducing inspiratory trigger sensitivity can help dissolve this problem. Double-triggering occurs when the ventilator inspiratory time is shorter than the patient's inspiratory time. The patient's effort is not completed at the end of the first cycle and triggers a second cycle. The solution is increasing the inspiratory time.

83.3.2 Poor Sleep Pattern

Repetitive hypoxia and hypercapnia and cortical arousals in OSA patients lead to abnormal sleep architecture and poor sleep quality. CPAP treatment may improve poor sleep pattern, but if CPAP treatment is insufficient, then residual sleepiness is a major consequence and may play a role in daytime sleepiness and chronic fatigue [4]. However, it is not a clear reason for deventilation dyspnea because it is a chronic challenge for OSA patients, and deventilation dyspnea is not seen after cessation of CPAP therapy.

83.3.3 Other Possible Reasons

Coexisting medical problems such as impaired lung function coexisting with chronic obstructive airway disease, central apnea, depression, and sedative drugs complicate treatment and CPAP compliance and may aggravate symptoms. However, they are not a likely cause of acute dyspnea after cessation of CPAP therapy. Further evaluation under PSG will help to determine the roles of these factors in deventilation syndrome.

Conclusion

The most common treatment for patients with OSA is CPAP. CPAP treatment presents some challenges for the patient, such as adjustment to the CPAP device, erroneous pressure level set-up, poor awareness about of the dead space and leak level of the device, and coexisting medical problems. These factors may play a role in hyperinflation under CPAP therapy, which causes deventilation syndrome. Deventilation syndrome is defined as severe morning dyspnea just after cessation of CPAP. The patient cannot get out of bed or perform daily activities for 30 min. In this period, the patient awakens and reverses the adverse effects of inaccurate CPAP application with an improvement in muscle tone and then goes on with daytime activities. To avoid the syndrome, it is important to determine the appropriate pressure level required by the patient, to keep in mind the leak levels and dead spaces present with the interfaces and the leak compensation capability of the CPAP device, and to be aware of the requirement of pressure changes during therapy. Deventilation syndrome is a new term and needs further research to clarify the mechanism and overcome the symptoms.

Key Major Recommendations

- CPAP is the key method for OSA treatment. Optimal monitoring always should be performed when titrating the optimum pressure level.
- Clinicians must be aware of the properties of the interfaces and their leak levels and the requirements for pressure changes during CPAP treatment.
- Deventilation syndrome should alert the clinician to check the ventilation parameters and coexisting medical challenges.
- The key to determining the optimum CPAP for the patient is taking into consideration the patient and ventilator properties so as to avoid deventilation syndrome.

References

1. Kielb SA, Ancoli-Israel S, Rebok GW, Spira AP. Cognition in obstructive sleep apnea-hypopnea syndrome (OSAS): current clinical knowledge and the impact of treatment. Neuromol Med. 2012;14:180–93.
2. Atwood Jr CW. Progress toward a clearer understanding of the role of bilevel positive airway pressure therapy for obstructive sleep apnea. J Clin Sleep Med. 2013;9(4):337–8.
3. Adler D, Perring S, Takahashi H, Espa F, Rodenstein D, Pepin JL, Janssens JP. Polysomnography in stable COPD under non-invasive ventilation to reduce patient–ventilator asynchrony and morning breathlessness. Sleep Breath. 2012;16(4):1081–90.
4. Esquinas AM, Ucar ZZ, Kirakli C. Deventilation syndrome in severe COPD patients during long-term noninvasive mechanical ventilation: poor sleep pattern, hyperinflation or silent chronic muscular fatigue? Sleep Breath. 2014;18:225–6.
5. Chan AS, Philips CL, Cistuli PA. Obstructive sleep apnoea – an update. Intern Med J. 2010;40:102–6.
6. Kushida CA, Chediak A, Berry RB, Brown LK, Gozal D, Iber C, PArthasarathy S, Quan SF, Rowley JA, Positive Airway Task Force; American Academy of Sleep Medicine. Clinical guidelines for the manual titration of positive airway pressure in patients with obstructive sleep apnea. J Clin Sleep Med. 2008;4(2):157–71.
7. Eckert DJ, Malhotra A. Pathophysiology of adult obstructive sleep apnea. Proc Am Thorac Soc. 2008;5(2):144–53.
8. Chao DC, Scheinhorn DJ, Stearn-Hassenpflug M. Patient-ventilator trigger asynchrony in prolonged mechanical ventilation. Chest. 1997;112:1592–9.
9. Mannarino MR, Di Filippo F, Pirro M. Obstructive sleep apnea syndrome. Eur J Intern Med. 2012;23(7):586–93.
10. Thille AW, Rodriguez P, Cabello B, Lellouche F, Brochard L. Patient-ventilator asynchrony during assisted mechanical ventilation. Intensive Care Med. 2006;32:1515–22.

Psychological Factors in Noninvasive Home Ventilation Users

84

Alicia Carissimi, Denis Martinez, and Cintia Zappe Fiori

Contents

A. Carissimi, PhD (✉)
Graduate Program in Medicine: Psychiatry, Universidade Federal do Rio Grande do Sul (UFRGS), Rio Grande do Sul (RS), Brazil

Cardiology Division, Hospital de Clínicas de Porto Alegre (HCPA), Ramiro Barcelos, 2350, Porto Alegre, RS, 90035-003, Brazil
e-mail: alicia.ufrgs@gmail.com

D. Martinez, MD, PhD
Graduate Program in Cardiology and Cardiovascular Sciences, Universidade Federal do Rio Grande do Sul (UFRGS), Rio Grande do Sul (RS), Brazil

Cardiology Division, Hospital de Clínicas de Porto Alegre (HCPA), Ramiro Barcelos, 2350, Porto Alegre, RS 90035-003, Brazil

Graduate Program in Medicine: Medical Sciences, Universidade Federal do Rio Grande do Sul (UFRGS), Porto Alegre, RS, Brazil
e-mail: denis@sono.com.br

C.Z. Fiori, PhD
Graduate Program in Cardiology and Cardiovascular Sciences, Universidade Federal do Rio Grande do Sul (UFRGS), Rio Grande do Sul (RS), Brazil

Cardiology Division, Hospital de Clínicas de Porto Alegre (HCPA), Ramiro Barcelos, 2350, Porto Alegre, RS, 90035-003, Brazil
e-mail: cintiazfiori@gmail.com

A.M. Esquinas (ed.), *Noninvasive Mechanical Ventilation: Theory, Equipment, and Clinical Applications*, DOI 10.1007/978-3-319-21653-9_84

Abbreviations

CPAP	Continuous positive airway pressure
OSA	Obstructive sleep apnea
POMS	Profile of Mood States

84.1 Introduction

Continuous positive airway pressure (CPAP), a noninvasive respiratory therapy technique, is the main treatment for obstructive sleep apnea (OSA). OSA is a common sleep breathing disorder, defined as recurrent episodes of obstructed breathing during sleep. Such episodes cause repeated arousals, sympathetic hyperactivity, and intermittent hypoxia. The influence of OSA on psychological factors is still debatable.

The consequences of OSA comprise serious anatomical damage to the brain, indicated by neuroimaging [1, 2]. In animal models of OSA, intermittent hypoxia causes neuronal apoptosis [3] and demyelination [4]. Despite such clear insult to the brain, no well-defined relationship between OSA and psychological symptoms has been recognized. The reversal of psychological symptoms after the elimination of apneas by CPAP would substantiate a causal relationship.

This chapter examines the response of the psychological symptoms after treatment with CPAP, searching for conclusive evidence on the of role apneas on OSA patients' mental health. As discussed below, this field of knowledge is far from settled.

84.2 Noninvasive Ventilation on Psychological Symptom

We performed a systematic literature search of the MEDLINE and Cochrane databases. We identified 187 articles, using MeSH (Medical Subject Headings) entry terms by the PICO strategy. We selected eligible studies according to our inclusion criteria (Table 84.1). The primary aim of the review was to find studies that evaluated the change in psychological symptoms after CPAP therapy in OSA patients. Twenty studies met inclusion criteria. Only three studies were randomized trials with adequate power to allow discussion.

Table 84.1 Search strategy

Population	Obstructive sleep apnea
Intervention	Continuous positive airway pressure
Outcome	Psychological or psychiatric symptoms
Design	Observational and experimental studies
Duration	Any follow-up length
Excluded	Review studies; adherence to CPAP therapy; age<18 years; animal studies; cognitive symptoms

84.3 Discussion

Improvement of psychological symptoms has been observed in several studies after CPAP use for treatment of OSA. Because most studies are not controlled, the overall results are inconclusive. In addition, many studies report negative results. Considering that an effect size of 0.2 could be clinically relevant, samples size in a randomized trial should be of at least 30 patients per group.

The studies with adequate design and sufficient number of subjects are reviewed in detail below. All were published in peer-reviewed journals.

In 2004, Barnes et al. [5] published a study of 80 patients undergoing 3-month CPAP and mandibular advancement splint treatment in a three-arm crossover trial, compared with placebo tablet. The depression scores evaluated by Beck Depression Inventory [6], did not improve significantly compared with placebo. Nevertheless, CPAP improved only general mood, compared with placebo, evaluated by Profile of Mood States (POMS) [7]. POMS consists of a 5-point scale with six factors. General mood score is calculated adding the scores for tension, depression, anger, fatigue, and confusion and subtracting the vigor score.

In 2007, Haensel et al. [8] studied 25 patients in CPAP and placebo groups over 2 weeks. Both groups showed improvement in POMS subscales: total score, tension, fatigue, and confusion after treatment. There was no significant interaction between time and treatment for any of the POMS subscales, indicating that this improvement was nonsignificantly different from placebo.

In a study published in 2012, with 71 patients using therapeutic and placebo CPAP during 3 weeks, 56 patients completed the study [9]. There were no significant changes in the Center for Epidemiologic Studies Depression Scale [10], POMS Depression, POMS Tension, and Brief Symptom Inventory of Depression and Anxiety scores [11]. No time × treatment interaction was found. The Center for Epidemiologic Studies Depression Scale is a screening test for depression and depressive disorder and contains 20 items in 9 different groups as defined by the American Psychiatric Association Diagnostic and Statistical Manual. The 53-item Brief Symptom Inventory is a short version of Symptom Check-list-90-Revised, and it was designed to assess levels of psychological distress.

We calculated the probability of beta error in accepting the null hypothesis in the three studies above. In the study of Barnes et al. [5], the POMS scale had an 81 % power and Beck Depression Inventory had a 76 % power to detect differences between treatments in a trial. In the other two studies mentioned, the psychological evaluation had a power of 5% and 40% to detect differences between treatments.

It was difficult to analyze the 20 studies obtained from the literature because 6 had uncontrolled design. They were performed with sample sizes varying from 5 to 30 in each group, used 14 types of instruments to assess the symptoms, and treatment follow-up ranged from 7 days to 1 year. Studies assessing the symptoms for a longer time are uncontrolled. Overall, the only significant result was that CPAP improved general mood evaluated by POMS compared with placebo [5]. This result represents insufficient evidence of a medically relevant relationship of OSA with mental health.

Before the role of OSA as a cause of mental distress can be accepted, the efficacy of CPAP to control psychological symptoms in patients with OSA needs to be investigated through randomized controlled trials with long-term follow-up and large sample size. In addition to being well designed and powered, research should address other dimensions of psychological distress, not being limited to scales of anxiety and depression, two disorders that seem to be unrelated to OSA or at least do not improve after OSA treatment. Depression and anxiety are common disorders as well as OSA. The coexistence of these conditions may be only a concomitance of events, without any causal connection.

In a nonrandomized controlled study performed by our group, we observed significant improvement in somatization scores after CPAP [12]. This suggests that OSA may be the cause of a variety of "functional" symptoms [13]. These symptoms have been attributed to psychological stress because, until now, a sleep study to rule out OSA is not considered part of the psychological assessment. It is necessary to explore unchartered dimensions of mental suffering before dismissing the OSA-psychological complaints link.

Considering that no study currently available is sufficiently powered and well designed as to allow accepting the negative results, it is difficult to reach any conclusion on this matter. Although highly plausible, the effect of OSA on mental health remains elusive.

Key Major Recommendations

- The indication of home noninvasive ventilation to treat psychological symptoms in OSA patients is not supported by the current literature.
- Additional well-designed and adequately powered clinical trials are needed to examine the response of the psychological symptoms to OSA treatment with CPAP.
- Future studies should address other dimensions of psychological distress, such as somatization, not being limited to scales of anxiety and depression.

References

1. Macey PM, Kumar R, Woo MA, Valladares EM, Yan-Go FL, Harper RM. Brain structural changes in obstructive sleep apnea. Sleep. 2008;31(7):967–77.
2. Morrell MJ, Jackson ML, Twigg GL, Ghiassi R, McRobbie DW, Quest RA, Pardoe H, Pell GS, Abbott DF, Rochford PD, Jackson GD, Pierce RJ, O'Donoghue FJ, Corfield DR. Changes in brain morphology in patients with obstructive sleep apnoea. Thorax. 2010;65(10):908–14.
3. Baronio D, Martinez D, Fiori CZ, Bambini-Junior V, Forgiarini LF, Pase da Rosa D, Kim LJ, Cerski MR. Altered aquaporins in the brains of mice submitted to intermittent hypoxia model of sleep apnea. Respir Physiol Neurobiol. 2013;185(2):217–21.
4. Kim LJ, Martinez D, Fiori CZ, Baronio D, Kretzmann NA, Barros HM. Hypomyelination, memory impairment, and blood-brain barrier permeability in a model of sleep apnea. Brain Res. 2015;9(1597):28–36.

5. Barnes M, McEvoy RD, Banks S, Tarquinio N, Murray CG, Vowles N, Pierce RJ. Efficacy of positive airway pressure and oral appliance in mild to moderate obstructive sleep apnea. Am J Respir Crit Care Med. 2004;170(6):656–64.
6. Beck AT, Ward CH, Mendelson M, Mock J, Erbaugh J. An inventory for measuring depression. Arch Gen Psychiatry. 1961;4:561–71.
7. McNair DM, Lorr M, Droppleman LF. POMS manual: profile of mood states. San Diego: Educational and Industrial Testing Service; 1992.
8. Haensel A, Norman D, Natarajan L, Bardwell WA, Ancoli-Israel S, Dimsdale JE. Effect of a 2 week CPAP treatment on mood states in patients with obstructive sleep apnea: a double-blind trial. Sleep Breath. 2007;11(4):239–44.
9. Lee IS, Bardwell W, Ancoli-Israel S, Loredo JS, Dimsdale JE. Effect of three weeks of continuous positive airway pressure treatment on mood in patients with obstructive sleep apnoea: a randomized placebo-controlled study. Sleep Med. 2012;13(2):161–6.
10. Radloff LS. The CES-D scale: a self-report depression scale for research in the general population. Appl Psychol Measur. 1977;1:385–401.
11. Derogatis L. BSI brief symptom inventory: administration, scoring, and procedure manual. 4th ed. Minneapolis: National Computer Systems; 1993.
12. Carissimi A, Martinez D, Kim LJ, Fiori CZ. Factors influencing the response of psychological symptoms to continuous positive airway pressure therapy. Sleep Breath. 2014;18(3):499–507.
13. Gold AR, Dipalo F, Gold MS, O'Hearn D. The symptoms and signs of upper airway resistance syndrome: a link to the functional somatic syndromes. Chest. 2003;123(1):87–95.

Ambulatory Model of Noninvasive Ventilation Adaptation: Implications for Health Care, Organization, and Outcome

85

Alessio Mattei, Cinzia Ferrero, and Giuseppe Tabbia

Contents

Abbreviations

ABG	Arterial blood gases
ALS	Amyotrophic lateral sclerosis
BURR	Back-up respiratory rate
COPD	Chronic obstructive pulmonary disease
HMV	Home mechanical ventilation
NIV	Noninvasive ventilation
NMDs	Neuromuscular diseases
OHS	Obesity hypoventilation syndrome
$PaCO_2$	Partial pressure of carbon dioxide in arterial blood
PEEP	Positive end-expiratory pressure
PFTs	Pulmonary function tests
PSG	Polysomnography

A. Mattei (✉) • C. Ferrero • G. Tabbia
Pulmonary Division, Cardiovascular and Thoracic Department,
Città della Salute e della Scienza, Molinette Hospital, C.so Bramante 88, Turin 10126, Italy
e-mail: mattei.alessio@virgilio.it; cinzia_ferrero@alice.it; gtabbia@cittadellasalute.to.it

A.M. Esquinas (ed.), *Noninvasive Mechanical Ventilation: Theory, Equipment, and Clinical Applications*, DOI 10.1007/978-3-319-21653-9_85

$PTCCO_2$	Transcutaneous CO_2 pressure
QoL	Quality of life
SpO_2	Peripheral capillary oxygen saturation

85.1 Introduction

Noninvasive home mechanical ventilation (HMV) is an effective treatment for hypercapnic respiratory failure due to restrictive thoracic diseases. It is also used in hypercapnic respiratory failure resulting from obstructive pulmonary disease (chronic obstructive pulmonary disease, COPD), although there is no strong evidence of efficacy [1–3].

Long-term HMV improves survival and quality of life (QoL) and reduces health-care costs. These effects are mainly due to a reduction in hospitalization for restrictive disorders [1, 4]. In Europe, about 6.6/100,000 inhabitants are ventilated, and most of them initiate HMV as hospital inpatients [3]. Time spent adapting to ventilation in the hospital leads to a delay in starting HMV, augmented infective risk, loss of work or study time for the patients and caregivers, increased health-care costs, and inappropriate occupation of hospital beds [5, 6]. Although adapting to HMV in the hospital is still considered the best approach for unstable patients, many studies have demonstrated that, in stable patients, it is possible to start HMV as outpatients.

85.2 Effectiveness of HMV Ambulatory Adaptation

Chatwin et al. [6] carried out a study randomizing ambulatory versus hospital adaptation in patients with neuromuscular and chest wall disease with nocturnal hypoventilation. They demonstrated the equivalence of the two groups for nocturnal and diurnal arterial blood gases (ABG), ventilator compliance, health-care professional contact time, and length of hospitalization.

Pallero et al. [5] performed a similar study randomizing ambulatory versus hospital adaptation in stable patients with chronic hypercapnic respiratory failure secondary to restrictive thoracic diseases, obesity hypoventilation syndrome (OHS), and slowly progressive neuromuscular diseases (NMDs). Ambulatory adaptation was as effective as hospital adaptation, however, its more accessible strategies reduced waiting time for starting HMV. Ambulatory adaptation represents a cost savings (71 % during initiation and 44 % during follow-up) and saves resources for the population requiring hospitalization.

Lujàn et al. [7], in a prospective observational study of only 16 patients, demonstrated the reduction in costs for ambulatory adaptation of HMV, with a cost savings of 53 %, but did not consider costs in follow-up. The authors studied not only patients with NMDs and OHS but also those with COPD with chronic hypercapnic respiratory failure. They demonstrated that there was no difference in clinical effectiveness or patient compliance.

Rabec et al. [8] proposed ambulatory initiation of HMV in stable patients with COPD, confirming that clinical effectiveness, improvement in QoL, and adherence to treatment are similar whether HMV is started in hospital or at home.

Sheers et al. [9] found better survival in patients with motor neuron disease in an ambulatory model of HMV implementation. They correlated the survival advantage in the ambulatory group to a shorter waiting period from the time of deciding to start HMV.

Hazenberg et al. [10] showed that home initiation of HMV in patients with chronic respiratory failure due to a neuromuscular or thoracic cage disease is as effective as hospital initiation for gas exchange and quality of life. In addition, they found that it is safe, technically feasible, and less expensive than hospital initiation. However, HMV initiation at home requires a qualified team with the possibility of home-telemonitoring.

85.3 Requirements for Ambulatory HMV

For ambulatory HMV, a pneumologist and respiratory nurses with experience in ventilation and possibly a physiotherapist are need. It the presence of a nurse in the role of case-manager to organize adaptation to ventilation, cough management, maintenance of equipment, and follow-up is also beneficial. The presence of a respiratory physiopathology laboratory is important, possibly integrated with the ambulatory ventilation, that performs pulmonary function tests (PFTs), ABG analysis, nocturnal pulse oximetry, and nocturnal cardiorespiratory monitoring/polysomnography (PSG). For HMV patients, it is also important to be able to perform fibrobronchoscopy if necessary. Good infrastructure, adequate equipment, and staff able to resolve any medical or technical problems that may arise will help to ensure the success of HMV. The equipment needed for ambulatory HMV is in Table 85.1.

85.4 Adaptation to Ambulatory HMV

Patients who fulfill the inclusion criteria (Table 85.2) must have recently performed PFTs, ABG analyses, and nocturnal pulse oximetry or PSG before starting ventilation. Before beginning HMV, the proper and personalized interface, ventilator, and

Table 85.1 Equipment for HMV ambulatory

Wide availability of interfaces
Wide availability of various models of domiciliary ventilators for correct adaptation to the characteristics of the patient
Possibility to use transcutaneous capnography ($PTCCO_2$) for the monitoring of ventilation during the adaptation and night monitoring in HMV
Built-in monitoring system to unload ventilation data (compliance, flow, pressure, leakages, volumes, etc.) and electronic archive

Table 85.2 Inclusion and exclusion criteria for ambulatory adaptation to HMV

Inclusion criteria	Exclusion criteria
Stable clinical condition	Unstable clinical condition or respiratory exacerbations
Residence in the urban area or within easy reach	Living far away from the HMV ambulatory
Adequate caregiver support or sufficient degree of autonomy to allow daily attendance at hospital	Inadequate caregiver support and/or insufficient autonomy
	Needs of frequent ambulatory controls

setting, including modality of ventilation, correct pressure support, positive end-expiratory pressure (PEEP), back-up respiratory rate (BURR), and oxygen supplementation, must be chosen. The patient should be monitored for peripheral oxygen saturation (SpO_2) and $PTCCO_2$. After an hour from the start of NIV, an ABG analysis should be performed. The session lasts about 2–3 h [5]. It is important to take into account the patient's tolerance to HMV. During the session of adaptation to HMV, the instructions to patients and caregivers regarding the use of the ventilator and interfaces are also carried out. Ventilation will be continued at home, with the recommendation that the patient and caregiver gradually increase use of the ventilator until reaching at least 4 h/night of ventilation.

The first ambulatory monitoring visit must be made within 30 days. During this visit, compliance, gas exchange, and built-in monitoring of ventilation data will be assessed. Before this visit, a nocturnal pulse oximetry or PSG during HMV should have been executed. The objective of this visit is to ensure compliance and check reduction of partial pressure of carbon dioxide in arterial blood ($PaCO_2$) while awake, increase in nocturnal saturation, and correction of nocturnal respiratory events. If these goals are not achieved, the settings should be changed and the monitoring visit rescheduled. The ambulatory HMV team is responsible for prescribing the ventilator and consumables at the end of adaptation.

85.5 Follow-Up

The follow-up should be modified according to the more or less progressive disease of the patient and the clinical severity. It must also be based on the patient's compliance and the training of patient and caregiver. The SomnoNIV group [11] proposed a decision flowchart for the follow-up of patients for optimizing HMV setting. They proposed evaluating the built-in monitoring data of the ventilator, the ABGs, and oximetry in NIV. Only if it is impossible to find solutions to the various problems in NIV (leaks, nocturnal hypoventilation, central and/or obstructive nocturnal respiratory events, presence of asynchronisms) do they recommended domiciliary polygraphy or PSG during NIV.

Follow-up is also useful to reinforce of patient and caregiver education, or to change or prescribe new consumables based on the actual needs of the patient and assessment of cough management. Above all, during follow up, any clinical instability in these patients requires accurate clinical evaluation to modify therapy if necessary.

Key Recommendations

- Ambulatory adaptation of HMV is possible only in clinically stable patients.
- Ambulatory adaptation of HMV may be carried out in all pathologies with indication to initiate HMV.
- The presence of a case manager is important to organize adaptation to ventilation.
- Ambulatory adaptation of HMV has efficacy equal to inpatient adaptation.
- Ambulatory adaptation of HMV will likely reduce health-care costs.

References

1. Simonds AK, Elliott MW. Outcome of domiciliary nasal intermittent positive pressure ventilation in restrictive and obstructive disorders. Thorax. 1995;50:604–9.
2. Consensus Conference. Clinical indications for noninvasive positive pressure ventilation in chronic respiratory failure due to restrictive lung disease, COPD, and nocturnal hypoventilation – a consensus conference report. Chest. 1999;116:521–34.
3. Lloyd-Owen SJ, Donaldson GC, Ambrosino N, et al. Patterns of home mechanical ventilation use in Europe: results from the Eurovent survey. Eur Respir J. 2005;25:1025–31.
4. Dave C, Turner A, Dretzke J, et al. Protocol for a systematic review and economic evaluation of the clinical and cost-effectiveness of non-hospital-based non-invasive ventilation (NIV) in patients with stable end-stage COPD with hypercapnic respiratory failure. Syst Rev. 2014;3:32.
5. Pallero M, Puy C, Güell R, et al. Ambulatory adaptation to noninvasive ventilation in restrictive pulmonary disease: a randomized trial with cost assessment. Respir Med. 2014;108:1014–22.
6. Chatwin M, Nickol AH, Morrell MJ, et al. Randomised trial of inpatient versus outpatient initiation of home mechanical ventilation in patients with nocturnal hypoventilation. Respir Med. 2008;102:1528–35.
7. Luján M, Moreno A, Veigas C, et al. Non-invasive home mechanical ventilation: effectiveness and efficiency of an outpatient initiation protocol compared with the standard in-hospital model. Respir Med. 2007;101:1177–82.
8. Rabec C, Gonzalez-Bermejo J, Arnold V, et al. Mise en route d'une ventilation non invasive au domicile: propositions du groupe de travail Casavni. Rev Mal Respir. 2010;27:874–89.
9. Sheers N, Berlowitz DJ, Rautela L, et al. Improved survival with an ambulatory model of non-invasive ventilation implementation in motor neuron disease. Amyotroph Lateral Scler Frontotemporal Degener. 2014;15:180–4.
10. Hazenberg A, Kerstjens HA, Prins SC, et al. Initiation of home mechanical ventilation at home: a randomised controlled trial of efficacy, feasibility and costs. Respir Med. 2014;108(9):1387–95.
11. Janssens JP, Borel JC, Pépin JL. Nocturnal monitoring of home non-invasive ventilation: the contribution of simple tools such as pulse oximetry, capnography, built-in ventilator software and autonomic markers of sleep fragmentation. Thorax. 2011;66:438–45.

Chronic Obstructive Pulmonary Disease and Obstructive Sleep Apnea, Known as the Overlap Syndrome: Indications for CPAP and BiPAP. Evidence and Key Practical Recommendations

86

Philippe Jaoude and Ali A. El Solh

Contents

86.1 Introduction

Chronic obstructive pulmonary disease (COPD) is a condition that primarily affects the lungs and is characterized by a progressive airway obstruction with ensuing airflow limitation. It is often associated with a variable degree of alveolar destruction and pulmonary vasculature attrition. These pathological changes are linked to important systemic features mediated by acute phase immune activation, leading, in some cases,

P. Jaoude, MD • A.A. El Solh (✉), MD, MPH
The Veterans Affairs Western New York Healthcare System, Buffalo, NY, USA

Division of Pulmonary, Critical Care, and Sleep Medicine, Department of Medicine, State University of New York at Buffalo School of Medicine and Biomedical Sciences and School of Public Health and Health Professions, Buffalo, NY, USA

Department of Social and Preventive Medicine, State University of New York at Buffalo School of Medicine and Biomedical Sciences and School of Public Health and Health Professions, Buffalo, NY, USA
e-mail: solh@buffalo.edu

A.M. Esquinas (ed.), *Noninvasive Mechanical Ventilation: Theory, Equipment, and Clinical Applications*, DOI 10.1007/978-3-319-21653-9_86

to weight loss, malaise, and fatigue. In 1985, Flenly coined the term "overlap syndrome" to define the coexistence of both COPD and obstructive sleep apnea (OSA) in a given patient. As may be intuitively expected, patients with overlap syndrome tend to have more severe inflammation and worse cardiovascular outcomes compared with patients with COPD or OSA alone. The daytime partial pressure of oxygen in arterial blood (PaO_2) is lower and nocturnal oxygen desaturation is greater in patients with overlap syndrome compared with patients with OSA or COPD alone. Daytime hypercapnia is also more commonly observed in overlap patients [1–3]. Alveolar hypoventilation is considered the prime culprit for most of the oxygen desaturation. Other causes include decreased ventilation–perfusion matching, respiratory muscle dysfunction, and decreased end-expiratory lung volume. The presence of an additive cardiovascular effect in overlap syndrome is reflected in an increased arterial stiffness [4], an increased right ventricular (RV) remodeling and RV mass [5], a more prevalent pulmonary hypertension, and a higher mortality compared with patients with COPD or OSA only. The treatment of overlap syndrome mainly consists of treating its constituents: COPD and OSA. Whereas treatment of COPD is essentially based on avoidance of risk factors, along with oxygen and symptomatic therapy, positive airway pressure (PAP) continues to be the mainstay of OSA treatment.

86.2 PAP Therapy in OSA and in COPD

Continuous positive airway pressure (CPAP) provides a constant airway pressure throughout the respiratory cycle. It is associated with an improvement in OSA symptoms such as snoring and excessive daytime sleepiness (EDS). There is also evidence that the use of CPAP reduces inflammatory markers and improves endothelial dysfunction in patients with OSA. Other research suggests that treatment of OSA with CPAP may improve glucose intolerance and hypertension. Although there are no randomized controlled trials to confirm a benefit in cardiovascular outcomes and mortality, it has been suggested that severe untreated OSA may be associated with increased mortality compared with treated severe or mild-to-moderate OSA and with controls [6].

Although no outcome benefit has been shown for bi-level positive airway pressure (BiPAP) compared with CPAP for treatment of OSA, BiPAP is still considered an alternative to CPAP when OSA is associated with hypoventilation during sleep, such as in obesity hypoventilation syndrome (OHS) or in neuromuscular disorders. It is also considered in patients who require high PAP pressures to treat their OSA, and who have difficulties tolerating such increased pressure [7].

The role of noninvasive positive pressure ventilation (NIPPV) in the management of chronic respiratory failure secondary to COPD has been controversial [8]. More recent evidence, however, seems to favor a positive impact of NIPPV on outcomes of hypercapnic patients with COPD. McEvoy and colleagues [9] randomized 144 stable hypercapnic patients with severe COPD to either long-term oxygen therapy (LTOT) alone or to LTOT with noninvasive ventilation (NIV). COPD patients who received the NIV + LTOT treatment had an improvement in adjusted mortality.

This benefit, however, was at the cost of a worsening in the quality of life. Similarly, Windisch and colleagues [10] reported an improvement in blood gases and lung function of patients with severe COPD and chronic hypercapnic respiratory failure after using NIPPV. A mortality benefit was also reported compared with historical controls. The PAP pressure used in the study, however, was very high and required in-hospital acclimatization.

86.3 CPAP and BiPAP in Overlap Syndrome

Although there are no studies comparing BiPAP to CPAP in overlap syndrome, different authors have used one or the other of the two modalities in addressing the effect of PAP on clinical outcomes.

86.3.1 Pulmonary Function Tests and Gas Exchange

Mansfield and Naughton [11] were among the first to examine the effect of CPAP in overlap syndrome. A cohort of 10 patients with OSA and COPD who were compliant with CPAP were followed for approximately 16.5 months. The average CPAP pressure was 10.2 cmH_2O with an estimated compliance of 4.8 h/night. The authors noted an increase in the forced expiratory volume in 1 s (FEV1) from 0.96 ± 0.13 to 1.10 ± 0.13 l ($p = 0.005$), and an improvement in the levels of awake arterial partial pressure of oxygen (PaO_2) and of carbon dioxide ($PaCO_2$). PaO_2 increased from 54.8 ± 3.8 to 63.2 ± 1.8 mmHg ($p = 0.015$), and $PaCO_2$ decreased from 58.0 ± 3.5 to 48.0 ± 2.9 mmHg ($p = 0.015$) on CPAP therapy.

A similar study included 55 patients, of whom 33 had hypercapnia (defined by $PaCO_2 \geq 45$ mmHg) who were placed on appropriate CPAP based on a titration study. After 6 months of PAP therapy, there were statistically significant increases in PaO_2, in FEV1, and forced vital capacity (FVC). There was also a statistically significant decrease in $PaCO_2$, in alveolar-arterial oxygen difference, and in serum bicarbonate level. These changes were associated with a significant decrease in body weight and body mass index (BMI). At 18 months follow-up, no further changes were observed in body weight, arterial blood gases, or pulmonary function. The response to CPAP was more prominent in the hypercapnic group. Although the results of the study suggest a beneficial effect of CPAP on lung function and blood gases in patients with overlap syndrome, these changes may have been related to weight loss [12]. Conversely, in a retrospective study, O'Brien and Whitman [13] reported worsening of FEV1 and FVC in patients with overlap syndrome who were compliant with CPAP, compared with those who were not compliant with CPAP. The results of this study could reflect a bias related to the fact that patients with most progressive disease and symptoms may have used CPAP the most. More recently, Toraldo et al. [16] examined the effect of PAP therapy in patients with coexistent severe OSA (apnea hypopnea index (AHI) >30) and mild to moderate COPD. At baseline, patients were hypercapnic, hypoxic, and obese, with a mean BMI of

34.2 ± 0.2. The authors assessed different variables at baseline and at 3, 12, and 24 months after starting treatment with CPAP. The variables included pulmonary function, maximum inspiratory pressure (Pimax), arterial blood gases, and echocardiographic mean pulmonary artery pressure (MPAP). Throughout the follow-up period, the CPAP pressure was 12.67 ± 0.24, with a mean use of 5.06 ± 0.14 h/night. A significant improvement was seen at 3 months and 12 months of CPAP therapy in $PaCO_2$, PaO_2, MPAP, FEV1, functional residual capacity (FRC), Pimax, and Epworth Sleepiness Scale (ESS). Whereas ESS, FEV1, and FRC continued to improve at 24 months follow-up, the remainder of the measures remained stable with no further improvement compared with 12 months prior.

The mechanism by which CPAP may improve pulmonary function and arterial blood gases in patients with overlap syndrome is not fully understood. It has been postulated that off-loading the respiratory muscles could decrease hypoventilation, oxygen consumption, and carbon dioxide production by the respiratory muscles. By improving upper airway irritation caused by recurrent airway collapse in OSA patients, CPAP may improve lower airway resistance. Alternatively, CPAP may offset intrinsic PEEP in severe COPD [14]. The net effect may be a better respiratory muscle function during wakefulness.

86.3.2 Exacerbations and Hospitalizations

The available data addressing the effect of CPAP on COPD exacerbations and hospitalizations in patients with overlap syndrome is limited, but seems to support a beneficial effect. In the study by Mansfield and Naughton [11], a decrease in the number of admissions per annum was observed from 3.85 in the 4 years preceding CPAP to 0.73 admissions per year following initiation of CPAP. The total inpatient days was also reduced from 25.6 to 5.1 days per annum after starting CPAP. The incidence of COPD exacerbations was reduced in those patients who were compliant with CPAP treatment. This finding occurred when the baseline reports of exacerbation were compared with results over a 9-year monitoring period for CPAP and non-CPAP groups. These groups were similar in many baseline characteristics (including BMI, smoking history, alcohol use, cardiac and respiratory medications, spirometry measurements, and AHI), and both groups received similar medical care and medications over the course of time [15].

Similar findings were reported by Toraldo et al. [16], who noted a reduction in the numbers of total COPD exacerbations per year, total hospital days, and in the number of yearly outpatient visits 2 years after starting CPAP therapy in patients with overlap syndrome.

86.3.3 Mortality

Long-term effects of CPAP treatment and particularly its effect on survival have been reported more recently. CPAP treatment was shown to have beneficial survival benefit, particularly in patients with moderate to severe OSA and concomitant COPD with hypoxia.

After a median follow-up of 9.4 years (range, 3.3–12.7), Marin et al. [6] showed a higher mortality in patients with overlap syndrome who were not treated with CPAP compared with patients with COPD only (relative risk, 1.79; 95 % confidence interval, 1.16–2.77). Patients with overlap syndrome treated with CPAP did not experience an increased mortality risk and had similar mortality to the COPD-only group. The most common cause of death in the untreated overlap patients was related to cardiovascular events. The nonrandomized nature of the study however, raises the issue that refusal of CPAP therapy may be a marker of noncompliance with general medical care, which may have contributed to the higher mortality in the untreated overlap syndrome group. The optimal prescription for CPAP was also unclear. The issue of whether there is a true threshold for optimal CPAP use remains unanswered by this study, as some patients had significant mortality reductions with CPAP use <4 h/night, which has previously been suggested as a minimal level needed for reductions in OSA morbidity. Nevertheless, recent studies have suggested near-linear improvements in sleepiness and cognitive function with increasing time on CPAP at night (2 versus 4 versus 6 h) [17]. This linear improvement on CPAP has been confirmed more recently by Antic and colleagues [18].

Machado et al. [19] studied hypoxemic COPD patients who were on LTOT for ≥6 months. Hypercapnia was also present in the group. Although all subjects who had moderate to severe OSA on polysomnography were prescribed CPAP therapy, not all the patients were able to use CPAP. The studied population was divided into two groups, those who used CPAP and those who did not use CPAP. The latter group included patients who refused CPAP, those who could not afford it, and those who were not adherent to CPAP. Adherence was defined as using CPAP ≥5 h per night on ≥5 nights per week. During a median follow-up of 41 months (range, 6–106 months), death occurred in 39 patients (41 % mortality). The 5-year survival estimate was 71 % (95 % confidence interval, 53–83 %) and 26 % (12–43 %) in the CPAP-treated and non-treated groups, respectively ($p<0.01$). The survival benefit persisted even after adjusting for several confounders, including age, FEV1, and comorbidities. Treatment with CPAP was associated with a significantly lower risk of death (hazard ratio HR) of death versus non-treated, 0.19 (0.08–0.48)). The lack of randomization of CPAP, and the fact that the group that did not use CPAP could have had financial challenges, may introduce a potential source of selection bias favoring the CPAP group.

A similar survival effect was reported by Stanchina et al. [20], who identified 227 patients with overlap syndrome, from an existing cohort database of 10,721 outpatient records. Death was reported in 7.4 % of patients with overlap syndrome. In a multivariate Cox proportional hazards analysis, only age (HR 1.14 (1.04–1.23), $p=0.003$) and CPAP nightly use (HR 0.71 [0.55–0.90], $p=0.004$) were significant predictors of mortality. Patients who used CPAP for an average 0–2 h per night had a decreased survival compared with groups who used CPAP for more than 2 h per night. The retrospective chart review nature of the study does not allow drawing of definite conclusions on a mortality benefit with the use of CPAP, as it is possible that patients who used CPAP more frequently have a better compliance with the treatment of other comorbidities, which may have affected their survival.

More recently, Jaoude et al. [21] examined all-cause mortality in 271 patients with overlap syndrome who were followed for a median of 71 months. Hypercapnia was present in 104 of the patients ($PaCO_2 = 51.6 \pm 4.3$ mmHg). Both normocapnic and hypercapnic patients had comparable AHI and similar adherence rates to CPAP (43 and 42 %, respectively, $p = 0.9$). Survival analysis revealed that hypercapnic patients who were adherent to CPAP had reduced mortality compared with nonadherent hypercapnic patients ($p = 0.04$). In contrast, the cumulative mortality rate for normocapnic patients was not significantly different between the adherent and the nonadherent group ($p = 0.42$). The results of this study suggest that patients with overlap syndrome who are hypercapnic may benefit the most from CPAP therapy.

86.3.4 Inflammation, Vascular Effect, and Pulmonary Hypertension

Various inflammatory and endothelial function markers have been examined in patients with overlap syndrome. Hypoxic and hypercapnic responses are reduced in the affected patients. After 6 weeks of treatment with BiPAP, the hypoxic response improved significantly but remained below normal range. In contrast to OSA patients who had their hypercapnic response normalized after 6 weeks of BiPAP use, there was no significant change in the hypercapnic response in patients with overlap syndrome [22].

Inflammatory markers such as C-reactive protein (CRP) and tumor necrosis factor (TNF)-α are increased in patients with overlap syndrome, but CPAP treatment is associated with an improvement in inflammation. The reduced inflammatory response appears to be similar in both patients with overlap syndrome and those with OSA only [23]. More importantly, there was an inverse relation between increased compliance with CPAP and the levels of the inflammatory mediators.

The altered chemoresponsiveness and inflammatory response in overlap syndrome is thought to modify the homeostatic pathways, resulting in endothelial dysfunction. Institution of BIPAP therapy improved vascular dysfunction even after 1 month of therapy [24]. This interplay between overlap syndrome and vascular dysfunction was highlighted by Perimenis et al. [25], who studied the effect of CPAP on erectile dysfunction (ED) in 48 men with overlap syndrome and concomitant ED. The reported improvement of ED was noted in 25 % of patients who were treated with CPAP.

86.3.5 Exercise and Quality of Life

There is scarce data on the effect of CPAP on exercise or quality of life. A small study suggested that CPAP improved exercise tolerance by 17 % in patient with overlap syndrome treated with CPAP [13]. Wang et al. [26] studied the effect of

CPAP on walking capacity in patients with COPD and patients with overlap syndrome. The sleep apnea in the study group was defined as an AHI >15, and the COPD group included patients with concomitant mild OSA. Both groups were treated with CPAP, and the incremental shuttle walking test (ISWT) was used to determine maximal walking capacity at baseline and after 2 days of CPAP treatment. Walking distance improved in both groups, but the improvement was significantly greater in the overlap syndrome than in the COPD patients. In addition, in patients with overlap syndrome, CPAP treatment significantly increased pre-exercise oxygenation, and significantly decreased pre-exercise Borg scale and heart rate. While the results are promising, the study did not address the long-term effects of CPAP on exercise tolerance and quality of life.

86.3.6 Other Considerations

Although the American Academy of Sleep Medicine (AASM) does not consider patients with significant lung disease as candidates for automatic CPAP titration, a small study by Guerrero et al. [27] showed that auto-CPAP titration may be appropriate in OSA patients with COPD. Comparing auto-CPAP titration in two groups of patients, one with OSA and COPD and the second with OSA only, no significant difference was observed in the residual AHI and in the optimal pressure between the two groups. There was, however, a significant increase in air leak in patients with OSA and COPD. Air leak was associated with a higher percentage of the night spent with oxygen saturation less than 90 % (CT90). Furthermore, the long-term effects of auto-CPAP titration on patient outcome were not addressed in this study. If auto-CPAP titration is to be used in patients with overlap syndrome, close attention should be paid to minimizing air leak, and a follow-up on nocturnal oxygen saturation should be conducted.

While NIPPV is often used to treat hospitalized patients presenting with COPD exacerbation, and has been investigated in the treatment of stable COPD, there is no evidence that BiPAP is superior to CPAP in treating patients with stable overlap syndrome. Patient tolerance of either modality may, however, be affected by the severity of the underlying COPD. Theerakittikul et al. [28] reported hyperinflation on a chest radiograph as a marker of decreased adherence to CPAP therapy in patients with overlap syndrome. When treating patients with overlap syndrome, the choice of PAP treatment modality may need to take into account other factors that could affect patients' tolerance and adherence.

Conclusion

Overlap syndrome is associated with increased morbidity and mortality. In addition to improving OSA, treatment with CPAP or BiPAP seems to have a beneficial effect on lung function and arterial blood gases. It may also improve survival and reduce COPD exacerbations and hospitalizations. Other favorable effects may be seen in inflammatory markers, vascular and endothelial function, pulmonary artery pressure, and exercise tolerance. There is no data to favor BiPAP over

CPAP in treatment of stable overlap syndrome, and the choice of PAP modality should be based on patient's tolerance and underlying factors such as the presence of lung hyperinflation or of hypoventilation during sleep. Future research should address the underlying mechanism that leads to worse outcomes in patients with overlap syndrome, compare BiPAP and CPAP in terms of effect, tolerance, and compliance, and focus on ways to improve patients' adherence to PAP therapy.

Key Recommendations

- Screening for overlap syndrome should be considered in patients with COPD, especially in the presence of worsening COPD symptoms, poor sleep quality, or symptoms of sleep apnea (snoring, excessive daytime sleepiness or fatigue).
- Discussion of potential benefits of PAP treatment on pulmonary function, gas exchange, mortality, and quality of life should be incorporated in the education process of patients with overlap syndrome.
- In-lab CPAP or BiPAP titration is the preferred modality for determining the appropriate PAP settings. If auto-PAP titration is considered, measures should be taken to minimize air leak, and nocturnal oxygen saturation should be assessed once the patient is using the PAP machine.
- The choice of PAP treatment modality largely depends on the patient's tolerance and preference. CPAP is the standard of care. BiPAP should be considered in patients with significant lung hyperinflation, who are not able to tolerate CPAP, or in patients with signs of hypoventilation during sleep.
- Patients with significant residual nocturnal oxygen desaturation on PAP therapy, despite adequate control of apnea and hypopnea events, should have combined nocturnal oxygen and PAP therapy.

Conflict of Interest None.

Financial Support Supported by a grant from the American Sleep Medicine Foundation (PJ) and a Merit Review Grant (CX000478) from the Department of Veterans Affairs (AES). The views expressed in this review do not communicate an official position of the Department of Veterans Affairs.

References

1. McNicholas WT. Chronic obstructive pulmonary disease and obstructive sleep apnea: overlaps in pathophysiology, systemic inflammation, and cardiovascular disease. Am J Respir Crit Care Med. 2009;180:692–700.
2. Chaouat A, Weitzenblum E, Krieger J, Ifoundza T, Oswald M, Kessler R. Association of chronic obstructive pulmonary disease and sleep apnea syndrome. Am J Respir Crit Care Med. 1995;151:82–6.

3. Lacedonia D, Carpagnano GE, Aliani M, et al. Daytime PaO_2 in OSAS, COPD and the combination of the two (overlap syndrome). Respir Med. 2013;107:310–6.
4. Shiina K, Tomiyama H, Takata Y, et al. Overlap syndrome: additive effects of COPD on the cardiovascular damages in patients with OSA. Respir Med. 2012;106:1335–41.
5. Sharma B, Neilan TG, Kwong RY, et al. Evaluation of right ventricular remodeling using cardiac magnetic resonance imaging in co-existent chronic obstructive pulmonary disease and obstructive sleep apnea. COPD. 2013;10:4–10.
6. Marin JM, Carrizo SJ, Vicente E, Agusti AG. Long-term cardiovascular outcomes in men with obstructive sleep apnoea-hypopnoea with or without treatment with continuous positive airway pressure: an observational study. Lancet. 2005;365:1046–53.
7. Nicolini A, Banfi P, Grecchi B, et al. Non-invasive ventilation in the treatment of sleep-related breathing disorders: a review and update. Rev Port Pneumol. 2014;20:324–35.
8. Kolodziej MA, Jensen L, Rowe B, Sin D. Systematic review of noninvasive positive pressure ventilation in severe stable COPD. Eur Respir J. 2007;30:293–306.
9. McEvoy RD, Pierce RJ, Hillman D, et al. Nocturnal non-invasive nasal ventilation in stable hypercapnic COPD: a randomised controlled trial. Thorax. 2009;64:561–6.
10. Windisch W, Haenel M, Storre JH, Dreher M. High-intensity non-invasive positive pressure ventilation for stable hypercapnic COPD. Int J Med Sci. 2009;6:72–6.
11. Mansfield D, Naughton MT. Effects of continuous positive airway pressure on lung function in patients with chronic obstructive pulmonary disease and sleep disordered breathing. Respirology. 1999;4:365–70.
12. de Miguel J, Cabello J, Sanchez-Alarcos JM, Alvarez-Sala R, Espinos D, Alvarez-Sala JL. Long-term effects of treatment with nasal continuous positive airway pressure on lung function in patients with overlap syndrome. Sleep Breath. 2002;6:3–10.
13. O'Brien A, Whitman K. Lack of benefit of continuous positive airway pressure on lung function in patients with overlap syndrome. Lung. 2005;183:389–404.
14. Nowinski A, Bielen P, Jonczak L, Sliwinski P. Influence of treatment with continuous positive airway pressure on respiratory muscle function and physical fitness in patients with obstructive sleep apnoea and overlap syndrome. Pneumonol Alergol Pol. 2007;75:46–56.
15. Marin JM, Soriano JB, Carrizo SJ, Boldova A, Celli BR. Outcomes in patients with chronic obstructive pulmonary disease and obstructive sleep apnea: the overlap syndrome. Am J Respir Crit Care Med. 2010;182:325–31.
16. Toraldo DM, De Nuccio F, Nicolardi G. Fixed-pressure nCPAP in patients with obstructive sleep apnea (OSA) syndrome and chronic obstructive pulmonary disease (COPD): a 24-month follow-up study. Sleep Breath. 2010;14:115–23.
17. Weaver TE, Maislin G, Dinges DF, et al. Relationship between hours of CPAP use and achieving normal levels of sleepiness and daily functioning. Sleep. 2007;30:711–9.
18. Antic NA, Catcheside P, Buchan C, et al. The effect of CPAP in normalizing daytime sleepiness, quality of life, and neurocognitive function in patients with moderate to severe OSA. Sleep. 2011;34:111–9.
19. Machado MC, Vollmer WM, Togeiro SM, et al. CPAP and survival in moderate-to-severe obstructive sleep apnoea syndrome and hypoxaemic COPD. Eur Respir J. 2010;35:132–7.
20. Stanchina ML, Welicky LM, Donat W, Lee D, Corrao W, Malhotra A. Impact of CPAP use and age on mortality in patients with combined COPD and obstructive sleep apnea: the overlap syndrome. J Clin Sleep Med: JCSM: Off Publ Am Acad Sleep Med. 2013;9:767–72.
21. Jaoude P, Kufel T, El-Solh AA. Survival benefit of CPAP favors hypercapnic patients with the overlap syndrome. Lung. 2014;192:251–8.
22. Wang HL, He ZM, Li J, et al. Effect of noninvasive ventilation on chemoresponsiveness in patients with sleep apnea and chronic obstructive pulmonary disease. Zhonghua yi xue za zhi. 2007;87:2193–7.
23. Wang Y, Su M, Zhang X. Effects of continuous positive airway pressure treatment of inflammatory factors in patients with overlap syndrome. Zhonghua yi xue za zhi. 2014;94:416–9.

24. Zhang XW, Cai W, Jin F, Zhang YQ, Zhang XL. Effect of bi-level positive airway pressure ventilator on the heart function and vascular endothelial function of patients with the overlap syndrome. Zhonghua jie he he hu xi za zhi =Zhonghua jiehe he huxi zazhi = Chin J Tuberc Respir Diseases. 2011;34:17–20.
25. Perimenis P, Karkoulias K, Konstantinopoulos A, et al. The impact of long-term conventional treatment for overlap syndrome (obstructive sleep apnea and chronic obstructive pulmonary disease) on concurrent erectile dysfunction. Respir Med. 2007;101:210–6.
26. Wang TY, Lo YL, Lee KY, et al. Nocturnal CPAP improves walking capacity in COPD patients with obstructive sleep apnoea. Respir Res. 2013;14:66.
27. Guerrero A, Montserrat JM, Farre R, Masa F, Duran J, Embid C. Automatic CPAP performance in patients with sleep apnea plus COPD. COPD. 2012;9:382–9.
28. Theerakittikul T, Hatipoglu U, Aboussouan LS. Hyperinflation on chest radiograph as a marker of low adherence to positive airway pressure therapy in the overlap syndrome. Respir Care. 2014;59:1267–74.

Continuous Positive Airway Pressure in Nonapneic Asthma

87

J. Navarro-Esteva and G. Juliá-Serdá

Contents

Abbreviations

AHR	Airway hyperresponsiveness
ASM	Airway smooth muscle
CPAP	Continuous positive airway pressure
eNO	Exhaled nitric oxide
FEV_1	Forced expiratory volume in 1 s
PEFR	Peak expiratory flow rate

87.1 Introduction

Airway smooth muscle (ASM) cells contribute in multiple ways to the pathogenesis of asthma, including direct causation of airflow obstruction through contraction and indirect promotion of airflow obstruction through airway remodeling and

J. Navarro-Esteva, MD (✉) • G. Juliá-Serdá, MD, PhD
Department of Pulmonary Medicine, Hospital Universitario Gran Canaria "Dr. Negrín", Las Palmas, Spain
e-mail: jnavest@gobiernodecanarias.org; jjulser@gobiernodecanarias.org

A.M. Esquinas (ed.), *Noninvasive Mechanical Ventilation: Theory, Equipment, and Clinical Applications*, DOI 10.1007/978-3-319-21653-9_87

modulating airway inflammation. Each of these processes interacts with the other. Among the contributing mechanisms to airway hyperresponsiveness (AHR), there are increased dynamic muscle stiffness, increased vagal tone, and cytokine-potentiated rises in intracellular free calcium. Studies at the micromechanic and molecular levels have repeatedly shown that stretching reduces the tone of ASM by lowering the number and cycling rate of cross bridges between actin and myosin filaments. However, there are other potentially important features that play a role in airway dynamics and include the nonlinear viscoelastic properties of the passive airway wall structures, mechanical coupling between the ASM and extracellular matrix, buckling of the epithelial basement membrane, and circumferential as well as radial stress distribution in the airway wall [1, 2].

In healthy people and in a few patients with asthma there is a breathing-induced reversal of bronchoconstriction and length adaptation likely due to perturbation in actin-myosin interactions. In most patients with asthma, however, the ability of deep breaths to reverse bronchoconstriction seems blunted [3]. One of the key mechanisms regulating airway caliber is provided by the changes in lung volume imposed by the respiratory pump. During lung inflation, airway caliber increases because airways and lung parenchyma are mechanically interdependent [4]. In the acute setting, there is evidence that bi-level positive airway pressure improves physiological variables in patients with severe asthma attacks [5]. Likewise, in the chronic setting, there is increasing interest in studying the effects of continuous positive airway pressure (CPAP) on AHR and asthma control.

87.2 Animal Studies

Zue et al. [6, 7] designed several studies in rabbits, ferrets, and mice, where CPAP versus sham CPAP was applied through a tracheostomy. In the first study, they showed that 4 days of external mechanical strain applied to the lungs resulted in lower AHR to acetylcholine in vivo. Decreased AHR was also observed in vitro. In the second study, the authors found that ferrets subjected to CPAP during 14 days had increased luminal areas of intrathoracic trachea and intraparenchymal airways and lower levels of myosin light-chain phosphorylation. These findings could account for the decreased AHR observed in vivo. In a new study, the authors proved that intermittent application of CPAP reduced AHR for at least 24 h. They also showed that CPAP suppressed AHR caused by ovoalbumin-induced airway inflammation. Two years later, the same authors showed that only 2 h of CPAP decreased airway resistance in vitro in the following 6 h, and CPAP was associated with downregulation of Akt phosphorylation, a mediator involved in AHR. This study led to speculation that, in humans, short application of CPAP could improve asthma control and be more acceptable than prolonged or nighttime CPAP treatment. The same group of investigators published in an abstract form that canine tracheal tissue stimulated with interleukin (IL)-13 produced significantly lower levels of eotaxin measured in the media of submucosa when subjected to CPAP.

87.3 Human Studies

Busk et al. [8] studied 16 patients with controlled mild asthma and performed baseline and follow-up methacholine challenge after 1 week of nocturnal CPAP, set at 8–10 cmH_2O. The control nonasthmatic group received sham CPAP. In the real CPAP group, AHR was clearly decreased (2.7-fold increase in the concentration of methacholine causing a 20 % fall in forced expiratory volume in 1 s (FEV_1)). No changes were found in FEV_1 or exhaled nitric oxide (eNO), but this was not expected since baseline FEV_1 was similar in both groups (86 % vs 89 %), and the asthma group was clinically stable from the outset. As a drawback, there are no data on body mass index or exclusion of sleep apnea, as AHR can be potentially influenced by those.

D'Amato et al. [9] studied 10 patients with noncontrolled severe asthma of longer than 25 years since diagnosis (mean FEV_1: 68 %, mean asthma control test score below 15). Automatic CPAP was applied during seven nights through a full face mask. Sleep apnea was excluded by polysomnography. The primary objective of this open unblinded pilot study was to determine the efficacy of automatic CPAP to achieve control of symptoms, reduce PEF variability, and improve quality of life. Measurements of lung function, asthma control, and quality of life were performed at baseline, during the treatment period, and within 1 month from baseline. Mean positive airway pressure applied was 5.3 ± 1.3 cmH_2O. The authors found that the variability of peak expiratory flow rate (PEFR) was reduced during treatment and the week after – W0 and W1 (Fig. 87.1). The asthma control score also improved significantly after automatic CPAP, mainly from decreased use of rescue $beta_2$ agonists. As limitations of this study, automatic CPAP was used instead of CPAP, and there was no control group.

Finally, Rondinel et al. [10] found that two daily sessions of respiratory exercises with incentive spirometry coupled to an expiratory airway pressure (EPAP) resistor

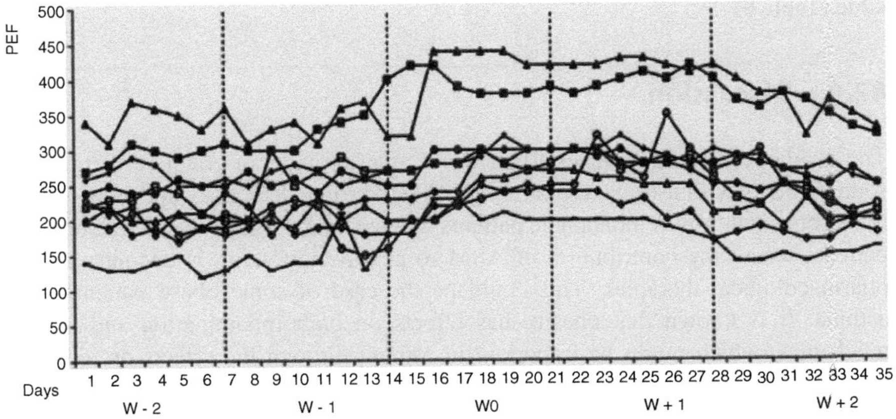

Fig. 87.1 Peak flow (individual) values measured throughout 5 weeks. CPAP was applied during the W0 period (shown with permission from the publisher)

Table 87.1 Studies in humans with nonexacerbated asthma and positive airway pressure. All the studies were carried on a limited number of patients

Study	Design	Intervention	Results	Commentary
Busk et al. (2013) [8]	Randomized controlled trial. Subjects: patients with mild asthma	Night CPAP 8–10 cmH_2O during 1 week. Metacholine challenge, FEV1 and eNO before and after intervention	CPAP decreases AHR. No changes in FEV_1 or eNO (expected)	Sleep apnea not ruled out
D'Amato et al. (2014) [9]	Noncontrolled study. Subjects: nonapneic patients with severe asthma	Night autoCPAP PEF values, control of symptoms, and quality of life before, during and after intervention	AutoCPAP (mean 5.3 cmH_2O) associated with higher PEF and better asthma control and reduced B_2 agonist use	Effects of CPAP on PEFR beyond time of application Limitation: noncontrolled study, autoCPAP used
Rondinel et al. (2014) [10]	Randomized controlled trial. Subjects: patients with severe asthma	Incentive spirometry coupled with EPAP. Twice daily sessions of 15 min during 5 weeks	EPAP titrated to 15 cmH_2O. Intervention group showed improvement in asthma control and quality of life	Monitoring of compliance with the device not done

were associated with clinically significant improvements in asthma control and quality of life. It was a randomized controlled trial that lasted 5 weeks on eight patients with severely uncontrolled asthma and six controls. Although it was not real CPAP, titration of EPAP from 5 to 15 cmH_2O was performed in the intervention group. In this case, no changes in pulmonary function were observed. As a limitation of the study, objective monitoring of compliance with the device was not feasible (Table 87.1).

87.4 Discussion

The available evidence suggests that CPAP may provide an effective therapy for some patients with asthma. Even though CPAP during sleep does not seem to be a reasonable solution for nonapneic patients with asthma, it could play a role in some patients where the contribution of ASM to airway narrowing is uncontrolled by pharmacological therapies. This could be the case of some obese patients with asthma. It is known that obesity has effects on both inflammation and airway mechanics, which might be important in asthma through the effects on airways' smaller caliber, muscle stiffness, and hyperresponsiveness exacerbated by the supine position. CPAP could be used as a "rescue" therapy in partially controlled or uncontrolled asthmatics through intermittent daily and/or nightly use.

There may be also a role of CPAP to assist in inhaled therapy and achieve a greater bronchodilation inasmuch as ventilation inhomogeneities are minimized at increased lung inflation [4]. However, there are several unresolved questions:

- It remains to be seen in humans whether application of CPAP induces reorganization of cytoskeletal and contractile proteins of ASM as well as extracellular matrix junctions found in animal studies.
- Duration of asthma should be accounted for in future studies because airway remodeling might blunt response to CPAP.
- Nasal intolerance is a frequent side effect occurring with CPAP, affecting as many as 50 % of treated patients with sleep apnea. Rhinitis is common in patients with asthma and might worsen with CPAP treatment.
- Potential interference of CPAP with sleep quality in the nonapneic patients with asthma might be a reason for noncompliance.
- PEF or FEV1 may not be the most reliable tools to assess the effect of CPAP on pulmonary function. They could have a role in some uncontrolled patients with asthma, but other tools such as measures of airway resistance, namely forced oscillometry or specific airway conductance, may be of help.
- Knowledge of the effects of CPAP in asthma's related comorbidities, that is, changes in inflammatory cytokines and gastroesophageal reflux, is limited.

Conclusion

Studies on induced AHR in animal models subjected to CPAP clearly indicate that application of positive airway pressure reduces AHR and has a lasting though limited effect. Results in human studies are hampered by the low number of patients but also point to a therapeutic effect of CPAP in AHR, control of symptoms, and possibly PEFR. A higher degree of evidence about the effects of CPAP on nonapneic asthmatic patients is needed. The trial "Effect of Positive Airway Pressure on Reducing Airway Reactivity in Patients with Asthma" is an ongoing, 12-week, randomized multicenter study with three arms (nocturnal sham CPAP, CPAP 5 cmH_2O, CPAP 10 cmH_2O) that will assess hyperresponsiveness to methacholine, clinical variables, and airway changes through computerized tomography. The results of this study could shed light on the role of this nonpharmacological treatment for asthma.

Key Major Recommendations

- Asthma is characterized by chronic airway inflammation and frequently reversible bronchoconstriction, where ASM cells play a prominent role.
- In animal models, there is a consistent effect on airway function when subjected to CPAP.
- In nonexacerbated patients with asthma, CPAP reduces the response to methacholine challenge and may improve control of asthma even after withdrawal.
- More studies are needed to explore both the effects of CPAP in stable asthma and strategies for its application and tolerance.

References

1. Fredberg JJ, Inouye D, Miller B, et al. Airway smooth muscle, tidal stretches, and dynamically determined contractile states. Am J Respir Crit Care Med. 1997;156:1752–9.
2. Doeing DC, Solway J. Airway smooth muscle in the pathophysiology and treatment of asthma. J Appl Physiol. 2013;114:834–43.
3. Skloot G, Permutt S, Togias A. Airway hyperresponsiveness in asthma: a problem of limited smooth muscle relaxation with inspiration. J Clin Invest. 1995;96:2393–403.
4. Pellegrino R, Pellegrino GM, Brusasco V. CPAP as a novel treatment for bronchial asthma? J Appl Physiol. 2011;111:343–4.
5. Carson KV, Usmani ZA, Smith BJ. Noninvasive ventilation in acute severe asthma: current evidence and future perspectives. Curr Opin Pulm Med. 2014;20:118–23.
6. Xue Z, Zhang L, Liu Y, Gunst SJ, Tepper RS. Chronic inflation of ferret lungs with CPAP reduces airway smooth muscle contractility in vivo and in vitro. J Appl Physiol. 2008;104:610–5.
7. Xue Z, Yu Y, Gao H, et al. Chronic continuous positive airway pressure (CPAP) reduces airway reactivity in vivo in an allergen-induced rabbit model of asthma. J Appl Physiol. 2011;111:353–7.
8. Busk M, Busk N, Puntenney P, et al. Use of continuous positive airway pressure reduces airway reactivity in adults with asthma. Eur Respir J. 2013;41:317–22.
9. D'Amato M, Stanziola AA, de Laurentiis G, et al. Nocturnal continuous positive airway pressure in severe non-apneic asthma. A pilot study. Clin Respir J. 2014;8:417–24.
10. Rondinel TZ, Corrêa IF, Hoscheidt LM, et al. Incentive spirometry combined with expiratory positive airway pressure improves asthma control and quality of life in asthma: a randomised controlled trial. J Asthma. 2014;2:1–7.

Chronic Heart Failure and Sleep-Disordered Breathing: Evidence for the Effect of Continuous Positive Airway Pressure and Key Practical Implications

88

Takatoshi Kasai

Contents

Abbreviations

AHI	Apnea-hypopnea index
ASV	Adaptive servo-ventilation
CANPAP	Canadian Continuous Positive Airway Pressure for Treatment of Central Sleep Apnea in Heart Failure
CHF	Chronic heart failure
CPAP	Continuous positive airway pressure
CSA	Central sleep apnea
CSR	Cheyne-Stokes respiration
LV	Left ventricular
LVEF	Left ventricular ejection fraction
OSA	Obstructive sleep apnea
$PaCO_2$	Arterial partial pressure of carbon dioxide

T. Kasai, MD, PhD
Cardiovascular Respiratory Sleep Medicine, Department of Cardiovascular Medicine, Juntendo University Graduate School of Medicine, 2-1-1 Hongo, Bunkyo-ku, Tokyo 113-8421, Japan
e-mail: kasai-t@mx6.nisiq.net

A.M. Esquinas (ed.), *Noninvasive Mechanical Ventilation: Theory, Equipment, and Clinical Applications*, DOI 10.1007/978-3-319-21653-9_88

REM	Rapid eye movement
RV	Right ventricular
SDB	Sleep-disordered breathing
SNA	Sympathetic nerve activity

88.1 Introduction

Patients with chronic heart failure (CHF) often have multiple concomitant diseases that complicate management and may adversely affect outcomes. Sleep-disordered breathing (SDB) is one of the common comorbidities in patients with CHF. More than 50 % of CHF patients have SDB [1]. Two types of SDB can be seen in patients with CHF: obstructive and central sleep apnea (OSA and CSA, respectively). OSA results from upper airway collapse, whereas CSA arises from reductions in the central respiratory drive in association with CHF. During OSA, the respiratory effort generated to overcome the narrowed upper airway causes the rib cage and abdomen to distort and move out of phase. In contrast, in CSA, respiratory movements are absent or attenuated, but in phase. In patients with CHF, CSA usually occurs as Cheyne-Stokes respiration (CSR), which is a form of periodic breathing characterized by a crescendo-decrescendo pattern of breathing followed by central apnea or hypopnea.

In patients with CHF, SDB may worsen their condition by exposing the heart to intermittent hypoxia, increased preload and afterload, and increased sympathetic nervous activity (SNA), and, in fact, the coexistence of SDB is associated with a poor prognosis [1–3]. However, clinical data suggest that treatment of SDB may attenuate these detrimental effects [1]. Thus, SDB may be a potential therapeutic target in patients with CHF. Continuous positive airway pressure (CPAP), which keeps the airway open and abolishes obstructive apnea and hypopnea, can be used for treating OSA in patients with CHF. In addition, several studies suggest that CPAP can suppress CSA in half of patients with CHF, possibly through cardiac unloading [4]. This chapter aims to highlight the effects of CPAP as a treatment for SDB, either OSA or CSA, in patients with CHF, in addition to the pathogenesis and pathophysiology of SDB. The discussion is confined to CHF due to left ventricular (LV) systolic dysfunction.

88.2 Pathogenesis of SDB in CHF

Patients with OSA generally have a narrow pharynx related to fat accumulation in the neck that compromises the pharyngeal lumen, to micrognathia, or to tonsillar hypertrophy. At sleep onset, loss of pharyngeal dilator muscle tone causes complete or partial pharyngeal collapse, causing obstructive apnea and hypopnea, respectively. Fluid accumulation in nuchal and peripharyngeal soft tissues can also cause pharyngeal narrowing and increase the likelihood of pharyngeal occlusion in patients predisposed to OSA. In addition, fluid accumulated in the legs while upright during the day can shift into the neck when recumbent during sleep. Such shifted fluid can cause edema of the peripharyngeal soft tissue that increases peripharyngeal tissue pressure, predisposing the patient to pharyngeal obstruction. These mechanisms can be more prominent in patients with CHF who may be more likely to have fluid overload [1]. A recent study, in which the craniofacial structures of OSA patients with CHF and age-, body mass index-, and severity-matched OSA patients without CHF were compared, found that OSA patients with CHF have more airway space while awake and upright, but they also have a more enlarged tongue, suggesting that an enlarged tongue may play a more prominent role in patients with CHF than in patients without CHF, and that alterations in upper airway condition during sleep or while recumbent may play a more prominent role in patients with CHF than in patients without CHF [5].

CSA appears to arise secondary to CHF. Patients with CHF tend to hyperventilate chronically owing to stimulation of pulmonary vagal irritant receptors by pulmonary congestion and to increased central and peripheral chemosensitivity [1]. When the arterial partial pressure of carbon dioxide ($PaCO_2$) falls below the apnea threshold because of an increase in the apnea threshold during the transition from wakefulness to sleep or an acute increase in ventilation that is triggered by a spontaneous arousal, CSA ensues [1]. Apnea persists until the $PaCO_2$ rises above the apnea threshold, and then ventilation will resume and ventilatory overshoot occurs. The $PaCO_2$ then decreases below the apnea threshold in association with arousal during the ventilatory phase and increased chemosensitivity, which is characteristic of CHF patients with CSA [1]. The length of the ventilatory phase following CSA is directly proportional to the lung-to-peripheral chemoreceptor circulation time, and inversely proportional to cardiac output, reflecting delayed transmission of changes in arterial blood gas tensions from the lungs to the chemoreceptors in association with impaired cardiac output in patients with CHF [1]. This could also contribute to the pathogenesis of CSA with the CSR pattern by facilitating ventilatory overshoot and undershoot. In addition to OSA, rostral fluid displacement from the legs at night can contribute to the pathogenesis of CSA. Some of the fluid might be redistributed into the lungs and cause pulmonary congestion that stimulates pulmonary vagal irritant receptors to elicit reflex hyperventilation, predisposing the patient to CSA [1].

88.3 Pathophysiology of SDB

In general, SNA, blood pressure (BP), heart rate (HR) fall and cardiac vagal activity increase during non-rapid eye movement (non-REM) sleep, which constitutes approximately 85 % of total sleep time [6]. In contrast, during REM sleep, intermittent surges in SNA, BP, and HR occur. However, in general, REM comprises only 15 % of total sleep time, and average BP and HR remain below waking levels. Thus, sleep is generally a state of cardiovascular quiescence [6]. SDB interrupts such cardiovascular quiescence, such that the sufferer may not enjoy the restorative effect of sleep.

During obstructive apnea, negative inspiratory intrathoracic pressure generated against the occluded pharynx increases LV transmural pressure (i.e., intracardiac minus intrathoracic pressure) and, consequently, LV afterload. It also increases venous return, augmenting right ventricular (RV) preload, while OSA-induced hypoxic pulmonary vasoconstriction increases RV afterload [6]. Consequent RV distension and leftward septal displacement during diastole impair LV filling [6]. The combination of increased LV afterload and diminished LV preload during obstructive apneas causes a progressive reduction in stroke volume and cardiac output [7]. This is a unique feature of OSA. Nevertheless, over months to years, these stresses can contribute to the progression of CHF.

Autonomic cardiovascular dysregulation, characterized by elevated SNA and parasympathetic withdrawal, is an important consequence of SDB, including both OSA and CSA [1, 6]. Intermittent hypoxia induced by apnea and hypopnea, the absence of breathing during apnea, which eliminates reflex inhibition of central sympathetic nerve traffic arising from pulmonary stretch receptors that are activated during normal breathing, and arousal from sleep augment SNA [1, 6]. In OSA, the baroreceptor reflex stimulated by reductions in stroke volume and cardiac output also augments SNA [1, 6]. Importantly, the adverse effects of SDB on the autonomic nervous system are not confined to sleep, but they may persist into wakefulness, although the mechanism of such daytime carryover effects remains unclear. Nevertheless, SDB may contribute to a worse prognosis in CHF, at least partly through autonomic dysregulation.

88.4 Effects of CPAP on OSA in CHF (Table 88.1)

CPAP is the standard treatment for OSA even in patients with CHF. As in patients without CHF, CPAP splints the pharynx and maintains its patency, thereby preventing apnea and hypopnea. In addition, independent from treating OSA, CPAP may have beneficial positive airway pressure effects on CHF, such as cardiac unloading. For instance, CPAP reduces LV transmural pressure and afterload in patients with CHF by increasing intrathoracic pressure. It also reduces LV preload and consequently LV end-diastolic volume and pressure. The acute response of cardiac output to CPAP therapy in awake patients with CHF is dependent on cardiac preload [8]. In patients with CHF and high LV filling pressure (i.e., $\geq$12 mmHg), CPAP of 5–10 cm H_2O generally augments cardiac output, but in patients with CHF and low LV filling pressure (i.e., <12 mmHg), it generally reduces cardiac output [8].

As an OSA treatment, in addition to the alleviation of OSA, one-night application of CPAP caused abolition of negative intrathoracic pressure swings and reductions in nocturnal BP that caused a dramatic reduction in LV afterload that was accompanied by a decrease in HR. [9] A recent study extended these findings by demonstrating that treatment of OSA by CPAP reversed overnight decreases in stroke volume and cardiac output and increases in peripheral resistance [7].

Other studies have shown that treatment of OSA by CPAP in CHF patients for 3–9 weeks improved the cardiac work metabolic index, indicating the energy-sparing effect of CPAP [10]. In a study in which subjects were randomized to

Table 88.1 Summary of clinical studies investigating the effects of OSA treatment by CPAP on cardiovascular outcomes in patients with CHF

Author (year)	Design	Duration	Outcome
Tkacova et al. (1998) [9]	Self-controlled	1 night	LV transmural pressure↓, systolic BP↓, HR↓
Kasai et al. (2015) [7]	Self-controlled	1 night	Attenuate overnight reduction in stroke volume and cardiac output and overnight increase in total peripheral resistance
Malone et al. (1991) [27]	Crossover	4 weeks	LVEF↑, but ↓ 1 week after withdrawal of CPAP
Johnson et al. (2008) [28]	Pre-post	7 weeks	LVEF↑, systemic vascular resistance index↓
Yoshinaga et al. (2007) [10]	Pre-post	3–9 weeks	LVEF↑, trend for reduced cardiac oxidative metabolism, work metabolic index↑
Kaneko et al. (2003) [12]	RCT	1 month	LVEF↑, systolic BP↓, HR↓
Usui et al. (2005) [13]	RCT	1 month	MSNA↓, systolic BP↓, HR↓
Ryan et al. (2005) [29]	RCT	1 month	Nocturnal ventricular ectopy↓, LVEF↑, systolic BP↓
Gliman et al. (2008) [17]	RCT	1 month	HF-HRV during wakefulness↑, LVEF↑
Ruttanaumpawan et al. (2008) [18]	RCT	1 month	Spontaneous BRS during wakefulness↑, LVEF↑, systolic BP↓, HR↓
Hall et al. (2014) [11]	RCT	6–8 weeks	Improved myocardial sympathetic nerve function
Mansfield et al. (2004) [15]	RCT	3 months	LVEF↑, urinary norepinephrine↓, improved quality of life
Smith et al. (2006) [16]	Randomized crossover	6 weeks	No differences in cardiovascular outcomes between CPAP and sham-CPAP groups
Egea et al. (2008) [14]	RCT	3 months	LVEF↑
Ferrier et al. (2008) [30]	Controlled, non-randomized	6 months	LVEF↑, left ventricular systolic volume↓, systolic BP↓
Wang et al. (2007) [2]	Observational	2.9 years (mean)	Trend for reduced mortality in the CPAP group
Kasai et al. (2008) [19]	Observational	2.1 years (mean)	Lower death and hospitalization risk in the CPAP group

BP blood pressure, *BRS* baroreflex sensitivity, *CHF* chronic heart failure, *CPAP* continuous positive airway pressure, *HF-HRV* high-frequency heart rate variability, *HR* heart rate, *LVEF* left ventricular ejection fraction, *MSNA* muscle sympathetic nerve activity, *OSA* obstructive sleep apnea, *RCT* randomized, controlled trial

receive either 6–8 weeks of CPAP therapy or not, cardiac positron emission tomography-derived indices of oxidative metabolism and cardiac sympathetic nerve presynaptic function were assessed in patients with CHF and OSA [11]. Although significant improvement in cardiac sympathetic nerve presynaptic function was observed in patients randomized to CPAP, oxidative metabolism was not improved with CPAP, probably due to the short time periods of CPAP treatment. However, it should be noted that improvement in oxidative metabolism with CPAP was observed in a subset of patients with more severe OSA.

In a 1-month randomized trial involving HF patients with severe OSA, fixed-pressure CPAP increased the LV ejection fraction (LVEF) by 9 % in association with reduced systolic BP and HR [12]. Considering that CPAP reduced sympathetic vasoconstrictor activity [13], it was suggested that this was a mechanism by which BP was lowered. Egea et al. [14] also reported that in 50 patients with CHF, fixed-pressure CPAP improved the LVEF after 3 months. In a 3-month randomized trial involving 40 patients with less severe CHF and OSA, Mansfield et al. [15] reported that fixed-pressure CPAP reduced urinary norepinephrine concentration and improved the LVEF and quality of life, but not BP. In another randomized trial, Smith et al. [16] found no improvement in the LVEF in CHF patients with OSA while on CPAP. In contrast to the previously mentioned trials, they used auto-titrating CPAP, and they did not confirm that it eliminated OSA in a sleep study at the end of the trial. Furthermore, short-term CPAP treatment increased high-frequency heart rate variability and baroreflex sensitivity, indicating an increase in parasympathetic modulation of the heart rate [17, 18].

These observations, along with the short-term beneficial effects on the LVEF and autonomic nervous system, suggest that CPAP may have beneficial effects on long-term clinical outcomes. In terms of long-term clinical outcomes, although there are no randomized, controlled trials, two observational studies exist. In a study involving 218 patients with CHF, of whom 51 had OSA and an apnea-hypopnea index (AHI) $\geq$15, there was a trend toward lower mortality in the 14 who accepted CPAP therapy than in the 37 who did not ($p=0.07$) over mean and maximum follow-up periods of 2.9 and 7.3 years, respectively [2]. In another study of 88 CHF patients with moderate to severe OSA, 65 CPAP-treated patients had significantly greater hospitalization-free survival than 23 untreated patients over mean and maximum follow-up periods of 2.1 and 4.8 years, respectively [19]. In the latter study, among the 65 CPAP-treated patients, the hospitalization-free survival rate was significantly higher in the more compliant group ($N=32$), whose average nightly usage was more than the median level (4.9 h), than in the less compliant group ($N=33$), whose average nightly usage was 4.9 h or less [19].

88.5 Effects of CPAP on CSA in CHF (Table 88.2)

Because CHF patients with CSA have increased LV filling pressures, CPAP has been used to augment cardiac output and improve hemodynamics. Indeed, some studies showed that, in patients with CHF, CPAP suppressed CSA [8]. However, the effects of CPAP on CSA have not been consistent. This is probably due to differences in how it is applied. When CPAP was applied acutely and at low pressure (i.e., 5–7.5 cmH_2O), CSA was not alleviated [8]. On the other hand, if CPAP were

Table 88.2 Summary of clinical studies investigating the effects of CSA treatment by CPAP on cardiovascular outcomes in patients with CHF

Author (year)	Design	Duration	Outcome
Javaheri (2000) [31]	Self-controlled	1 night	Ventricular ectopy↓
Davies et al. (1993) [32]	Randomized crossover	2 weeks	No differences in cardiovascular outcomes between CPAP of 1.5 and 7.5 cm H_2O
Naughton et al. (1994) [20]	Controlled, non-randomized	1 month	$PtcCO_2$↑, tidal volume↓ and minute ventilation↓ during stage 2 sleep, LVEF↑, NYHA class↓
Naughton et al. (1995) [21]	RCT	1 month	Plasma and urine norepinephrine↓, LVEF↑, NYHA class↓
Takasaki et al. (1989) [22]	Crossover	3 months	LVEF↑, but ↓ 1 week after withdrawal of CPAP NYHA class↓
Naughton et al. (1995) [23]	RCT	3 months	LVEF↑, NYHA class↓, improved quality of life
Granton et al. (1996) [24]	RCT	3 months	Maximal inspiratory pressure↑, LVEF↑, NYHA class↓
Tkacova et al. (1997) [25]	RCT	3 months	Mitral regurgitant fraction↓, plasma atrial natriuretic peptide↓, LVEF↑, NYHA class↓
Arzt et al. (2007) [33]	Controlled, non-randomized	3 months	Ventilatory efficiency during exercise (V_E / V_{CO_2} -slope)↓, LVEF↑
Sin et al. (2000) [26]	Subgroup analysis of RCT	2.2 years (median)	Better transplant-free survival rate in the CPAP group
Bradley et al. (2005) [34]	RCT (Multicenter)	2 years (mean)	No difference in transplant-free survival rate. Plasma norepinephrine↓, LVEF↑, distance in 6 min walk test↑ in CPAP group.
Arzt et al. (2007) [4]	Post-hoc analysis of RCT (Multicenter)	23 months (mean)	LVEF↑, better transplant-free survival rate in patients whose AHI following CPAP was <15 compared with control subjects. Lower death and hospitalization risks in the CPAP group

BP blood pressure, *BRS* baroreflex sensitivity, *CHF* chronic heart failure, *CPAP* continuous positive airway pressure, *CSA* central sleep apnea, *HR* heart rate, *LVEF* left ventricular ejection fraction, *NYHA* New York Heart Association, *RCT* randomized, controlled trial

gradually initiated with pressures of 8–12.5 cmH_2O, the AHI was reduced by >50 % [8]. In addition, CPAP alleviated CSA in association with an increase in the $PaCO_2$ [20], a reduction in SNA [21], and improvements in cardiopulmonary functions, including increases in the LVEF [22, 23], inspiratory muscle strength [24], reductions in functional mitral regurgitation, and daytime plasma atrial natriuretic peptide concentrations [25]. In one small randomized trial in HF patients with and without CSA, CPAP had no effect on either the LVEF or the composite of mortality and cardiac transplantation in those without CSA [26]. However, in those with CSA, CPAP improved the LVEF at 3 months and showed a trend toward a reduced event rate ($p=0.059$, median follow-up period, 2.2 years). In particular, a subgroup of patients who were compliant with CPAP had a significant reduction in the event rate ($p=0.017$).

The Canadian Continuous Positive Airway Pressure for Treatment of Central Sleep Apnea in Heart Failure (CANPAP) trial sought to determine whether CPAP would improve CSA, morbidity, mortality, and cardiovascular function in CHF patients with CSA receiving contemporary medical therapy for CHF. The CANPAP trial, which included 258 patients with CHF and CSA (130 in a control group and 128 in a CPAP-treated group), reproduced previous findings that CPAP attenuates CSA, improves the LVEF, and lowers SNA. However, there were no significant differences in transplant-free survival between the two groups (mean follow-up duration, 2-years). Because reversal of CSA itself appears to be one means by which CPAP could improve cardiovascular outcomes, and as it was suggested that there are some CHF patients whose CSA cannot be attenuated by CPAP, a post hoc analysis of the CANPAP trial was carried out [4]. It suggested that patients whose AHI was reduced below 15 by CPAP at 3 months have a significantly better transplant-free survival rate compared with control groups. The results of the CANPAP trial do not support routine use of CPAP for CHF, but the post hoc analysis implies the potential for the effective suppression of CSA (i.e., AHI <15). Given this perspective, a newer type of noninvasive positive airway pressure, adaptive servo-ventilation (ASV), which can suppress CSA more effectively than CPAP, has been the focus of attention. A detailed description of ASV is beyond the scope of this chapter, and, thus, it should be discussed elsewhere. Findings from the CANPAP trial also suggest that if patients were successfully treated by CPAP (i.e., AHI <15), they could show a significant improvement in transplant-free survival rate. Therefore, in CHF patients with CSA, CPAP should be tried first, and then, if AHI ≥ 15 even for CPAP, ASV may be considered.

Conclusions

In patients with CHF, OSA has adverse effects on cardiac function and could be associated with progression of CHF, and CSA worsens the prognosis. In short-term or non-randomized studies, treatment of SDB using CPAP appeared to have beneficial effects on long-term outcomes in patients with CHF.

ASV, a newer type of noninvasive positive airway pressure, can more effectively suppress SDB than CPAP in patients with CHF. Two ongoing, large-scale, randomized trials investigating the effects of ASV in CHF patients with SDB on long-term clinical events will provide further information on the SDB treatment strategy in patients with CHF.

Key Major Recommendations

- Because OSA is frequently observed in patients with CHF, and coexisting OSA promotes the progression of cardiac dysfunction and increased mortality through the generation of exaggerated negative intrathoracic pressure during obstructive apnea and sympathetic nervous system overactivation, in association with intermittent hypoxia and reoxygenation, identifying OSA is recommended in patients with CHF.
- Because CSA is also frequently observed in patients with CHF, and coexisting CSA increases sympathetic nervous activity and is also associated with an increased risk of death in patients with CHF, identifying CSA is also recommended in patient with CHF.
- In CHF patients with OSA, abolition of OSA by CPAP improves underlying cardiac dysfunction and may contribute to improvement of long-term outcomes; therefore, CPAP therapy for OSA is recommended in CHF patients with OSA.
- Although treatment options of CSA vary compared with OSA treatment, in patients with CSA, CPAP can also improve underlying cardiac dysfunction and may contribute to the improvement of long-term outcomes (if CSA is suppressed as AHI <15). Thus, treatment of CSA by CPAP can be considered.

References

1. Kasai T, Floras JS, Bradley TD. Sleep apnea and cardiovascular disease: a bidirectional relationship. Circulation. 2012;126:1495–510.
2. Wang H, Parker JD, Newton GE, et al. Influence of obstructive sleep apnea on mortality in patients with heart failure. J Am Coll Cardiol. 2007;49:1625–31.
3. Javaheri S, Shukla R, Zeigler H, et al. Central sleep apnea, right ventricular dysfunction, and low diastolic blood pressure are predictors of mortality in systolic heart failure. J Am Coll Cardiol. 2007;49:2028–34.
4. Arzt M, Floras JS, Logan AG, et al. Suppression of central sleep apnea by continuous positive airway pressure and transplant-free survival in heart failure: a post hoc analysis of the Canadian Continuous Positive Airway Pressure for Patients with Central Sleep Apnea and Heart Failure Trial (CANPAP). Circulation. 2007;115:3173–80.
5. Inoshita A, Kasai T, Takahashi M, et al. Craniofacial anatomical risk factors in men with obstructive sleep apnea and heart failure: a pilot study. Sleep Breath. 2014;18:439–45.
6. Kasai T, Bradley TD. Obstructive sleep apnea and heart failure: pathophysiologic and therapeutic implications. J Am Coll Cardiol. 2011;57:119–27.
7. Kasai T, Yumino D, Redolfi S, et al. Overnight effects of obstructive sleep apnea and its treatment on stroke volume in patients with heart failure. Can J Cardiol. 2015;31(7):832–8.
8. Arzt M, Bradley TD. Treatment of sleep apnea in heart failure. Am J Respir Crit Care Med. 2006;173:1300–8.

9. Tkacova R, Rankin F, Fitzgerald FS, et al. Effects of continuous positive airway pressure on obstructive sleep apnea and left ventricular afterload in patients with heart failure. Circulation. 1998;98:2269–75.
10. Yoshinaga K, Burwash IG, Leech JA, et al. The effects of continuous positive airway pressure on myocardial energetics in patients with heart failure and obstructive sleep apnea. J Am Coll Cardiol. 2007;49:450–8.
11. Hall AB, Ziadi MC, Leech JA, et al. Effects of short-term continuous positive airway pressure on myocardial sympathetic nerve function and energetics in patients with heart failure and obstructive sleep apnea: a randomized study. Circulation. 2014;130:892–901.
12. Kaneko Y, Floras JS, Usui K, et al. Cardiovascular effects of continuous positive airway pressure in patients with heart failure and obstructive sleep apnea. N Engl J Med. 2003;348:1233–41.
13. Usui K, Bradley TD, Spaak J, et al. Inhibition of awake sympathetic nerve activity of heart failure patients with obstructive sleep apnea by nocturnal continuous positive airway pressure. J Am Coll Cardiol. 2005;45:2008–11.
14. Egea CJ, Aizpuru F, Pinto JA, et al. Cardiac function after CPAP therapy in patients with chronic heart failure and sleep apnea: a multicenter study. Sleep Med. 2008;9:660–6.
15. Mansfield DR, Gollogly NC, Kaye DM, et al. Controlled trial of continuous positive airway pressure in obstructive sleep apnea and heart failure. Am J Respir Crit Care Med. 2004;169:361–6.
16. Smith LA, Vennelle M, Gardner RS, et al. Auto-titrating continuous positive airway pressure therapy in patients with chronic heart failure and obstructive sleep apnoea: a randomized placebo-controlled trial. Eur Heart J. 2007;28:1221–7.
17. Gilman MP, Floras JS, Usui K, et al. Continuous positive airway pressure increases heart rate variability in heart failure patients with obstructive sleep apnoea. Clin Sci (Lond). 2008;114:243–9.
18. Ruttanaumpawan P, Gilman MP, Usui K, et al. Sustained effect of continuous positive airway pressure on baroreflex sensitivity in congestive heart failure patients with obstructive sleep apnea. J Hypertens. 2008;26:1163–8.
19. Kasai T, Narui K, Dohi T, et al. Prognosis of patients with heart failure and obstructive sleep apnea treated with continuous positive airway pressure. Chest. 2008;133:690–6.
20. Naughton MT, Benard DC, Rutherford R, et al. Effect of continuous positive airway pressure on central sleep apnea and nocturnal PCO_2 in heart failure. Am J Respir Crit Care Med. 1994;150:1598–604.
21. Naughton MT, Benard DC, Liu PP, et al. Effects of nasal CPAP on sympathetic activity in patients with heart failure and central sleep apnea. Am J Respir Crit Care Med. 1995;152:473–9.
22. Takasaki Y, Orr D, Popkin J, et al. Effect of nasal continuous positive airway pressure on sleep apnea in congestive heart failure. Am Rev Respir Dis. 1989;140:1578–84.
23. Naughton MT, Liu PP, Bernard DC, et al. Treatment of congestive heart failure and Cheyne-Stokes respiration during sleep by continuous positive airway pressure. Am J Respir Crit Care Med. 1995;151:92–7.
24. Granton JT, Naughton MT, Benard DC, et al. CPAP improves inspiratory muscle strength in patients with heart failure and central sleep apnea. Am J Respir Crit Care Med. 1996;153:277–82.
25. Tkacova R, Liu PP, Naughton MT, et al. Effect of continuous positive airway pressure on mitral regurgitant fraction and atrial natriuretic peptide in patients with heart failure. J Am Coll Cardiol. 1997;30:739–45.
26. Sin DD, Logan AG, Fitzgerald FS, et al. Effects of continuous positive airway pressure on cardiovascular outcomes in heart failure patients with and without Cheyne-Stokes respiration. Circulation. 2000;102:61–6.
27. Malone S, Liu PP, Holloway R, et al. Obstructive sleep apnoea in patients with dilated cardiomyopathy: effects of continuous positive airway pressure. Lancet. 1991;338:1480–4.

28. Johnson CB, Beanlands RS, Yoshinaga K, et al. Acute and chronic effects of continuous positive airway pressure therapy on left ventricular systolic and diastolic function in patients with obstructive sleep apnea and congestive heart failure. Can J Cardiol. 2008;24:697–704.
29. Ryan CM, Usui K, Floras JS, et al. Effect of continuous positive airway pressure on ventricular ectopy in heart failure patients with obstructive sleep apnoea. Thorax. 2005;60:781–5.
30. Ferrier KA, Neill AM, O'Meeghan T, et al. Continuous positive airway pressure in heart failure patients with obstructive sleep apnoea. Intern Med J. 2008;38:829–36.
31. Javaheri S. Effects of continuous positive airway pressure on sleep apnea and ventricular irritability in patients with heart failure. Circulation. 2000;101:392–7.
32. Davies RJ, Harrington KJ, Ormerod OJ, et al. Nasal continuous positive airway pressure in chronic heart failure with sleep-disordered breathing. Am Rev Respir Dis. 1993;147:630–4.
33. Arzt M, Harth M, Luchner A, et al. Enhanced ventilatory response to exercise in patients with chronic heart failure and central sleep apnea. Circulation. 2003;107:1998–2003.
34. Bradley TD, Logan AG, Kimoff RJ, et al. Continuous positive airway pressure for central sleep apnea and heart failure. N Engl J Med. 2005;353:2025–33.

Part X

Non Invasive Ventilation in Long-Term Applications

Long-Term Noninvasive Ventilation Application in COPD: Determinants and Lessons Learned

89

Nicolino Ambrosino

Contents

Chronic respiratory failure (CRF) is frequent in the end stage of the natural progression of chronic obstructive pulmonary disease (COPD). Among other factors, in these patients, inspiratory muscle dysfunction caused by pulmonary hyperinflation leads to ineffective alveolar ventilation, resulting in chronic hypercapnia [1]. Whether chronic hypercapnia is adversely associated with overall prognosis is still the subject of discussion, at least in patients on long-term oxygen therapy (LTOT) [2].

Long-term noninvasive positive pressure ventilation (NPPV) is well established and increasingly used in patients with CRF cause by restrictive thoracic (RTD) and neuromuscular diseases (NMD) as well as in those with obesity hypoventilation syndrome. There is evidence that in COPD patients with chronic hypercapnia, long-term (nighttime) NPPV may improve physiological and clinical parameters such as daily arterial blood gases, exercise capacity, and, with conflicting results, health-related quality of life (HRQL) when evaluated with appropriate questionnaires [3, 4]. Furthermore, it has been reported that, in these patients, compared with LTOT alone, addition of long-term NPPV is associated with fewer hospital admissions [3] and lower overall treatment costs [5]. Nevertheless, the role of NPPV in improving survival in COPD patients with CRF remains uncertain [6].

As shown by a one meta-analysis [7], most of the earlier and more recent large randomized controlled trials (RCTs) of addition of NPPV to LTOT did not show any substantial improvement in survival compared with LTOT alone [3, 7, 8]. Although

N. Ambrosino
Auxilium Vitae, Volterra, Italy
e-mail: nico.ambrosino@gmail.com

A.M. Esquinas (ed.), *Noninvasive Mechanical Ventilation: Theory, Equipment, and Clinical Applications*, DOI 10.1007/978-3-319-21653-9_89

the small sample size of the evaluated studies prevents definite conclusions, in the meta-analysis [7], nighttime home NPPV for at least 3 months in stable hypercapnic patients with COPD showed no consistent clinically or statistically significant effect on arterial blood gases, exercise tolerance, HRQL, lung function, respiratory muscle function, or sleep efficiency. One RCT showed a small significant survival benefit, which, however, was associated with worsening in HRQL [4].

The “negative” results in survival benefit reported by these studies have been challenged by a German RCT and ascribed to the applied inspiratory pressures that were considered “low” and, as such, unable to improve hypercapnia [9]. This one-year randomized, prospective, multicenter RCT of NPPV addition to standard treatment versus standard treatment alone was performed over many years in patients with stable GOLD (Global Initiative on Obstructive Lung Disease) stage IV COPD and daytime carbon dioxide tension ($PaCO_2$) of 51.9 mmHg or higher. NPPV was targeted to reduce baseline $PaCO_2$ by at least 20 % or to achieve $PaCO_2$ values lower than 48.1 mmHg. One-year mortality was 12 % in the intervention group and 33 % in the control group. The authors concluded that the addition of long-term NPPV to standard treatment improves survival of patients with hypercapnic, stable COPD when inspiratory pressure is targeted to greatly reduce hypercapnia [9].

The results of the study [9] differ from those of another study [8] that has investigated whether nighttime home NPPV in patients admitted to hospital for acute respiratory failure (ARF) prolongs the time to readmission for respiratory causes or death in the following 12 months. Although daytime $PaCO_2$ was significantly improved in NPPV versus standard treatment alone, as was night transcutaneous PCO_2, 1 year after discharge, 65 % of patients treated with NPPV versus 64 % of patients in standard treatment were readmitted to hospital for respiratory causes or had died, and time to event was not different. Furthermore, the number of exacerbations, lung function, mood state, daily activity, and severity or dyspnea were not significantly different. Only HRQL showed a trend in favor of NPPV. Therefore, these authors could not demonstrate any improvement in time to readmission or death by adding NPPV for 1 year in COPD patients with prolonged hypercapnia after an episode of ARF treated with NPPV. This author agrees with these investigators that there is no reason to believe the NPPV was not effective, inasmuch as daytime $PaCO_2$ and nighttime PCO_2 improved.

These two studies are conflicting. It seems that, despite the effectiveness in reducing daytime $PaCO_2$ and transcutaneous nighttime PCO_2 in one study [8], NPPV was unable to improve prognosis of these patients. In addition, the other study [3] was unable to improve 2-year survival, despite the ability to improve daytime $PaCO_2$ (while breathing oxygen), and HRQL and to reduce readmissions. Therefore, it is not probable that differences in 1-year survival between the German study and the others is the result of the claimed “high inspiratory pressures” applied or whatever ability to reduce $PaCO_2$ levels was obtained in that study [9]. Furthermore, the control population of the German study suffered from a high mortality rate, which was significantly higher than in population also treated with NPPV [9]. This may indicate that severity of the patients’ disease rather than correction of hypercapnia or any other supposed effect of “high inspiratory pressures” may be the reason for differences in survival in patients treated with NPPV in different studies. The claim that chronic hypercapnia is associated with worse survival is questionable, at least in the patients undergoing oxygen therapy [2], and should be evaluated with specific studies. Furthermore, there is growing evidence that mortality of patients with COPD is related to many other factors, such as exercise capacity, comorbidities, and inflammatory status [10].

Conclusion

NPPV may reduce readmissions and, with less evidence, mortality in patients with COPD after acute hypercapnic respiratory failure. The question of when to select patients with prolonged hypercapnia needs further assessment. Once stable hypercapnia is proven, NPPV may improve survival and, again, with less evidence, HRQL. As a consequence, in spite of studies that have added to the comprehension of the role of long-term NPPV, this author believes that there is not enough evidence for a widespread generalized use of this therapeutic approach in stable hypercapnic patients with COPD. This modality should be reserved for individual cases.

Key Points

- Chronic respiratory failure is frequently in the final stage of the natural progression of COPD.
- Whether chronic hypercapnia is adversely associated with overall prognosis remains uncertain.
- The role of long-NPPV in improving survival in COPD patients with CRF is still under discussion.
- Long-term nighttime noninvasive ventilation in these patients has some physiological and clinical benefits.
- Long-term noninvasive ventilation should be reserved for individual patients.

References

1. Ambrosino N, Guarracino F. Respiratory failure. In: Palange P, Simonds AK, editors. ERS handbook of respiratory medicine. 2nd ed. Sheffield: ERS; 2013. p. 162–5.
2. Aida A, Miyamoto K, Nishimura M, et al. Prognostic value of hypercapnia in patients with chronic respiratory failure during long-term oxygen therapy. Am J Respir Crit Care Med. 1998;158:188–93.
3. Clini E, Sturani C, Rossi A, et al. The Italian multicentre study on noninvasive ventilation in chronic obstructive pulmonary disease patients. Eur Respir J. 2002;20:529–38.
4. McEvoy RD, Pierce RJ, Hillman D, et al. Nocturnal non-invasive nasal ventilation in stable hypercapnic COPD: a randomized controlled trial. Thorax. 2009;64:561–6.
5. Clini EM, Magni G, Crisafulli E, et al. Home non-invasive mechanical ventilation and long-term oxygen therapy in stable hypercapnic chronic obstructive pulmonary disease patients: comparison of costs. Respiration. 2009;77:44–50.

6. Ambrosino N. The history of home ventilation: what have we learned? The Buyer's guide. 2014–2015, 31–4.
7. Struik FM, Lacasse Y, Goldstein R, et al. Nocturnal non-invasive positive pressure ventilation for stable chronic obstructive pulmonary disease. Cochrane Database Syst Rev. 2013;(6):CD002878.
8. Struik FM, Sprooten RT, Kerstjens HA, et al. Nocturnal non-invasive ventilation in COPD patients with prolonged hypercapnia after ventilatory support for acute respiratory failure: a randomised, controlled, parallel-group study. Thorax. 2014;69:826–34.
9. Köhnlein T, Windisch W, Köhler D, et al. Non-invasive positive pressure ventilation for the treatment of severe stable chronic obstructive pulmonary disease: a prospective, multicentre, randomised, controlled clinical trial. Lancet Respir Med. 2014;2:698–705.
10. Stolz D, Meyer A, Rakic J, et al. Mortality risk prediction in COPD by a prognostic biomarker panel. Eur Respir J. 2014;44:1557–70.

90 Long-Term Noninvasive Ventilation Among Chronic Respiratory Failure Diseases (Cystic Fibrosis and Other Diseases) Awaiting Lung Transplantation: Key Determinants and Practical Implications

Ana Souto Alonso, Pedro Jorge Marcos Rodriguez, and Carlos J. Egea Santaolalla

Contents

90.1 Introduction

Lung transplant prevalence continues to increase in spite of the recent advances that have been made in the knowledge and treatment of lung diseases in recent years. Today, it is a therapeutic option for patients with end-stage lung disease with poor prognosis in 2 year's time to improve their chance of survival and quality of life.

A. Souto Alonso (✉) • P.J. Marcos Rodriguez
Respiratory Service, Instituto de Investigación Biomédica de A Coruña (INIBIC), Complejo Hospitalario Universitario de A Coruña (CHUAC), Sergas, Universidade da Coruña (UDC), Corunna, Spain
e-mail: Ana.Souto.Alonso@sergas.es

C.J. Egea Santaolalla
Sleep Unit, Araba University Hospital, Basque Country University, School of Medicine, Ciberes, BioaAraba Project, Vitoria-Gasteiz, Spain

A.M. Esquinas (ed.), *Noninvasive Mechanical Ventilation: Theory, Equipment, and Clinical Applications*, DOI 10.1007/978-3-319-21653-9_90

In Spain in 2014, according to the National Transplantation Office Annual Report [1], interstitial lung disease (ILD, 38 %), chronic obstructive pulmonary disease (COPD, 35 %), and cystic fibrosis (CF, 11 %) are the three most frequent principal diagnoses among patients awaiting lung transplantation. Other indications include bronchiectasis, pulmonary hypertension, and retransplantation [1]. This distribution is similar in the international registry [2].

It is important to highlight the difference between the time the patient is referred to evaluation by the multidisciplinary transplantation team and the time to be placed to wait for lung transplantation [3, 4]. There are national and international consensus recommendations to manage this situation, and we must acknowledge that the decision to include a patient on the waiting list for lung transplant is complex and involves taking into account specific program and regional factors that affect such a decision [3, 4].

In 2014, 262 patients out of 601 listed underwent lung transplantation in Spain [1]. The average and median number of days spent on the waiting list were 241 (standard deviation (SD) 221) and 178 (range 75–329), respectively. The waiting list global mortality rate was 3.9 %. Nearly 1 out of 10 transplantation procedures was under emergency code, and the most common diseases were ILD (45 %) and CF (28 %). Mortality under emergency code has remained between 6 and 11 % during the past few years.

Although every country has its own transplant waiting list management system, territorial distribution criteria together with severity index and anthropometric features are taken into account for most of them. The Lung Allocation Score (LAS) is a statistical model used in some countries that considers both urgency and post-transplant survival and prioritizes listing and transplantation for high risk patients.

The treatment of symptomatic chronic respiratory failure (CRF) continues to be the cornerstone of the management of critically ill patients, and noninvasive ventilation (NIV) is the key element to its success. Initially, it was used as a bridge to lung transplantation strategy instead of invasive mechanical ventilation [5]. Gradually, its use has adopted a long-term view with the aim of stabilizing critically ill patients to improve access to lung transplantation as pre-transplant life expectancy increases, and to improve the probability of success as the patient undergoes surgery in better condition [3, 6–8]. Currently, the need for ventilatory support is an element of severity to be assessed while the patient is being evaluated to be a lung transplant candidate, and it is not considered as a contraindication [3, 4]. Nor does it bias the prioritization scales used in some countries. What determines a change in consideration and in priority is the beginning of invasive ventilation.

In spite of the spread of its use, the scientific evidence that supports long-term NIV for patients awaiting lung transplantation relies on observational studies. This is due to the ethical difficulty of designing a randomized trial for these patients. This chapter reviews the most representative studies of long-term NIV within this context.

90.2 Long-Term NIV in Patients with Chronic Respiratory Failure Diseases Awaiting Lung Transplantation

The long-term NIV approach for patients on a waiting list lung for transplantation is a situation that is mainly seen in patients with CF and COPD, as it is irrelevant to the pathogenesis and course of lung interstitial and vascular diseases. The role of invasive and noninvasive ventilation for CF patients was initially evaluated as a bridge to lung transplantation in patients with respiratory failure and severe advanced disease. It was then considered as a treatment option for respiratory failure in very advanced disease, irrespective of the patient's status as a lung transplant candidate. The difficulty of not having randomized studies means that the scientific evidence for this approach is based on observational series alone. There are no data about short-term NIV or treating exacerbations. There are no clinical guidelines for how to start and adapt ventilation in these patients. Each team has its own program based on the available evidence and on its proven experience.

The highest level of evidence to support the use of NIV is achieved in the treatment of COPD patients with hypercapnic respiratory failure exacerbation. Benefits in survival, less orotracheal intubation (OTI), and hospital length of stay have been proven. However, its role in respiratory failure outside the context of an exacerbation scenario is more controversial. Nevertheless, after several scientific studies there is favorable evidence for its use in a group of patients with stable hypercapnic chronic respiratory failure. We have not found any specific studies about long-term NIV in COPD designed in the lung transplant context.

90.2.1 Cystic Fibrosis

Pulmonary alteration in patients with CF is characterized by bronchiectasis that damages lung parenchyma and by progressive bronchial obstruction due to bronchial wall inflammation and mucous plugs. Hart et al. [9] observed that, in children and young adults with CF and stable advanced lung disease, there was a correlation between forced expiratory volume in 1 s (FEV1) fall and muscle respiratory load rise. As a result, these patients develop a compensatory mechanism of rapid shallow breathing pattern. Although this respiratory strategy succeeds in maintaining the level of ventilation, pCO_2 eventually increases, and the efficiency of the respiratory muscle pump in eliminating CO_2 diminishes. Supportive treatment with NIV alleviates the muscle respiratory load and, therefore, respiratory muscle performance can be preserved. Despite this physiopathological basis, more studies are required to determine for whom, when, and how this therapy is proven to be beneficial.

In 2002, Madden et al. [6] produced the first and most extensive retrospective report on 113 patients with end-stage CF receiving nasal ventilation. Indication for ventilatory support was established when clinical condition and arterial blood gases where judged to be a severe risk to survival. They studied 23 non-transplant candidates and 90 patients who were either waiting for or being evaluated for a lung transplant. They looked after most patients on a general ward or at home. The mean duration of NIV support was 61 days (range 1–600) for those on the lung transplant waiting list, 53 days (range 1–279) for patients under evaluation and 45 days (range 0–379) among those patients who were not being considered for a lung transplant. They described their experience in treating respiratory failure until transplantation with NIV for advanced patients who are actually on the lung transplant waiting list or being evaluated for it. They also recommend caution in its use among non-candidate patients as it may unnecessarily delay the inevitable and prolong suffering.

There are few references to long-term NIV therapy. This chapter focuses on two more recent works. One is a French study based on the analysis of data from the CF National Register Centre, and the second is an English study that reviewed 20 years of clinical practice in a lung transplant center with a multidisciplinary team.

The aim of the study of Faroux et al. [7] was to evaluate the respiratory function of patients with CF following 1 year of NIV. The study selected 41 out of 89 patients who had initiated long-term NIV between 1999 and 2001 and had been monitored during the following 2 years. Reasons for exclusion were lung transplantation, death, no match available, and lack of follow-up. For each ventilated patient, a control match from the same center was included. They were comparable in terms of age, anthropometric data, lung function (±10 % of pred%FEV1 (percentage of predicted value)), genotype, and equal follow-up period. Anthropometric data, lung function, gas analyses, antibiotic prescription, inhaled and oral corticosteroid therapy, insulin treatment, nutritional support, and oxygen therapy were compared between both groups through 3 years of study. Initiation of NIV was based on functional and clinical signs that reflected an accelerated decline of respiratory status, with moderate hypercapnia at the beginning of therapy. Ventilated patients experienced during the previous year of NIV a greater decline in pulmonary function than the control group patients. After 1 year of NIV, the reduction in pulmonary function was comparable in both groups. Thus, data has shown that long-term NIV was related to the stabilization of pulmonary function in patients with advanced CF. Nevertheless, the authors pointed out that in the year when treatment was initiated and in the previous year, ventilated patients were treated in a more intensive way and had received intravenous antibiotic for more days and were prescribed nutritional support and oxygen more frequently, and this may have contributed to their stabilization. The study was not designed to assess survival and the authors mention that more studies with a larger number of patients and a longer follow up period are needed.

Flight et al. [8] analyzed the data of all domiciliary NIV prescriptions in patients with CF in their center between 1991 and 2010. Out of 47 patients, 10 had started NIV between 1991 and 2000, and 37 since 2001. The average length of NIV was 16 months (range 2–90). Twenty-four (51 %) patients were on the lung transplant waiting list while they were on NIV. Predicted %FEV1 was significantly lower in the 17 patients who underwent lung transplantation than in those who died while on NIV (17.1 % vs 24.9 %; $p=0.0015$). Nine out of 10 patients received pressure mode (either spontaneous or controlled) and all of them used a nasal mask. Persistent diurnal hypercapnia and/or inability to maintain oxygenation in a safe way with available devices were the NIV starting criteria. The authors found a variable response among patients, where those with more rapid decline suffering from the most severe level of disease and the worst lung function were more likely to respond. The main limitations of the study were related to its retrospective design, its limited number of patients, and the absence of a control group, meaning that their results cannot being generalized to the whole CF population. Considering the results and the limitations of the study, they also suggest that NIV might slow down or even reverse the decline of lung function in adults with advanced CF. Compared with the previous year, and because every patient received the same intensive therapy for their respiratory failure (physiotherapy, antibiotics, nebulized medication, diabetes treatment, and nutritional support), and this care was maintained throughout the years, the authors suggest that the improvement in pulmonary function is related to the use of NIV. However, they highlighted the need for extensive multicenter prospective studies to clarify the effects of NIV in CF and to determine the optimal starting time.

90.2.2 COPD

COPD is the most frequent indication for lung transplantation worldwide [2]. However, it is still challenging to define which patients benefit from it and to define the most accurate procedure time. Therefore, it is essential for these patients to be evaluated within the framework of a multidisciplinary lung transplant program.

The main goal of transplantation is to increase survival rates and improve quality of life. Thus, short- or medium-term survival probability supports the candidate selection to referral and waiting list placing criteria. Tools such as the BODE (for Body-mass index, airflow Obstruction, Dyspnea, and Exercise) score have been developed to assess prognosis in COPD patients [10]. Despite not being designed in the lung transplant setting, it has been used to guide the referral and listing time [3, 4]. It is recommended that patients with BODE >5 should be referred to be evaluated, and those with BODE >7 and holding another circumstance that affects prognosis will be placed on the waiting list. These situations include any acute hypercapnic exacerbation that needs hospital admission [3, 4]. Patients with BODE between 7 and 10 have a 52-month overall mortality of 80 % [10], and a 2-year survival after hospitalization for acute hypercapnic exacerbation of 49 % [11]. In contrast, overall survival after transplantation from COPD is 5.5 years [2].

The worldwide utilization of NIV to treat hypercapnic respiratory failure in the context of COPD exacerbation is based on strong scientific evidence that it is proven to decrease mortality rates, OTI need, and hospital admission length [12, 13]. To date, this level of evidence does not exist with regard to its use in hypercapnic stable patients. However, some recent studies have shown beneficial effects that have led to the inclusion of some suggestions in current clinical practice guidelines, such as the one from the National Institute for Health and Care Excellence (NICE) [14]. Referral to a specialized center is recommended for COPD patients with hypercapnic chronic respiratory failure disease who had ventilatory support during an exacerbation or have hypercapnia or acidosis with long-term oxygen therapy (LTOT) [14].

In the latest Global Strategy for Diagnosis, Management and Prevention of COPD update, the wide use of NIV in patients with stable, very severe COPD is acknowledged [13]. The authors report that, in a subset of patients with pronounced daytime hypercapnia, the combination of NIV and LTOT may be of some use, although they also say that there is not sufficient evidence to make a recommendation.

Patients with very severe disease for whom acute or chronic hypercapnia might mean their inclusion on the lung transplant waiting list may be treated with NIV in an attempt to decrease premature mortality and to increase transplantation survival.

90.2.3 NIV Modalities and Operating Procedures

NIV is a sign that objectively denotes the gravity of the disease. Therefore, the sooner patients and their family have information about the possibility of starting the therapy in the near future the better. This could occur in an acute exacerbation context or it could be planned when the clinical condition recommends it. Sometimes, in poor prognosis cases, if the transplant is not carried out in the short term, the line between curative and palliative intention becomes blurred. So, patients must be supported throughout the whole process to decide on the measures they may want to adopt.

Successful NIV requires that patients are appropriately selected and informed, and that the selection of the kind of ventilation, interface, and accessories is suitable for their specific clinical condition. Most of the studies refer to using nasal masks, which usually interfere less with speech and oral intake, induce less gastric distension, and allow coughing and expectoration. In any case, different types of interfaces should be available to provide comfort and meet each patient's needs, as these will enhance long-term ventilation compliance.

Although most of the studies and series have used spontaneous or controlled positive pressure ventilators, it is important to take into account that it may be necessary to use another kind of respiratory support for a given patient. In addition, this may vary over the months or years, thus close follow-up and monitoring is required.

It is crucial to establish the treatment goals at each stage, and to consider that equipment with other functions might be needed. One must be prepared to deal with different types of asynchrony that might be associated with the trigger sensitivity and the respiratory cycling time, which may vary among different devices. If ventilatory support is required for at least 16 h, it is recommended to have a backup machine and an independent energy supply as well. In addition, the use of an appropriate humidification system in these patients is a valuable way to prevent the adverse effects of cold, dry air in the epithelial wall [15].

It is essential that the starting clinical environment is adequate, usually in a hospital ward, with a highly specialized team composed of doctors, nurses, and physiotherapists with professional skills in the management of ventilation for these patients. The standard operating procedure must include how to succeed in adapting to NIV, the patient's education, and the monitoring process. One fundamental aspect that provides the guarantee of receiving adequate health care is the availability of access to this professional team around the clock, 365 days of the year, if any changes or decline occurs.

90.2.3.1 Clinical Key Points When Employing NIMV on These Patients

It is preferable to start this therapy in an inpatient setting. However, if close monitoring and safety concerns can be addressed, an outpatient controlled initiation and titration of NIV is possible When considering NIV, even in the clinically stable patient, it is important to assess a very recent chest radiograph to identify any contraindications to ventilation (e.g., pneumothorax).

Initially, short daytime trials that increase gradually in duration are implemented so that the patient becomes accustomed to the machine and the interface. Experienced personnel should adjust the interface to assure a good seal with minimal air leakage, which is necessary to achieve effective ventilation and to assure the well-being of the patient and improve compliance. A nasal mask is usually tried first because it is generally well tolerated. Oral-nasal masks are useful for patients who have excessive oral air leaks or poorly fitting nasal masks, though it should be used with caution among patients with either high sputum volume or needs for intensive chest physiotherapy, such as patients with CF.

90.2.4 Advantages of NIV

Although NIV has the drawbacks of an unprotected airway and it provides no access for tracheal suction, we believe that the advantages outweigh the disadvantages. When the patient is not ill enough to require special monitoring or treatment, the use of NIV facilitates handling the patient outside the intensive care unit in a regular ward, a respiratory care unit, or even at home, becomes a cost-effective solution.

With NIV, patients are able to communicate, eat, be active during chest physiotherapy and have their nutrition and general physical condition optimized while receiving this treatment. Depending on patient condition, NIV will be applied in a wide range of situations, from continuously, in more severe cases, to only at night for nocturnal hypoventilation.

For selected patients, NIV provides a useful but limited period of extra time in which suitable donor organs may be found. Moreover, it may also reduce the risk of infection and ischemia of the airway after transplantation, classically associated with patients under invasive mechanical ventilation.

Some patients will require NIV after lung transplantation, mainly after extubation, and so the employment of this treatment before the surgical procedure may help the patient to become familiarized with it and to tolerate it better because NIV is usually well tolerated when it is reintroduced [6].

Conclusion

NIV appears to be a safe option for managing patients with hypercapnic respiratory failure awaiting lung transplantation. Most of the data comes from observational isolated experiences. In this context, although we understand that there are ethical difficulties in carrying out randomized studies that could bring scientific evidence to support the use of pretransplant NIV, more specific designed studies are needed to determine in which circumstances and to which patients this therapy should be offered.

An common international approaching procedure needs to be defined. This should incorporate the evaluation and the positioning of all therapies that have been developed so far to manage hypercapnic respiratory failure, such as extracorporeal lung assistance and NIV.

Key Recommendations

- NIV for candidates for a lung transplant allows them to avoid invasive mechanical ventilation and increases the probability of receiving an organ under optimal conditions.
- Long-term domiciliary NIV may be considered for COPD patients with chronic hypercapnic respiratory failure who experience progressive destabilization despite optimal non-ventilatory treatment and after a first hypercapnic exacerbation while awaiting lung transplantation.
- NIV is now an established treatment for CF patients with respiratory failure and plays a role in maintaining lung health while awaiting lung transplantation.
- Most of the evidence for NIV effectiveness for patients with COPD or CF awaiting lung transplantation comes from observational retrospective studies.
- Extensive multicenter prospective studies are necessary to clarify the role of NIV for patients with CF and COPD and to determine its optimum starting time.

References

1. Organización Nacional de Trasplante. Memoria de actividad donación y trasplante pulmonar. España. 2014.
2. Yusen RD, Edwards LB, Kucheryavaya AY, Benden C, Dipchand AI, for the International Society for Heart and Lung Transplantation. The Registry of the International Society for Heart and Lung Transplantation: thirty-first adult lung and heart-lung transplant report – 2014; focus theme: retransplantation. J Heart Lung Transplant. 2014;33:1009–24.
3. Weill D, Benden C, Corris PA, Davies RD, et al. A consensus document for the selection of lung transplant candidates: 2014 – an update from the Pulmonary Transplantation Council of the International Society for Heart and Lung Transplantation. J Heart Lung Transplant. 2015;34:1–15.

4. Roman A, Ussetti P, Solé A, Zurbano F, Borro JM, et al.; Normativa SEPAR. Normativa para la selección de pacientes candidatos a trasplante pulmonar. Arch Bronconeumol. 2011;47(6):303–9.
5. Hodson ME, Madden BP, Steven MH, Tsang VT, Yacoub MH. Non-invasive mechanical ventilation for cystic fibrosis patients – a potential bridge to transplantation. Eur Respir J. 1991;4:524–7.
6. Madden BP, Kariyawasam H, Siddiqi AJ, Machin A, et al. Noninvasive ventilation in cystic fibrosis patients with acute or chronic respiratory failure. Eur Respir J. 2002;19:310–3.
7. Flight WG, Shaw J, Johnson S, Webb AK, et al. Long-term non-invasive ventilation in cystic fibrosis – experience over two decades. J Cyst Fibros. 2012;11:187–92.
8. Faroux B, Le Roux E, Ravilly S, Bellis G, Clément A. Long-term noninvasive ventilation in patients with cystic fibrosis. Respiration. 2008;76:168–74.
9. Hart N, Polkey MI, Clément A, Boulé M, et al. Changes in pulmonary mechanics with increasing disease severity in children and young adults with cystic fibrosis. Am J Respir Crit Care Med. 2002;166:61–6.
10. Celli BR, Cote CG, Marin JM, Casanova C, et al. The body-mass index, airflow obstruction, dyspnea, and exercise capacity index in chronic obstructive pulmonary disease. N Engl J Med. 2004;350:1005–12.
11. Connors Jr AF, Dawson NV, Thomas C, Harrell Jr FE, et al. Outcomes following acute exacerbation of severe chronic obstructive lung disease. Am J Respir Crit Care Med. 1996;154:959–67.
12. Brochard L, Mancebo J, Wysocki M, et al. Non-invasive ventilation for acute exacerbations of chronic obstructive pulmonary disease. N Engl J Med. 1995;333:817–22.
13. Global Initiative for Chronic Obstructive Lung Disease. The global strategy for diagnosis, management and prevention of COPD (updated 2015). http://www.goldcopd.org.
14. National Institute of Clinical Excellence. Chronic obstructive pulmonary disease: management of chronic obstructive pulmonary disease in adults in primary and secondary care. 2010. http://www.nice.org.uk. Accessed 2 Feb 2015.
15. Esquinas Rodriguez AM, et al. Clinical review: humidifiers during non-invasive ventilation – key topics and practical implications. Crit Care. 2012;16:203.

Home Mechanical Ventilation and Quality of Life in Neuromuscular Patients During Noninvasive Mechanical Ventilation: New Trends and Key Practical Topics

91

Catarina Ferreira and Joaquim Moita

Contents

Abbreviations

ALS	Amyotrophic lateral sclerosis
CO_2	Carbon dioxide
DMD	Duchenne muscular disease
FVC	Forced vital capacity
NIV	Noninvasive ventilation
NMD	Neuromuscular disease
$PaCO_2$	Partial pressure of carbon dioxide

C. Ferreira (✉) • J. Moita
Pulmonology Department, Centro Hospitalar e Universitário de Coimbra – Hospital Geral, Coimbra, Portugal
e-mail: catfer24@hotmail.com; joaquimmoita@gmail.com

A.M. Esquinas (ed.), *Noninvasive Mechanical Ventilation: Theory, Equipment, and Clinical Applications*, DOI 10.1007/978-3-319-21653-9_91

PaO_2	Partial pressure of oxygen
PCF	Peak cough flow
PEG	Percutaneous endoscopy gastrostomy
PSG	Polysomnography
REM	Rapid eye movement
SpO_2	Peripheral oxygen saturation
VC	Vital capacity

91.1 Introduction

The neuromuscular respiratory system is divided into three main areas of function: ventilator function determined predominantly by the inspiratory muscles; cough function determined by inspiratory, expiratory, and bulbar muscles; and swallowing and airway protection determined by glottic muscles [1]. Many chronic neuromuscular disorders (NMD) lead to progressive respiratory muscle dysfunction, which in turn can lead to respiratory failure and death. When and how to ventilate these patients are relevant issues in the evaluation and monitoring of neuromuscular disease. The answers are based on the knowledge of the natural history of respiratory failure that in neuromuscular disease has specific contours [2].

91.2 Discussion and Analysis Main Topic

Patients with neuromuscular diseases can have rapidly progressive disease with muscle impairment that worsens over months and results in death within a few years, such as amyotrophic lateral sclerosis (ALS) and some forms of spinal muscular atrophy. Duchenne muscular disease (DMD) is considered a relatively rapidly progressive NMD, resulting in muscle impairment within a few years and death in young adulthood. Other myopathies, such as Becker muscular dystrophy, facioscapulohumeral muscular dystrophy, limb-girdle muscular dystrophy, and myotonic dystrophy are slowly progressive diseases, resulting in slow reduction in muscular function and only mildly reduced life expectancy. Respiratory failure is the most common cause of morbidity and morbility in patients with chronic or rapidly progressive neuromuscular diseases [3].

Neuromuscular diseases are the oldest and one of the most successful indications for noninvasive mechanical ventilation (NIV). Modern NIV, based in positive pressure portable ventilators and noninvasive interfaces, emerged in the 1980s. The expansion benefited from the technology developed to treat respiratory sleep disorders, with modern masks and ventilators [2]. Respiratory failure is the most common cause of morbidity and mortality in patients with chronic or rapidly progressive neuromuscular diseases [3].

Molecular biology now allows identification of the genetic defects present in many neuromuscular conditions, and there is hope that, in the future, gene therapy could be used for the treatment of some conditions such as DMD [4]. In parallel with the pharmacological research, we are witnessing today a quiet revolution provided by NIV. An increasing number of children with congenital NMDs reach adulthood. And even when survival is not significantly prolonged, as in end-stage ALS, NIV has a tangible palliative benefit [2].

91.2.1 Chronic Respiratory Failure in Neuromuscular Diseases

Chronic respiratory failure in neuromuscular diseases results from progressive inspiratory muscle weakness (mainly the diaphragm), leading to restrictive ventilatory impairment with decreased inspiratory capacity and breathing pattern with low tidal volumes and increased respiratory rate. There is an increased dead space ratio/tidal volume, resulting in the inability to maintain alveolar ventilation at a level that prevents the appearance of hypercapnia.

This progressive respiratory muscle weakness also results in mechanical respiratory system changes with reduced lung and chest wall distensibility (compliance) and musculoskeletal chest deformation, with progressive decline in vital capacity (VC) and increase in muscle work of breathing and increased risk of muscle fatigue. A rapid-shallow breathing pattern is also associated with increased work of breathing and inability to breathe deeply, leading to chronic microatelectasis and decreased lung and thorax compliance. Furthermore, these patients may also present changes in the respiratory center (drive), with loss of sensitivity of central and peripheral chemoreceptors.

Alveolar hypoventilation in neuromuscular disease typically appears during the rapid eye movement (REM) sleep stage. In REM sleep, there is respiratory muscular weakness with hypotonia of intercostal muscles and pharyngeal dilators, with relative excess loading of the diaphragm, and also instability of the upper airway due to weakness of the bulbar muscles. Breathing becomes asynchronous, faster, and less effective. This phenomenon, which is physiological, is amplified with decreased muscle strength and compliance seen in NMD, which may result in severe alveolar hypoventilation leading to sustained oxygen desaturation and hypercapnia.

NMD may also be associated with obstructive apneas particularly during REM sleep. $PaCO_2$ increases and PaO_2 decreases, which is not compensated because, in REM sleep, paradoxically, the response of the respiratory center (drive) to these chemical stimuli is decreased. The possible adaptive response is in the form of frequent arousals that allow regaining characteristic control of the wakefulness phase. Arousals cause sleep fragmentation, with decreased sleep efficiency and sleep deprivation; this in turn increases the hypotonia of the upper airway and further reduces the capacity of the drive respond to respiratory stimuli.

Thus, a vicious circle is perpetuated, leading to a progressive and sustained increase of hypercapnia, which in turn reduces the sensitivity of chemoreceptors to subsequent changes in $PaCO_2$ (with depression of the respiratory center). The chronic respiratory failure that began in REM phase then extends progressively to non-REM and finally to wakefulness. That is, the nighttime alveolar hypoventilation, changes in control of ventilation, and change in breathing pattern ultimately lead to daytime alveolar hypoventilation. The development of pulmonary hypertension and premature death depend in part on the severity of desaturation during sleep.

Chronic respiratory failure in NMD is predominantly hypercapnic. Hypoxia is a secondary and late-onset alveolar hypoventilation manifestation but may be relevant in the presence of changes in ventilation/ perfusion, with infections and atelectasis (predominantly basal) being the most frequent causes of involvement of the lung parenchyma in these patients. Frequently, respiratory failure occurs acutely in the context of a respiratory infection secondary to retention of secretions by ineffective cough or aspiration. The weakness of the expiratory, abdominal, and intercostal muscles results in ineffective cough, with failure to remove respiratory secretions, affecting the pulmonary defense mechanisms and facilitating the emergence of respiratory infections [1, 2, 4–7].

91.2.2 Home Noninvasive Mechanical Ventilation in Patients with Neuromuscular Disease

Long-term NIV improves quality of life in most patients with neuromuscular disease and improves survival in some patients, allowing patients with slowly progressive neuromuscular diseases to live to nearly normal life expectancy. It extends survival by many years in patients with other conditions such as DMD. In patients with forms of rapidly progressive disease, as happens in ALS, symptoms can be palliated even if mortality is not reduced [4].

The best accepted indication to start nocturnal noninvasive ventilator assistance in neuromuscular disease is symptomatic hypoventilation with diurnal hypercapnia ($PaCO_2$ >45 mmHg) or nocturnal desaturation with peripheral oxygen saturation (SpO_2) <88 % for 5 consecutive minutes. However, it is now recognized that international recommendations to initiate NIV in neuromuscular diseases are questionable for other symptoms. In the early stage of the disease, the patient does not value the symptoms consistent with sleep-disordered breathing and hypoventilation such as nocturnal awakenings, nocturia, vivid nightmares, fatigue, morning headaches, daytime sleepiness, depression, decreased concentration and/or memory and diminished daytime performance [1].

Symptoms become evident only when diurnal hypercapnia appears, and at that time a poor outcome is expected. In patients with symptomatic hypercapnia with advanced disease, NIV reduces the work of breathing muscles and corrects alveolar hypoventilation, but the results of this late treatment, however, are limited in terms of quality of life and survival. Therefore, symptoms should be carefully researched and NIV during the sleep period should be scheduled earlier, in normocapnic patients, when the nocturnal hypoventilation is identified. Under these circumstances, NIV enhances chemosensitivity to CO_2 changes, increasing ventilatory response of the respiratory center and stabilizing the structure of sleep [4].

Some authors recommend starting NIV as soon as nighttime hypoventilation is identified, which requires the systematic realization of a polygraph sleep study [2, 4]. Guidelines list severe restriction with forced vital capacity (FVC) <50 % of predicted or maximum inspiratory pressure (MIP) <60 mmHg as a criterion for initiation of NIV.

Patients with slowly progressive conditions, such as limb-girdle muscular dystrophy, may not become symptomatic or hypoventilate until FVC falls well below 50 %. On the other hand, this criterion may be sensible for patients with rapidly progressive neuromuscular syndromes such as DMD, allowing time to adapt to NIV before impairment becomes severe. In ALS, NIV should be started early when FVC is <70 % of predicted because, in this disease, when FVC is no longer normal its decline is rapid and unpredictable. Volume loss is preceded by a decrease in muscular strength (MIP) [4].

Sleep-disordered breathing and nocturnal hypoventilation usually precede the onset of diurnal hypoventilation in neuromuscular patients. Partly because of their inability to maintain physical activity, patients with NMD are often unaware of dyspnea or other respiratory symptoms, even when they have severe restriction [6]. For patients who have hypercapnia despite adequate nocturnal therapy, dyspnea during the daytime or hypoxemia due to recurrent respiratory infections associated with atelectasis, daytime ventilation may also be needed [1].

Noninvasive ventilation and cough-assist techniques may also be indicated to manage some acute exacerbations of NMD caused by bronchitis and pneumonia and acute respiratory failure in the home and to reduce the need for hospitalization. Thus, the combination of NIV with cough-assist techniques decreases pulmonary morbidity and hospital admissions [1].

91.2.3 NIV Versus Tracheostomy Ventilation

Consensus opinion consistently supports that home NIV is preferred to tracheostomy and invasive mechanical ventilation for the long-term ventilatory support of patients with neuromuscular disease. The reasons are many, including ease of administration of care, less strain on caregivers, more comfort for patient, greater portability, lower cost, more security, lower airway complications, fewer infections, and reduced need for hospitalization. Tracheostomy ventilation may be necessary when patients have severe bulbar dysfunction and intolerance to NIV or with copious secretions and uncontrolled aspiration, which is reflected in permanent desaturation under NIV [1].

91.2.4 Duchenne Muscular Dystrophy

DMD is an X-linked recessive disease caused by a mutation of the dystrophin gene and is the most common muscular dystrophy of childhood. Chronic respiratory failure is an expected complication of the disease and, without ventilatory support, death occurred on average at 19 years. These arise as a result of progressive loss of expiratory muscles strength, which occurs in parallel with the inspiratory muscle weakness with respiratory insufficiency, ineffective cough, and inevitable accumulation of secretions.

The well-conducted NIV, associated with assisted cough, changed the natural history of the disease, and children with DMD are now surviving to adulthood with the aid of ventilatory support. Today, patients tend to die of cardiac complications of the disease: abnormal electrical conduction or decompensated cardiomyopathy, associated with lack of dystrophin. The management of heart disease is the major challenge in the future.

NIV should be initiated when there is nighttime hypoventilation, even if the symptoms associated with it are not visible [5]. The slow vital capacity (VC) and FVC are classic indicators of the evolution of DMD. Hypoventilation, predominantly in REM, can arise when the VC drops below 60 %. At this time, registration of sleep-disordered breathing should be performed, ideally by polysomnography (PSG), and at least with oximetry and capnography registration. PSG has the additional advantage of identifying obstructive apneas that are common in DMD, which affect the way in which the ventilation is conducted. PSG is also helpful in determining pressure settings.

Patients with DMD have poor sleep quality, with fragmented sleep due to a high number of arousals and low mean SpO_2, even in the absence of relevant respiratory events. Arousals can be seen as a compensatory mechanism to sleep hypoventilation and may contribute to clinical diurnal manifestations, such as excessive daytime sleepiness and poor quality of life [8].

The NIV, initiated and conducted based on the identification and characterization of nocturnal hypoventilation, seems to stabilize the decline in FVC [9]. Thus, NIV has clearly demonstrated its usefulness, significantly increasing the survival and quality of life of these patients. NIV stabilizes vital capacity, increases PaO_2, decreases $PaCO_2$, and improves the quality of sleep. The use of long-term home NIV can significantly decrease pulmonary morbidity and the incidence of respiratory hospitalizations, reduce the number of days of hospitalization, and prolong survival in DMD patients without resort to tracheostomy. These findings may impact the decision to initiate NIV at earlier stages.

91.2.5 Amyotrophic Lateral Sclerosis

ALS is a disease characterized by signs of loss of function of the upper and lower motor neurons at the spinal and bulbar level. ALS often affects the respiratory muscles, including those for airway protection and cough [1]. Bulbar symptoms (drooling, difficulty in speech, aspiration of secretions, and chronic respiratory failure) may not be present at presentation but are invariably present in the late stage of the disease.

Respiratory infections and respiratory failure are the leading cause of death in ALS. Sleep-disordered breathing associated with respiratory muscle weakness is common in ALS and increases in frequency with the progress of the disease. Monitoring pulmonary function is critical in these patients. In ALS patients, NIV should be considered when FVC is less than 70 % of predicted or sleep studies show desaturation or sleep-disordered breathing. As in the other NMDs, sleep studies are important to confirm hypoventilation overnight because nocturnal desaturation correlates directly with mortality [8].

Home NIV increases survival and improves quality of life, sleep-related symptoms, and functional scores, especially in patients without bulbar dysfunction. Patients with severe bulbar dysfunction are often intolerant to NIV and have no survival benefit, but in tolerant patients, sleep-related symptoms and some domains of quality of life improved. Thus, a trial of NIV is justified, even in these patients, but when it is not effective tracheostomy and long-term invasive ventilation should be considered.

More than in any other neuromuscular pathology, in ALS, NIV should be complemented by other supportive measures [9]. The introduction of insufflation-exsufflation cough-assist is mandatory when the peak cough flow (PCF) is less than 160 l/min, a level that reflects the patient's inability to mobilize bronchial secretions. Some authors recommend its use with PCF below 270 l/min, because viral infections decrease muscle strength. Regular use of cough-assist significantly improves the ability of cough. However, when there is deep bulbar involvement, it may have the perverse effect of bringing about the dynamic collapse of the upper airway in exsufflation phase [10].

Muscle cachexia and malnutrition are serious problems directly related with mortality in patients with ALS. The situation is aggravated by frequent choking (particularly liquid) and dysphagia in patients bulbar. Percutaneous endoscopic gastrostomy (PEG) should not be delayed in these patients. Its placement should preferably be done in patients with higher FVC 50 %. It is a fast and safe procedure even in severe patients and can be done with the support of NIV. Administration of botulinum toxin in the parotid glands and submaxillary is safe and effective, dramatically reducing drooling [11].

91.2.6 Starting Home Mechanical Ventilation

Before starting NIV, the most appropriate type of noninvasive ventilator and interfaces should be chosed, based on the patient's needs and lifestyle factors, the patient's preference, the patient's tolerance of the treatment, the risk and possible consequences of ventilator failure, the power supply required, including battery back-up, how easily the patient can get to hospital, whether a humidifier is required, and issues relating to secretion management.

91.2.7 Ventilators

There are two types of positive pressure ventilators for home use: volume-controlled (volume target ventilators) and pressure-controlled (pressure target ventilators). Some newer hybrid systems have the capacity for regulation of volume and pressure.

The bi-level ventilator is a type of pressurimetric ventilator that is widely used for the treatment of chronic respiratory failure in patients with neuromuscular diseases. At home, these ventilators are usually set to work in pressure-support and assisted-controlled mode. The management is facilitated by algorithms that adapt the ventilator to the patient's respiratory pattern and leak compensation. Inasmuch as the objective is to maintain pressure during inspiration, if there is any leakage, flow is automatically incremented to achieve pressurization. Pressurimetric ventilators increase the patient's comfort with sensitive triggers (especially when it is for flow), deliver volume through a decelerating flow that fits the patient's best effort, and, finally, the breathing pattern is not as fixed. However, ventilation regulated by pressure has a limited ability to ventilate patients with low thoracopulmonary compliance [2].

Currently, there is some preference for volume-programmed ventilation. In this type of ventilation, when a certain volume or a certain inspiratory time is reached, the inspiratory valve is closed and the exhalation valve opens. No evidence has been found of a difference between pressure and volume programmed ventilators in patients with chronic respiratory failure. However, patient tolerance is better with pressure-limited modes [6].

Hybrid ventilators allow the patient to be ventilated during the day in volume mode and during the night in pressure mode. The ventilation in volume mode ensures a predefined tidal volume ventilation to correct alveolar hypoventilation and facilitates air stacking during the day. In sleep, pressure ventilation is more comfortable and the leaks are compensated [2].

AVAPS (average volume-assured pressure support) is a more recent additional technology for bi-level NIV. AVAPS combines characteristics of ventilation regulated by pressure and volume to effectively manage the ventilation of the patient and to adapt to the evolution of the disease, automatically adapting pressure support to the changing needs of the patient, to ensure a predefined tidal volume target.

Finally, the best ventilator is the one that responds to the individual needs of the patient.

91.2.8 Interfaces

There are many interfaces used to deliver NIV: oronasal masks, full face masks, nasal masks, nasal pillows, and mouth pieces, with different sizes and different materials. Nasal masks are often better tolerated than oronasal masks for long-term ventilation. Facial masks are indicated in the presence of uncontrollable leakage or nasal obstruction.

In general, the complications and adverse effects of NIV are not serious and relatively rare if patients are appropriately selected and managed. The most common complications are related to the interface, airflow, pressure, or the ventilator itself and are preventable. These include mask discomfort, claustrophobic reactions, nasal or oral congestion or dryness and eye irritation due to air leakage, gastric insufflation, and nasal bridge redness and ulceration. These problems are treated with local measures, including refitting of masks or headgear, using alternative interfaces, or adjusting delivered pressures or volumes [6].

The patient on permanent ventilation can combine more than one interface using nasal or face mask during sleep and nasal pillows or mouthpieces during the day to facilitate reading and social interaction. This solution also allows the variation of pressure points and therefore prevents skin ulceration [2].

Conclusion

Patients with chronic neuromuscular disorders have progressive respiratory muscle dysfunction with hypoventilation and respiratory failure, cough dysfunction, and respiratory infections, leading to death. Home NIV as a treatment for neuromuscular disease has several benefits and improves quality of life. It has been shown to decrease work of breathing and improve blood gases, symptoms of fatigue, daytime sleepiness, and morning headaches. NIV should be started earlier in the course of neuromuscular diseases. The future of NIV is to provide more life to life.

Key Major Recommendations

- Patients with chronic NMDs have progressive respiratory muscle dysfunction with hypoventilation and respiratory failure, cough dysfunction, and respiratory infections and eventual death.
- Noninvasive mechanical ventilation in neuromuscular diseases should be started earlier in the course of the disease when patients present symptomatic hypoventilation with diurnal hypercapnia ($PaCO_2$ >45 mmHg) or nocturnal desaturation with peripheral oxygen saturation (SpO_2) <88 % for 5 consecutive minutes.
- In patients with DMD, NIV should be considered when FVC is <50 % of predicted or MIP is <60 mmHg. In ALS, NIV should be started when FVC is <70 % of predicted.
- Noninvasive mechanical ventilation in neuromuscular diseases improves symptoms of fatigue, daytime sleepiness, and morning headaches as well as blood gas exchange, thus improving quality of life.
- Appropriate selection of ventilators, ventilation mode and parameters, and interfaces is crucial to the success of NIV and patient comfort.

References

1. Benditt JO, Boitano LJ. Pulmonary issues in patients with chronic neuromuscular disease. Am J Respir Crit Care Med. 2013;187(10):1046–55.
2. Moita J, Martins V, Guimarães C. Ventilação mecânica não invasiva na patologia neuromuscular. In Princípios da Ventilação Mecânica Não Invasiva – do Hospital ao Domicilio. Ed. Esquinas AM. Gasin Mèdica. Gasin Médica; 2011;196–203.

3. Ambrosino N, Carpenè N, Gherardi M. Chronic respiratory care for neuromuscular diseases in adults. Eur Respir J. 2009;34:444–51.
4. Simonds AK. Recent advances in respiratory care for neuromuscular disease. Chest. 2006;130:1879–86.
5. Ward S, et al. Randomised controlled trial of non-invasive ventilation (NIV) for nocturnal hypoventilation in neuromuscular and chest wall disease patients with daytime normocapnia. Thorax. 2005;60:1019–1024.
6. Hill NS. Ventilator management for neuromuscular disease. Semin Respir Crit Care Med. 2002;23(3):293–306.
7. Shneerson JM, Simonds AK. Non invasive ventilation for chest wall and neuromuscular disorders. Eur Respir J. 2002;20:480–7.
8. Ferreira C, et al. How sleep studies are important to initiate noninvasive ventilation in Duchenne muscular dystrophy. Sleep Med. 2013;14S:e123.
9. Marques A, et al. Pulmonary function in Duchenne muscular dystrophy patients before and after noninvasive ventilation. Eur Respir J. 2005;26 Suppl 49:85s.
10. Miller RG, et al. Practice parameter update: the care of the patient with amyotrophic lateral sclerosis: drug, nutritional and respiratory therapies (an evidence-based review): report of the Quality Standards Subcommittee of the American Academy of Neurology. Neurology. 2009;73(15):1218–26.
11. Sancho J, et al. Efficacy of mechanical insufflation-exsufflation in medically stable patients with amyotrophic lateral sclerosis. Chest. 2004;125(4):1400–5.

European Models of Home Noninvasive Mechanical Ventilation: What Have We Learned? Evidence and Key Determinants

92

Francisco J. Ribas-Solís, Julia A. Garcia-Fuertes, and Carlos J. Egea-Santaolalla

Contents

Abbreviations

ALS	Amyotrophic lateral sclerosis
COPD	Chronic obstructive pulmonary disease
HMV	Home mechanical ventilation
NIV	Noninvasive ventilation

F.J. Ribas-Solís (✉) • J.A. Garcia-Fuertes
Respiratory Department, Araba University Hospital, Vitoria-Gasteiz, Spain
e-mail: xevi_ribas@yahoo.es; juliaamaranta.garciafuertes@osakidetza.net

C.J. Egea-Santaolalla
Multidisciplinary Sleep Unit, Araba University Hospital, Vitoria-Gasteiz, Spain
e-mail: carlosjavier.egeasantaolalla@osakidetza.net

A.M. Esquinas (ed.), *Noninvasive Mechanical Ventilation: Theory, Equipment, and Clinical Applications*, DOI 10.1007/978-3-319-21653-9_92

92.1 Introduction

In the history of mechanical ventilation over the last 100 years, from 1928, when an iron lung was first used at the Children's Hospital of Boston (Massachusetts), through its highest level of use in the 1940s and 1950s during the poliomyelitis epidemics, until our current times, we realize it is a two-speed journey. The fast track was taken in the 1950s, when iron lungs started to be replaced by positive airway pressure through intubation, and the second track started when the facial mask started to be used as a noninvasive ventilation method. Thus, the possibility of avoiding long hospital stays became a reality with the creation of the first home mechanical ventilation (HMV) programs.

The prevalence rate of HMV has considerably increased in Europe in recent years, both in countries that traditionally had low prevalence rates like Switzerland [1] and the Netherlands [2], in those that had the highest rates, such as France (data source is ANTADIR) [3], and also in countries such as Australia and New Zealand (9.9–12/100,000) [4].

In the beginning, most patients (70 %) were invasively ventilated with positive pressure mechanical ventilators through a tracheostomy tube, and the rate of patients whose ventilation was noninvasive was low. The interfaces used for these were either mouth or nasal pieces (16 %), or negative pressure ventilators (14 %). In the 1980s, nasal masks started to be used in patients with Duchenne's disease, and negative pressure ventilators were limited to exceptional use [5].

After that time, the use of noninvasively implemented mechanical ventilators spread quickly as the technique of choice among patients with restrictive respiratory failure. Patients adapted to the ventilator in a hospital setting and there were later followed-up in their homes; this is when the first positive pressure noninvasive ventilation (NIV) home programs appeared. In 1994, Leger et al. [6] published the first series of patients treated with positive pressure NIV at home, with a follow-up of 276 patients during 5 years. In this study, the benefit for patients with kyphoscoliosis or sequelae from tuberculosis or Duchenne's disease was clear. Moreover, the study showed that patients with chronic obstructive pulmonary disease (COPD) and bronchiectasis also benefited from this method. In 1992, the first pressure support ventilator was created and, since then, the technology has improved and different ventilation methods have appeared.

HMV programs have evolved in recent years and, at the same time, technological progress has allowed for an increase in home monitoring of patients on NIV. Moreover, HMV program implementation aims to bring NIV as close to patients' homes as possible.

92.2 HMV Prevalence in Europe

HMV's introduction into Europe has been uneven and has differed according to country. In 2001 and 2002, to assess the pattern of HMV use in Europe, questionnaires were sent to 483 centers in 16 European countries. A total of 329 replied, which amounts to between 62 and 79 % of HMV users in Europe. This data was published in the EUROVENT [7] study. The average prevalence in Europe was estimated at 6.6 patients/100,000 citizens, although there was a large variation between countries: France was the country with the highest prevalence (17/100,000) whereas Poland had the lowest (0.1/100,000) (Table 92.1). Prevalence variation could be related partly to the average years since NIV started to be implemented. Differences in the relative proportion of patients with obstructive disease, rib cage pathology, and neuromuscular disease were also made clear.

In fact, it is highly likely that data obtained from EUROVENT is not up to date. This is the case with Poland, which went from a 0.1/100,000 prevalence in 2002, to 2.5/100,000 in 2010, with a reduction from over 80 % of neuromuscular patients in 2002 to 51 % in 2010 as a result of the increase in the number of patients with respiratory disease [8].

A similar case is that of the Spanish region of Valencia. Spain showed a prevalence of HMV in 1999 of 4.59/100,000 according to a study by De Lucas et al. [9], and of 6.3/100,000 in 2002 according to the EUROVENT study (close to the European average) [7]. In 1999, the Valencia region showed a prevalence of 4.83 [5]. In a study carried out in 2007 by Chiner et al. [10] in the Valencia region, HVM prevalence was proven to have risen to 29/100,000. Although this is data from just one region in Spain, it can probably be extrapolated to the rest of the country.

Table 92.1 Estimated prevalence of users in HMV programs in 16 European countries (2001–2002)

	Estimated prevalence per 100,000 (2001–2002)
Austria	3.8
Belgium	5.0
Denmark	9.6
Finland	8.7
France	17.0
Germany	6.5
Greece	0.6
Ireland	3.4
Italy	3.9
Netherlands	5.6
Norway	7.8
Poland	0.1
Portugal	9.3
Spain	6.3
Sweden	10.0
United Kingdom	4.1
All countries	6.6

92.3 HMV Models

NIV use in patients with chronic respiratory failure is covered by national health systems, however, only a few countries have clear guidelines about how NIV should be started and in which patient groups. Public national health systems and private insurance companies usually hire private home therapy companies to provide and maintain NIV equipment prescribed by patients' doctors to use when patients are at home. These companies have paramedical staff that can train patients and their families to correctly use NIV. The frequency of visits depends on the type of ventilator prescribed for each patient; the interface type can be adjusted and humidifiers can be provided. In some cases, these companies can also offer other home services, for instance $SatO_2$ night monitoring can be provided. If problems arise at patients' homes, they are communicated to the prescribing doctor; good coordination with the reference hospital is key [11].

Sometimes, the relationship between these companies and the national health systems is poor and often there is no formal infrastructure. Thus, a European study that was carried out in 16 countries including more than 20,000 ventilated patients showed that, in 62 % of centers, an external company carried out services provided to patients. It also showed that the maintenance frequency ranged between 3 and 12 months; that interaction between the service-providing companies and the hospitals was scarce; that the participation of hospitals in the quality control of equipment was poor; and that there were important differences not only between countries but also within the same country [10, 12].

An outstanding exception is France's HMV program. The French model's efficacy is partly attributed to local and regional services, which get support from a specialized center. The services network is effectively maintained as a result of the national capacity to gather data to advance and support the service assessment and research [13].

92.4 NIV Adaptation in HMV Programs

NIV adaptation can take place during a programmed hospital stay, although it can also be effectively implemented in day hospitals, outpatient settings, and even at the patient's home. Pallero et al. [14] carried out a multicenter, randomized, prospective study to compare efficacy and costs according to whether the HMV program was started in a hospital setting or an outpatient setting, with patients who had stable chronic respiratory failure with NIV indication. The main study variable was the $PaCO_2$ drop 6 months after NIV initiation. They found a significant decrease in both groups, although they did not find significant differences between them. Direct costs of both interventions were estimated. The hospital setting intervention was estimated to have a cost of 2692 euros, whereas the outpatient setting intervention had a cost of 1500 euros. Therefore, the conclusion was that, because adapting NIV in the outpatient setting is equivalent to doing it in the hospital setting from a therapeutic perspective, adaptation in the outpatient setting could lead to cost-savings for the health system.

92.5 HMV Programs Follow-Up

There are no data on how frequently patients should see their specialized center doctor, and it depends on different factors such as the patient's pathology, how they adapt to NIV, and how easy it is for them to travel to the hospital. If a private home services company is involved, some of the follow-up can be done in patients' homes. The information can be transmitted to the prescribing doctor who, every 3 months, can systematically check the patients' approximate symptoms, quality of life, ventilation-related side effects, and compliance. After receiving this information, the doctor will be able to determine whatever adjustments are needed.

Some of the tests can only be carried out in the hospital; therefore, it seems that some kind of hospital follow-up is necessary. Generally, the average number of outpatient visits per year is three. Follow-up complementary tests during these visits include arterial blood gas, chest X-rays, and respiratory function tests. The nocturnal evaluation is carried out at home, if possible, or in the hospital to control ventilation quality during the night, and, if possible, in the 3 months following NIV initiation. Patient nocturnal follow-up during the HMV program's first year includes monitoring O_2 saturation, if possible with capnography, respiratory polygraphy, polysomnography, and arterial blood gas first thing in the morning. For many of the more restrictive patients, once they are stable, the supervision required is minimal. Unstable patients or patients who are insufficiently stabilized with NIV need closer follow-up (e.g., those with rapidly progressing neuromuscular diseases such as amyotrophic lateral sclerosis (ALS), and to a lesser extent, patients with muscular dystrophy caused by Duchenne's disease or COPD) [11].

92.6 Telemonitoring

Telemonitoring can be used to check a ventilator's compliance and performance. Although not widely available at the moment, the situation is likely to improve in the future. In 2010, Pinto et al. [15] published a prospective study on 40 patients with ALS who were divided into two groups. In the intervention group, the ventilator data was received by modem, whereas in the control group, compliance and ventilator parameters were checked on official visits. The study did not find differences between groups regarding compliance, although the number of visits to the doctor and to the ER was significantly lower in the group in which telemonitoring was carried out ($p<0.0001$). Moreover, although there were no significant differences, survival showed a positive trend in the group with telemonitoring ($p=0.13$), the conclusion being that telemonitoring reduces the need to use health services and probably has a favorable impact on costs, survival, and performance status.

Telemonitoring might also be useful for patients other than those with ALS. In 2015, Borel et al. [16] published a study that observed that an increase in the breathing rate and the percentage of respiratory cycles caused by the patient were predictive of a COPD exacerbation. Both parameters can be registered by NIV software.

Conclusions

A progressive increase of the NIV prevalence rate by all European Union member states demands cost-effective schemes to manage patients on HMV. Moreover, telemonitoring these patients should be the first option to effectively solve this public health issue, although prospective, multicenter studies that ensure its feasibility are still needed.

Key Major Recommendations

- The exponential and global growth, in Europe, of patients on HMV programs generates a key area for development.
- There is a need for European guidelines on home assistance management models.
- Unique quality indicators for the HMV model are needed.
- The cost-efficiency of telemonitoring programs requires assessment.

References

1. Janssens JP, Derivaz S, Breitenstein E, De Muralt B, Fitting JW, Chevrolet JC, Rochat T. Changing patterns in long-term noninvasive ventilation: a 7-year prospective study in the Geneva Lake area. Chest. 2003;123:67–79.
2. Hazenberg A, Cobben NA, Kampelmacher MJ, Rischen J, Wijkstra PJ. Home mechanical ventilation in the Netherlands. Ned Tijdschr Geneeskd. 2012;156:A3609.
3. Antadir. www.antadir.com. 2014.
4. Garner DJ, Berlowitz DJ, Douglas J, Harkness N, Howard M, McArdle N, Naughton MT, Neill A, Piper A, Yeo A, Young A. Home mechanical ventilation in Australia and New Zealand. Eur Respir J. 2013;41:39–45.
5. Diaz Lobato S, Mayorales AS. Modern non-invasive mechanical ventilation turns 25. Arch Bronconeumol. 2013;49:475–9.
6. Eger P, Bedicam JM, Cornette A, Reybet-Degat O, et al. Nasal intermittent positive pressure. Long-term follow-up in patients with severe chronic respiratory insufficiency. Chest. 1994;105:100–5.
7. Lloyd-Owen SJ, Donaldson GC, Ambrosino N, et al. Patterns of home mechanical ventilation use in Europe: results from the Eurovent survey. Eur Respir J. 2005;25:1025–31.
8. Nasiłowski J, Wachulski M, Trznadel W, et al. The evolution of home mechanical ventilation in Poland between 2000 and 2010. Respir Care. 2015;60:577–85.
9. De Lucas Ramos P, Rodríguez González-Moro JM, Paz González L, et al. Estado actual de la ventilación domiciliaria en España: resultados de una encuesta de ámbito nacional. Arch Bronconeumol. 2000;36:545–50.
10. Chiner E, Llombart M, Martínez-García MA, Fernández-Fabrellas E, et al. Noninvasive mechanical ventilation in Valencia, Spain: from theory to practice. Arch Bronconeumol. 2009;45:118–22.
11. Leger P, Laier-Groeneveld G. Infrastructure, funding and follow-up in a programme of noninvasive ventilation. Eur Respir J. 2002;20:1573–8.
12. Farré R, Lloyd-Owen SJ, Ambrosino N, et al. Quality control of equipment in home mechanical ventilation: a European survey. Eur Respir J. 2005;26:86–94.

13. Stuart M, Weinrich M. Integrated health system for chronic disease management – lessons learned from France. Chest. 2004;125:695–703.
14. Pallero M, Puy C, Güell R, et al. Ambulatory adaptation to noninvasive ventilation in restrictive pulmonary disease: a randomized trial with cost assessment. Respir Med. 2014;108:1014–22.
15. Pinto A, Almeida JP, Pinto S, Pereira J, Oliveira AG, de Carvalho M. Home telemonitoring of non-invasive ventilation decreases healthcare utilisation in a prospective controlled trial of patients with amyotrophic lateral sclerosis. J Neurol Neurosurg Psychiatr. 2010;81:1238–42.
16. Borel JC, Pelletier J, Taleux N, et al. Parameters recorded by software of non-invasive ventilators predict COPD exacerbation: a proof-of-concept study. Thorax. 2015;70:284–5.

Telemonitoring of CPAP Compliance: Key Technical Topics and Clinical Implications

93

Sevinc Sarinc Ulasli and Aylin Ozsancak Ugurlu

Contents

Abbreviations

AHI	Apnea/hypopnea index
ALS	Amyotrophic lateral sclerosis
APAP	Automated positive airway pressure
COPD	Chronic obstructive pulmonary disease
CPAP	Continuous positive airway pressure
HMV	Home mechanical ventilation
NIV	Noninvasive ventilation
NMD	Neuromuscular disease

S.S. Ulasli, MD (✉)
Faculty of Medicine, Department of Pulmonary Diseases,
Afyon Kocatepe University, Afyon, Turkey
e-mail: sevincsarinc@gmail.com

A.O. Ugurlu, MD
Department of Pulmonary Medicine, Baskent University Hospital, Istanbul, Turkey
e-mail: aozsancak@hotmail.com

A.M. Esquinas (ed.), *Noninvasive Mechanical Ventilation: Theory, Equipment, and Clinical Applications*, DOI 10.1007/978-3-319-21653-9_93

OSAS	Obstructive sleep apnea syndrome
$PaCO_2$	Arterial carbon dioxide pressure
TLC	Telephone-linked communications

93.1 Introduction

Telemonitoring provides close follow-up of patients by ensuring transmission of clinical and physiologic data and by supporting prompt medical intervention before deteriorations of patients' conditions occur. It has been used for the management and close follow-up of several chronic diseases (such as diabetes, hypertension, cardiac diseases, etc.) with improved access to health care, reduced waiting times for appointments, and increased patient adherence to chronic illness treatment plans [1]. In the setting of respiratory medicine, telemonitoring has been used in the management of patients with asthma, chronic obstructive pulmonary disease (COPD), obstructive sleep apnea syndrome (OSAS), and pulmonary transplantation [2]. In this chapter, the role of telemonitoring for improving the adherence of patients with OSAS to continuous positive airway pressure (CPAP) therapy is discussed.

93.2 Discussion and Analysis

93.2.1 Definition and Types of Telemedicine and Telemonitoring

Chronic diseases such as COPD, diabetes, hypertension, and OSAS represent a significant burden of disease. These affect both the patients themselves and the health-care systems with imposition of huge costs for management. Telemedicine, defined as "the use of information and communication technology to deliver health services, expertise and information over distance, geographic, time, social and cultural barriers" [3], involves various technologies to potentially enhance quality of care and reduce health-care costs, especially in these chronic disorders.

Telemedicine encompasses diverse patient care services such as telepsychiatry, teleradiology, teledermatology, and teleophthalmology [2, 3]. The main roles of telemedicine in management of chronic diseases includes providing education (to improve self-care), enabling information transfer (e.g., telemonitoring), facilitating contact with medical professionals (e.g., telephone interviews and follow-ups), and improving medical records [4].

Three different models exist in telemedicine:

1. *Store-and-forward telemedicine (asynchronous)* involves acquiring medical data (e.g., medical images, biosignals, etc.) and then transmitting recorded data to a health professional at a convenient time for assessment offline. It does not require the presence of both parts at the same time. A properly structured medical record, preferably in electronic form, is the major component of this transfer. The store-

and-forward process requires the clinician to rely on a history report and audio/video information in lieu of a physical examination.

2. *Remote monitoring*, also known as self-monitoring or testing, enables medical professionals to monitor a patient remotely using various technological devices. This method is primarily used for managing chronic diseases or specific conditions, such as cardiovascular diseases, diabetes mellitus, or asthma.
3. *Interactive telemedicine services (synchronous)* provide real-time interactions between patient and provider (e.g., telephone or videoconference, online communication) with or without physiological monitoring, Many activities such as history review, physical examination, psychiatric evaluations, and ophthalmology assessments can be conducted comparably to those done in traditional face-to-face visits [2, 3].

"Telemonitorization" is a rapidly evolving domain of telemedicine focused on providing care in a home setting with the primary intent of supporting the patient rather than the health professionals [5]. The term *home telemonitoring* is used in a more restrictive sense and encompasses the use of audio, video, and other telecommunication technologies to monitor patient status at a distance.

93.2.2 Telemonitoring for Respiratory Disorders

Respiratory disorders have significant effects and burdens on society. In patients with chronic respiratory diseases, underlying disorders, the level of dependency on caregivers, the hours spent under mechanical ventilation, the presence of tracheostomy, distance from home to hospital, and hospital access are parts of the care burden both for the family and health-care systems. These patients need education, self-monitoring, and close management to ensure better outcomes and improve survival. Patient-, ventilator-, or interface-related problems (e.g., patient-ventilator asynchrony, re-breathing, or leaks) should be detected so that the most appropriate ventilator settings and interface in patients receiving home mechanical ventilation (HMV) can be selected. Home telemonitoring presents an alternative tool for close follow-up of patients by ensuring timely transmission of clinical and physiologic data to estimate detrimental events in patients treated with HMV during day and night. Subsequent rapid troubleshooting of potential problems may improve adherence to HMV therapy.

93.2.2.1 Types of Telemonitorization Used for Respiratory Diseases

Electronic diary and spirometer systems were widely used methods for telemonitoring of respiratory diseases in the 1990s, whereas more recent studies introduced more sophisticated technologies such as handheld devices, digital technology, and wireless networks [6]. Telephone short messaging services, internet-based monitoring systems and electronic diaries are commonly used methods for data transmission of patients with respiratory diseases. Despite variability in the technologies used and their sophistication over the years, the modalities were similar across studies in relation to the types of transmitted data and frequency of transmission.

Telemonitorization for Sleep-Related Breathing Disorders

OSAS is a highly prevalent sleep-related breathing disorder with high morbidity and mortality, defined as presence of five or more predominantly obstructive respiratory events per hour of sleep during polysomnography. This chronic disease mainly leads to cardiovascular complications (e.g., coronary artery disease, heart failure, arrhythmias, stroke, systemic and pulmonary hypertension), neuropsychiatric complications (e.g., cognitive and memory impairment, depression), impotence, socioeconomic problems, and metabolic complications. CPAP, the first-line medical treatment in adults with OSAS, effectively improves sleep architecture, reduces the apnea-hypopnea index (AHI), normalizes oxyhemoglobin saturation, and decreases neurocognitive and cardiovascular sequences. However, adherence to CPAP limits its overall effectiveness among all age groups [4].

CPAP adherence is defined as using CPAP for an average of 4 h a night for at least 70 % of the nights. The importance of adherence to treatment has been demonstrated with the return of sleepiness and impairment in simulated driving ability in as little as one night off CPAP. Furthermore, CPAP withdrawal resulted in a rapid recurrence of apneic events, daytime sleepiness, increased blood pressure, and increased heart rate [7].

Factors affecting CPAP compliance include the severity of the disorder, air leak, side effects, therapeutic response, claustrophobia, patient's perception of disease seriousness, family support, and cost. Strategies to improve adherence to CPAP that have been tested are broadly categorized as educational, technological, psychosocial, pharmacological, and multidimensional. Heated humidification, mask optimization, and topical nasal therapy can increase adherence.

Adherence can also be significantly improved by comprehensive support programs and timely interventions by health professionals. Therefore, to increase patients' understanding of the expected benefits of CPAP use, and to motivate using this therapy, to determine side effects, and to monitor and promote adherence to CPAP therapy at the beginning of use are needed to improve CPAP adherence.

CPAP adherence can be evaluated with self- report measures including diaries and verbal recall, hour meter readings, and CPAP devices that measure night-by-night and mask-on CPAP application at effective pressure over each 24-h period. This recent CPAP technology allows CPAP adherence data to be transmitted to practice sites by several vehicles, including modem, smartcard, or web portal, depending on the manufacturer. In this way, CPAP adherence can be assessed more reliably.

Previous studies related to different telemonitoring options have demonstrated variable effectiveness in CPAP adherence of OSAS patients. Telephone-linked communications (TLC) systems offer an effective, low-cost, and convenient way of providing information, advice and counseling to improve patient adherence. Sparrow et al. [8] revealed improvement of CPAP adherence with the use of a telemedicine intervention with TLC in a relatively large randomized controlled study (250 patients with OSAS from two different centers); therefore, they indicated a potentially useful role for telemedicine in the management of patients with OSAS. Telemedicine intervention with an automated TLC system designed around the concepts of motivational interviewing, a patient-centered approach to increase motivation to engage in health behavior by addressing the themes of perceived importance of using CPAP, was applied. Every week for the first month (beginning from 3 days after initiating CPAP therapy) and every month thereafter for a 12-month period, patients called the system and reported perceptions and experiences with OSAS and CPAP (including compliance) from the previous week. The computer system called the participants if they did not make a call at the expected times. The intervention arm received tailored feedback and counseling to increase motivation of patients to use CPAP. The control arm received general health information through the TLC system. At 12 months, median CPAP use was significantly higher in the telemedicine group (2.98 h vs 0.99 h/night).

Taylor et al. [9] randomized 114 patients with OSAS to either a telemedicine arm or traditional care. In the intervention arm, questionnaires (including questions related to CPAP use, hours of sleep, and quality of sleep) were sent to patients via computer. The patients' responses were monitored by the sleep medicine practitioner, and the patient telephoned if required. They did not find a significant difference in the hours of CPAP use between two groups (4.22 vs 4.29 h night; $p=0.87$). However, only self-reported data was provided to the health-care provider; objective compliance and detailed physiological information were lacking.

Fox et al. [10] randomized 75 patients with OSAS to either standard care with an auto-titrating positive airway pressure (APAP) machine or an APAP machine that transmitted physiologic information such as adherence, air leak, residual AHI daily to a website that could be reviewed. If any problems were detected from information on the website, the patient was contacted by phone. APAP adherence after 3 months was significantly higher in the intervention arm than the standard arm (191 min per day vs 105 min per day; $p=0.006$). On days when APAP was used, mean adherence was 321 min in the telemedicine arm and 207 min in the standard arm (difference = 113 min, 95 % CI: 62–164 min, $p<0.0001$). So, APAP adherence was improved with the use of a web-based telemedicine system at the initiation of treatment.

From the patients' point of view, telemedicine seems to be an effective time and cost-saving method in the care of sleep medicine. A survey study investigating the patients' perspectives of telemonitoring in sleep medicine revealed that video telemedicine was considered as an option for care of patients with OSAS, despite the fact that none of the respondents had any personal experience with video telemedicine. Patients with OSAS described challenges about in-person visits, such as time away from work or school and cost associated with travel, gas, parking, or missed work [11].

Telemonitorization for Other Chronic Respiratory Disorders

Telemonitoring with home spirometry assists in early identification and treatment of deterioration, organ rejection, and complications (e.g., bronchiolitis obliterans syndrome, etc.) in the health-care status of patients after lung transplantation. Home telemonitoring ensures the diagnosis of asthma and also improves the management of asthma with the identification of early signs of deterioration and control of acute exacerbations. Patients with COPD and respiratory failure also seem to utilize telemonitoring [6]. Vitacca et al. [12] evaluated the effectiveness of a tele-assistance program supported by the continuous availability of a 24-h call center and pulse oxygen device, as compared with the usual outpatient follow-up regimen in 240 patients requiring long-term oxygen therapy or home mechanical ventilation. Reduction in home exacerbations, emergency room admissions, and urgent general practitioner calls were tested. A nurse-centered tele-assistance program in that study was found to be effective in preventing hospitalizations, home acute exacerbations, and urgent general practitioner calls, and especially patients with COPD and respiratory failure received more benefit from this program. These positive outcomes can improve patients' adherence to medical and long-term oxygen treatment and NIV.

Telemonitoring, especially associated with remotely controlling the settings of ventilator, may be useful in patients with neuromuscular diseases (NMD) receiving NIV. In a prospective controlled trial by de Almeida et al. [13], compliance with NIV in patients with amyotrophic lateral sclerosis (ALS) was assessed with a telemonitoring device that was able to act as a digital recorder of parameters exported from the NIV device via wireless modem. The authors remotely monitored home-ventilated ALS patients and tuned the settings of the respiratory ventilator according to the patients' needs. The number of office and emergency room visits and in-hospital admissions was lower and daily hours of ventilation use was higher in the telemonitoring intervention arm. So, it was useful to improve management and compliance of ALS patients receiving NIV at home. Moreover, cost analysis revealed that telemedicine was cost effective.

Finally, an important problem during the initiation of HMV has been the lack of professional supervision in the home environment and nighttime observation during sleep. Hazenberg et al. [14] investigated whether or not initiation of HMV at home in a selective group of patients with chronic respiratory failure resulting from NMD or thoracic cage disorder by using telemonitoring is non-inferior to an in-hospital based setting. Patients were randomized into two groups (38 patients in the home group; 39 patients in the hospital group) and the primary outcome measure was the arterial carbon dioxide ($PaCO_2$), and quality of life and costs were secondary outcome measurements. Telemonitoring was performed every morning during the initiation period of HMV at home. The data of ventilator settings, respiratory rate, and carbon dioxide and oxygen saturation levels were sent to the hospital. The nurse practitioner receiving the anonymous digital data by email called the patient to evaluate the results. A software program especially developed for the study started the data collection from the ventilator and transcutaneous monitor automatically, and data was transferred to the hospital. $PaCO_2$ and quality of life were not significantly different between groups. Initiation of HMV at home, using telemonitoring, was safe, feasible, and less expensive than the initiation of mechanical ventilation at the hospital. From the patients' view, initiation of HMV at home by using a mobile connection without technical delays is an ideal treatment option; there is no need for hospital admission and highly individualized care can be maintained at the beginning of HMV.

93.2.3 Limitations of Telemonitorization

Many questions remain before telemedicine can be considered for broad application. Multicenter studies of telemedicine technologies in a broad range of academic and community sleep centers are needed to address this issue, and the cost implications of this technology (e.g., cost per additional quality-adjusted life year saved) should be clarified. Most importantly, most crucial telemedicine components improving adherence need to be better understood so that the most efficient system can be designed. In addition, it is not known whether regular automated telephone follow-ups or more advanced technology (monitoring CPAP pressures, leaks, and objective compliance and sending this information to the practitioner on a daily basis) will improve adherence the most. How to integrate telemedicine in the daily practice of patients receiving NIV in the most cost-efficient way needs to be determined.

Conclusion

Further exploration of methods of telemedicine are needed to improve NIV compliance. The potential benefits of telemonitoring (such as early intervention for problems, patient education, improving adherence, and outcomes) should be considered more important than technology costs.

Key Major Recommendations

- Telemonitoring, supporting early identification of deteriorations in patients' conditions and increasing NIV adherence, represents a promising patient management approach that is well received by patients.
- Initiation of HMV can be ensured by the use of telemonitoring to transmit digital data and to provide clinical health care outside the hospital.
- Despite minimal evidence of its economic viability, preliminary studies demonstrate promising results and the affordability of telemonitoring to improve NIV compliance.

References

1. Chaudhry SI, Phillips CO, Stewart SS, et al. Telemonitoring for patients with chronic heart failure: a systematic review. J Card Fail. 2007;13:56–62.
2. Darkins AW, Cary MA. Telemedicine and telehealth principles, policies, performance and pitfalls. 1st ed. New York: Springer; 2000. p. 1–321.
3. Meystre S. Telemedicine and e-Health. Telemed J E Health. 2005;11(1):63–9.
4. Sawyer AM, Gooneratne N, Marcus CL, et al. A systematic review of CPAP adherence across age groups: clinical and empiric insights for developing CPAP adherence interventions. Sleep Med Rev. 2011;15:343–56.

5. Paré G, Jaana M, Sicotte C. Systematic review of home telemonitoring for chronic diseases: the evidence base. J Am Med Inform Assoc. 2007;14(3):269–77.
6. Jaana M, Paré G, Sicotte C. Home telemonitoring for respiratory conditions: a systematic review. Am J Manag Care. 2009;15:313–20.
7. Schwab RJ, Badr SM, Epstein LJ, et al. An official American Thoracic Society statement: continuous positive airway pressure adherence tracking systems. The optimal monitoring strategies and outcome measures in adults. Am J Respir Crit Care Med. 2013;188:613–20.
8. Sparrow D, Aloia M, Demolles DA, Gottlieb DJ. A telemedicine intervention to improve adherence to continuous positive airway pressure: a randomised controlled trial. Thorax. 2010;65:1061–6.
9. Taylor Y, Eliasson A, Andrada T, et al. The role of telemedicine in CPAP compliance for patients with obstructive sleep apnea syndrome. Sleep Breath. 2006;10:132–8.
10. Fox N, Hirsch-Allen AJ, Goodfellow E, et al. The impact of a telemedicine monitoring system on positive airway pressure adherence in patients with obstructive sleep apnea: a randomized controlled trial. Sleep. 2012;35:477–81.
11. Kelly JM, Schwamm LH, Bianchi MT. Sleep telemedicine: a survey study of patient preferences. ISRN Neurol. 2012;135329. doi:10.5402/2012/135329.
12. Vitacca M, Bianchi L, Guerra A, et al. Tele-assistance in chronic respiratory failure patients: a randomised clinical trial. Eur Respir J. 2009;33:411–8.
13. de Almeida JP, Pinto A, Pinto S, et al. Economic cost of home-telemonitoring care for BiPAP-assisted ALS individuals. Amyotroph Lateral Scler. 2012;13:533–7.
14. Hazenberg A, Kerstjens HA, Prins SC, et al. Initiation of home mechanical ventilation at home: a randomised controlled trial of efficacy, feasibility and costs. Respir Med. 2014;108:1387–95.

Psychological Factors as a Determinant of Noninvasive Ventilation Compliance: Key Practical Aspects and Topics

94

Marie-Christine Rousseau and Stéphane Pietra

Contents

94.1 Introduction

Noninvasive mechanical ventilation (NIV) is a useful procedure in the management of patients with chronic respiratory failure with hypercapnia resulting from motor neuron disease, spinal cord injury, neuromuscular diseases, or post-polio syndrome [1–4]. NIV relieves respiratory symptoms and reduces energy expenditure in patients with amyotrophic lateral sclerosis (ALS) [5]; several studies have suggested that NIV leads to a longer survival time and better health-related quality of life and physiological parameters in patients with ALS or chronic respiratory failure [2, 3, 5–7]. In spite of these benefits, NIV is rejected by a large proportion of patients because of psychological factors.

M.-C. Rousseau, MD (✉) • S. Pietra
Hôpital San Salvadour (Assistance Publique Hôpitaux de Paris), BP 30080, Hyeres 83407, France
e-mail: marie-christine.rousseau@ssl.aphp.fr; stephane.pietra@ssl.aphp.fr

A.M. Esquinas (ed.), *Noninvasive Mechanical Ventilation: Theory, Equipment, and Clinical Applications*, DOI 10.1007/978-3-319-21653-9_94

94.2 Discussion

Outcome for patients with ALS who are dependent on mechanical ventilation is similar to that of patients with locked-in-syndrome: both categories have a healthy brain locked into a paralyzed body. Studies show that patients receiving NIV report good perceived health, despite severe physical limitations, and NIV is becoming more popular, considering the great benefits that it represents [7].

Several studies have demonstrated the positive effect of NIV on patients' wellbeing, including improvement in night sleep, tiredness, and daily activity, decrease of shortness of breath and orthopnea, and amelioration of cognitive functions [4, 8]. NIV has a positive impact on social activities, too, and the physical benefits induced by NIV have a positive impact patients' psychological condition.

Contraindications for the use of NIV in motor neuron diseases are cognitive impairment, neurobehavioral dysfunctions, social isolation, and rapidly progressive disease [9]. Factors associated with acceptance of NIV are cognitive and educational status and level of executive functions.

Psychological factors have a great influence on patient compliance with NIV. Fear of death has been reported to be a facilitator for the initiation of and the adherence to NIV. Others psychological factors associated with NIV acceptance are a focus by the patient on perceived benefits from NIV and a positive coping style. NIV may also be used in patients who have declined tracheal intubation and is also applied in other chronic encephalopathies with hypercapnia.

Patients' NIV acceptance and compliance depends also on how family caregivers can develop resilience and coping through the situation [10]. Although NIV increases the caregivers' burden and may negatively affect their physical function (which appear through signs of exhaustion such as insomnia, anxiety disorders, or loss of attention) it shows good acceptance by them [6]. This emphasizes the importance of informing caregivers regarding the effects and the value of NIV on survival, respiratory symptoms, and patient's quality of life (QOL). Caregivers should also be involved in the planning of care and should receive therapeutic education training. Psychological interventions for caregivers are necessary to help them to cope with this challenge.

Although NIV can benefit survival and quality of life, it is rejected by a substantial proportion of people with motor neuron disease [10]. However, its application in chronically ill and dependent patients with chronic respiratory failure requires taking into consideration a range of disorders and psychological mechanisms and possible impact on patients' QOL. Psychological factors in patients with life-threatening situations are the consequence of a number of diverse psychological disorders. These disorders are linked to a potentially fatal disease, or to a condition so severe that, psychologically, it cannot be assumed because the evolution of the disease defeats the psychological defense mechanisms and can lead to a collapse of these ones and a severe depression.

In the study of Ando et al. [8] on patients with motor neuron disease, about a third of patients declined NIV ventilation. Psychological reasons for patient disengagement with NIV include threat to the self, sense of loss of control, anxiety, negative perceived impact of NIV on dignity and quality of life, and negative experience with health-care services. NIV may also not be accepted by patients for fear of prolonged survival and increasing disability. This emphasizes the importance of sustained psychological support for this category of patients.

In our experience, for patients with a significant level of anxiety when NIV is proposed, the use of hypnosis sessions performed as the patient is wearing the mask allow a reduction of anxiety and enhance the acceptance of NIV. Support with hypnotherapy treatment at the frequency of one session per day generally yields good compliance after a week, on average.

In several studies, these factors (psychological support) were more important to patients than prolonging life in its current form [8]. During long-term use of NIV in patients with motor neuron disease, patients' perceptions of NIV evolve over time and have an impact in their adherence to NIV. The study of Ando et al. [8] suggested that a positive coping style, adaptation, and hope are key factors for psychological well-being of patients with NIV.

Conclusion

It is important to control psychological factors of NIV acceptance because better compliance with NIV is related to better survival, and good QOL is associated with the desire to live longer and consequently with NIV compliance.

Key Major Recommendations

- Caregivers should be involved in the planning of care of patients on NIV.
- Clinicians must inform patients of benefits from NIV on QOL, respiratory symptoms, and survival.
- Psychotherapy support, performed before starting the NIV, helps to reduce defense mechanisms.
- Sustained psychological support for patients on NIV should always be provided.

References

1. Markström A, Sundell K, Lysdahl M, Andersson G, Schedin U, Klang B. Quality-of-life evaluation of patients with neuromuscular and skeletal diseases treated with noninvasive and invasive home mechanical ventilation. Chest. 2002;122(5):1695–700.
2. Bach JR, Bakshiyev R, Hon A. Noninvasive respiratory management for patients with spinal cord injury and neuromuscular disease. Tanaffos. 2012;11(1):7–11.
3. Aboussouan LS, Khan SU, Meeker DP, et al. Effect of non-invasive positive-pressure ventilation on survival in amyotrophic lateral sclerosis. Ann Intern Med. 1997;127:450–3.
4. Piepers S, Van Den Berg JP, Kalmijn S, Van Der Pol WL, Wokke JHJ, Lindeman E, Van Der Berg LH. Effects of non-invasive ventilation on survival, quality of life, respiratory function and cognition: a review of the literature. Amyotroph Lateral Scler. 2006;7:195–200.

5. Georges M, Morélot-Panzini C, Similowski T, Gonzalez-Bermejo J. Noninvasive ventilation reduces energy expenditure in amyotrophic lateral sclerosis. BMC Pulm Med. 2014;14:17.
6. Mustfa N, Walsh E, Bryant V, Lyall RA, Addington-Hall J, Goldstein LH, Donaldson N, Polkey MI, Moxham J, Leigh PN. The effect of noninvasive ventilation on ALS patients and their caregivers. Neurology. 2006;66(8):1211–7.
7. Tsolaki V, Pastaka C, Kostikas K, Karetsi E, Dimoulis A, Zikiri A, Koutsokera A, Gourgoulianis KI. Noninvasive ventilation in chronic respiratory failure: effects on quality of life. Respiration. 2011;81(5):402–10. doi:10.1159/000317138.
8. Ando H, Williams C, Angus RM, Thornton EW, Chakrabarti B, Cousins R, Piggin LH, Young CA. Why don't they accept non-invasive ventilation?: insight into the interpersonal perspectives of patients with motor neurone disease. Br J Health Psychol. 2014;20:341–59.
9. O'Neill CL, Williams TL, Peel ET, McDermott CJ, Shaw PJ, Gibson GJ, Bourke SC. Non-invasive ventilation in motor neuron disease: an update of current UK practice. J Neurol Neurosurg Psychiatry. 2012;83(4):371–6.
10. Cousins R, Ando H, Thornton E, Chakrabarti B, Angus R, Young C. Determinants of accepting non-invasive ventilation treatment in motor neurone disease: a quantitative analysis at point of need. Health Psychol Behav Med. 2013;1(1):47–58.

Part XI

Non Invasive Ventilation Pediatric

95 Interfaces for Acute and Long-Term Noninvasive Positive Pressure Ventilation in Children: Key Technical Elements and Clinical Implications

Brigitte Fauroux, Adriana Ramirez,
and Alessandro Amaddeo

Contents

B. Fauroux, MD, PhD (✉)
Pediatric Noninvasive Ventilation and Sleep Unit,
AP-HP, Hôpital Necker-Enfants Malades, Paris, France

Paris Descartes University, Paris, France

Inserm U 955, Team 13, Creteil, France
e-mail: brigitte.fauroux@nck.aphp.fr

A. Ramirez, MSc
ADEP Assistance, Suresnes, France

Pediatric Noninvasive Ventilation and Sleep Unit,
AP-HP, Hôpital Necker-Enfants Malades, Paris, France
e-mail: adriana.ramirez@adepassistance.com

A. Amaddeo, MD
Pediatric Noninvasive Ventilation and Sleep Unit,
AP-HP, Hôpital Necker-Enfants Malades, Paris, France

Paris Descartes University, Paris, France
e-mail: alessandro.amaddeo@nck.aphp.fr

A.M. Esquinas (ed.), *Noninvasive Mechanical Ventilation: Theory, Equipment, and Clinical Applications*, DOI 10.1007/978-3-319-21653-9_95

Abbreviations

CPAP	Continuous positive airway pressure
NPPV	Noninvasive positive pressure ventilation
PICU	Pediatric intensive care unit
OSAS	Obstructive sleep apnea syndrome

95.1 Introduction

Noninvasive positive pressure ventilation (NPPV) is increasingly used in children, both in the acute and the chronic setting. Indeed, acute or chronic respiratory failure or various origins may be improved or cured by means of NPPV. NPPV is now recommended as a first-line therapy in the pediatric intensive care unit (PICU) for bronchiolitis [1–5], acute respiratory exacerbations caused by neuromuscular disease, cystic fibrosis [6–8], pneumonia [9, 10], or sickle cell disease [11], and upper airway obstruction [12–14]. The number of children treated at home with long term NPPV for neuromuscular or lung disease, or various causes of upper airway obstruction is also growing rapidly [15–17]. However, respiratory mechanics and maxillofacial development are different in children as compared to adults, which justify age-adapted ventilators, interfaces, and headgears.

This chapter presents the different types of interfaces available for children in the acute and chronic setting, their advantages and limitations, how to choose the optimal interface, and how to monitor the tolerance of the interface.

95.2 Interfaces for Children

Noninvasive interfaces can be classified as follows (Figs. 95.1, 95.2, 95.3, 95.4, 95.5, 95.6, 95.7, 95.8, and 95.9):

- Nasal pillows or plugs (which occlude the outer part of the nostrils),
- Nasal masks, which cover the nose
- Nasobuccal masks, which cover the nose and the mouth
- Full face masks, which cover the mouth, the nose, and the eyes
- Mouthpieces or oral masks
- And the helmet, which covers the entire head.

Nasal pillows or plugs are minimal-contact interfaces that are available for patients weighing more than 30 kg, but small sizes can be used in children of 6–8 years (Fig. 95.1). They have the major advantage of exerting no pressure contact on the child's face. The acceptance of these interfaces is generally excellent in school-aged children in whom they are proposed as first-line interfaces for NPPV [18]. Because of the minimal dead space, the patient may sometimes have the impression that the level of positive pressure is higher with nasal pillows than with another

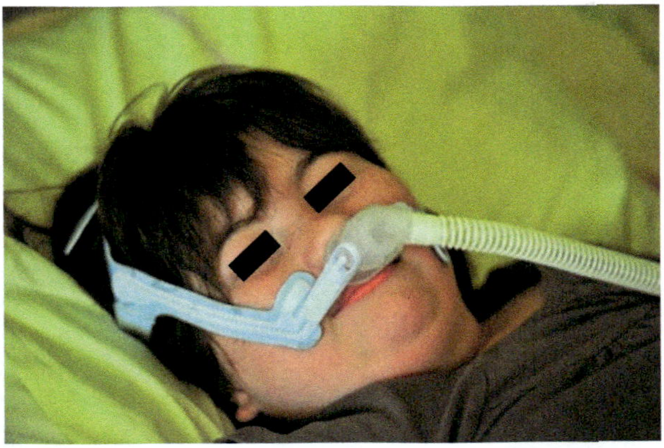

Fig. 95.1 Nasal pillows or plugs

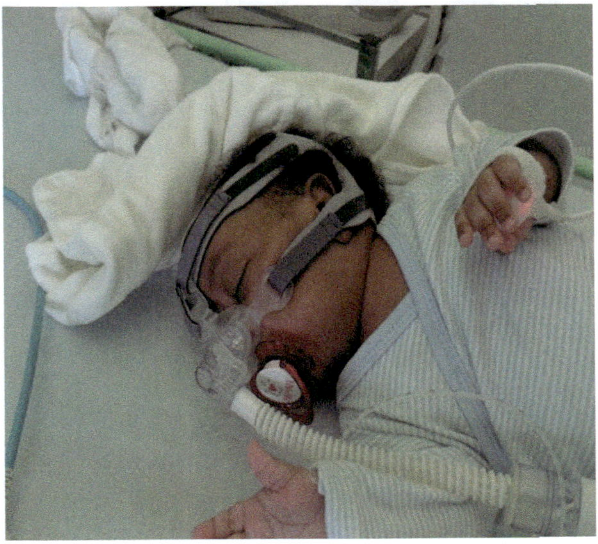

Fig. 95.2 Nasal mask on an infant

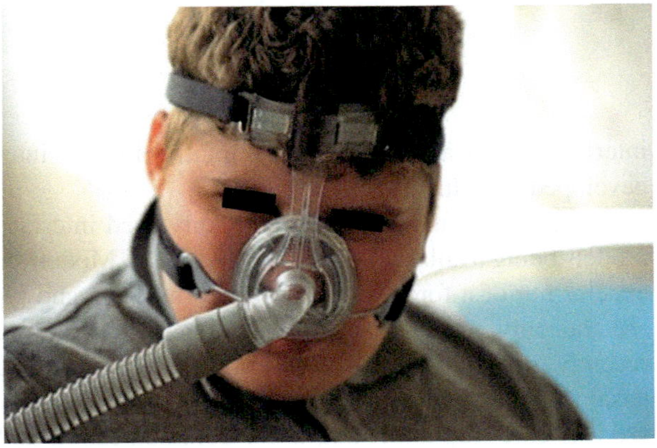

Fig. 95.3 Nasal mask on a boy with Prader Willi syndrome

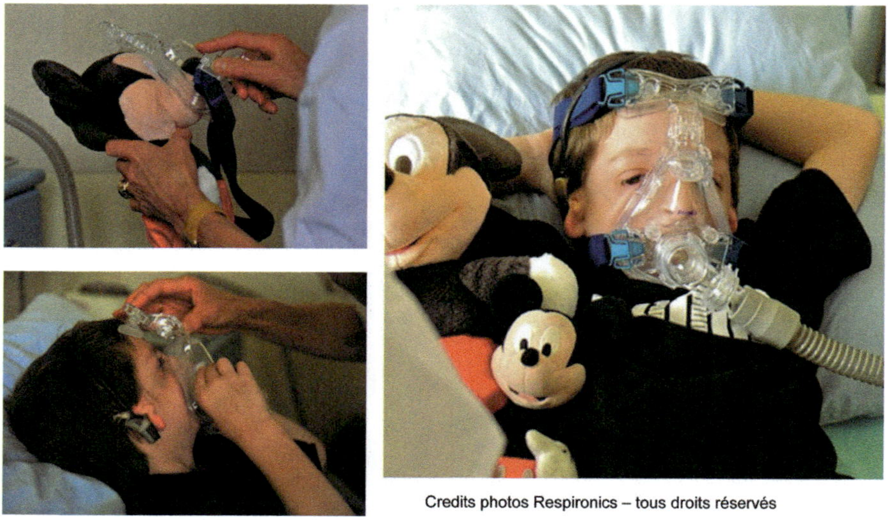

Fig. 95.4 Nasobuccal mask on a boy with Treacher Collins syndrome

Fig. 95.5 Full face mask

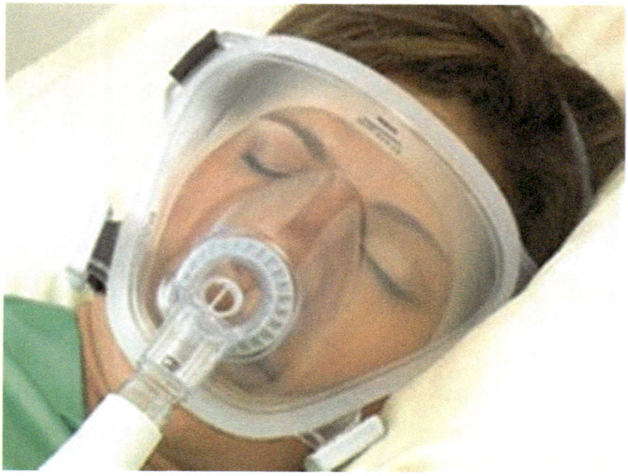

interface. The headgear may be a limitation in these interfaces that have been mainly developed for adults.

Nasal masks are the most commonly used interfaces, with numerous different models being available (Figs. 95.2 and 95.3). Models differ with regard to the presence or not of a forehead support, internal flap, and type of fixation. These masks are the only industrially available interfaces for preschool children and, more recently, infants and neonates (weight >3–3.5 kg) (Fig. 95.2). In young children, nasal masks are preferred to larger masks because they have less static dead space, are less claustrophobic, and allow communication and expectoration more easily

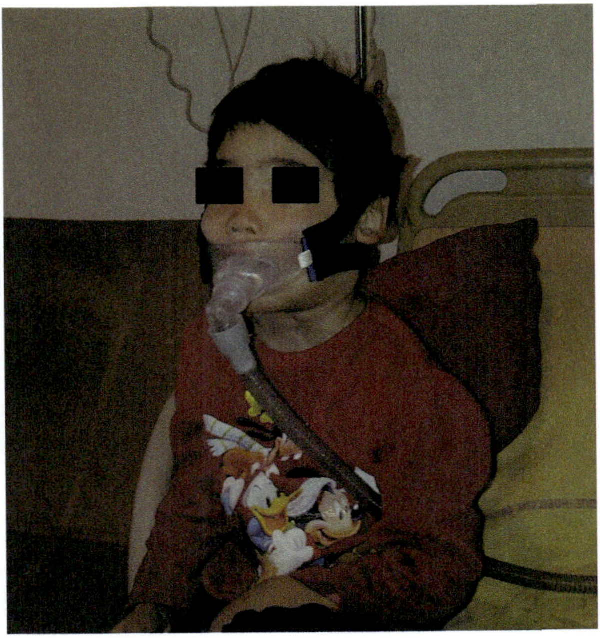

Fig. 95.6 Oral mask on a child with severe obstructive sleep apnea and total obstruction of the nasal airways

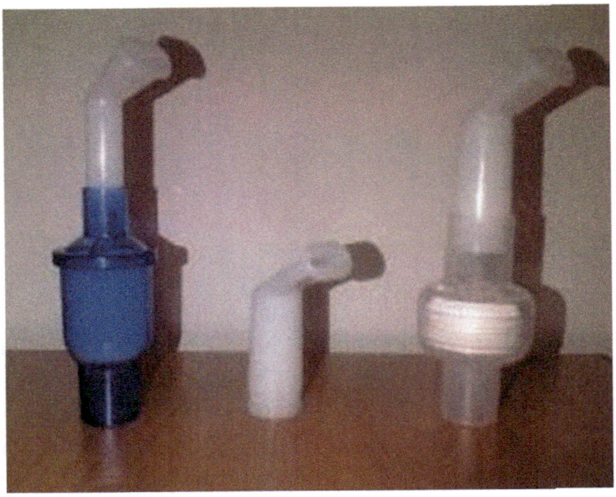

Fig. 95.7 Mouthpieces for mouthpiece ventilation

than nasobuccal or full face masks. Nasal masks also allow the use of a pacifier in infants, which may contribute to a better acceptance of NPPV and the reduction of mouth leaks (Fig. 95.2). New models integrating thin internal flaps that inflate with the airway pressure are associated with a better skin tolerance because of a reduction in the pressure forces.

Nasobuccal masks cover the nose and the mouth and are indicated in case of mouth breathing during sleep (Fig. 95.4). These interfaces are larger, have a greater

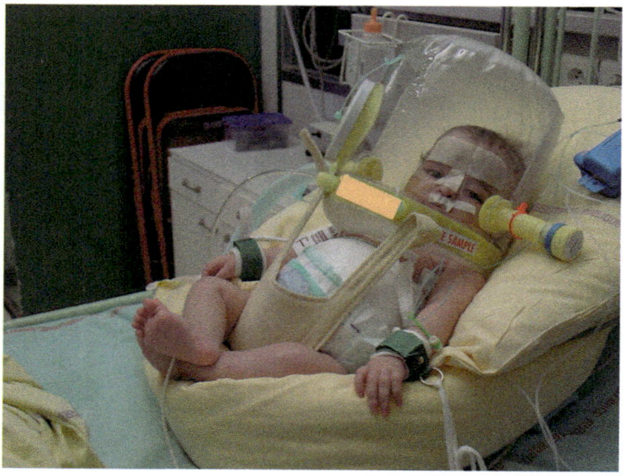

Fig. 95.8 Helmet on an infant in the pediatric intensive care unit

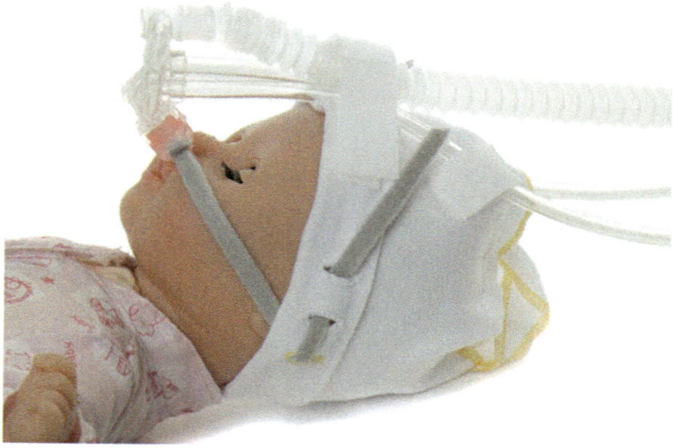

Fig. 95.9 Infant nasal cannula

dead space, and are heavier than nasal masks. Some have a forehead support. These interfaces are contraindicated in case of esogastric reflux and when the child is not able to remove the interface by himself because of the potential risk of inhalation.

Full face masks cover the mouth, the nose, and the eyes (Fig. 95.5). They are used as last-choice masks, in case of intolerance or non-acceptance of all the other interfaces. They may cause claustrophobia and, as with the nasobuccal masks, are not recommended in case of reflux.

Mouthpiece and oral masks allow ventilation through the mouth (Figs. 95.6 and 95.7). Mouthpieces are generally used on demand during daytime in patients with neuromuscular disease as a daytime extension of nocturnal ventilation with another interface [19, 20]. They have been exceptionally used in children with total nasal obstruction and severe obstructive sleep apnea syndrome (OSAS) [21].

The helmet is a commonly used interface in the PICU (Fig. 95.8). This interface is composed of a plastic transparent bag that covers the entire head of the patient and that is sealed around the neck by a hermetic collar. Two ports act as an inlet (upper) and outlet (lower) of the gas flows. This interface can be used for continuous positive airway pressure (CPAP) or bilevel ventilation. Its use has been evaluated during acute exacerbations of neuromuscular disease in children in the PICU [22, 23]. The helmet has proved to be an efficient alternative to a nasal or a face mask but its large dead space and the risk of asphyxia in case of power failure or other technical problems restricts its use to the PICU. Also, the quality of the ventilatory support may be less optimal with this interface compared with a nasobuccal mask or a tracheal cannula [24]. In premature infants or neonates, nasal cannula or nasal masks can be used to deliver oxygen, CPAP, or humidified high-flow oxygen, which creates a low CPAP level, in the neonatal ICU (Fig. 95.9).

Interfaces can be vented or non-vented, that is, with or without intentional leaks. The choice of non-vented interfaces is more limited than that of vented interfaces. Vented interfaces need a minimal positive end-expiratory pressure, which is generally 4 cmH_2O. In adult patients, the importance of manufacturer intentional leaks on the mask may influence the quality of NPPV. Indeed, a first bench study showed that the type of interface and importance of leaks did not influence trigger performances [25]. However, the ability to achieve and maintain inspiratory positive airway pressure was significantly decreased with all ventilators and in all simulated lung conditions when intentional leaks increased (especially when leaks > 40 l/min). Another study showed that the importance of manufacturer intentional leaks on the mask was able to modify patient-ventilator synchronization, ventilator performance, and risk of rebreathing [26]. Such studies have not been performed in children. However, a systematic clinical evaluation of every mask change is recommended, checking and eventually adjusting the inspiratory trigger sensitivity and pressurization, and checking the absence of rebreathing [27].

For all types of interfaces, the headgear is of crucial importance. Indeed, the face and skull of children requiring ventilatory support differ from healthy children [18]. An inappropriate headgear may compromise the use of a well-adapted interface in children. The most important qualities of a headgear are the appropriate size, stability, and the ease with which it can be put on and removed.

95.3 Side Effects and Monitoring of the Interface

The interface represents a crucial determinant of the success of NPPV. The patient will be unable to tolerate and accept NPPV in case of facial discomfort, skin injury, or significant unintentional leaks. The evaluation of the short- and long-term tolerance of the nasal mask is thus an essential component of NPPV [28] (Figs. 95.10, 95.11 and 95.12).

Interfaces for NPPV need to be adapted to the facial anatomy and physiognomy of children. In the chronic setting, a growing number of young patients are treated with NPPV. These patients represent a heterogeneous group, not only with regard to the underlying disease, but also with regard to age, weight, and maxillofacial physiognomy [15, 18, 29–31]. Numerous children have genetic diseases associated with facial deformities, such as, for example, Treacher Collins syndrome, Goldenhar

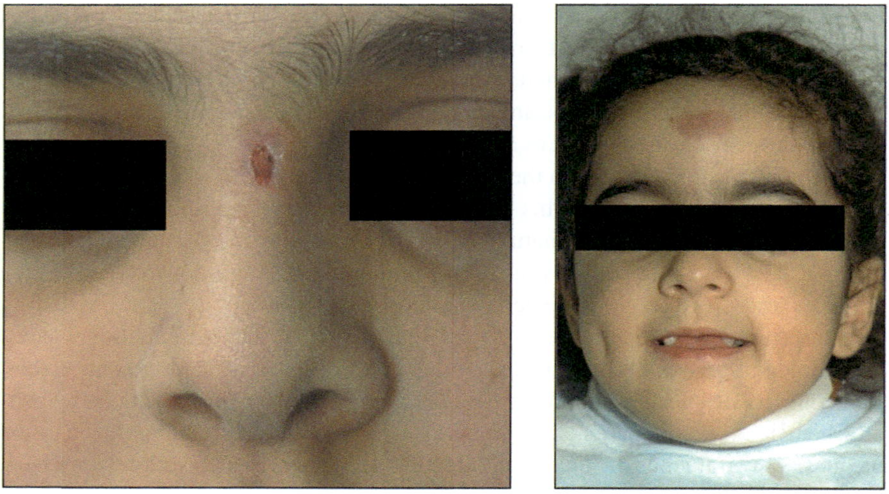

Fig. 95.10 Skin injury caused by a nasal mask

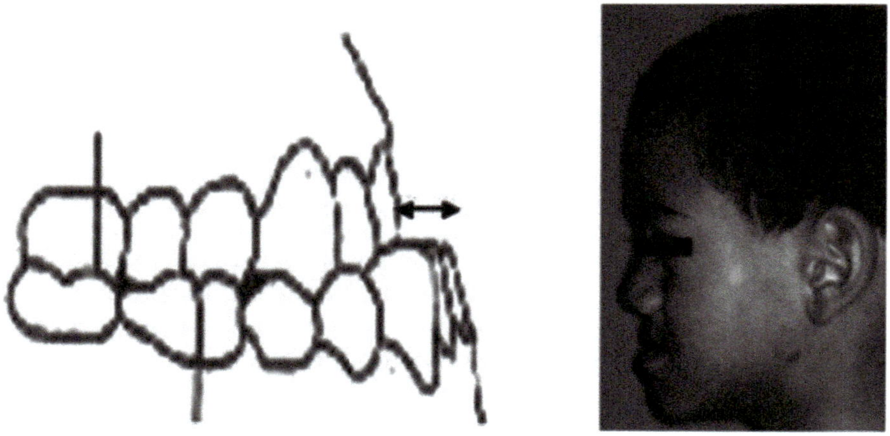

Fig. 95.11 Maxilla retrusion in a boy ventilated since 3 years for severe laryngomalacia

syndrome, Pierre Robin syndrome, achondroplasia, or osteogenesis imperfecta. Individually adapted interfaces are thus mandatory for these patients. In our experience, children with OSAS resulting from maxillofacial deformity represented the group that needed the greatest number of mask changes [18].

The soft tissue beneath the skin is thinner in children compared with adults. Children are thus at greater risk of skin injury during NPPV than adults (Fig. 95.10). Skin injury occurs as a consequence of pressure sores, which are defined as a lesion on any skin surface that occurs as a result of pressure. The principal causative factor is the application of localized pressure to an area of skin not adapted to the magnitude and duration of such external forces. Tissue damage will occur if both a critical pressure threshold and a critical time are exceeded. Because young children may need NPPV during extended periods including nocturnal sleep and daytime naps, they are at increased risk of skin injury [28]. The effect of repetitive loading on skin and bone tissue is also of major importance, which is the case during NPPV. The anatomy of the facial bones and the proportions between the facial elements differ in children compared with adults. The anatomy of the maxillofacial structures changes continuously during growth, which is particularly rapid during the two first years of life. Facial growth occurs predominantly in an anterior and sagittal axis in children. NPPV hinders this normal facial growth and may cause facial deformity (Figs. 95.11 and 95.12). Indeed, NPPV is always used during sleep, which can represent the major part of the day in young infants. In these young patients, there is thus a potential risk of facial flattening and maxilla retrusion, caused by the pressure applied by the mask on growing facial structures. Facial flattening and maxilla retrusion are commonly observed in children receiving long-term NPPV by means of nasal or nasobuccal masks, which justifies a systematic evaluation and follow-up by a pediatric maxillofacial surgeon before and during NPPV [28]. When possible, alternative use of different interfaces to vary the pressure forces may reduce these side effects.

Monitoring of the facial side effects of interfaces is of crucial importance in young children in whom interfaces need to be changed frequently because of the rapid growth of the facial structures. The caregivers and the child (if old enough) should be informed about the need to alert the NPPV team about any facial side effect or poor or non-tolerance of the interface.

95.4 How to Choose the Optimal Interface?

The choice of the interface depends on:

- The patient's age and weight
- The facial (and skull) anatomy and adaptability of the headgear
- The presence of mouth breathing and nasal permeability
- The ventilatory mode, requiring a vented or non-vented interface
- The patient's autonomy with regard to the removal of the interface (e.g., in patients with neuromuscular disease)
- The patient's comfort with the mask and the level of unintentional leaks
- The patient's tolerance with regard to skin injury and facial deformity
- The clinical situation: in an acute setting, mouth breathing is common, which explains the greater use of nasobuccal or full face masks in the PICU than in the home setting. Pressure sores are also more common in the ICU because of the greater instability of the patients.

Figure 95.13 shows an updated algorithm of mask choice. Indeed, because of the availability of industrial nasal masks for newborns and infants, we did not need to make any custom-made masks in our unit over the last year [18].

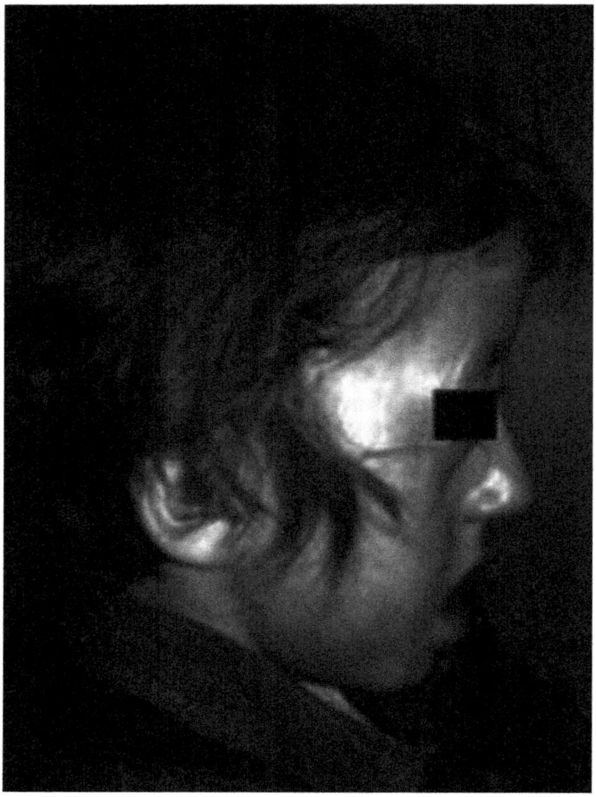

Fig. 95.12 Facial flattening in a girl with spinal muscular atrophy ventilated with a nasal mask

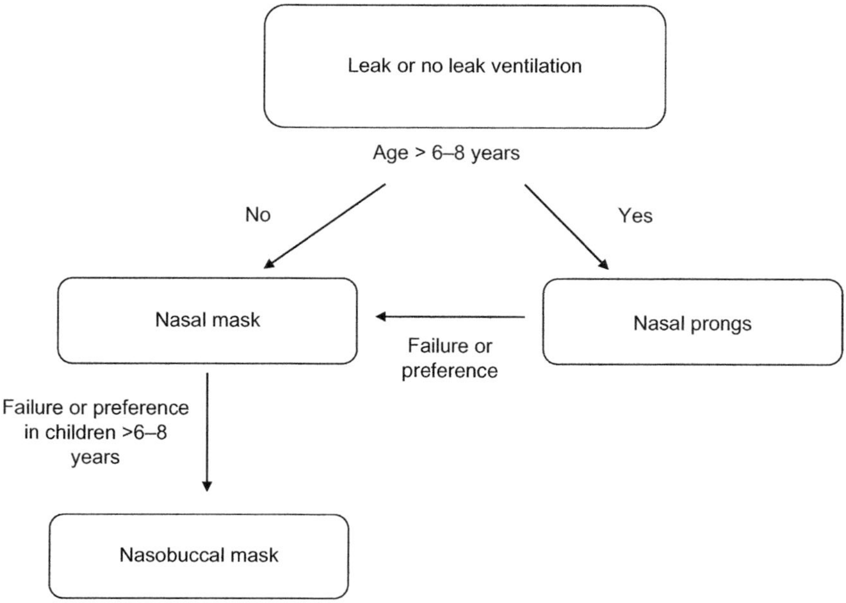

Fig. 95.13 Algorithm for mask choice

Compliance with NPPV can be excellent with any type of interface when the choice of the interface is appropriate. Indeed, our experience, objective compliance reached almost a mean night use of 8:30 in a consecutive cohort of 62 children treated with long-term NPPV at home [18]. Objective compliance was not related to the age, gender, duration of home NPPV, or type of interface. Of note, compliance was similarly excellent in adolescents using nasal pillows or plugs, underlining the interest in this type of interface for this age group.

Conclusion

Important improvements have been made in interfaces for children. Nasal masks for young infants are now available and several comfortable nasal masks are available for older children, Nasal plugs or pillows are well accepted by older children. However, headgears could be improved and the availability of nasal plugs or prongs and nasobuccal interfaces for young children would constitute further progress (Table 95.1).

Table 95.1 Advantages, limitations, and side effects of the different types of interfaces available for NPPV in children

Interface	Advantages	Limitations	Side effects
Nasal pillows or plugs	Small, light No pressure sores	Not available for infants Not to be used when mouth breathing	Nasal irritation
Nasal mask	Small volume Large choice	Not to be used when mouth breathing	Pressure sores
Nasobuccal mask	Prevents mouth leaks	Large volume Not available for infants	Pressure sores
Full face mask	Prevents mouth leaks	Large volume, claustrophobic	Pressure sores
Helmet	No pressure sores	Large dead space, claustrophobic For the PICU only Can decrease the sensibility of the ventilator's trigger	Noise, pressure around the head (eyes)

Abbreviations: *PICU* pediatric intensive care unit

Key Major Recommendations

- The choice of an interface should take into account the type of ventilation, the child's facial anatomy, the type of breathing, and the acceptance and comfort of the child.
- A change in the interface can modify the efficacy of NPPV.
- The choice of headgear is as important as that of the interface.
- Every child on NPPV should be monitored closely for potential interface-related side effects such as skin injury or facial deformity.
- Objective compliance with NPPV can be excellent with every type of interface when appropriately chosen.

References

1. Pirret AM, Sherring CL, Tai JA, et al. Local experience with the use of nasal bubble CPAP in infants with bronchiolitis admitted to a combined adult/paediatric intensive care unit. Intensive Crit Care Nurs. 2005;21:314–9.
2. Shah PS, Ohlsson A, Shah JP. Continuous negative extrathoracic pressure or continuous positive airway pressure for acute hypoxemic respiratory failure in children. Cochrane Database Syst Rev. 2008;23(1):CD003699.
3. Javouhey E, Barats A, Richard N, Stamm D, Floret D. Non-invasive ventilation as primary ventilatory support for infants with severe bronchiolitis. Intensive Care Med. 2008;34:1608–14.
4. Thia LP, McKenzie SA, Blyth TP, et al. Randomised controlled trial of nasal continuous positive airways pressure (CPAP) in bronchiolitis. Arch Dis Child. 2008;93:45–7.
5. Essouri S, Durand P, Chevret L, et al. Optimal level of nasal continuous positive airway pressure in severe viral bronchiolitis. Intensive Care Med. 2011;37:2002–7.
6. Ellaffi M, Vinsonneau C, Coste J, et al. One-year outcome after severe pulmonary exacerbation in adults with cystic fibrosis. Am J Respir Crit Care Med. 2005;171:158–64.
7. Sood N, Paradowski LJ, Yankaskas JR. Outcomes of intensive care unit care in adults with cystic fibrosis. Am J Respir Crit Care Med. 2001;163:335–8.
8. Texereau J, Jamal D, Choukroun G, et al. Determinants of mortality for adults with cystic fibrosis admitted in intensive care unit: a multicenter study. Respir Res. 2006;7:14–24.
9. Fortenberry JD, Del Toro J, Jefferson LS, Evey L, Haase D. Management of pediatric acute hypoxemic respiratory insufficiency with bilevel positive pressure (BiPAP) nasal mask ventilation. Chest. 1995;108:1059–64.
10. Padman R, Lawless S, Von Nessen S. Use of BiPAP by nasal mask in the treatment of respiratory insufficiency in pediatric patients: preliminary investigation. Pediatr Pulmonol. 1994;17:119–23.
11. Essouri S, Durand P, Chevret L, et al. Physiological effects of noninvasive positive ventilation during acute moderate hypercapnic respiratory insufficiency in children. Intensive Care Med. 2008;34:2248–55.
12. Fauroux B, Pigeot J, Polkey MI, et al. Chronic stridor caused by laryngomalacia in children. Work of breathing and effects of noninvasive ventilatory assistance. Am J Respir Crit Care Med. 2001;164:1874–8.
13. Essouri S, Nicot F, Clement A, et al. Noninvasive positive pressure ventilation in infants with upper airway obstruction: comparison of continuous and bilevel positive pressure. Intensive Care Med. 2005;31:574–80.
14. Khirani S, Ramirez A, Aloui S, et al. Continuous positive airway pressure titration in infants with severe upper airway obstruction or bronchopulmonary dysplasia. Crit Care (London, England). 2013;17:R167.
15. Fauroux B, Boffa C, Desguerre I, Estournet B, Trang H. Long-term noninvasive mechanical ventilation for children at home: a national survey. Pediatr Pulmonol. 2003;35:119–25.
16. Paulides FM, Plötz FB, Verweij-van den Oudenrijn LP, van Gestel JP, Kampelmacher MJ. Thirty years of home mechanical ventilation in children: escalating need for pediatric intensive care beds. Intensive Care Med. 2012;38:847–52.
17. McDougall CM, Adderley RJ, Wensley DF, Seear MD. Long-term ventilation in children: longitudinal trends and outcomes. Arch Dis Child. 2013;98:660–5.
18. Ramirez A, Delord V, Khirani S, et al. Interfaces for long term noninvasive positive pressure ventilation in children. Intensive Care Med. 2012;38:655–62.
19. Toussaint M, Steens M, Wasteels G, Soudon P. Diurnal ventilation via mouthpiece: survival in end-stage Duchenne patients. Eur Resp J. 2006;28:549–55.
20. Khirani S, Ramirez A, Delord V, et al. Evaluation of ventilators for mouthpiece ventilation in neuromuscular disease. Respir Care. 2014;59:1329–37.

21. Khirani S, Kadlub N, Delord V, Picard A, Fauroux B. Nocturnal mouthpiece ventilation and medical hypnosis to treat severe obstructive sleep apnea in a child with cherubism. Pediatr Pulmonol. 2013;48:927–9.
22. Piastra M, Antonelli M, Chiaretti A, et al. Treatment of acute respiratory failure by helmet-delivered non-invasive pressure support ventilation in children with acute leukemia: a pilot study. Intensive Care Med. 2004;30:472–6.
23. Piastra M, Antonelli M, Caresta E, et al. Noninvasive ventilation in childhood acute neuromuscular respiratory failure: a pilot study. Respiration. 2006;73:791–8.
24. Moerer O, Fischer S, Hartelt M, et al. Influence of two different interfaces for noninvasive ventilation compared to invasive ventilation on the mechanical properties and performance of a respiratory system: a lung model study. Chest. 2006;129:1424–31.
25. Borel JC, Sabil A, Janssens JP, et al. Intentional leaks in industrial masks have a significant impact on efficacy of bilevel noninvasive ventilation: a bench test study. Chest. 2009;135:669–77.
26. Louis B, Leroux K, Isabey D, Fauroux B, Lofaso F. Effect of manufacturer-inserted mask leaks on ventilator performance. Eur Respir J. 2010;35:627–36.
27. Paiva R, Krivec U, Aubertin G, et al. Carbon dioxide monitoring during long-term noninvasive respiratory support in children. Intensive Care Med. 2009;35:1068–74.
28. Fauroux B, Lavis JF, Nicot F, et al. Facial side effects during noninvasive positive pressure ventilation in children. Intensive Care Med. 2005;31:965–9.
29. Khirani S, Ramirez A, Aloui S, et al. CPAP titration in infants with severe airway obstruction. Crit Care. 2013;17:R167.
30. Caldarelli V, Borel JC, Khirani S, et al. Polygraphic respiratory events during sleep with non-invasive ventilation in children: description, prevalence, and clinical consequences. Intensive Care Med. 2013;39:739–46.
31. Amaddeo A, Caldarelli V, Fernandez-Bolanos M, et al. Polygraphic respiratory events during sleep in children treated with home continuous positive airway pressure: description and clinical consequences. Sleep Med. 2015;16:107–12.

Part XII

Non Invasive Ventilation, Epidemiology, Health Care Organization, Education and Ethics

Epidemiology, Practice and New Trends in Noninvasive Mechanical Ventilation: What Are We Learning?

96

Claudia Crimi and Annalisa Carlucci

Contents

Abbreviations

AECOPD	Acute exacerbation of chronic obstructive pulmonary disease
ACPE	Acute cardiogenic pulmonary edema
ARF	Acute respiratory failure
CHF	Congestive heart failure
DNI	Do-not-intubate
DNR	Do-not-resuscitate
ED	Emergency department
ICU	Intensive care unit
NIV	Noninvasive ventilation

C. Crimi, MD, PhD
Respiratory Intensive Care Unit,
Azienda Ospedaliera per l'Emergenza Cannizzaro, Catania, Italy
e-mail: claudia.crimi@aoec.it

A. Carlucci, MD (✉)
Respiratory Intensive Care Unit and Pulmonary Rehabilitation,
Fondazione Salvatore Maugeri-IRCCS, Pavia, Italy
e-mail: annalisa.carlucci@fsm.it

A.M. Esquinas (ed.), *Noninvasive Mechanical Ventilation: Theory, Equipment, and Clinical Applications*, DOI 10.1007/978-3-319-21653-9_96

96.1 Epidemiology of Noninvasive Ventilation in the Acute-Care Setting

96.1.1 Introduction

Noninvasive ventilation (NIV) represents one of the most important advances in the field of pulmonary and critical care medicine of the last 30 years. The efficacy of NIV in appropriately selected patients with acute respiratory failure (ARF) has been widely confirmed by several randomized controlled trials and meta-analyses. Strong evidence supports the application of NIV as a first-line treatment in patients with acute exacerbation of chronic obstructive pulmonary disease (AECOPD) and acute cardiogenic pulmonary edema (ACPE). Moreover, NIV has also been proven to be beneficial in patients with respiratory failure following solid organ transplantation and in those who are immunocompromised and to wean chronic obstructive pulmonary disease (COPD) patients from invasive ventilation [1] (Table 96.1).

Although the compelling evidence for the benefit of NIV has been shown by the literature, the implementation of this innovative tool in clinical practice found several barriers, initially. The increasing number of research articles published on the topic, year in and year out, highlighted physicians' interest on this new tool that, although very attractive, has a substantial learning curve and important prerequisites for successful implementation.

96.1.2 Discussion and Analysis

96.1.2.1 The Surveys: How Much NIV Is Used in Real Life

Several surveys have explored the pattern of NIV use and awareness among clinicians at various institutions in different geographic areas. These studies overall, showed a heterogeneous distribution of NIV practices among different countries that has been changing over time [2].

Table 96.1 Patient selection for NIV

Absolute contraindications
Coma (not attributed to CO_2 narcosis)
Cardiac arrest
Respiratory arrest (apnea or agonal respirations)
Any other condition requiring immediate intubation
Relative contraindications (exceptions should be reviewed on a case–by-case basis)
Cardiac instability (shock, vasopressor requirements, cardiac instability due to dysrhythmias, complicated myocardial infarction)
Gastrointestinal bleeding (hemodynamic instability, hematemesis)
Potential upper airway obstruction (head and neck tumor, angioedema)
Inability to protect airway due to depressed sensorium, inability to cough or clear secretions (cerebrovascular accident, advanced neuromuscular disease, severe drug overdose)
Status epilepticus

One of the first surveys, conducted in 1998, assessed NIV use and availability in 268 acute care hospitals in the United Kingdom and found that, at that time, NIV was available in only half of the surveyed hospitals (especially in the intensive care units (ICUs)) and, when available, was underutilized (used >60 patients/year in only 7 % of hospitals). A similar result was highlighted by Vanpee and coworkers in 2002 when exploring the availability and use of NIV for the treatment of AECOPD in an emergency department (ED) in Belgium[2].

The estimated utilization rate of NIV in acute care settings was also relatively low (20 %) among North American (Massachusetts and Rhode Island) respiratory therapists, with great regional variations, as pointed out by a survey published in 2006 [2]. In all of these studies, lack of physician knowledge or training, equipment, and financial limitations were the main declared barriers to NIV use. Similar results of a low penetration of NIV for the treatment of AECOPD throughout Canadian urban hospitals were registered in another survey conducted during in 2004 [2] (Table 96.2).

Table 96.2 Clinical conditions suitable for management with noninvasive ventilation

Established efficacy (for most patients, multiple studies)
Chronic obstructive pulmonary disease (COPD) exacerbations
Cardiogenic pulmonary edema (CPE)
Efficacy in selected patients (effective in subgroups or experience limited)
Asthma
Post-extubation; following discontinuation of mechanical ventilation (COPD and hypercapnia)
Community acquired pneumonia (and COPD)
Immunocompromised state and infiltrates (known cause of infiltrates)
Solid organ transplants
Febrile neutropenic patients
Postoperative respiratory distress and respiratory failure
Atelectasis
Postoperative lung resection
Rib fractures
Trauma with nonpenetrating chest injury; flail chest
Decompensated obstructive sleep apnea/cor pulmonale
Efficacy promising or limited (limited reports)
Acute respiratory distress syndrome (ARDS)
Do not intubate status
Cystic fibrosis
Interstitial lung disease
Neuromuscular respiratory failure (better in chronic than acute respiratory failure); best to avoid if upper airway issues
Kyphoscoliosis
Muscular dystrophy
Post-polio syndrome
Severe acute respiratory distress syndrome (SARS)
Mild *Pneumocystis jiroveci* pneumonia

The stunning dissemination of scientific literature on the utility of NIV has likely been able to overcome the initial barriers to the technique, and NIV has started to become more widely available in hospitals, but, again, important regional differences have been registered. In fact, a postal survey published in 2005 [2] aimed at exploring physicians' stated practices regarding the use of bi-level NIV for ARF in Ontario, Canada, showed the availability of NIV and protocols or guidelines for its application in 12 out of the 15 interviewed hospitals, with a great variation in NIV utilization among physician specialties (critical care, pulmonology, and internal and emergency medicine).

Devlin and coworkers, in their international web-based survey of intensivists published in 2007, reported a marked regional variation in stated use of NIV in ARF. Overall, Europeans were more likely to use NIV than North American physicians and preferably in AECOPD, congestive heart failure (CHF), and obesity hypoventilation syndrome. On the contrary, they pointed out that North American physicians were more inclined to use sedatives (41 % vs 24 %), analgesics (48 % vs 35 %), and hand restraints (27 % vs 16 %) during NIV treatment compared with the Europeans [2].

The results of a questionnaire distributed to North American physicians and respiratory therapists working in EDs, published in 2009, pointed out that 90 % of respiratory therapists and 64 % of physicians stated that they were very familiar with NIV and that its use in the ED is more common for AECOPD and CHF; moreover, the study confirms the already known barriers to a greater application of this technique such as: physician familiarity, equipment availability in EDs, and the human cost and raises the important problem of the availability of respiratory therapists (RTs) [3]. Another study published in 2009 [4] showed a wide availability of NIV in the American Veterans Affairs health-care system, where NIV can be accessible in both monitored (ICU, step-down, EDs) and unmonitored settings; however, its use and perceived efficacy among the interviewed clinicians was low, with a success rate of >50 % noted by only 29 % of respondents.

The setting where the scientific evidence had largely influenced everyday clinical practice, resulting in an extensive application of NIV in real life, seems to be with patients with do-not-resuscitate (DNR) orders. The Canadian group of Sinuff and coworkers [2] showed that NIV is a quite frequently considered option for this cohort of patients and that >80 % of clinicians initiate NIV mainly in DNR patients with COPD or CPE. Fewer (59 % of physicians, 69 % of RTs) stated using NIV for DNR patients with underlying malignancy or for patients choosing comfort measures only (40 % of physicians, 51 % of RTs). The study also showed that pulmonologists were more likely than intensivists to use NIV in the management of do-not-intubate (DNI) patients.

Data on frequency of NIV use and availability of resources for its delivery were also recorded in Spain [5] with a study published in 2008 showing quite high NIV utilization rate among Spanish ICUs, respiratory medicine departments, and EDs (100 %, 88 % and 69 % of respondents, respectively) and a relatively low percentage of use in internal medicine departments (37 %) and other wards (11 %), with a great heterogeneity in terms of type of patients and equipment and lack of protocols.

Another European survey published in 2010 [6] showed a relatively high utilization rate of NIV, with considerable differences based on the underlying disease of respiratory failure (mainly AECOPD), with an overall greater utilization of the technique mainly by pulmonologists (52.9 % reported >20 % of patients treated with NIV/year vs 34.3 % of intensivists/anesthesiologists). The study showed that pulmonologists were more likely to use NIV in the treatment of AHRF compared with intensivists (58.9 % vs 35.2 %). Conversely the latter were more likely to use NIV in patients with ACPE (18.7 % vs 7.2 %), hypoxic respiratory failure (19.1 % vs 6.2 %), and weaning from invasive ventilation (14.4 % vs. 8.5 %) ($p<0.05$). For all the physicians interviewed, the preferred equipment for NIV was dedicated NIV ventilators and an oronasal interface.

In conclusion, the clinical application of NIV has slowly but significantly increased in the last 10 years in ICUs as well as in respiratory medicine departments and EDs. Its use seems to be in line with scientific evidence. However, differences between European and North American practices are still evident, the latter being less prone to use NIV, even in clinical situations with strong evidence for its use.

96.1.2.2 Observational Studies: Clinical Results in Real-Life

The accumulating evidence for the efficacy of NIV has increased its use in clinical practice over time, as shown by observational studies based on on-site data collection at selected hospitals rather than on clinicians' estimates of use in response to questionnaires [2].

In 2003, Girou et al. published a retrospective study analyzing the clinical data of their 26-bed medical ICU from 1994 through 2001. The authors found a gradual and significant increase in NIV for similar patients admitted for AECOPD or ACPE over the 8-year period with a positive impact on patients' outcome due to a reduction in complications related to invasive mechanical ventilation, such as nosocomial infections, either pneumonia and urinary, and catheter-related infections. Also, mortality rates in these subgroups of patients significantly improved over the years, probably as a consequence of the reduction of infections [2].

A larger survey [2] involving 42 ICUs in Europe (France, Switzerland, Belgium, and Spain) and Tunisia aimed to prospectively follow all consecutive admissions for ARF over an observation period of 3 weeks. A total of 1,337 patients were admitted over that period for ARF (hypoxic (48 %), hypercapnic (15 %), coma (30 %), CHF (7 %)). Among the 689 patients requiring ventilatory support, NIV was used as initial ventilation approach in 108 (16 %) and was discontinued in 52 (48 %) due to lack of arterial blood gas improvement (46 %), inability to manage copious secretions in 32 %, patient's refusal to continue NIV in 22 %, and full dependence on ventilatory support in 11 %. The 28-days hospital mortality was significantly higher in those who needed IMV, compared with those who received NIV (41 % vs 22 %). The incidence of ventilator-associated pneumonia was as low as 2 % in patients who were successfully managed with NIV compared with 19 % in those who needed IMV.

Five years later, a new version of the same survey was performed in French ICUs with the aim of evaluating a possible change in the NIV use and success rate over time [2]. The authors showed an increased utilization of NIV from 16 to 23 % of the total ventilated patients and from 35 to 52 % of patients not intubated before ICU admission. Significant increases in NIV use were noted mainly for acute-on-chronic respiratory failure (50 % vs 64 %) and hypoxic respiratory failure (14 % vs 22 %), with an unchanged success rate.

A similar trend in increasing use of NIV to treat ARF was also described in a large survey on 349 ICUs in 23 countries. Comparing with a cohort study published in 1998, Esteban et al. showed a change in the use of NIV from 4 to 11 % in 2008. Despite strong evidence coming from the literature, the absolute percentage of NIV use remains low. As in the French survey, no differences in outcomes were found [2].

Similar results were shown in an epidemiological study performed in the United States by Stefan and coworkers [7], who found a steady increase in the number of hospitalizations over the period from 2001 to 2009 with a discharge diagnosis of ARF identified using the ICD-9 coding system. The study highlighted a decrease in inpatient mortality and a significant shift toward the use of NIV that increased significantly from 3.8 to 10.1 %, with a decrease in the rates of invasive mechanical ventilation use (Table 96.3).

96.1.2.3 NIV Outside the ICU

The majority of studies on NIV have been conducted in the ICU, which is certainly the ideal setting for an effective and safe use of this technique in acute and potentially fatal episodes of respiratory failure. Nevertheless, the emerging scientific evidences on the benefit of NIV in several common clinical scenarios such as AECOPD, ACPE, and acute respiratory failure in immunocompromised patients, also made NIV an appealing and attractive tool in clinical practice outside the ICU setting, especially in general wards [8].

Paus-Jenssen [9] described the feasible use of NIV outside the critical care setting in a single center in Canada, observing all consecutive patients hospitalized for ARF (AECOPD, hypoxic respiratory failure, hypercapnic respiratory failure, CHF, and patients with shortness of breath) over a 5-month period. The author found no

Table 96.3 Predictors of response to NIV

Severity of illness (moderate to severe)
Hypercapnic respiratory acidosis (pH 7.20–7.34); lower limit of effectiveness not known
APACHE II (Acute Physiology and Chronic Health Evaluation) score <25
Glasgow Coma Scale >11
Respiratory rate ≤35
Combination may further identify poor candidates
Trial of therapy (response to 1–2 h trial)
Improvement in respiratory parameters (respiratory rate, oxygenation, dyspnea)
Improvement in pH (increase by ≥0.06)
Improvement in $PaCO_2$ (decline by ≥8 mmHg)

difference in outcome and mortality compared with data from controlled studies performed in more aggressively monitored patients.

An international survey published in 2015 explored the use of NIV outside the ICU, in general non-monitored ward evaluating settings and modalities of NIV application and monitoring, estimated outcomes, technical and organizational aspects, and observed complications [10]. NIV application in general wards was reported by nearly 66 % of the respondents and perceived as feasible and effective. Limited training and economic resources were highlighted as possible limitations to NIV application.

The possibility of using NIV even in the pre-hospital setting was studied by Bruge et al., who reported the results of a 2-year prospective observational investigation of NIV in pre-hospital care, in emergency-response vehicles equipped with bi-level ventilators with favorable and appealing results [8].

96.1.3 New Trends in NIV

96.1.3.1 Bronchoscopy

The use of NIV during diagnostic and therapeutic bronchoscopy has been reported as a feasible and safe strategy but further studies need to address its impact on mortality and intubation rate in critically ill patients [11]. NIV-assisted bronchoscopy may be useful in obtaining lung biopsy or bronchoalveolar lavage in patients with severe hypoxemia and lung infiltrates, but, although there are several reports on the feasibility of this application, NIV during bronchoscopy should be performed only in centers with a wide experience (Table 96.4).

Table 96.4 Intubation guidelines

Intubation criteria (any one of the following):
Cardiac or respiratory arrest
Loss of consciousness
Hemodynamic instability with systolic blood pressure <70 mmHg
PaO_2 <45 mmHg despite oxygen
Intubation criteria (two or more in the context of respiratory distress):
Respiratory rate >35/min or <6/min
Tidal volume <5 ml/kg
Oxygen desaturation <90 % despite adequate supplemental oxygen
pH <7.20 and decreasing on NIV support
Hypercapnia ($PaCO_2$ >10 mm increase) or acidosis (pH decline >0.08) from baseline
Increase in encephalopathy or decreased level of consciousness
Abdominal paradox

Modified from Refs. [1, 9]

96.1.3.2 Interventional Procedures

NIV may represent a great opportunity for patients with a high risk of undergoing general anesthesia due to old age and/or co-morbidity or orthopnea due to severe lung-disease [11]. Boitano et al. [12] used bi-level NIV to support five patients with amyotrophic lateral sclerosis and forced vital capacity that ranged from 21 to 44 % of predicted during percutaneous endoscopic gastrostomy tube placement, without experiencing any complications.

NIV advantages have also been described in case series, during the performance of continuous transesophageal echocardiograph examination in lightly sedated patients with severe aortic valve stenosis and orthopnea, through a modified face mask, avoiding intubation and general anesthesia without complications [11]. In another report of the literature [13], patients with severe pulmonary disease and considerable orthopnea uneventfully underwent percutaneous implantation of an aortic bioprosthesis for severe valve stenosis during NIV with conscious sedation.

A case report on the successful use of pressure support during urgent coronary angiography and stent implantation in an 86-year-old women with ARF due to myocardial infarction complicated by ACPE was published by Rucci and colleagues [14].

96.1.3.3 Chest Trauma

The use of NIV has also been reported in patients with chest trauma with the goal of preventing or treating respiratory failure and a recent meta-analysis grouping 10 studies on chest trauma patients showed a significant benefit in the NIV group of patients compared with the control group, with an improvement of oxygenation and a reduction of endotracheal intubation, ICU length of stay, and mortality (3 % vs. 22.9 %) [11].

96.1.3.4 Palliative Treatment

NIV may represent a chance to reduce and alleviate respiratory symptoms, reducing the amount of sedation need, in patients with a nonreversible cause of respiratory failure. The use of NIV in patients with DNI orders was reported by almost 50 % of European physicians [11].

96.1.3.5 Postoperative Respiratory Failure

The application of NIV after complex surgical procedures in patients with high risk for postoperative acute respiratory failure (e.g., obesity) has been described. Several studies showed that it may be helpful in preventing and treating ARF after major surgery (abdominal and lung), reducing patients' intubation rate compared to oxygen treatment [11]. Jaber et al. suggested that the two potential goals of NIV in the postoperative period are to prevent acute respiratory failure (prophylactic treatment) and to treat acute respiratory failure and avoid re-intubation (curative treatment). The use of prophylactic CPAP for at least 6 h following extubation compare to standard treatment was tested by Zarbock et al. The authors found a lower incidence of pneumonia, re-intubation rate, and ICU readmission in the intervention group, suggesting a positive effect of CPAP in preventing postoperative atelectasis [11].

96.1.3.6 Pandemics

Some reports on the successful use of NIV during major pandemics such as SARS and H1N1 are available, but the safety of its use in these clinical situations has generated some concerns. Cheung et al. reported their experience with NIV and SARS in Hong Kong, showing that NIV was able to avoid intubation and to reduce ICU length of stay compared with intubated patients. The major debate is on the safety of NIV, because, during exhalation, infectious droplets can be spread into the ambient air through the exhalation ports of the NIV mask or tubing, enhancing the risk of contamination for the caregiver. A bench study of aerosol dispersion during NIV showed a dispersion that ranged up to 0.5 m from the mask; therefore, clinicians might be at high risk of contamination. We suggest that health-care workers providing NIV, working close to an infected patient, should have a higher level of respiratory protection. In fact, two reports showed no evidence of viral contamination to caregivers when appropriate precautions were adopted [11].

Conclusion

NIV represents one of the major advances in pulmonary and critical care medicine of the last three decades that has proven to change dramatically the outcome of some patients with respiratory failure. Although there is striking evidence proving its utility in clinical practice, its actual use in real life, as reported by surveys and observational studies, is still heterogeneous. Nevertheless, the literature suggests that NIV use increases as clinicians become more familiar with its use and human and economic resources are available. As with every innovation, a more even dissemination of NIV requires hard work, problem solving, thinking "outside the box," not fearing failure, and being comfortable with unknown. Moreover, undoubtedly NIV requires the knowledge of some technical aspects that can appear complex to the naïve user. Educational programs in some places are judged inadequate and need to be implemented.

Indeed, NIV is probably more art than science, and requires a considerable learning curve, the need of team work and dedicated staff, and the possibility of having a selection of devices and interfaces. Adequate training and educational programs for medical students, residents, and attending physicians of different specialties and also hospital staff on evidence-based learning objectives to guide NIV instructions is strongly suggested to further expand the use of this valuable technique in clinical practice and to optimize its success. We expect a more widespread use in coming years, with the advances in ventilator and mask technology, and increasing experience and skill at acute care centers.

Key Major Recommendations

- NIV should always be used, when clinically indicated, as a first-line method of ventilation, before invasive mechanical ventilation is considered, but in some institutions it remains underutilized.
- Barriers to greater use at low-utilizing institutions include lack of education of the staff and lack of appropriate equipment.

- Educational programs are likely to remove some of these barriers and further expand NIV diffusion.
- Overall, the use of NIV in real life has been increasing over the past decade both inside and outside the ICU, in selected subgroups of respiratory failure, according to data from the literature.
- New trends in the application of NIV are emerging and seem promising, but further larger studies need to confirm its safety.

References

1. Nava S, Hill N. Non-invasive ventilation in acute respiratory failure. Lancet. 2009;374(9685):250–9.
2. Pierson DJ. History and epidemiology of noninvasive ventilation in the acute-care setting. Respir Care. 2009;54(1):40–52.
3. Hess DR, Pang JM, Camargo Jr CA. A survey of the use of noninvasive ventilation in academic emergency departments in the United States. Respir Care. 2009;54(10):1306–12.
4. Bierer GB, Soo Hoo GW. Noninvasive ventilation for acute respiratory failure: a national survey of Veterans Affairs hospitals. Respir Care. 2009;54(10):1313–20.
5. Chiner E, Llombart M, Martinez-Garcia MA, et al. Noninvasive mechanical ventilation in Valencia, Spain: from theory to practice. Arch Bronconeumol. 2009;45(3):118–22.
6. Crimi C, Noto A, Princi P, et al. A European survey of noninvasive ventilation practices. Eur Respir J. 2010;36(2):362–9.
7. Stefan MS, Shieh MS, Pekow PS, et al. Epidemiology and outcomes of acute respiratory failure in the United States, 2001 to 2009: a national survey. J Hosp Med. 2013;8(2):76–82.
8. Boldrini R, Fasano L, Nava S. Noninvasive mechanical ventilation. Curr Opin Crit Care. 2012;18(1):48–53.
9. Paus-Jenssen ES, Reid JK, Cockcroft DW, Laframboise K, Ward HA. The use of noninvasive ventilation in acute respiratory failure at a tertiary care center. Chest. 2004;126(1):165–72.
10. Cabrini L, Esquinas A, Pasin L, et al. An international survey on noninvasive ventilation use for acute respiratory failure in general non-monitored wards. Respir Care. 2015;60(4):586–92.
11. Ambrosino N, Guarracino F. Unusual applications of noninvasive ventilation. Eur Respir J. 2011;38(2):440–49.
12. Boitano LJ, Jordan T, Benditt JO. Noninvasive ventilation allows gastrostomy tube placement in patients with advanced ALS. Neurology. 2001;56(3):413–4.
13. Guarracino F, Cabrini L, Baldassarri R, Petronio S, De Carlo M, Covello RD, et al. Noninvasive ventilation for awake percutaneous aortic valve implantation in high-risk respiratory patients: a case series. J Cardiothorac Vasc Anesth. 2011;25(6):1109–12.
14. Rucci G, Casale T, Nava S. First use of noninvasive ventilation during urgent coronary stenting in acute myocardial infarction complicated by pulmonary edema. Intensive Care Med. 39(6):1166–7.

Determinants of Utilization of Noninvasive Mechanical Ventilation in Hospitals: Key Technical and Nontechnical Issues

97

Guy W. Soo Hoo

Contents

Positive pressure noninvasive ventilation (NIV) delivered through a mask interface has become a mainstay in the management of patients with acute respiratory failure since the initial reports of its efficacy a little more than 25 years ago [1]. Indications have expanded beyond exacerbations of chronic obstructive pulmonary disease (COPD) to most causes of acute respiratory failure [2, 3]. However, despite widespread endorsement and evidence-based support for its efficacy, utilization of NIV remains quite variable. In Europe, NIV use in respiratory failure due to COPD

G.W. Soo Hoo, MD, MPH
Pulmonary and Critical Care Section (111Q),
West Los Angeles VA Healthcare Center, VA Greater Los Angeles
Healthcare System, Geffen School of Medicine at UCLA, Los Angeles, CA, USA
e-mail: Guy.soohoo@va.gov

A.M. Esquinas (ed.), *Noninvasive Mechanical Ventilation: Theory, Equipment, and Clinical Applications*, DOI 10.1007/978-3-319-21653-9_97

approaches 50 %, but the utilization in the United States has been reported to be in the 5–15 % range. There is a similar disparity in NIV utilization within countries and states where local or regional use has been high. Although there is an overall trend of increasing NIV use, actual application of NIV remains lower than the pool of potential candidates for treatment [4, 5]. Unlike some critical care interventions that only require limited engagement, a successful NIV program requires coordination and the support of the entire critical care infrastructure.

The most basic description of NIV involves the provision of ventilatory support for patients with acute respiratory distress or respiratory failure through a mask interface, thereby avoiding the "invasive" introduction of an endotracheal or tracheostomy tube into the tracheal bronchial tree. This "noninvasive" approach virtually eliminates the potential complications and discomforts associated with invasive ventilation. Although NIV provides ventilatory support, it may not be viewed as the same level of life support as invasive ventilation. Other advantages include the preservation of speech, oral function, and, in some cases, oral intake, while providing an easier transition on and off ventilator support than invasive ventilation. On the other hand, NIV requires a little more staff vigilance for signs of ineffective or failing therapy. Patients who fail therapy may be candidates for intubation. The timing of intubation is often imperfect and may increase the risk of adverse outcomes. The following provides an overview of the critical clinical (nontechnical) and technical elements that influence utilization of NIV in the hospitalized patient.

97.1 Patient Selection

Proper patient selection is crucial for successful application of NIV. This requires recognition of the severity of illness as well as the disease conditions best suited for NIV. NIV is not well suited for patients with immediately life-threatening critical illness. Since it uses a removal mask interface to deliver ventilatory support, it is ineffective for those who need airway protection or those with shock and multiorgan dysfunction. Those critically ill patients are better treated with immediate endotracheal intubation and mechanical ventilation, bypassing treatment with NIV. Other concomitant conditions that are better suited for invasive ventilation through an endotracheal tube include active gastrointestinal bleeding, those with upper airway obstruction, and patients with an inability to protect their airway (Table 97.1).

Once it is determined that the patient does not require immediate intubation, careful consideration should be made of the underlying disease causing respiratory failure. The vast majority of success with NIV has been accumulated in patients with exacerbations of COPD, and these patients remain the best suited for NIV. Cardiogenic pulmonary edema is another condition that readily responds to NIV. Although these are the two best-suited conditions for NIV, there has been expansion of NIV use into other causes of respiratory failure and in circumstances where NIV has not been traditionally applied (Table 97.2).

The next step in patient selection is to determine the severity of their respiratory illness because this may influence their ability to be managed with NIV. This has been

Table 1 Patient selection for noninvasive ventilation (NIV)

Absolute contraindications
Coma (not attributed to CO_2 narcosis)
Cardiac arrest
Respiratory arrest (apnea or agonal respirations)
Any other condition requiring immediate intubation
Relative contraindications (exception should be reviewed on a case-by-case basis)
Cardiac instability (shock, vasopressor requirements, cardiac instability due to dysrhythmias, complicated myocardial infarction)
Gastrointestinal bleeding (hemodynamic instability, hematemesis)
Potential upper airway obstruction (head and neck tumor, angioedema)
Inability to protect airway due to depressed sensorium, inability to cough or clear secretions (cerebrovascular accident, advanced neuromuscular disease, severe drug overdose)
Status epilepticus

Table 2 Clinical conditions suitable for management with noninvasive ventilation

Established efficacy (for most patients, multiple studies)
Chronic obstructive pulmonary disease (COPD) exacerbations
Cardiogenic pulmonary edema (CPE)
Efficacy in selected patients (effective in subgroups or experience limited)
Asthma
Post-extubation, following discontinuation of mechanical ventilation (COPD and hypercapnia)
Community acquired pneumonia (and COPD)
Immunocompromised state and infiltrates (known cause of infiltrates)
Solid organ transplants
Febrile neutropenic patients
Postoperative respiratory distress and respiratory failure
Atelectasis
Postoperative lung resection
Rib fractures
Trauma with nonpenetrating chest injury; flail chest
Decompensated obstructive sleep apnea/cor pulmonale
Efficacy promising or limited (limited reports)
Acute respiratory distress syndrome (ARDS)
Do not intubate status
Cystic fibrosis
Interstitial lung disease
Neuromuscular respiratory failure (better in chronic than acute respiratory failure); best to avoid if upper airway issues
Kyphoscoliosis
Muscular dystrophy
Post-polio syndrome
Severe acute respiratory distress syndrome (SARS)
Mild *Pneumocystis jiroveci* pneumonia

Table 3 Predictors or response to NIV

Severity of illness (moderate to severe)
Hypercapnic respiratory acidosis (pH 7.20—7.34); lower limit of effectiveness not known
*APACHE II score <25
*Glasgow Coma Scale >11
*Respiratory rate ≤35
*combination may further identify poor candidates
Trial of therapy (response to 1–2 h trial)
Improvement in respiratory parameters (respiratory rate, oxygenation, dyspnea)
Improvement in pH (increase by ≥0.06)
Improvement in $PaCO_2$ (decline by ≥8 mmHg)

most extensively studied in patients with COPD exacerbations. NIV is best suited for those with decompensated COPD who have a moderate to moderately severe illness, defined by the severity of hypercapnic respiratory acidosis starting with a pH<7.35. Those with a pH≥7.35 have not been demonstrated to derive any benefit from the addition of NIV to standard therapy. However, increasing respiratory acidosis does increase the possibility of intubation as it falls below 7.25 and especially below 7.20. The lowest threshold of effectiveness is not well defined inasmuch as comatose patients with severe hypercapnic respiratory acidosis, CO_2 narcosis, and pH as low as 6.93 have been successfully treated with NIV. Although hypoxemia is one of the hallmarks of cardiogenic pulmonary edema, those who also have a hypercapnic respiratory acidosis may represent a group most responsive to management with NIV. These and other factors used in patient selection are presented in Table 97.3. None of these values are absolute contraindications to NIV, but should be factored into the decision to institute NIV, as well as determining failure of therapy and need for endotracheal intubation. Some have identified a combination of factors, including severity of illness (Acute Physiology and Chronic Health Evaluation (APACHE) II), neurologic status (Glasgow Coma Score), and respiratory rate as predictive of failure and, therefore, patients who may be poorly suited for NIV [6].

97.2 Location of Therapy

NIV was restricted to the intensive care unit (ICU) when first used to treat patients with respiratory failure. There was a learning curve that required frequent monitoring by nursing and respiratory staff and the ventilator devices initially used for NIV were not well suited for this application. There was also concern for possible respiratory failure requiring intubation and, therefore, NIV was best administered in a location where there would be rapid transition to invasive mechanical ventilation. However, with staff education, experience, and smaller NIV dedicated ventilators, it became evident that NIV could be provided in an unmonitored ward setting with staff specially trained in the nuances of NIV. In the ensuing years, the location of NIV has become less of an issue as NIV is routinely provided for patients in a step-down unit setting, emergency room, and even an unmonitored ward. The ward still represents a third or fourth-line option for its applications (behind the ICU, step-down unit, and emergency department), but this is changing as providers gain experience and are more comfortable with NIV in a ward setting [7].

97.3 Trial of Therapy

The other approach that has been used to determine the utility of NIV has been a time-limited trial of therapy. Most patients who are treated with NIV are able to tolerate a trial of therapy. However, some patients fail NIV in minutes or within an hour of initiation. This group represents about 15 % of all patients treated with NIV. For the remainder, the response to a short 1–2 h trial of therapy is often predictive of successful treatment. This is often clinically evident at the bedside, manifested as a reduction in respiratory rate and accessory muscle use. Arterial blood gases before and after the trial provide further evidence of efficacy with decreasing $PaCO_2$ and increasing pH, objective markers that reflect effective patient synchrony and ventilation. A short trial is useful to identify not only those effectively treated with NIV but also to identify those with a poor response to NIV, thereby invoking consideration for intubation and mechanical ventilation [6, 8]. Extended trials without significant improvement only delay intubation and mechanical ventilation with a risk of other adverse events at the time of intubation. Failure of NIV usually occurs early, within 4–12 h of initiation, but there are those that fail after 24–48 h and others with late failure, after 48 h of NIV, some in spite of initial response to therapy. Failure to improve sensorium or respiratory acidosis after 24 h of NIV is another marker of eventual failure. Although this experience has been mostly accumulated in COPD patients, this clinical experience should hold for other conditions treated with NIV.

97.4 Health-Care Staff

Staff experience is another factor that can influence utilization of NIV. As with any therapy, there is a learning curve for staff whenever NIV is introduced into use, and this involves physicians, nurses, and respiratory therapists. Early experience with NIV was tempered by some nursing and respiratory therapy staff who experienced difficulties in its application, thereby limiting its effectiveness. These issues dissipated with increasing staff education and experience, and NIV generally does not require significantly more time for initiation and maintenance than invasive ventilation using an endotracheal or tracheostomy tube. When surveyed, the vast majority spend <30 min with initiation and maintenance of NIV, a good portion reported <15 min, but, of course, some patients may require an hour of time for satisfactory NIV. As may be expected, larger centers with more patients have more frequent use of NIV and also report greater success rates. It is difficult to discern whether patient volume or operator expertise best explains the differences in institutional utilization and outcomes, as both factors are inexorably related. Prior education and experience with NIV also influences its utilization, which may partially explain some of the global differences in utilization between Europe and North America. NIV utilization is much higher in Europe, where there has been long-standing experience with NIV.

97.5 Technical Issues

97.5.1 Masks

The mechanics of NIV application may also impact on its efficacy. Even though NIV can be used to treat comatose, hypercapnic COPD patients, the ideal patient needs to be sufficiently cooperative to allow proper mask fitting and synchronization with the ventilator. Agitated and uncooperative patients are unlikely to tolerate NIV. The type of mask interface between the patient and ventilator may facilitate patient adherence to NIV. Nasal or face (oronasal) masks are the most common types of masks used in NIV. The severity of illness may identify the mask best suited for use, as less severely ill patients better tolerate the nasal mask, which requires a little more cooperation, but are subject to more leaks, whereas the face mask is better suited for the patient who may not be able to cooperate [2, 8]. There has been no significant difference in the efficacy of NIV in head-to-head comparisons of the masks. On the other hand, there is individual variability and the optimal mask interface is the one that is best tolerated by the patient.

The masks do have to be fitted tightly for proper administration of NIV and pressure necrosis attributed to the mask can occur. Loosening of the mask without exacerbating leaks, changing the type of mask, using facial pads, and providing time off NIV are the main approaches to address this complication. Sedation has been used by some to assist in coordination and ventilator synchrony, but it is not clear whether this uniformly facilitates tolerance to NIV, and there is always a risk for excessive sedation and respiratory failure.

Other mask interfaces include mouthpieces, nasal pillows, full face mask, and helmets [8]. These other masks were used or developed because patients were not able to tolerate the more common nasal or oronasal mask or because of concerns with facial pressure necrosis as a result of tight-fitting masks. Although all have demonstrated efficacy, mouthpiece masks do require more cooperation by the patient, especially to avoid excessive leaks in the ventilator system. Less patient cooperation is required for application of the full face or helmet masks, and there may be fewer instances of facial pressure necrosis with these masks.

The proper mask interface is crucial for successful NIV. A properly fitted mask facilitates delivery of NIV, which in turn translates into effective treatment and recovery from acute respiratory failure. The mask also facilitates the trial of therapy, which is often used to gauge the potential success of NIV. It is self-evident that poor mask fit or intolerance of the mask will doom NIV and is an important limitation to its use.

97.5.2 Ventilators

The ventilators used to provide NIV have evolved since the initial reports, which primarily utilized the same bedside ventilators used in endotracheally intubated patients using both volume- and pressure-cycled ventilation. Generally, these ventilators were not optimal for NIV and were often plagued by mask leaks and alarms. Addressing these technical issues has led to the development of specialty ventilators, specifically designed to deliver NIV [1, 9]. Over time there has been a blurring of the distinction between these and bedside ventilators, as modern devices have the versatility to support both NIV and traditional mechanical ventilation through an endotracheal tube or tracheostomy tube. These ventilators have also expanded the modes of ventilation that can be delivered to patients administered NIV as well as traditional invasive ventilation.

97.5.3 Modes of Ventilation

The first devices designed for NIV were based on the continuous positive airway pressure (CPAP) devices used to treat obstructive sleep apnea. This mode remains available and has been demonstrated to be especially effective in treating patient with cardiogenic pulmonary edema. CPAP effectively recruits lung for ventilation and also has the dual effect of treating cardiogenic pulmonary edema by decreasing cardiac preload and afterload. However, higher CPAP pressures can be difficult to tolerate. Experience with traditional volume cycle ventilation was tempered by leaks and often high pressures. Inefficient patient-ventilator coordination, dyssynchrony, and breath stacking could limit effective ventilation. Pressure-cycled ventilators delivering pressure support ventilation provide comparable ventilatory support but have advantages of better leak compensation and patient control of inspiratory flow, which in turn produces better patient-ventilator synchrony. Volume delivery was more variable, but better tolerance of pressure-cycled ventilators made these more effective devices. It should be noted that neither mode has been demonstrated to be superior to the other.

This led to a ventilator with a proprietary name of BiPAP, which has become synonymous with NIV. Two levels of support are provided, one inspiratory positive airway pressure (IPAP) and the other expiratory positive airway pressure (EPAP). The difference between the two represents the amount of pressure provided to the patient, and it can be considered similar to a bedside ventilator mode of pressure support and PEEP. The ventilators have become more sophisticated, with a focus on improving patient ventilator synchrony. This has produced machines with improved signal processing technology and speed, which permits faster response times.

The newer ventilator modes often have proprietary names, and nomenclature can be confusing. Proportional assist ventilation (PAV) or proportional pressure ventilation (PPV) has been used in NIV and provides ventilator support with adjustments in inspiratory flow and pressure to match the patient's spontaneous efforts. This provides support proportional to the patient's efforts and thereby better matches their needs and facilitates patient-ventilator synchrony. Its efficacy is comparable but has not been demonstrated to be superior to the more commonly used BiPAP mode.

Another increasingly used variation of BiPAP is the average volume-assured pressure support (AVAPS) mode. This adjusts for variations in inspiratory pressure by changing pressure support levels to achieve a targeted tidal volume. This modality may be especially useful in patients with neuromuscular or thoracic cage respiratory disorder to deliver a target tidal volume and ensure a target minute ventilation. It has also been used in COPD patients and may be better suited for the patient with an advanced hypercapnic respiratory acidosis and CO_2 narcosis.

Advances in mask interfaces and noninvasive ventilators have greatly improved the patient's ability to tolerate and respond to NIV. These no longer limit optimal NIV, as may have been the case in the past, but there are still some nuances to be aware of involving these devices that may impact a patient's ability to tolerate NIV.

97.5.4 Ventilator Settings

Irrespective of the mask interface and device, the goals of NIV remain adequate ventilation with a reduction in work of breathing. Gas exchange disturbances must be also be corrected. The approach to ventilator settings has remained relatively unchanged. Fraction of inspired oxygen (FiO_2) can be adjusted to achieve target oxygen saturation, but blood gases are essential to track the overall response in gas exchange. Because most NIV patients have a hypercapnic respiratory acidosis, ventilator settings are set to achieve adequate tidal volume and minute ventilation to achieve normocapnia. Inspiratory and end-expiratory pressures are the most common targets for ventilator settings. These pressure-cycled settings permit a target volume of 5–7 ml/kg with inspiratory pressures increased to match that goal. Generally, in patients with a hypercapnic respiratory acidosis, the inspiratory pressures are increased to permit an increase in tidal volume to facilitate clearance of CO_2. This pressure also represents the amount of pressure support provided by the ventilator. IPAP of 10 cmH_2O and EPAP of 5 cmH_2O are frequently used as initial pressures. Further adjustments to the ventilator should be based on the response to therapy. Persistent hypercapnia can be treated with increasing minute ventilation, with an increase in frequency and/or tidal volume.

In hypoxemic patients without hypercapnia, changes in the ventilator settings are made to both the inspiratory and expiratory pressures. This effectively increases the positive end-expiratory pressure (PEEP) in the system and helps recruit lung and improve oxygenation. Volume cycle ventilation can be used with NIV, but is tempered by inadequate volume delivery in the setting of mask leaks or patient dyssynchrony with the ventilator.

97.6 Medication Delivery

Inasmuch as one of the goals of NIV is to avoid intubation in those with respiratory distress and impending respiratory failure, optimizing medication delivery during NIV may facilitate recovery. Because successful application of NIV will further its utilization, it is important to recognize that there is the potential for enhanced bronchodilator therapy with NIV. NIV can increase patient tidal volume and decrease respiratory rate, factors that can enhance aerosol delivery of bronchodilators. There is evidence that demonstrates greater improvement in the measure of lung function when bronchodilators are delivered with NIV compared with a standard nebulizer. However, the magnitude of this benefit has not been extensively studied.

97.7 Complications of NIV

The spectrum of complications associated with NIV differs from invasive ventilation but may still be of sufficient magnitude to limit its use. The most common complications involve pressure necrosis associated with the mask at its contact points with the skin. The pressure ulcers can be quite large and deep, thereby limiting effective delivery of ventilatory support. Options in management have been previously outlined in the section on masks, and include the use of different types of masks including large full face masks and helmets. Alternating the size of the mask and type of mask is another option as well as dressings to minimize the pressure of the mask on the face. The goal is to relieve and minimize the facial pressure by the mask, thereby reducing the risk of pressure ulcers.

Other complications associated with NIV mirror the complications also seen with invasive mechanical ventilation [10]. These include barotrauma, hemodynamic compromise due to increased intrathoracic pressure, and infectious complications. Barotrauma is related to the pressures used and generated during ventilator support. The pressures delivered to the airway and eventually the alveoli are often limited to less than 20 cmH_2O, as higher pressures are typically not used or not tolerated during NIV. Leaks inherent with any mask also limit pressure. Nevertheless, there are instances during patient-ventilator dyssynchrony where the pressures may approach or exceed plateau pressures of 30 cmH_2O, which in turn places the lung at risk for barotraumas. The treatment of complications that occur during NIV mirrors the treatment of complications related to positive pressure ventilation during invasive mechanical ventilation. Barotrauma that causes a pneumothorax typically warrants tube thoracostomy. Barotrauma can be minimized by a reduction in airway pressures with lower volume targets for ventilator support. Hemodynamic compromise is also addressed with lower pressure setting, but patients can also be supported with intravenous fluids, which will help ameliorate the adverse hemodynamic effects of positive pressure ventilation. Nosocomial respiratory infections occur at a much lower rate during NIV compared with invasive ventilation. However, patients may be at risk for gastric insufflations and subsequent aspiration event. This specifically differs from invasive ventilation as airflow in NIV is delivered to the entire oropharynx with subsequent flow down the esophagus as well as the tracheobronchial tree. Excess pressures can overcome the lower esophageal sphincter, generating gastric distension and increasing the risk of reflux, aspiration, and pneumonia. Local measures such as head-of-bed elevation, breaks between NIV support, and frequent breaks off NIV may reduce that risk. Antimicrobial therapy remains a mainstay of therapy.

All of the aforementioned complications are manageable and should not preclude the use of NIV in the appropriate patient. Utilization of NIV may require some modification, but should not be limited by these complications.

97.8 Discontinuation of NIV

One of the advantages of NIV over invasive ventilation is its ease of application and discontinuation. As noted previously, it is a noninvasive approach to ventilator support and requires less advanced technical skill than intubation and mechanical ventilation for initiation. Similarly, the discontinuation of NIV is not as complicated as with invasive ventilation. Extubation is always tempered by the possibility of recurrent respiratory distress and need for reintubation. The timing of extubation is an imperfect science and may be preceded by several weaning trials. NIV is typically provided as intermittent ventilator support and broken up by approximate hour breaks over the course of a day. Each time it is discontinued, a patient's clinical status should be evaluated. Respiratory distress may have resolved and subjects may no longer require ongoing ventilator support. Objective measures of response to therapy include resolution of physical signs of increased work of breathing (accessory muscle use, wheezing, tachypnea, diaphoresis, diaphragmatic paradox), along with improvement or resolution of hypoxemia, hypercapnia, and hypercapnic respiratory acidosis.

97.9 Failure of NIV

Conversely, patients may not respond to NIV and there may need to be consideration for invasive ventilation. Of course, in some patients, because of advanced underlying disease, NIV will represent the extent of life-support therapies. In the others, there needs to be vigilance of findings that would portend progression of respiratory failure to a point where intubation would be indicated. Table 97.4 provides some objective findings that can be used to signify failure of NIV and the need to proceed with intubation and mechanical ventilation. The early, sometimes preemptive intubation in patients failing NIV is of the utmost importance as these patients have been demonstrated to have worse outcomes and higher mortality than those who are successfully treated with NIV [5]. It is important to incorporate these measures of NIV failure (as well as success) in written guidelines to minimize any confusion among staff with respect to therapy as well as to standardize treatment [2].

Table 4 Intubation guidelines

Intubation criteria (any one of the following):
Cardiac or respiratory arrest
Loss of consciousness
Hemodynamic instability with systolic blood pressure <70 mmHg
PaO_2 <45 mmHg despite oxygen
Intubation criteria (two or more in the context of respiratory distress):
Respiratory rate >35/min or <6/min
Tidal volume <5 ml/kg
Oxygen desaturation <90 % despite adequate supplemental oxygen
pH <7.20 and decreasing on NIV support
Hypercapnia ($PaCO_2$ >10 mm increase) or acidosis (pH decline >0.08) from baseline
Increase in encephalopathy or decreased level of consciousness
Abdominal paradox

Modified from Refs. [1, 9]

Conclusion

In summary, positive pressure NIV has dramatically changed the management of patients with respiratory distress and respiratory failure. It is considered a first-line option for the management of acute exacerbations of COPD with hypercapnic respiratory distress and cardiogenic pulmonary edema. The determinants for utilization have been separated into clinical (nontechnical) and technical issues associated with NIV. Each area is important and, along with provider education and experience, are major factors in its utilization.

References

1. Brochard L, Mancebo J, Wysocki M, Lofaso F, Conti G, Rauss A, et al. Noninvasive ventilation for acute exacerbations of chronic obstructive pulmonary disease. N Engl J Med. 1995;333(13):817–22.
2. Soo Hoo GW. Noninvasive ventilation in adults with acute respiratory distress: a primer for the clinician. Hosp Pract (Minneap). 2010;38(1):16–25.
3. Keenan SP, Sinuff T, Burns KE, Muscedere J, Kutsogiannis J, Mehta S, et al. Clinical practice guidelines for the use of noninvasive positive-pressure ventilation and noninvasive continuous positive airway pressure in the acute care setting. CMAJ. 2011;183(3):E195–214.
4. Schnell D, Timsit JF, Darmon M, Vesin A, Goldgran-Toledano D, Dumenil AS, et al. Noninvasive mechanical ventilation in acute respiratory failure: trends in use and outcomes. Intensive Care Med. 2014;40(4):582–91.
5. Walkey AJ, Wiener RS. Use of noninvasive ventilation in patients with acute respiratory failure, 2000–2009: a population-based study. Ann Am Thorac Soc. 2013;10(1):10–7.
6. Confalonieri M, Garuti G, Cattaruzza MS, Osborn JF, Antonelli M, Conti G, et al. A chart of failure risk for noninvasive ventilation in patients with COPD exacerbation. Eur Respir J. 2005;25(2):348–55.

7. Cabrini L, Esquinas A, Pasin L, Nardelli P, Frati E, Pintaudi M, et al. An international survey on noninvasive ventilation use for acute respiratory failure in general non-monitored wards. Respir Care. 2014;60(4):586–92.
8. Nava S, Hill N. Non-invasive ventilation in acute respiratory failure. Lancet. 2009;374(9685):250–9.
9. Bott J, Carroll MP, Conway JH, Keilty SE, Ward EM, Brown AM, et al. Randomised controlled trial of nasal ventilation in acute ventilatory failure due to chronic obstructive airways disease. Lancet. 1993;341(8860):1555–7.
10. Carron M, Freo U, BaHammam AS, Dellweg D, Guarracino F, Cosentini R, et al. Complications of non-invasive ventilation techniques: a comprehensive qualitative review of randomized trials. Br J Anaesth. 2013;110(6):896–914.

Influence of Staff Training on the Outcome of Noninvasive Ventilation

98

Bárbara M.E.M.A. Seabra

Contents

Abbreviations

AHRF Acute hypercapnic respiratory failure
COPD Chronic obstructive pulmonary disease
CRF Chronic respiratory failure
NIV Noninvasive ventilation

98.1 Introduction

Since its introduction into clinical practice, noninvasive ventilation (NIV) has progressively gained a major role in the treatment of acute and chronic respiratory failure of multiple etiologies. Despite the "relative simplicity" of its concept and mechanism, the generalized use of NIV does not guarantee overall treatment success. Several studies have suggested the importance of staff training in the outcome of NIV. However, training goes well beyond acquisition of theoretical knowledge. In fact, its subtle specificities require, in addition to the latter, consistent "hands-on"

B.M.E.M.A. Seabra, MD
Department of Respiratory, Hospital Pedro Hispano, Matosinhos, Portugal
e-mail: barbara.seabra@ulsm.min-saude.pt; antmesquinas@gmail.com

A.M. Esquinas (ed.), *Noninvasive Mechanical Ventilation: Theory, Equipment, and Clinical Applications*, DOI 10.1007/978-3-319-21653-9_98

experience for increasingly efficient and speedy treatment adjustments, in accordance with each particular setting. This chapter discusses and analyzes the role of staff training in the outcome of NIV in its most commonly used modality: positive pressure noninvasive ventilation.

98.2 Staff Training in Noninvasive Ventilation

There are several aspects of staff training in NIV that have not been clarified:

- Definition of adequate staff training in NIV or its aims
- Which teachings contribute to an efficient training program
- Adequate duration of initial training
- Desirable frequency and contents during "maintenance" training
- Objective influence of staff training in NIV both in acute and chronic settings

98.2.1 NIV Staff Training – Definition

Despite the fact that most, if not all, medical centers where NIV takes place have a local NIV training protocol, the definition of adequate NIV staff training has not been globally established. Staff training may be defined as all the educational preparation, both theoretical and practical, delivered to NIV team constituents with the goal of improving the general and specific skills of each member. This allows the delivery of progressively more efficient and correct patient treatment. Training should probably be continuous and shaped according to local and individual needs. Training may take place both actively (through active article and guideline research, theoretical updates, participating in practical courses, etc.) and "passively" (through daily handling of this technique).

98.2.2 NIV Staff Training – Methods

Efficient staff training has not been clearly established, although the generally adopted and recommended formation includes [1, 2]:

- regular local educational courses for doctors, nurses, and physical therapists;
- elaborating and teaching local protocols of action in NIV;
- updates on locally available ventilators and interfaces, adequate use, and maintenance;
- attending national and international NIV courses;
- "hands-on" experience in progressively more differentiated or acute settings; and
- discussion of local practical aspects and difficulties on a regular basis, searching for learning and improvement opportunities.

98.2.3 NIV Staff Training – Contents

All members of the NIV team, especially the medical coordinator, should be aware and ideally absolutely comfortable with different variables continuously handled during this procedure: technical knowledge, staff roles and capabilities, available ventilators and their potential, patient profile, current interactions between the intervenients (patient–ventilator–staff–coordinator), and so on. Some of these variables are briefly listed in Table 98.1. Generally speaking, addressing this content in staff training may bring benefits to clinical practice and NIV success.

Doctors, nurses, and physical therapists may share a common background but should develop specific skills according to their activities in the NIV team. Differentiated training and education according to the role played by each staff member is desirable and may make a difference in critical patients. Once again, the content and the duration of what is considered an adequate training program have not been defined. As a general rule, each NIV center has developed its own training programs according to what is considered locally needed.

98.3 Current Evidence on Staff Training in NIV

When handling a patient with either acute or chronic respiratory failure, NIV – mainly positive pressure NIV – may be among several treatment options available to a medical team. Having its benefits widely identified in specific settings, its generalized use should not be taken lightly.

NIV treatment consists of a complex network where the main actors – the patient, the medical coordinator, staff (including doctors, nurses, and physical therapists), and the NIV in itself – are dynamically interrelated (Fig. 98.1). Each intervenient plays its specific role during this procedure, and the resulting method of ventilation contributes largely to the patient's acceptance and compliance with this treatment option, which is essential for a positive outcome [3].

Staff training and expertise in NIV are essential for successful NIV treatment, especially in the acute hypercapnic respiratory failure (AHRF) setting. However, medical and paramedical expertise is generally difficult to evaluate and has been poorly studied, including in NIV [4].

The complexity and subtlety of NIV demand generalized knowledge, both theoretical and practical, of several aspects of this treatment modality. It seems logical to assume that respiratory physiopathology, NIV basic knowledge, and updated NIV guidelines are the essential pillars on which all NIV techniques may be developed with regular clinical practice.

Available publications specifically addressing NIV staff training are scarce, mainly approach positive pressure NIV and its use in AHRF, and have limited statistical evidence. However, the general importance of staff training in the outcome of NIV has been repeatedly stressed.

Table 98.1 Multiple variables handled by the medical coordinator and staff in NIV

Technical knowledge (theoretical and practical)	Medical coordinator – staff/patient interaction	Medical coordinator – staff/ventilator interaction	Ventilator/patient interactions	Other variables
Indications/contraindications for NIV Intubation and mechanical ventilation criteria NIV physiopathology NIV mechanisms NIV particularities according to diagnosis Treatment aims Alarm signs	Adequate Bilateral communication – understanding and meeting patients' needs Getting across a sense of safety and reassurance to the patient Early identification of alarm signs	Knowledge of available ventilators (potential and limitations, advantages and disadvantages) General ventilator maintenance Ventilation modes How to manipulate the ventilator How to adjust settings Interpreting data and pressure/flow waveforms	Assure patient comfort Causes of disadaptation Patient/ventilator asynchrony Adjusting: Mask and headgear Leaks Trigger/cycling Humidification	Staff capabilities and limitations Staff's confidence in NIV results Patient profile Proximity to the ICU

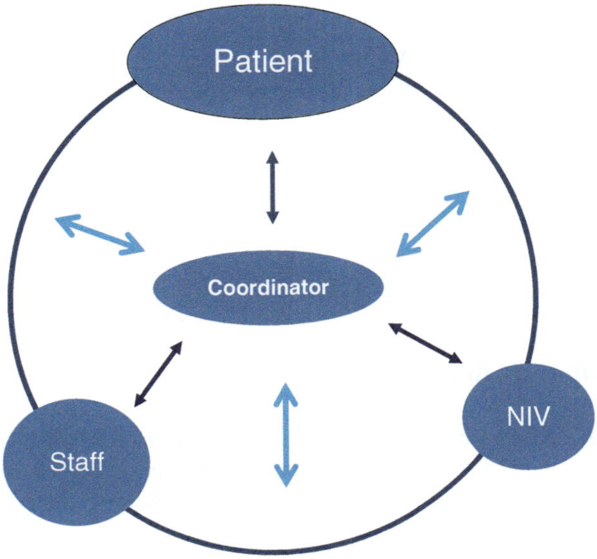

Fig. 98.1 Network of intervenients in NIV and respective interrelationships. Although successful patient treatment is the main aim of this network, the medical coordinator holds the central role in its attainment, observing, receiving continuous feedback, and coordinating all activity leading to NIV success and better patient outcome

Although it is difficult to correctly evaluate staff training, several studies have led to the conclusion that the level of experience of the team conditions the result of NIV. Some studies aiming to identify the ideal location for NIV in the acute setting reached the conclusion that the main factor associated with different location treatment outcomes was local team expertise in NIV [1]. Lopez-Campos et al. [4] suggested that the use of NIV by inexperienced personnel led to a high NIV failure rate. On the other hand, with adequate staff training, earlier and adequate NIV treatment may even be attained in a general ward, contributing to a better patient prognosis (although this treatment location is not generally recommended) [2].

Reports have shown that maintaining and, most of all, initiating NIV is time consuming, usually demanding close attention and staff dedication for adequate adaptation and treatment success. However, progressive staff training contributes to consistently diminished time expenditure and patient/nurse and patient/doctor ratio needs [1], favoring treatment of increasingly more severe patients without significantly changing success rate [2, 4]. It is even suggested that the cumulative experience acquisition deriving from regular handling of NIV over the years may modify clinical practice and improve patient outcome [2].

Table 98.2 Possible consequences of inadequate staff training in NIV in the CRF setting

Short term	Medium term	Long term
Inability to reassure patient initiating NIV	Patient disadaptation/discomfort	More episodes of ARF over CRF
Inability to motivate patient to adhere to NIV	Patient NIV low compliance	More hospital admissions
Inability to correctly adjust NIV settings for patient comfort	Patient NIV refusal	Higher morbidity and mortality related to CRF

98.3.1 NIV in the Chronic Respiratory Failure Setting

There is a considerable range of patients with indications for NIV who may initiate this treatment in an outpatient setting, during stable disease. Patients diagnosed with obesity -hypoventilation syndrome, chest wall deformities, some neuromuscular diseases, overlap syndrome, and certain patients with chronic obstructive pulmonary disease are within this group.

Most publications and recommendations concentrate on the importance of staff training in NIV in the acute respiratory failure setting, possibly due to the more immediate consequences of its failure. Studies reflecting the importance of staff training in chronic respiratory failure (CRF) are lacking. However, clinical practice suggests that one may generally draw the same conclusions in this setting. Although the negative consequences of lack of staff training in this setting may not be as obvious in the short term, they may surface sooner or later (Table 98.2).

As a general rule, one may deduce that inexperienced NIV teams, aware of their own technical limitations, may have more difficulties in reassuring and motivating a patient initiating NIV. If this is not the case, inability to correctly adjust the ventilator and interfaces may cause patient discomfort and disadaptation. In the short term, this may lead to non-adherence to treatment which, in the long term, may consequently lead to more episodes of acute respiratory failure over CRF, higher hospital admission rates, and increased patient morbidity and mortality.

As the complexity of these patients, higher dependency, and specific requirements from NIV increase, the impact of staff training in better patient care may be progressively higher. Patients with neuromuscular disease and amyotrophic lateral sclerosis, in particular, are a paradigmatic example of this situation, requiring progressively more differentiated and expert care as their disease and needs evolve.

Once again, solid background theoretical knowledge and practical experience of each intervenient in NIV contributes to patients' acceptance of NIV in the chronic setting, to an adequate response to patients' needs, and possibly to the motivation of treatment adherence, preventing long-term consequences of untreated CRF.

Conclusions

NIV involves continuously handling several complex variables, frequently in borderline situations. Adequate staff training plays a major part in the success of NIV. Its impact in NIV has been identified mainly in the AHRF setting, however, its influence in CRF is probably not negligible.

Current evidence on NIV staff training suggests the followin:

- Medical and paramedical expertise is generally difficult to evaluate and has been poorly studied, including in NIV.
- Staff training and expertise will influence the resulting method of ventilation, largely contributing to the patient's acceptance and compliance with this treatment option.
- The main factor associated with different location treatment outcomes is local team expertise in NIV.
- The use of NIV by inexperienced personnel may lead to a high NIV failure rate.
- Progressive staff training contributes to consistently diminished time expenditure and patient/nurse and patient/doctor ratio needs and may allow for caring for increasingly more severe patients without significantly changing the treatment success rate.

Staff training should ideally include theoretical formation generously complemented with regular NIV practice and learning experiences, although training duration and contents have not yet been defined. Today, the multitude of indications for NIV and the ever-growing number of ventilators, ventilatory modes and settings, interfaces, and so on demand a continuous update in this area.

Key Major Recommendations

- Staff training in NIV seems to improve general outcome of patients in AHRF and to diminish time expenditure and doctor/patient and nurse/patient ratios needs and should therefore be widely promoted. Staff regularly handling patients in need of NIV should be adequately trained.
- Theoretically, practical training and regular updates in NIV are essential to provide the best treatment to patients and improve their prognosis.
- Staff training should be continuous and adapted to local and individual needs.
- Objective NIV training protocols with proven efficacy (for both the acute and chronic settings) are yet to be established and should be addressed in future studies.

References

1. Elliot MW, Confalonieri M, Nava S. Where to perform noninvasive ventilation? Eur Respir J. 2002;19:1159–66.
2. Nava S, Fracchia C, Rubini F, et al. Changes in the practice of non-invasive ventilation in treating COPD patients over 8 years. Intensive Care Med. 2003;29:419–25.
3. Nava S, Ceriana P. Causes of failure of noninvasive mechanical ventilation. Respir Care. 2004;49(3):295–303.
4. Lopez-Campos JL, Garcia Polo C, Leon Jimenez A, et al. Staff training influence on non-invasive ventilation outcome for acute hypercapnic respiratory failure. Monaldi Arch Chest Dis. 2006;3:145–51.

Quality of Life during Long-Term Mechanical Ventilation in Hypercapnic Respiratory Failure: Main Determinants and Evidence

99

Graham T. Atkins and Alex H. Gifford

Contents

Abbreviations

ALS	Amyotrophic lateral sclerosis
CF	Cystic fibrosis
CFQ	Cystic fibrosis questionnaire
COPD	Chronic obstructive pulmonary disease
CPAP	Continuous positive airway pressure
DMD	Duchenne muscular dystrophy
EPAP	Expiratory positive airway pressure
ESS	Epworth sleepiness scale
IPAP	Inspiratory positive airway pressure

G.T. Atkins, MBChB, MRCP(UK) • A.H. Gifford, MD (✉)
Section of Pulmonary and Critical Care Medicine, Dartmouth-Hitchcock Medical Center, One Medical Center Drive, Lebanon, NH, USA
e-mail: Alex.H.Gifford@hitchcock.org

A.M. Esquinas (ed.), *Noninvasive Mechanical Ventilation: Theory, Equipment, and Clinical Applications*, DOI 10.1007/978-3-319-21653-9_99

NIPPV	Noninvasive positive pressure ventilation
NMD	Neuromuscular disease
OHS	Obesity hypoventilation syndrome
$PaCO_2$	Arterial partial pressure of carbon dioxide
QoL	Quality of life
RCT	Randomized controlled trial
SAQLI	Calgary sleep apnea quality of life index
SF-36	Medical outcomes study Short Form 36 quality of life questionnaire
SGRQ	St George's respiratory questionnaire

99.1 Introduction

Considerable evidence supports the use of noninvasive positive pressure ventilation (NIPPV) to manage acute hypercapnic respiratory failure. Questions remain regarding the utility of NIPPV in chronic hypercapnic respiratory failure, including whether it can improve quality of life (QoL) for all or certain subsets of patients. Common causes of chronic hypercapnic respiratory failure include chronic obstructive respiratory disease (COPD), obesity hypoventilation syndrome (OHS), cystic fibrosis (CF), and neuromuscular diseases (NMD) such as amyotrophic lateral sclerosis (ALS) and Duchenne muscular dystrophy (DMD). In this chapter, we review selected studies that question whether NIPPV, usually administered nocturnally, can improve QoL for these patients. Sleep-disordered breathing may co-exist with COPD, inevitably occurs in NMD, and by definition is present in OHS. Most investigations in this area have sought to identify a mortality benefit of NIPPV in chronic hypercapnic respiratory failure and employed dyspnea scores or health-related QoL questionnaires as secondary outcome measures. Selected commonly used QoL and

Table 99.1 Selected quality of life and symptom scoring systems [1]

Medical Outcomes Study SF – 36	Short Form 36 question health related quality of life questionnaire that scores from 0 to 100 in 8 categories. A mental health and physical health summary score (MCS and PCS), also from 0 to 100, are generated. Higher scores indicate greater perceived quality of life
St George's Respiratory Questionnaire (SGRQ)	50 items are measured to generate scores in two distinct areas: (1) symptoms and (2) activity and limitations. Scores are on a 0–100 scale with higher scores indicating worse symptoms and limitations
Calgary Sleep Apnea Quality of Life Index (SAQLI)	35 item measurement, scored 1–7 in 5 domains, including an assessment of the negative quality of life impact that treatment may have
Epworth Sleepiness Scale (ESS)	8 questions on a 4 point scale to measure sleepiness
Cystic Fibrosis Questionnaire – Revised (CFQ/CFQ-R)	Disease-specific instrument designed to measure impact on overall health, daily life, perceived well-being, and symptoms

symptom scoring systems are listed in Table 99.1 [1]. QoL, rather than mortality, may be a more appropriate metric by which to evaluate the efficacy of NIPPV in some patients with end-stage pulmonary or neurological diseases. The questions regarding QoL and the use of NIPPV in hypercapnic respiratory failure that are addressed in this chapter include:

- Does noninvasive ventilation (NIV) improve or preserve QoL for all patients with hypercapnic respiratory failure, or only for patients with specific diseases?
- Do patients need to have evidence of sleep-disordered breathing to benefit from nocturnal NIPPV?
- Does NIPPV have any negative effects on QoL?
- Is normalizing the arterial partial pressure of carbon dioxide ($PaCO_2$) important and what NIPPV settings should be used for patients with chronic hypercapnia?

99.2 NIPPV for Hypercapnic Respiratory Failure

The disease-specific literature is reviewed below, but there is some evidence to suggest that NIPPV can improve QoL for all patients with hypercapnic respiratory failure. In a prospective study, a cohort of 85 patients with mean $PaCO_2 > 50$ mmHg commenced 1 year of home NIPPV with the aim of normalizing $PaCO_2$ [2]. The study population included those with COPD, restrictive thoracic disease, NMD, and OHS. Mean inspiratory airway pressure (IPAP) and expiratory airway pressure (EPAP) were > 20 cmH_2O and 2 cmH_2O, respectively. Mean NIPPV use was 7.3 h per day, and mean $PaCO_2$ was <45 mmHg after 1 year of treatment. The authors found that health-related QoL had improved at 1 month and that this improvement was sustained at 1 year, with an approximate 5-point increase in the SF-36 mean MCS and PCS. Frequently reported adverse effects (37–22 % of the study population) included dry throat, facial soreness, sleep disruption, nasal congestion, and abdominal distension. Although there was no control group in this study, the small but significant improvement in quality life scores is striking.

99.3 Hypercapnic Respiratory Failure Due to Neuromuscular Disease

A Cochrane review of nocturnal mechanical ventilation for chronic hypoventilation due to neuromuscular or chest wall disorders showed that mechanical ventilation improved symptoms up to 1 year after commencing NIPPV [3]. The two subgroups for which the strongest evidence exists are patients with ALS and DMD. In both disorders, patients develop sleep-disordered breathing followed by nocturnal hypercapnia and then daytime hypercapnia as respiratory muscle function deteriorates. A randomized controlled trial (RCT) of NIPPV in 41 patients with ALS showed that NIPPV preserved QoL scores (SAQLI and SF-36 MCS) at 75 % of baseline for longer than supportive care (median comparisons: 173 vs 99 days for SAQLI and 168 vs 99 days for SF-36 MCS) [4]. Although statistically significant, this 11 week greater preservation of QoL may not be clinically meaningful; however, in patients with good bulbar function, QoL was preserved for around 6 months longer with NIPPV [4]. A review of mechanical ventilation in patients with DMD considered whether 24-h NIPPV or home ventilation via a tracheostomy might be more beneficial to QoL [5]. Tracheostomy allows clearance of secretions, which is often required as the disease progresses but may necessitate care in an institution rather than at home. Patients with a tracheostomy expressed fewer positive statements regarding QoL than those receiving NIPPV. The finding that those with milder disease derived a longer period of maintained QoL raises the question of when to commence NIPPV in patients with ALS and DMD. Early initiation of NIPPV in neuromuscular disease, for instance, when patients demonstrate nocturnal but not daytime hypercapnia, is an approach that may improve quality of life based on the results of a single RCT [6].

99.4 Hypercapnic Respiratory Failure Due to Obesity Hypoventilation Syndrome

OHS is characterized by obesity, daytime hypercapnia ($PaCO_2$>45 mmHg), and sleep-disordered breathing. Japanese investigators compared the effect of nocturnal continuous positive airway pressure (CPAP) in three groups of patients: those with OHS, obese patients with obstructive sleep apnea (OSA) but daytime normocapnia, and non-obese patients with OSA and daytime normocapnia [7]. The duration, compliance, and the pressure settings of CPAP used were not specified but CPAP was titrated to abolish apnea and maintain saturations of >90 %. Improvements in all domains of the SF-36 QoL score and the ESS were seen post treatment [7]. All improvements were statistically significant, with the exception of SF-36 bodily pain scale in OHS patients and SF-36 physical function and emotional limitation scales in non-obese patients with OSA. It is not known whether $PaCO_2$ improvements occurred for the OHS population during this study. These data suggest that nocturnal NIPPV can improve QoL for patients with OHS but that this improvement is likely mediated through an improvement in OSA.

99.5 Hypercapnic Respiratory Failure Due to Cystic Fibrosis

Progressive decline in lung function and QoL is seen in patients with CF. Young et al. [8] conducted a randomized crossover trial of nocturnal NIPPV in patients with daytime hypercapnia and nocturnal hypoxia. They found that NIPPV without supplemental oxygen, compared with air delivered at 2 l/min via nasal cannula, improved chest symptoms at 6 weeks as measured using the CFQ (71 vs 64)

[7]. NIPPV use was not associated with significant changes in physical functioning or emotional response domains of the CFQ, nor did it affect scores on the ESS or the MRC dyspnea scale. NIPPV was well tolerated during the 6-week intervention period.

99.6 Hypercapnic Respiratory Failure Due to COPD

Tsolaki et al. [9] reported that hypercapnic patients without sleep-disordered breathing, apnea hypopnea index (AHI) <10, showed a mean increase of 9 points on the SF-36 score after 1 year with NIPPV. This was not a RCT, but the control group patients who could not tolerate NIPPV had no change or even a decrease in their QoL metrics at 1 year. The relatively high mean IPAP, 15.3 cmH_20, and mean 9 h of daily NIPPV use were notable. When RCTs were conducted, the beneficial effect of NIPPV on QoL was not observed. A trial of 144 hypercapnic COPD patients by McEvoy et al. [10] in Australia randomized to receive NIPPV with oxygen or oxygen alone showed slightly lower SF-36 scores in patients receiving NIPPV. A 2014 Cochrane review of RCTs (which included the study by McEvoy et al.) showed no significant differences in quality of life when NIPPV was used for 3–12 months in hypercapnic patients with COPD [11]. When the RCT of McEvoy et al. is compared to the study by Tsolaki et al., the patients appear similar in terms of their degree of hypercapnia and airflow obstruction, but the treatment intervention has significant differences. In the RCT by McEvoy et al. the levels of IPAP are lower, there is no significant change in $PaCO_2$, and patients used NIPPV for a much shorter period of time each day (mean of 4.5 h vs 9 h). One could hypothesize that normalizing hypercapnia, through the use of relatively high IPAP, is important to achieve a QoL improvement.

With this in mind, a European study by Köhnlein et al. [12] randomized 195 patients with COPD with mean $PaCO_2$ of 58 mmHg to 1 year of NIV titrated to reduce $PaCO_2$ by 20 % or to <48 mmHg. There was no assessment or exclusion of patients with sleep-disordered breathing. Mean IPAP was 21.6 cmH_2O and mean EPAP was 4.8 cmH_2O. Mean daily NIPPV use was 5.9 h. There were small but significant QoL differences between the NIPPV and control groups, in favor of NIPPV treatment. There was an 8.6 point improvement in the SF-36 general health perception subscale, a 6.2 point improvement in the SGRQ summary score, and a 5.6 point improvement in the SRI summary scale score, all statistically better than changes in the control group ($p<0.05$).

99.7 Cost of NIV and Admissions to Hospital

Some data suggest that in-home NIV for patients with hypercapnic respiratory failure may be a cost-effective therapeutic intervention. In a trial of 13 hypercapnic patients with COPD, in-home NIPPV provided a cost saving by reducing the frequency and duration of hospital admissions [13]. Admissions to hospital are associated with lower QoL scores for patients with hypercapnic respiratory failure [14].

Conclusions

NIPPV appears to improve QoL for hypercapnic patients with NMD, CF, and OHS. The studies suggest that the majority of these patients have sleep-disordered breathing, and an improvement in sleep quality is a contributor to the overall improvements in quality of life. There is conflicting literature regarding NIPPV to improve QoL in hypercapnic COPD patients. If NIPPV is used for patients with COPD, relatively high levels of support (i.e., IPAP > 15 mmHg), 6 or more hours of daily NIPPV use, and a ventilation strategy targeted to normalize $PaCO_2$ are the factors associated with increased QoL. It is notable that, in all the studies of NIPPV, patients were hospitalized for 3–12 days to establish NIPPV and that there was close follow-up throughout. It is not clear whether strict adherence to this methodology is required for patients to derive improvement from NIPPV in clinical practice. In one study, NIPPV appeared to be associated with a reduced QoL and observed adverse effects from NIPPV include skin breaks at the site of the mask, facial soreness, dry throat, and abdominal distension. Thus, the possibility of these untoward events should be discussed with patients and their families prior to the initiation of treatment.

Key Recommendations

To improve QoL for patients with hypercapnic respiratory failure we recommend:

- Identify the etiology of hypercapnic respiratory failure, establish goals of care, and screen for sleep-disordered breathing.
- Use a QoL measurement before initiating NIPPV and repeat at 4–6 weeks to assess whether NIPPV is having a beneficial effect on QoL.
- Titrating IPAP to normalize daytime hypercapnia may lead to the greatest improvements in QoL, and may be mandatory in patients with COPD to improve QoL.
- Adjust mask fit and pressure settings as needed to reduce the adverse effects of NIPPV that may occur, such as facial soreness, dry mouth, sore throat, and abdominal distension.
- Treat patients at home rather than in a hospital setting if possible, as this is associated with greater QoL scores.

References

1. American Thoracic Society. Quality of life resource 2007. http://qol.thoracic.org/sections/instruments/index.html.
2. Windisch W, et al. Impact of home mechanical ventilation on health-related quality of life. Eur Respir J. 2008;32:1328–36.

3. Annane D, Orlikowski D, Chevret S. Nocturnal mechanical ventilation for chronic hypoventilation in patients with neuromuscular and chest wall disorders. Cochrane Database Syst Rev. 2014;(12):CD001941.
4. Bourke SC, et al. Effects of non-invasive ventilation on survival and quality of life in patients with amyotrophic lateral sclerosis: a randomized controlled trial. Lancet Neurol. 2006;5:140–7.
5. Toussaint M, Chatwin M, Soudon P. Mechanical ventilation in Duchenne patients with chronic respiratory insufficiency: clinical implication of 20 years published experience. Chron Respir Dis. 2007;4:167–77.
6. Ward S, et al. Randomized controlled trial of non-invasive ventilation (NIV) for nocturnal hypoventilation in neuromuscular and chest wall disease patients with daytime normocapnia. Thorax. 2005;60(12):1019–24.
7. Hida W, et al. Nasal continuous positive airway pressure improves quality of life in obesity hypoventilation syndrome. Sleep Breath. 2003;7:3–12.
8. Young AC, et al. Randomised placebo controlled trial of non-invasive ventilation for hypercapnia in cystic fibrosis. Thorax. 2008;63:72–7.
9. Tsolaki V, et al. One-year non-invasive ventilation in chronic hypercapnic COPD: effect on quality of life. Respir Med. 2008;102:904–11.
10. McEvoy RD, et al. Nocturnal non-invasive nasal ventilation in stable hypercapnic COPD: a randomized controlled trial. Thorax. 2009;64:561–6.
11. Struik FM, et al. Nocturnal non-invasive positive pressure ventilation for stable chronic obstructive pulmonary disease. Cochrane Database Syst Rev. 2013;(6):CD002878.
12. Köhnlein T, et al. Non-invasive positive pressure ventilation for the treatment of severe stable chronic obstructive pulmonary disease: a prospective, multicenter, randomized, controlled clinical trial. Lancet Respir Med. 2014;2:698–705.
13. Tuggey JM, Plant PK, Elliott MW. Domiciliary non-invasive ventilation for recurrent acidotic exacerbations of COPD: an economic analysis. Thorax. 2003;58:867–71.
14. López-Campos JL, et al. Factors related to quality of life in patients receiving home mechanical ventilation. Respir Med. 2008;102:605–12.

Ethics: Decision Making in Noninvasive Ventilation

100

Andrea Purro

Contents

100.1 Introduction

Ethics: a set of principles that people use to decide what is right and what is wrong.

Invasiveness of interventions, complexity of diseases, and patients' age are increasing in intensive care medicine. Ethical and legal issues are particularly challenging at the end of life of critically ill patients. At the borderline between intensive care and palliative medicine, a significant number of patients suffer from respiratory failure. Modern modes of mechanical ventilation may be able to improve ventilation and quality of life. On the other hand, they may oppose a dignified death at the end of a long-lasting chronic disease and prolong the suffering.

In contrast to endotracheal intubation and invasive mechanical ventilation, noninvasive ventilation (NIV) enables patients to participate in the decision making process. Under normal circumstances, ethical standards dictate that patients themselves participate in the medical decision making process. Patients with indications for NIV can be categorized into three groups: those who want all possible treatments and life-support; those who have elected specific limits on life-support and

A. Purro, MD
Emergency Department, Gradenigo Hospital, Turin, Italy
e-mail: andrea.purro@gmail.com

A.M. Esquinas (ed.), *Noninvasive Mechanical Ventilation: Theory, Equipment, and Clinical Applications*, DOI 10.1007/978-3-319-21653-9_100

treatments, such as patients with do-not-intubate (DNI) orders; and patients very near the end of life who will receive comfort measures only (CMO) [1].

100.2 Discussion and Main Topics

Over the last 20 years, the majority of the literature on NIV for acute respiratory failure (ARF) has focused on patients who want all possible life support and treatments. Randomized controlled trials have described the settings where NIV is effective.

Many patients who set limits on life support and treatments have had poor experiences with intubation and have chronic disease and a poor prognosis. CMO patients may desire only to minimize discomfort and ease the dying process.

Clearly, the goals of therapy differ in the three care categories. The main ethical concern about NIV for ARF in DNI and CMO patients is informed consent, which is necessary but can be problematic, because not all patients with terminal diseases have discussed end-of-life issues with their physicians, and many physicians are reluctant to discuss advance directives with their patients. Johnston et al. [2] surveyed 329 adult outpatients, 282 residents, and 272 practicing physicians (response rates 75 %, 76 %, and 65 %, respectively) for their opinions about advance directives. The patients believed that discussions regarding advance directives should occur earlier in the course of disease and earlier in the patient-physician relationship than did the physicians. Both physician and patients thought it was the physician's responsibility to initiate the discussions about advance directives. Despite literature that indicates patients' desire to discuss advance directives and a mandate by regulatory agencies, many patients with end-stage disease, and the elderly, have not formalized their treatment wishes with advance directives. Many patients at end of life who are transferred to acute-care hospitals do not have advance directives [3].

Because standard advance directives are not commonly found in patients' medical records, it can be difficult to know whether a patient at end of life has discussed NIV. Recent statements about palliative care from societies whose focus is patients with chronic pulmonary diseases do not discuss NIV in the sections on the standard of care for patients with cardiopulmonary disease at end of life [4]. Thus, it is up to the clinician to determine whether the patient has consented to NIV. The patient should be educated to the fact that NIV is a form of life support, but is noninvasive, and that the patient can discontinue NIV at any time. Ideally, a discussion about NIV should occur long before the patient is near the end of life. The ideal is to provide precise direction to all caregivers regarding the patient's wishes. NIV is an ethical approach to managing a patient at end of life if the patient provides informed consent. The literature on the application of NIV to DNI and CMO patients is limited, and there have been no randomized controlled trials. In addition, underlying primary diagnosis was an important determinant of survival. Patients with congestive heart failure had significantly better survival than any of the other groups.

Little information is available on clinicians' perspectives on NIV in DNI and CMO patients. Sinuff et al. [5] surveyed pulmonologists, intensivists, and respiratory therapists (RTs) in 18 Canadian and 2 US institutions on the use of NIV in patients with ARF near the end of life. The survey asked about factors associated with the use of NIV in DNI and CMO patients. Overall, 104 (57 %) of 183 physicians and 290 (61 %) of 473 RTs responded. Sixty-two percent of the physicians indicated that they include NIV in DNI discussions at least part of the time. Eighty-seven percent of the RTs indicated that NIV should be included in these discussions. Regarding CMO patients, fewer respondents thought NIV should be included in the discussion. Forty-nine percent of the physicians indicated that at least some of the time they include NIV in the discussion, whereas 41 % of the RTs thought that NIV should be part of the discussion. The RTs indicated that they were asked to initiate NIV on DNI and CMO patients more frequently than the physicians indicated they ordered it. Both physicians and RTs indicated they used NIV more frequently in DNI patients than in CMO patients. The physicians were more likely than the RTs to believe that NIV relieves dyspnea and facilitates communication in DNI and CMO patients. The RTs more commonly than physicians indicated that NIV was used so that the patient's family had time to come to terms with their loved one's death. Physicians more commonly than RTs indicated that NIV was used so that patients would have time to get their personal affairs in order. Both physicians and RTs indicated that NIV at end of life for either DNI or CMO was more likely in patients with COPD or congestive heart failure than in patients with end-stage cancer.

These data clearly indicate an inconsistency of practice between physicians and RTs with regard to NIV at the end of life. Additional study is needed on the use of NIV in DNI and CMO patients, and about those patients' perspectives on NIV.

NIV has been well recognized as a palliative tool, merely aimed to treat dyspnea when acute respiratory distress or failure ensues [6]. The need for mechanical support is theoretically the main intervention when an organ is failing beyond a point at which any pharmacological intervention is ineffective or partially effective. This is true for the kidney, lung, and even the heart. The problem is understanding in clinical practice when mechanical support may be futile. Failure of weaning from invasive mechanical ventilation is one of the major clinical problems in patients with COPD. In one study [7], these "chronically critically ill" patients, representing only 3 % of the total number of patients admitted to the ICU, used almost 40 % of the total patient days of care.

The manner in which this relatively small population cuts into hospital costs has drawn the attention of experts in the field. Thus, Seneff et al. [7] have openly stated that, "there is some level of costs of acute care that is beyond our society's economic capacity." Does this mean that a patient with advanced COPD always "deserves" an end-of-life care decision? The general perception is that the outcome of COPD patients requiring mechanical ventilation is poor, despite several studies in which invasive ventilation or NIV was employed to demonstrate an acceptable survival rate. With the introduction of NIV to treat acute respiratory failure of different etiologies 20 years ago, classical outcome measures such as hospital mortality, need for endotracheal intubation, complications of invasive ventilation, and length of hospital stay have been drastically improved. The feasibility and usefulness of NIV in the palliative care of patients with acute respiratory failure near the end of their lives is still not well demonstrated.

Frequently, NIV is also used for those patients with terminal diseases to help alleviate respiratory distress and attempt to provide some additional time to say goodbye to their relatives and friends or to solve some administrative issues, but most clinicians are unclear about the goals of care. For example, it has been highlighted that NIV may be inappropriate in this context because of an increased use of medical resources, prolongation of the dying process, and intensification of suffering. So there is a need to facilitate the decision concerning NIV or any other form of mechanical ventilation.

When patients are well informed, they are generally satisfied with the decision that has been made and do not change their mind later. Therefore, the decision to commence mechanical ventilation in end-stage COPD needs the active participation of the patient. Physicians and educators should target patients with COPD to improve patients' education about diagnosis and the disease process, and to explain the treatments, prognosis, what dying might be like, and advance care planning. To address these issues, Dales et al. [8] developed and tested an aid to assist patients with decisions about mechanical ventilation. A scenario-based decision aid was developed, consisting of an audiocassette and a booklet describing intubation and mechanical ventilation and its possible outcomes. From this study it may be concluded that, when discussed and explained in detail, an end-of-life decision is stable in time and the patients achieve satisfaction and confidence. Proxy decisions were incongruent, especially when made by family members; however, the strong sex effect suggested a call for further investigation.

When used as life-support, NIV for ARF should be applied in the intensive care unit (ICU), in an intermediate care unit, or in the emergency department. Curtis et al. [9] defined NIV as life support when the patient is unable to sustain spontaneous breathing for at least 1 h without NIV. However, DNI and CMO patients have been successfully sustained on NIV outside the ICU. A general medical/surgical unit's staff must understand the risks and benefits of NIV, and patients must be appropriately monitored, including alarms for ventilator disconnect, pressure-loss, high airway pressure, pulse oximetry, and cardiovascular monitoring, which should all annunciate in the hall and nursing station to rapidly alert staff of changes in patient status or ventilator malfunction. All categories of patients who require NIV can be safely and effectively managed on general medical units, given proper staff training and patient monitoring.

The best setting for NIV in older patients with DNI orders is the subject of some debate [10]. Whereas the use of NIV in patients with acute respiratory failure without preset limitations on life-sustaining treatment may be implemented in different settings (ICUs, respiratory ICUs (RICUs), and emergency rooms), depending on the typology of acute syndrome and the likelihood of success, the ideal care for "DNI patients" is likely to be more appropriate outside the ICU. In fact, for these patients for whom endotracheal intubation is questionable or care is centered largely on symptom palliation or both, NIV failure requires to increase of comfort measures only, adequately performed in totally or partially "open" environments. The option of NIV in end-of-life decisions is emerging in European RICUs, where a large majority of DNI patients are treated by pulmonologists. This is not surprising, as RICUs differ substantially from ICUs in terms of patient population, staffing, monitoring, and use of NIV as the preferred ventilator approach [4]. Furthermore, a recent American survey showed that the stated use of NIV and the confidence in its utility in end-of-life patients were greater for pulmonologists than for intensivists. A pulmonologist's point of view may be influenced by caring for end-stage respiratory patients over the entire spectrum of the illness as opposed to the greater focus on acute care among intensivists.

In conclusion, the assignment of older patients with DNI orders to an environment, such as the ICU, that was originally designed to treat patients without preset limitations of care (i.e., invasive mechanical ventilation) raises financial and ethical concerns, namely (a) the questionable cost-utility ratio of allocating the precious, limited ICU resources for patients whose needs may be met by lower levels of care (i.e., nurse workload) and (b) the inappropriateness of a "closed environment" for managing respiratory patients who would like to spend the end of their lives near their friends and family. Hospital administrators should identify, in expert pulmonology units, the optimal setting for implementing NIV within the DNI and end-of-life context to achieve economic and ethical benefits that surpass those of the ICU.

Conclusion

NIV can benefit patients who have elected specific limits on life support and treatments (e.g., DNI) and patients who will receive comfort measures only. The critical ethical issue with regard to NIV for DNI and CMO patients is informed consent. The risks and potential benefits of NIV must be clearly discussed. Data from terminal cancer patients suggest that is important to patients retaining control over end-of-life care decisions and having adequate time to prepare for death. If control over care decisions is assured, NIV may be able to reverse an ARF that is not necessarily a life-terminating event, or improve patient comfort, or sustain life until the patient can put his or affairs in order.

Key Major Recommendations

- NIV can be useful in DNI and CMO patients.
- The critical ethical issue with regard to NIV for DNI and CMO patients is informed consent.
- Hospital administrators should identify the optimal setting for implementing NIV within the DNI and end-of-life context.

References

1. Kacmarek RM. Should noninvasive ventilation be used with the do-not-intubate patient? Respir Care. 2009;54:223–9.
2. Johnston SC, Pfeifer MP, McNutt R. The discussion about advance directives. Patient and physician opinions regarding when and how it should be conducted. Arch Intern Med. 1995;155(10):1025–30.
3. Selecky PA, Elisson AH, Hall RI, et al. Palliative and end of life care for patients with cardiopulmonary diseases: American College of Chest Physicians Position Statement. Chest. 2005;128:3599–610.
4. Carlucci A, Guerrieri A, Nava S. Palliative care in COPD patients: is it only an end-of-life issue? Eur Respir J. 2012;21:347–54.
5. Sinuff T, Cook DJ, Keenan SP, et al. Noninvasive ventilation for acute respiratory failure near the end of life. Crit Care Med. 2008;36(3):789–94.
6. Nava S, Sturani C, Hartl S, et al. End-of-life decision-making in respiratory intermediate care units: a European survey. Eur Respir J. 2007;30:156–64.
7. Seneff MG, Wagener D, Thompson D, et al. The impact of long-term acute-care facilities on the outcome and cost of care for patients undergoing prolonged mechanical ventilation. Crit Care Med. 2000;28:342–50.
8. Dales RE, O'Connor A, Hebert P, Sullivan K, et al. Intubation and mechanical ventilation for COPD: development of an instrument to elicit patient preferences. Chest. 1999;116:792–800.
9. Curtis JR, Cook DJ, Sinuff T, White DB, Hill N, Keenan SP, et al. The SCCM Palliative NPPV Task Force. Noninvasive positive pressure ventilation in critical and palliative care settings: understanding the goals of therapy. Crit Care Med. 2007;35(3):932–39.
10. Scala R, Esquinas A. Noninvasive mechanical ventilation for very old patients with limitations of care: is the ICU the most appropriate setting? Crit Care. 2012;16:429.

Index

A.M. Esquinas (ed.), *Noninvasive Mechanical Ventilation: Theory, Equipment, and Clinical Applications*, DOI 10.1007/978-3-319-21653-9

T

9783319793573